Spinal Tumor Surgery

Daniel M. Sciubba
Editor

Spinal Tumor Surgery

A Case-Based Approach

Springer

Editor
Daniel M. Sciubba, MD
Department of Neurosurgery
Johns Hopkins University
Baltimore, MD
USA

ISBN 978-3-319-98421-6 ISBN 978-3-319-98422-3 (eBook)
https://doi.org/10.1007/978-3-319-98422-3

Library of Congress Control Number: 2018965499

This Springer imprint is published by the registered company Springer Nature Switzerland AG
The registered company address is: Gewerbestrasse 11, 6330 Cham, Switzerland

Foreword

Surgery for the treatment of primary and metastatic tumors requires considerable thought, planning, and a multidisciplinary approach. This book provides a case-based approach to surgery for spinal tumors—striking a balance between surgical atlas and informative text. The book delves into treatment indications, regional, and tumor-specific considerations for the surgical management of spinal neoplasms.

Although metastatic spine disease outweighs primary spinal neoplasms, it is important to recognize the operative approaches and goals of treatment for both. Many technical descriptions of spinal surgery have focused on the surgical exposure for a broad range of conditions, including degenerative, deformity, and tumor. Previous spinal oncology texts illustrate oncologic principles, predictive analytics, and management guidelines to inform multidisciplinary treatment. However, the present text is unique in that it describes the surgical planning and approach to spinal tumor surgery, specifically. As such, it is meant to serve as a stepwise technical guide for surgeons treating patients with neoplastic spine disease.

Optimal care relies upon surgeon familiarity with the various surgical approaches to the spinal column and an understanding of established treatment goals. The chapters are outlined by experts in the field, relative to spinal region of pathology, and compartment (i.e., extradural, intradural extramedullary, and intramedullary). Notably, the authors pay particular attention to patient evaluation, indications for surgery, preoperative planning, surgical technique, and complex spinal reconstruction. This text is an invaluable resource for surgeons, encompassing the biomechanic and anatomic complexity of spine tumor surgery, with detailed case descriptions and beautiful artist illustrations.

Ziya L. Gokaslan, MD, FAANS, FACS
Gus Stoll, MD Professor and Chair, Department of Neurosurgery
The Warren Alpert Medical School of Brown University
Neurosurgeon-in-Chief, Rhode Island Hospital and The Miriam Hospital
Clinical Director, Norman Prince Neurosciences Institute
President, Brown Neurosurgery Foundation
Providence, RI, USA

Preface

The operative techniques, treatment goals, biomechanical considerations, and indications for surgery are of particular importance to surgeons in the treatment of patients with spinal tumors. Unlike the operative management of traumatic injury, deformity or degenerative conditions, surgery for spinal tumors requires multifaceted consideration of prognosis, systemic burden, clinical presentation, tumor etiology, and options for neoadjuvant, adjuvant, or conservative treatment.

Surgical texts in this field have commonly grouped approaches applicable to the broad spectrum of spinal disorders, and spinal oncology texts focus on treatment guidelines. As such, there is limited informative material unifying the oncologic principles and technical aspects of spinal tumor surgery. The purpose of this book is to address this gap, serving as an educational resource for trainees, fellows, and attending spine surgeons.

Spinal Tumor Surgery: A Cased-Based Approach contains 28 chapters, organized by location—spanning from pathologies of the craniocervical region to sacral and intradural pathologies. Chapters are structured to describe the anatomy and biomechanics of a specific region, patient evaluation, essential oncologic principles, decision-making process, and technical steps of surgery. A representative case illustration is provided at the end of each chapter, exemplifying pertinent concepts described. With emphasis on surgical technique and artist illustration, this book is meant to serve as a tool for spinal surgeons, focusing specifically on the operative management of spinal tumors.

Baltimore, MD, USA | Daniel M. Sciubba, MD

Acknowledgments

With gratitude to Karrie, Hayley, Camryn, and Duncan, for all of their love and support; to Karim, for his selfless work ethic to get this book completed; and to Ziya, for introducing me to the world of spinal oncology and for mentoring me along the way.

Contents

Part I Anterior Approaches

Contributors

A. Karim Ahmed, BS, MD Department of Neurosurgery, The Johns Hopkins Hospital, Baltimore, MD, USA

Christopher Pearson Ames, MD University of California, San Francisco, Department of Neurosurgery, San Francisco, CA, USA

Ali Baaj, MD New York Presbyterian, Weill Cornell Brain and Spine Center, Department of Neurological Surgery, New York, NY, USA

Ori Barzilai, MD Memorial Sloan Kettering Cancer Center, Department of Neurosurgery, New York, NY, USA

Deb A. Bhowmick, MD University of North Carolina Healthcare, Department of Neurosurgery, Chapel Hill, NC, USA

Mark H. Bilsky, MD Memorial Sloan Kettering Cancer Center, Department of Neurosurgery, New York, NY, USA

Department of Neurological Surgery, Weill Cornell Medical College, New York, NY, USA

Shanda H. Blackmon, MD, MPH Mayo Clinic, Department of General Thoracic Surgery, Rochester, MN, USA

Stefano Boriani, MD IRCCS Galeazzi Orthopedic Institute, Spine Surgery Unit, Milan, Italy

Étienne Bourassa-Moreau, MD, MSc, FRCSC Hôpital du Sacré-Coeur de Montréal, Department of Orthopaedic Surgery, Montreal, Canada

Eric Bourekas, MD, MBA, FACR Ohio State University Wexner Medical Center, Department of Radiology, Columbus, OH, USA

Ali Bydon, MD The Johns Hopkins Hospital, Department of Neurosurgery, Baltimore, MD, USA

Dean Chou, MD University of California, San Francisco, Department of Neurosurgery, San Francisco, CA, USA

Michelle J. Clarke, MD, MA Mayo Clinic, Department of Neurologic Surgery, Rochester, MN, USA

Ian Cote, MD Jackson Memorial Hospital/University of Miami Hospital, Department of Neurological Surgery, Miami, FL, USA

Cecilia L. Dalle Ore, BA University of California, San Francisco, Department of Neurological Surgery, San Francisco, CA, USA

Juan Del Castillo-Calcáneo, MD National Autonomous University of Mexico, Department of Neurosurgery, Mexico City, Mexico

Chikezie I. Eseonu, MD Johns Hopkins Hospital, Department of Neurosurgery, Baltimore, MD, USA

Charles G. Fisher, MD, MHSc, FRCSC Vancouver General Hospital, Department of Orthopaedics, Division of Spine, Vancouver, BC, Canada

Jared Fridley, MD Department of Neurosurgery, Rhode Island Hospital, Warren Alpert School of Medicine at Brown University, Providence, RI, USA

Joel Gagnon, MD, FRCSC Vancouver General Hospital, Department of Vascular Surgery, Vancouver, BC, Canada

Gary Gallia, MD, PhD Johns Hopkins University, Department of Neurosurgery, Baltimore, MD, USA

Ziya L. Gokaslan, MD Department of Neurosurgery, Rhode Island Hospital, Warren Alpert School of Medicine at Brown University, Providence, RI, USA

C. Rory Goodwin, MD, PhD Duke University Medical Center, Department of Neurosurgery, Durham, NC, USA

Barth A. Green, MD Jackson Memorial Hospital/University of Miami Hospital, Department of Neurological Surgery, Miami, FL, USA

Mari L. Groves, MD Johns Hopkins Hospital, Department of Neurosurgery, Baltimore, MD, USA

James S. Harrop, MD Department of Neurological Surgery, Thomas Jefferson University Hospital, Philadelphia, PA, USA

Roger Härtl, MD New York Presbyterian, Weill Cornell Brain and Spine Center, Department of Neurological Surgery, New York, NY, USA

Wataru Ishida, MD The Johns Hopkins Hospital, Department of Neurosurgery, Baltimore, MD, USA

Masaru Ishii, MD Johns Hopkins University, Department of Otolaryngology, Baltimore, MD, USA

George Jallo, MD Johns Hopkins All Children's Hospital, Department of Neurosurgery, St. Petersburg, FL, USA

Thomas Kosztowski, MD Department of Neurosurgery, Rhode Island Hospital, Warren Alpert School of Medicine at Brown University, Providence, RI, USA

Darryl Lau, MD Department of Neurological Surgery, University of California, San Francisco, San Francisco, CA, USA

Ilya Laufer, MD Memorial Sloan Kettering Cancer Center, Department of Neurosurgery, New York, NY, USA

Department of Neurological Surgery, Weill Cornell Medical College, New York, NY, USA

Xun Li, MD Department of Neurosurgery, Rhode Island Hospital, Warren Alpert School of Medicine at Brown University, Providence, RI, USA

Sheng-fu Larry Lo, MD, MHS Johns Hopkins University School of Medicine, Department of Neurosurgery, Baltimore, MD, USA

James G. Malcolm, MD, PhD Emory University, Department of Neurosurgery, Atlanta, GA, USA

Hani Malone, MD Scripps Clinic, Division of Neurosurgery, San Diego, CA, USA

Rex A. W. Marco, MD Musculoskeletal Oncology and Reconstructive Spine Surgery, Houston Methodist Hospital, Houston, TX, USA

Kyle L. McCormick, BA Neurosurgery Department, Columbia University Medical Center, New York, NY, USA

Ehud Mendel, MD, MBA, FACS The Ohio State Neurological Society, Columbus, OH, USA

OSU Spine Research Institute, Columbus, OH, USA

Wexner Medical Center at The Ohio State University/The Arthur James Cancer Hospital, Columbus, OH, USA

Katherine Miller, MD Houston Methodist, Department of Orthopedics and Sports Medicine, Houston, TX, USA

Ahmed Mohyeldin, MD, PhD Ohio State University Medical Center, Department of Neurosurgery, Columbus, OH, USA

Michael K. Moore, MD, MS Emory University, Department of Neurosurgery, Atlanta, GA, USA

Rodrigo Navarro-Ramirez, MD New York Presbyterian, Weill Cornell Brain and Spine Center, Department of Neurological Surgery, New York, NY, USA

John E. O'Toole, MD, MS Rush University Medical Center, Department of Neurological Surgery, Chicago, IL, USA

Courtney Pendleton, MD Department of Neurological Surgery, Thomas Jefferson University Hospital, Philadelphia, PA, USA

Zach Pennington, BS, MD The Johns Hopkins Hospital, Department of Neurosurgery, Baltimore, MD, USA

Daniel Refai, MD Emory University, Department of Neurosurgery and Orthopaedics, Atlanta, GA, USA

Peter S. Rose, MD Mayo Clinic, Department of Othopaedic Surgery, Rochester, MN, USA

George N. Rymarczuk, MD Department of Neurological Surgery, Thomas Jefferson University Hospital, Philadelphia, PA, USA

Meic H. Schmidt, MD, MBA Brain and Spine Institute, Department of Neurosurgery, Westchester Medical Center at the New York Medical College, Valhalla, NY, USA

Joseph H. Schwab, MD, MS Massachusetts General Hospital, Department of Orthopaedic Surgery, Boston, MA, USA

Daniel M. Sciubba, MD Department of Neurosurgery, The Johns Hopkins Hospital, Baltimore, MD, USA

Akash A. Shah, MD Massachusetts General Hospital, Department of Orthopaedic Surgery, Boston, MA, USA

Daniel L. Shepherd, MD Mayo Clinic, Department of Neurosurgery, Rochester, MN, USA

Ian Suk, BSC, BMC Department of Neurosurgery, The Johns Hopkins Hospital, Baltimore, MD, USA

Nicholas Theodore, MD Department of Neurosurgery, The Johns Hopkins Hospital, Baltimore, MD, USA

Christian B. Theodotou, MD Jackson Memorial Hospital/University of Miami Hospital, Department of Neurological Surgery, Miami, FL, USA

Brian D. Thorp, MD Department of Otolaryngology-Head and Neck Surgery, University of North Carolina School of Medicine, Chapel Hill, NC, USA

Luis M. Tumialán, MD Department of Neurosurgery, Barrow Neurological Institute, St. Joseph's Hospital and Medical Center, Phoenix, AZ, USA

Feng Wei, MD Peking University Third Hospital, Department of Orthopedics, Beijing, China

Ulas Yener, MD Ohio State University Medical Center, Department of Neurosurgery, Columbus, OH, USA

Zoe Zhang, MD Ohio State University Medical Center, Department of Neurosurgery, Columbus, OH, USA

Corinna C. Zygourakis, MD Johns Hopkins Hospital, Department of Neurosurgery, Baltimore, MD, USA

Part I

Anterior Approaches

Anterior Cranio-Cervical Approach: Transnasal

1

Chikezie I. Eseonu, Gary Gallia, and Masaru Ishii

Case Presentation

A 37-year-old male presented with several months of persistent headaches that were getting progressively worse. The physical examination was unremarkable. A magnetic resonance imaging (MRI) of the brain showed a T2 hyperintense, enhancing 1.2 × 2.8 × 2.5-cm lesion centered at the mid and lower clivus with involvement of the cranio-cervical junction (CCJ, Fig. 1.1). The lesion extended intradurally, abutting the vertebral arteries and medulla. An endoscopic endonasal transclival and transcranial cervical junction approach was planned for resection of the clival mass.

The patient was positioned in the supine position, with the head fixated in the neutral position with a skull clamp. Stereotactic imaging was registered, and the nasal cavities were treated with vasoconstrictor spray and prepped with a clindamycin wash. The right middle turbinate was resected, and right maxillary antrostomy and ethmoidectomy were performed. A nasoseptal flap (NSF) was elevated on the right side with a monopolar electrocautery needle tip and tucked into maxillary sinus. Posterior septectomy and large bilateral sphenoidectomy were performed, and the sphenoid sinus mucosa was removed. The pharyngobasilar fascia and superior pharyngeal constrictor muscle were opened at the midline. The pharyngeal mucosa incision was extended inferiorly down to C1. The longus capitis muscles were dissected off laterally to expose C1 inferiorly and laterally. The perimeter aspects of the tumor were identified along the clivus and cranio-cervical junction and resected using angled endoscopes and instruments. The subsequent resection cavity was reconstructed with an inlay and onlay dural substitute button graft. Fibrin glue was placed on the edges of the onlay graft circumferentially. An abdominal fat graft was then harvested and placed on top of the onlay graft to obliterate the dead space along with absorbable gelatin compressed sponges (Gelfoam, Pfizer, New York, NY) wrapped in oxidized cellulose (Surgicel, Ethicon, Somerville, NJ). The longus capitis muscles and superior pharyngeal muscles were closed over the resection cavity and covered with a nasoseptal flap. Postoperative imaging showed a gross total resection and the patient did well after surgery (Fig. 1.2).

C. I. Eseonu (✉)
Johns Hopkins Hospital, Department of Neurosurgery, Baltimore, MD, USA
e-mail: ceseonu1@jhmi.edu

G. Gallia
Johns Hopkins University, Department of Neurosurgery, Baltimore, MD, USA

M. Ishii
Johns Hopkins University, Department of Otolaryngology, Baltimore, MD, USA

D. M. Sciubba (ed.), *Spinal Tumor Surgery*, https://doi.org/10.1007/978-3-319-98422-3_1

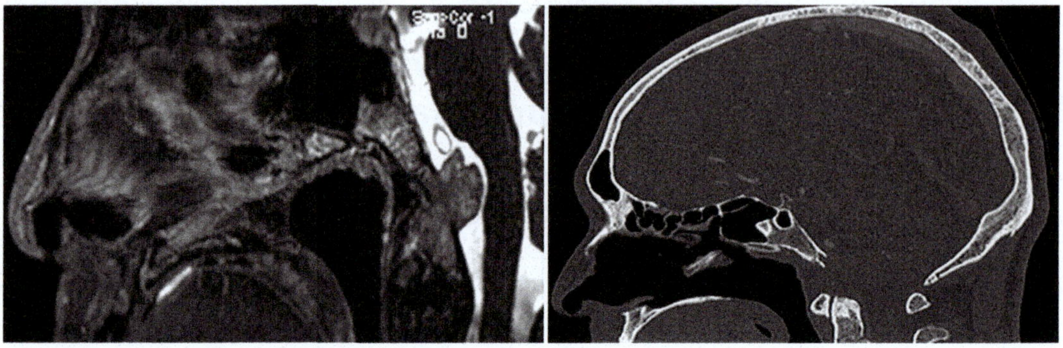

Fig. 1.1 T2 hyperintense mildly enhancing tumor centered within the mid and lower clivus with extraosseous extension into the premedullary cistern seen on sagittal (left) CISS and (right) CT sequence

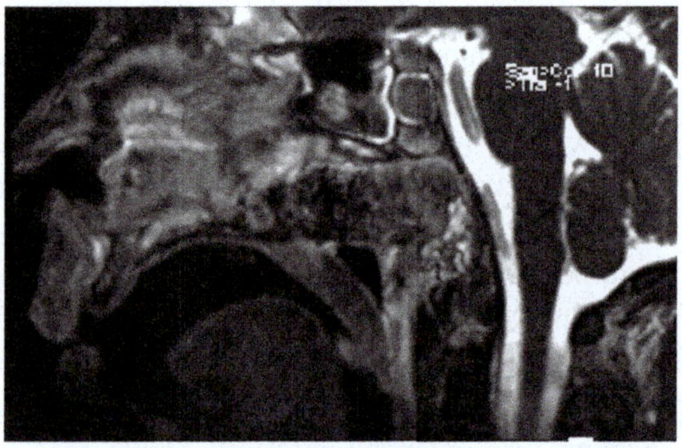

Fig. 1.2 Sagittal CISS MRI status after a transnasal approach for resection of a mid/lower clival tumor. No definite residual tumor is present. Fat packing was used for the skull base reconstruction

Introduction

Anterior and anterolateral cranio-cervical lesions present challenging operative cases given their proximity to vital neurovascular structures. Several pathologies can affect the cranio-cervical junction including neoplasms, rheumatologic disease, fibroconnective tissue disease, congenital disease, infections, and traumatic and degenerative disorders [1]. Numerous approaches have been employed to gain access to this region, including the transcervical, transnasal, transoral, and variations of the far-lateral approach. Traditionally, the transoral approach had been used to provide a direct route to the cranio-cervical junction (CCJ); however, this approach can be susceptible to contamination given the surgical exposure to the bacterial flora of the oral cavity [2–4]. In addition, limited surgical range of motion can be found in patients with a smaller oral cavity, which may require splitting the soft and/or hard palate that may cause damage to the oral cavity and lead to airway edema and extended postoperative intubation time [5, 6].

The transnasal approach for the cranio-cervical region was first shown by Kassam et al. [7]. It provides an alternative approach that allows for good visualization of the CCJ while limiting the number of complications. The use of endoscopy for the transnasal approach provides a panoramic view that can provide improved lighting and resolution compared to the operative microscope [2, 3, 8, 9]. It also provides direct access to the anterior and anterolateral CCJ without needing to mobilize the surrounding neurovasculature. This chapter describes the transnasal surgical approach to the anterior cranio-cervical junction.

Preoperative Planning

Preoperative imaging is required for the assessment of the CCJ pathology as well as any anatomical variations. A thin-cut (1 mm) maxillofacial computed tomography (CT) can evaluate the bony anatomy and orientation of the nasal sinuses. T1 magnetic resonance imaging (MRI)

with and without gadolinium and a constructive interference in steady state (CISS) sequence are used to evaluate the relationship between the pathology and the cranial nerves. Neuronavigation is also utilized intraoperatively for these cases.

The sinonasal anatomy of the patient should also be evaluated to determine whether there are any deviations, perforations, or spur formations of the nasal septum. The nasal anatomy of the middle and inferior turbinates and the nasal septum can also limit the range of motion of the operative instruments, and although resecting these turbinates can resolve this problem, it may lead to increased nasal crusting and infections of the upper airway [2, 3, 10]. Preoperative swallow evaluations or laryngoscopic evaluation of the vocal cords may be warranted in patients with swallowing or vocal symptoms to establish a preoperative baseline [11].

Measurement to Evaluate Accessibility to the Cranio-Cervical Junction

Multiple methods can be used to evaluate whether the transnasal approach will provide adequate accessibility to the CCJ including the nasopalatine line (NPL) and the naso-axial line (NAxL, Fig. 1.3).

The nasopalatine line can be used to predict whether there would be adequate access to the ventral cranio-cervical junction. By drawing a line from the rhinion to the ventral spinal column that incorporates the posterior end of the hard palate on a sagittal view, an estimate of the inferior surgical extent that is accessible by the endoscope can be determined [12]. Studies related to the NPL have reported that the visual limit of the cranio-cervical junction with the endoscopic-assisted transnasal approach allows for direct visualization of the odontoid and clivus, while its inferior limit is around the base of C2 [3, 12, 13].

The naso-axial line is another method to evaluate CCJ accessibility that is similar to the NPL, except it measures from the midpoint between the rhinion and the anterior nasal spine to the ventral vertebral body. This line attempts to account for the structural limitations to the endoscope imposed by the nares and predicts the inferior extent of the endoscope, using a straight 0-degree scope, to around the upper half of C2 [14].

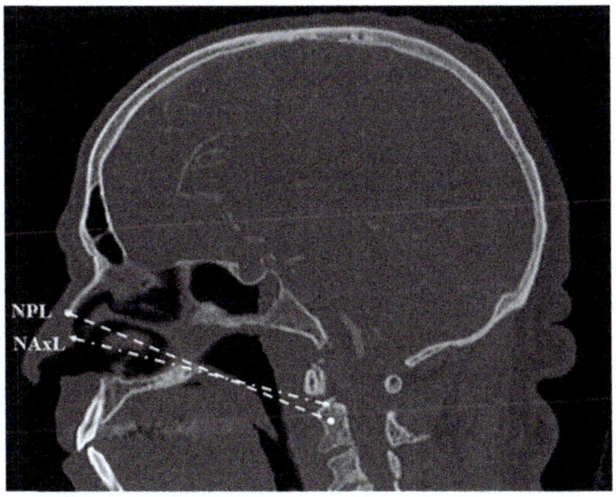

Fig. 1.3 Methods to estimate the inferior extent of a transnasal approach. Nasopalatine line (NPL) and naso-axial line (NAxL)

Patient Positioning

The patient is placed in the supine position with the body at the upper right edge of the bed and the arms tucked to the side, thereby allowing access to the abdomen for potential harvesting of the abdominal fat (Fig. 1.4). The endotracheal tube is placed to the patient's left side of the mouth in addition to an orogastric tube to prevent blood collection in the stomach as well as reflux into the surgical field. A three-point fixation device is used to secure the head in the appropriate position, with transclival cases requiring a neutral position, whereas slight flexion is utilized for odontoidectomy or upper cervical approaches to facilitate an easier surgical trajectory.

Intraoperative neuromonitoring can be used to evaluate somatosensory evoked potentials (SSEP) and electroencephalography (EEG). Motor evoked potentials (MEP), neural integrity monitor electromyogram, and monitoring of the lower cranial nerves may also be useful for particular cases [11, 15].

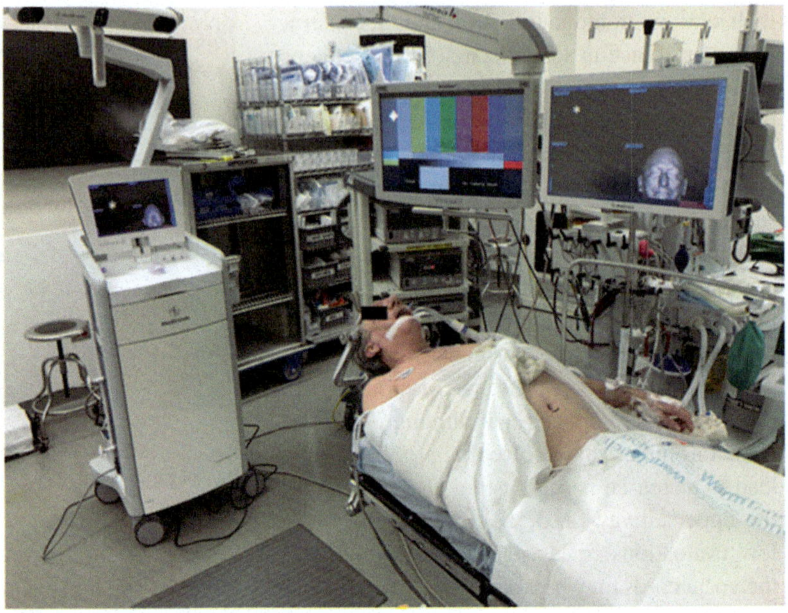

Fig. 1.4 Patient positioning for the endoscopic transnasal approach. The patient is positioned supine with exposure of the abdomen for potential abdominal fat harvesting. Monitors for neuro-navigation (*) and the endoscope (♦) are placed in the working view of the surgeon

Surgical Approach

Transnasal Approach

A 0-degree endoscope is used for visualization during the opening of the procedure. The nasal mucosa is injected with 1% lidocaine with 1:100,000 epinephrine, and Afrin®- or cocaine-soaked pledgets are placed within both nostrils for 5 min. A right-sided middle turbinectomy is performed to provide a larger corridor for the endoscope. If surgical access is needed in the patient's far-left lateral corridor, then the left turbinate is also displaced laterally. A maxillary antrostomy is then performed on the ipsilateral side of the patient by resecting the uncinate process and expanding the natural os of the maxillary sinus in order to prevent iatrogenic sinus disease. A right-sided spheno-ethmoidectomy is then performed in order to provide a corridor laterally for the endoscope and instrumentation.

The choana is then identified in the nasopharynx, and the sphenoid ostium is identified medial to the superior turbinate. A nasoseptal flap can be harvested by identifying the sphenopalatine artery that serves as the pedicle for the flap. A monopolar electrocautery needle tip is then used to make an inferior cut that extends from the posterior sphenopalatine foramen and moves anteriorly, above the choana, along the posterior part of the vomer down to the floor of the nasal cavity and is extended anteriorly to the head of the inferior turbinate. The superior cut is made slightly below the sphenoid sinus os and continues anteriorly at this level until it passes the olfactory epithelium. The incision is then curved superiorly, 1 cm below the nasal roof, to incorporate the septal body prior to joining the anterior incision made just behind the nasal valve. The nasoseptal flap can be elevated, on the side that most favors the skull base reconstruction, and can be tucked within the ethmoid or maxillary sinus for preservation until needed for reconstruction, depending on the extent of the CCJ that will need to be visualized. If a nasoseptal flap is not needed, then an inferior posterior septectomy can be done, which spares the pedicle of the nasoseptal flap and can be used for later harvest if needed.

An extensive sphenoidotomy is performed based on the size of the pathology, and the posterior nasal septum is detached from the rostrum of the sphenoid bone. The face of the sphenoid bone is drilled off to open the sphenoid sinus, and 1–2 cm of the posterior septum is also removed. The pituitary fossa and carotid protuberances are then identified.

For access to the lower clival and upper cervical region, the Eustachian tubes, soft palate, and fossa of Rosenmüller are visualized bilaterally. A midline incision is then made in the nasopharyngeal mucosa and pharyngobasilar fascia. The prevertebral fascia is then dissected, and the surrounding muscle is elevated. Avoiding incisions into the oropharynx when possible helps in reducing long-term intubation and postoperative parenteral nutritional supplement [1]. This also avoids exposure to the saliva and oral flora that can contaminate the surgical field [16]. The floor of the sphenoid sinus is drilled down further to connect the sphenoid sinus with the nasopharynx. The mucosa and the muscle on the nasopharynx are lateralized, exposing the fascial layer of the nasopharynx, which is also elevated off the clivus. Additional muscle (i.e., longus capitis, longus colli, or anterior atlanto-occipital membrane) can be lateralized off the occipital, C1, or odontoid bone as needed.

Transclival Approach

For tumor resection within the clival region, an endonasal transclival approach can be used (Fig. 1.5). Pathologies such as foramen magnum meningiomas and clival chordomas may be treated by this method.

Following the endonasal opening, as mentioned in the transnasal approach, the clivus can be drilled. The clival corridor is limited superiorly by the lacerum segment of the internal carotid artery (ICA) and inferiorly by the occipital condyles. If the tumor invades lateral to the occipital condyle, then the anterior medial portion of the condyle can be removed to expand lateral access.

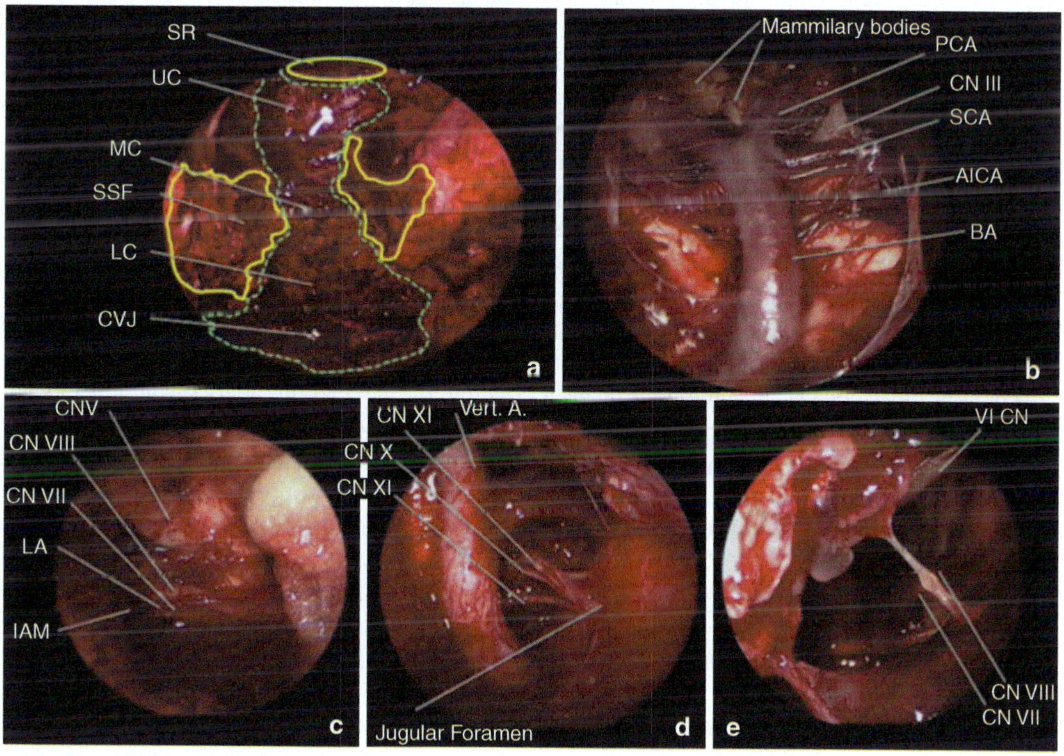

Fig. 1.5 Intraoperative images following the removal of a clival chordoma. (**a**) 0-degree scope. (**b–e**) 30°. AICA anterior inferior cerebellar artery, BA basilar artery, CVJ craniovertebral junction, IAM internal acoustic meatus, LA labyrinthine artery, LC lower clivus, MC middle clivus, PCA posterior cerebral artery, SCA superior cerebellar artery, SR sellar region, SSF sphenoid sinus floor, UC upper clivus, Vert. A. vertebral artery. (Reproduced with permission from Zoli et al. [17])

This is achieved by exposing the atlanto-occipital joint by dissection of the rectus capitis anterior and the capsule of the atlanto-occipital joint. The occipital condyle can then be drilled up to the hypoglossal canal. The inferior aspect of the condyle should be left intact, as this portion of the bone connects with the alar ligament and can affect the stability of the occipito-atlantal region [18, 19].

Skull Base Reconstruction

The main complication with transnasal approaches is the postoperative cerebrospinal fluid (CSF) leak; however, reconstruction methods with nasoseptal flaps have significantly reduced the incidence of this complication [20, 21]. Nasoseptal flaps for the CCJ require a flap that is large enough to reach the caudal extent of the surgical defect. Often, in cases where a CSF leak has been found, an inlay dural substitute or autologous free graft is used followed by the vascularized nasoseptal onlay flap. The NSF must be placed on the bony edges that surround the resection cavity and have been stripped off the mucosa. Absorbable gelatin compressed sponges (Gelfoam, Pfizer, New York, NY) wrapped in oxidized cellulose (Surgicel, Ethicon, Somerville, NJ) are placed onto the NSF onlay for reinforcement, and fibrin glue (Evicel, Ethicon, Somerville, NJ) is then placed along the edge of the NSF.

For large clival defects, an autologous fat graft can be used to obliterate the dead space of the resection cavity. The nasal cavity is then packed with bioresorbable nasal packing (NasoPore, Stryker, Kalamazoo, MI), and nasal stents may also be used.

Postoperative Management

For patients who experience high-flow CSF leaks following surgery, the patient is kept on bedrest for at least 24 h with the head of the bed elevated. Absorbable nasal packing tends to be left in the nose to bolster the skull base reconstruction. If a nasoseptal flap is used, then Doyle Open Lumen Splints are left in the nares, bilaterally, for 5–7 days, and then removed in the outpatient setting. Patients are encouraged to not use straws; to avoid bending, straining, or bearing down; as well as to avoid sneezing and coughing with an open mouth for 4 weeks following surgery. Postoperative nasal crusting can be treated with nasal saline spray in the short term, followed by nasal irrigation once the reconstruction is integrated.

Complications

Systemic literature reviews show very few complications and mortalities associated with the use of the transnasal approach, with mortality being at 1.4–3.5%, infections at 0–1.2%, and cerebral spinal fluid leak at 0–3.5% [1, 22].

Postoperative CSF leak following transnasal surgery can often be addressed by using a lumbar drain or surgical intervention to repair the CSF leak. Intrathecal fluorescein can be used to identify the CSF fistula during intraoperative re-exploration.

Carotid injury can also be a major complication with the transnasal approach. Operating in a controlled manner by utilizing anatomical landmarks to orient your surgical position is important for approaching the carotid. Preoperative imaging can also allow for the localization of the internal carotid arteries and early identification of the carotid arteries, intraoperatively, using stereotactic-guided navigation, and micro-Doppler can help in visualizing the segments of the carotid in proximity to the tumor of interest. If carotid injury occurs, controlling the surgical field becomes paramount. Large-bore suctioning (10F) should be used to suction the blood from the surgical field, and this helps in identifying the site of carotid injury. Oftentimes, two surgeons are needed in this case, with one diverting blood flow and the other attempting to get hemostasis. Hemostasis can be achieved by compression from packing, suture repair, or a bipolar cautery to weld the carotid defect shut. Packing has been described to occur with Teflon, fibrin glue, oxidized cellulose packing thrombin-gelatin material, methyl methacrylate patch, and crushed muscle patch [23]. In situations where the vessel injury is not enclosed with the bone and there is adequate access to the vessel injury, then direct closure can be attempted. For intradural procedures, packing alone is insufficient for hemostasis since the blood can travel into the subdural space [24]. In cases where hemostasis cannot be achieved, endovascular angiography can be used to assess the extent of injury to the carotid and the development of a pseudoaneurysm. Endovascular intervention can then be used to occlude the vessel of interest.

Damage to the lower brainstem and cranial nerves is also a potential risk with transnasal surgery in the CCJ. The use of intraoperative neuromonitoring and careful dissection of cranial nerves can help reduce traction injury from manipulation of the cranial nerves. A gross total resection may also not be possible for tumors that are adherent to vital neurovascular structures.

Advantages and Limitations of the Approach

Advantages

The transnasal approach allows for preservation of the soft palate and retropharyngeal soft tissues, thus allowing patients to resume an oral diet as early as postoperative day 1 [3, 25, 26]. This also avoids excess exposure to the oral flora, which can help reduce risks with infection [16]. The transnasal approach also avoids retraction of vital structures around the brainstem, which would be required for posterior lateral approaches.

Limitations

The transnasal approach provides a minimally invasive technique that avoids making skin incisions. The nasal cavity provides some natural anatomic barriers that limit the surgeon's range of motion with the instruments. The hard palate and nasal bone in the nasal cavity can also limit the operative range of motion inferiorly and superiorly, respectively [27]. Intraoperative issues with vascular injury can be difficult to manage with the endoscope as pooling blood in the operative field can hinder the view of scope, thus making it difficult to achieve hemostasis. The endoscopic approach also requires a significant learning curve in order to become facile with the technique while limiting the amount of complications [11, 28].

References

1. Fujii T, Platt A, Zada G. Endoscopic endonasal approaches to the craniovertebral junction: a systematic review of the literature. J Neurol Surg B Skull Base. 2015;76(6):480–8.
2. Lee A, Sommer D, Reddy K, Murty N, Gunnarsson T. Endoscopic transnasal approach to the craniocervical junction. Skull Base. 2010;20(3):199–205.
3. Ponce-Gomez JA, Ortega-Porcayo LA, Soriano-Baron HE, Sotomayor-Gonzalez A, Arriada-Mendicoa N, Gomez-Amador JL, et al. Evolution from microscopic transoral to endoscopic endonasal odontoidectomy. Neurosurg Focus. 2014;37(4):E15.
4. Yu Y, Hu F, Zhang X, Ge J, Sun C. Endoscopic transnasal odontoidectomy combined with posterior reduction to treat basilar invagination: technical note. J Neurosurg Spine. 2013;19(5):637–43.
5. Hankinson TC, Grunstein E, Gardner P, Spinks TJ, Anderson RC. Transnasal odontoid resection followed by posterior decompression and occipitocervical fusion in children with Chiari malformation Type I and ventral brainstem compression. J Neurosurg Pediatr. 2010;5(6):549–53.
6. Patel AJ, Boatey J, Muns J, Bollo RJ, Whitehead WE, Giannoni CM, et al. Endoscopic endonasal odontoidectomy in a child with chronic type 3 atlantoaxial rotatory fixation: case report and literature review. Childs Nerv Syst. 2012;28(11):1971–5.
7. Kassam AB, Snyderman C, Gardner P, Carrau R, Spiro R. The expanded endonasal approach: a fully endoscopic transnasal approach and resection of the odontoid process: technical case report. Neurosurgery. 2005;57(1 Suppl):E213; discussion E213.
8. Eseonu CI, ReFaey K, Rincon-Torroella J, Garcia O, Wand GS, Salvatori R, et al. Endoscopic versus microscopic transsphenoidal approach for pituitary adenomas: comparison of outcomes during the transition of methods of a single surgeon. World Neurosurg. 2017;97:317–25.
9. Cavallo LM, Cappabianca P, Messina A, Esposito F, Stella L, de Divitiis E, et al. The extended endoscopic endonasal approach to the clivus and craniovertebral junction: anatomical study. Childs Nerv Syst. 2007;23(6):665–71.
10. Alfieri A, Jho HD, Tschabitscher M. Endoscopic endonasal approach to the ventral cranio-cervical junction: anatomical study. Acta Neurochir. 2002;144(3):219–25. discussion 225

11. Kshettry VR, Thorp BD, Shriver MF, Zanation AM, Woodard TD, Sindwani R, et al. Endoscopic approaches to the craniovertebral junction. Otolaryngol Clin N Am. 2016;49(1):213–26.
12. de Almeida JR, Zanation AM, Snyderman CH, Carrau RL, Prevedello DM, Gardner PA, et al. Defining the nasopalatine line: the limit for endonasal surgery of the spine. Laryngoscope. 2009;119(2):239–44.
13. Baird CJ, Conway JE, Sciubba DM, Prevedello DM, Quinones-Hinojosa A, Kassam AB. Radiographic and anatomic basis of endoscopic anterior craniocervical decompression: a comparison of endonasal, transoral, and transcervical approaches. Neurosurgery. 2009;65(6 Suppl):158–63; discussion 63-4.
14. Aldana PR, Naseri I, La Corte E. The naso-axial line: a new method of accurately predicting the inferior limit of the endoscopic endonasal approach to the craniovertebral junction. Neurosurgery. 2012;71(2 Suppl Operative):ons308–14; discussion ons314.
15. Atlas G, Lee M. The neural integrity monitor electromyogram tracheal tube: anesthetic considerations. J Anaesthesiol Clin Pharmacol. 2013;29(3):403–4.
16. Laufer I, Greenfield JP, Anand VK, Hartl R, Schwartz TH. Endonasal endoscopic resection of the odontoid process in a nonachondroplastic dwarf with juvenile rheumatoid arthritis: feasibility of the approach and utility of the intraoperative Iso-C three-dimensional navigation. Case report. J Neurosurg Spine. 2008;8(4):376–80.
17. Zoli M, Milanese L, Bonfatti R, Faustini-Fustini M, Marucci G, Tallini G, et al. Clival chordomas: considerations after 16 years of endoscopic endonasal surgery. J Neurosurg. 2018;128:329–38.
18. Panjabi M, Dvorak J, Crisco JJ 3rd, Oda T, Wang P, Grob D. Effects of alar ligament transection on upper cervical spine rotation. J Orthop Res. 1991;9(4):584–93.
19. Panjabi M, Dvorak J, Crisco J 3rd, Oda T, Hilibrand A, Grob D. Flexion, extension, and lateral bending of the upper cervical spine in response to alar ligament transections. J Spinal Disord. 1991;4(2):157–67.
20. Hadad G, Bassagasteguy L, Carrau RL, Mataza JC, Kassam A, Snyderman CH, et al. A novel reconstructive technique after endoscopic expanded endonasal approaches: vascular pedicle nasoseptal flap. Laryngoscope. 2006;116(10):1882–6.
21. Kassam AB, Thomas A, Carrau RL, Snyderman CH, Vescan A, Prevedello D, et al. Endoscopic reconstruction of the cranial base using a pedicled nasoseptal flap. Neurosurgery. 2008;63(1 Suppl 1):ONS44–52; discussion ONS52–3.
22. Fang CH, Friedman R, Schild SD, Goldstein IM, Baredes S, Liu JK, et al. Purely endoscopic endonasal surgery of the craniovertebral junction: a systematic review. Int Forum Allergy Rhinol. 2015;5(8):754–60.
23. Padhye V, Valentine R, Wormald PJ. Management of carotid artery injury in endonasal surgery. Int Arch Otorhinolaryngol. 2014;18(Suppl 2):S173–8.
24. Solares CA, Ong YK, Carrau RL, Fernandez-Miranda J, Prevedello DM, Snyderman CH, et al. Prevention and management of vascular injuries in endoscopic surgery of the sinonasal tract and skull base. Otolaryngol Clin N Am. 2010;43(4):817–25.
25. Kassam A, Snyderman CH, Mintz A, Gardner P, Carrau RL. Expanded endonasal approach: the rostrocaudal axis. Part II. Posterior clinoids to the foramen magnum. Neurosurg Focus. 2005;19(1):E4.
26. Mazzatenta D, Zoli M, Mascari C, Pasquini E, Frank G. Endoscopic endonasal odontoidectomy: clinical series. Spine (Phila Pa 1976). 2014;39(10):846–53.
27. Messina A, Bruno MC, Decq P, Coste A, Cavallo LM, de Divittis E, et al. Pure endoscopic endonasal odontoidectomy: anatomical study. Neurosurg Rev. 2007;30(3):189–94; discussion 194.
28. Eseonu CI, ReFaey K, Pamias-Portalatin E, Asensio J, Garcia O, Boahene K, et al. Three-hand endoscopic endonasal transsphenoidal surgery: experience with an anatomy-preserving mononostril approach technique. Oper Neuros. 2017;14:158–165.

Contemporary Transoral Approach for Resection of Craniocervical Junction Tumors

2

Brian D. Thorp and Deb A. Bhowmick

Introduction

Tumors of the odontoid process and the second cervical vertebra or axis present unique challenges for adequate resection, neural element decompression, and reconstruction for the spine surgeon. As the tumors differ in shape and location from the subaxial spine, routine retropharyngeal approaches to the axis are difficult and technically challenging due to the lack of significant visualization and impedance of facial structures. The transoral approach to the odontoid process and the axis was invented and popularized by Crockard [1] as a more direct and easily maintained surgical corridor for masses in the odontoid process and retro-odontoid space. Since its introduction, multiple improvements and technical modifications to the transoral approach have been made to improve visualization and resection of masses involving the atlantoaxial complex. These advances include palate- and jaw-splitting extensions of the approach as well as the use of innovative combined approaches to the skull base and the subaxial spine that allow for adequate tumor resection and reconstruction [2].

Advantages of the transoral approach are balanced by the unique complications that come with the disruption of important airway and swallowing structures, the use of a contaminated surgical corridor, and the need for appropriate reconstruction that is resistant to atlanto-occipital motion forces. Retropharyngeal abscess, cerebrospinal fluid (CSF) leaks, and hardware failures are not easily tolerated or managed in patients with transoral approaches. Furthermore, routine postoperative care, even for uncomplicated resections, can still result in extended intubation or long-term alimentary diversion [3]. Many of these complications or routine postoperative issues are not managed well by a singular spinal surgeon. Thus, a multidisciplinary team of anesthesiologists, otorhinolaryngologists, intensivists, as well as speech therapists and nutritionists are needed for intraoperative and postoperative care for nearly all of these patients.

While there exist no absolute indications for a transoral approach for the treatment of craniocervical spine masses, reasonable guidance would be to consider the approach for the resection of masses that cannot be easily resected or decompressed from neural structures through a dorsal approach only. Other candidates for transoral approaches are patients that have failed or progressive disease with dorsal resection, those with suspected primary tumors of the vertebra, and those with radio-insensitive tumors causing pathological fractures or deformity. Relative contraindications to the approach would be the

B. D. Thorp
Department of Otolaryngology-Head and Neck Surgery, University of North Carolina School of Medicine, Chapel Hill, NC, USA

D. A. Bhowmick (✉)
University of North Carolina Healthcare, Department of Neurosurgery, Chapel Hill, NC, USA
e-mail: deb_bhowmick@med.unc.edu

D. M. Sciubba (ed.), *Spinal Tumor Surgery*, https://doi.org/10.1007/978-3-319-98422-3_2

presence of significant scarring or radiation to the posterior pharynx, inability to provide appropriate dorsal fixation points for reconstruction, as well as the presence of effective alternative non-surgical treatment options if the patient is neurologically intact.

Preoperative assessment of patients suspected of needing transoral vertebral resections would include appropriate imaging, functional swallowing and airway assessments, and assessment of prognosis and postoperative treatment options by a multidisciplinary oncological team (Fig. 2.1). Due to the significant risk of morbidity and likely lengthy interruption of systemic treatment, a minimal prognosis of 1 year of life expectancy is required in most centers prior to offering operative treatment of this nature. Exceptions, however, are commonly made for progressive quadriparesis or impending brainstem compression from craniocervical deformity or tumor. Thus, an extensive discussion of common complications of the treatment should be had with the patient and his or her caregivers. Furthermore, innovative modifications of the traditional transoral approach can be considered to decrease morbidity and postoperative complications.

At minimum, preoperative MRI and CT of the upper cervical spine are required prior to surgery. This delineates the margins of the tumor as well as the extent of bony destruction. Furthermore, the location of carotid and vertebral arteries needs to be definitively visualized on preoperative films or dedicated vascular imaging to avoid injury during exposure or reconstruction. When alternative or additive approaches are being utilized, including transnasal and mandible splitting

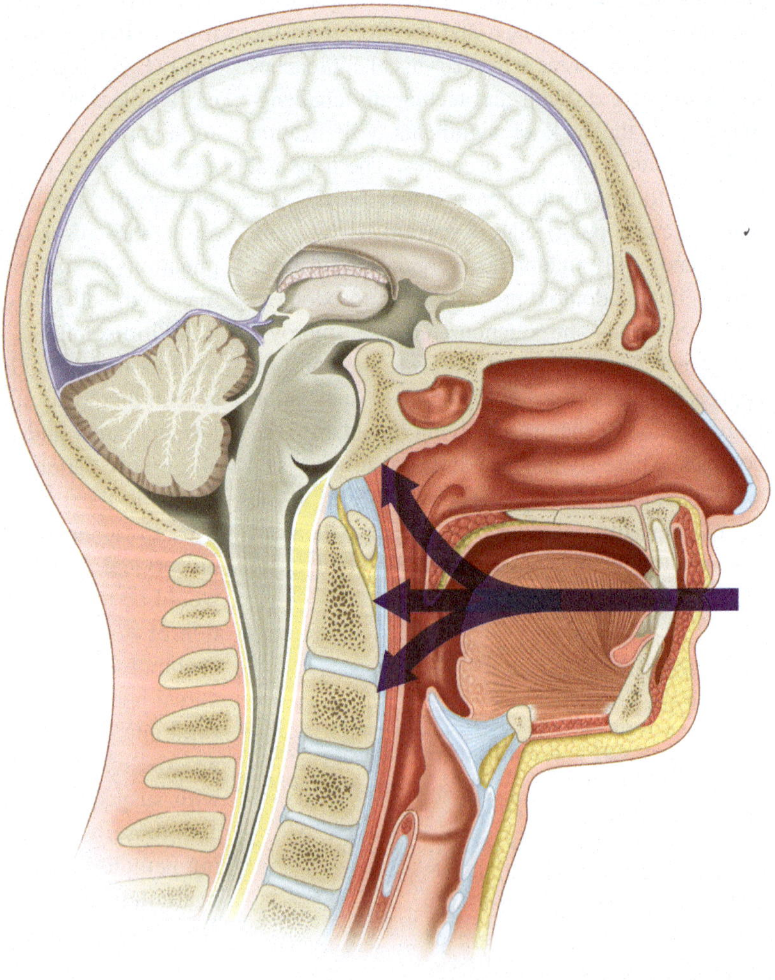

Fig. 2.1 Transoral surgical trajectory. (Reproduced with permission from Pasztor et al. [4])

techniques, it is usually necessary to also obtain a CT of the facial, nasal, and sinus structures. Upright cervical X-rays are also helpful when kyphosis or need for occipitocervical fixation is required so that a baseline measurement of cervical parameters, including chin-brow angle, atlantoaxial, and subaxial sagittal vertical axis, can be obtained prior to surgery.

Surgical Technique

The transoral approach traditionally requires the use of multiple self-retaining retractors to maintain the oral opening as well the posterior pharyngeal dissection. This can be done using a Dingman retractor with tongue and tonsil depression attachments to maintain the oral opening, or if only a small pharyngeal opening is needed, a hand-held tongue retractor with a simple dental cheek retractor inset is all that is needed. For larger exposures, especially if tumor plains must be maintained for en bloc resection, a Crockard pharyngeal retractor is used to retract the posterior pharyngeal constrictors during surgery. The airway is maintained orally through an armored endotracheal tube, which may be retracted laterally during the surgery. Prior to incision, an oral chlorhexidine wash is used to minimize gross contamination from oral particulates.

Typically, a midline incision in the posterior oral mucosa is made from just inferior to the pharyngeal tubercle to the expected inferior portion of the C2 mass within the visualized operative field (Fig. 2.2). The size of the incision may be guided by intraoperative fluoroscopy or image

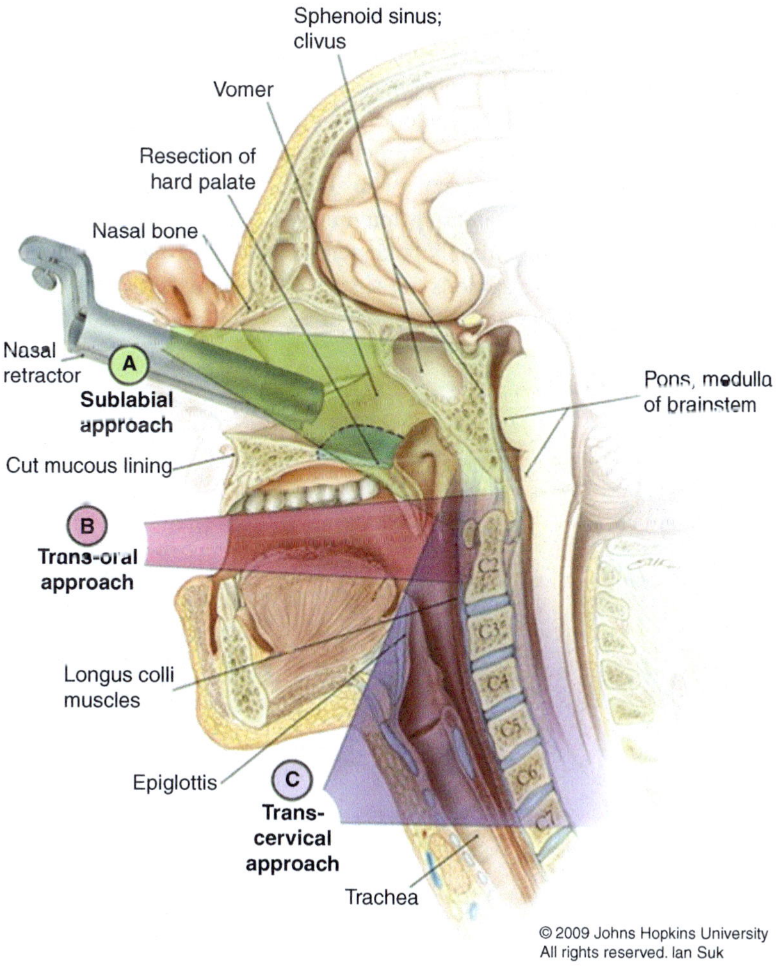

Fig. 2.2 Transoral, sublabial, and transcervical operative corridors. (Reproduced with permission from Bettegowda et al. [5])

guidance to minimize mucosal disruption. The uvula and attached soft palate may be retracted upward through the nasopharynx, with a suture passed through the uvula, and then nasally to aid in visualization. In extreme situations, the soft palate may be split to gain greater cranial exposure (Fig. 2.3). However, soft palate disruption should not be taken lightly, as it significantly affects postoperative swallowing function [3]. If the posterior oral anatomy is significantly affected by mass effect, it is always advisable to obtain preoperative vascular imaging and consider use of an intraoperative Doppler probe to avoid incursion into the carotid arteries.

Sharp dissection is then followed through the relatively avascular pharyngeal raphe. Bleeding points can easily be controlled with pressure and retraction. Cautery is limited to bipolar tips to avoid unneeded injury to the superior pharyngeal constrictors. The buccopharyngeal fascia is often adherent to the raphe and is commonly opened incidentally with cautery or retraction to reveal a thin translucent layer of retropharyngeal fascia and the brightly white-colored anterior longitudinal ligament of the spine below. Tumors of the spine rarely traverse these fascial plains; thus, judicious opening of the anterior longitudinal ligament with cautery should only be undertaken if a primary tumor of the spine is not suspected, to allow for appropriate circumferential resection. Once the mass is entered, any number of tools, including drills, aspirators, and sonicators, may be utilized to resect the mass and decompress any neural structure. It must be pointed out that tumors of the C2 vertebra rarely traverse the relatively thick apical craniocervical ligaments but are more likely to cause neural compression asymmetrically around or through the lower posterior longitudinal ligament.

Reconstruction of the transoral opening is relatively simple, using a few interrupted sutures to close the pharyngeal raphe and the mucosal opening. Adjuncts to closure can be very useful to avoid unnecessary long-term contamination of the operative field. Often, fat grafting, use of fascia lata, fibrin glue, or AlloDerm™ is underlaid the muscular closure to provide an additional sealing barrier from mouth contents. Intraoperative antibiotics with oral flora coverage are usually continued for 72 h in our center however, may not be needed.

The use of modifications to the traditional open technique has largely been reported in a few case reports and series [2, 6–9]. However, in our center, we have found the need for traditional large-opening transoral resections to be decreasing in numbers. This is due to the advent of advanced visualization through transnasal endoscopic tools and less invasive transnasal and transoral mucosal openings, no longer

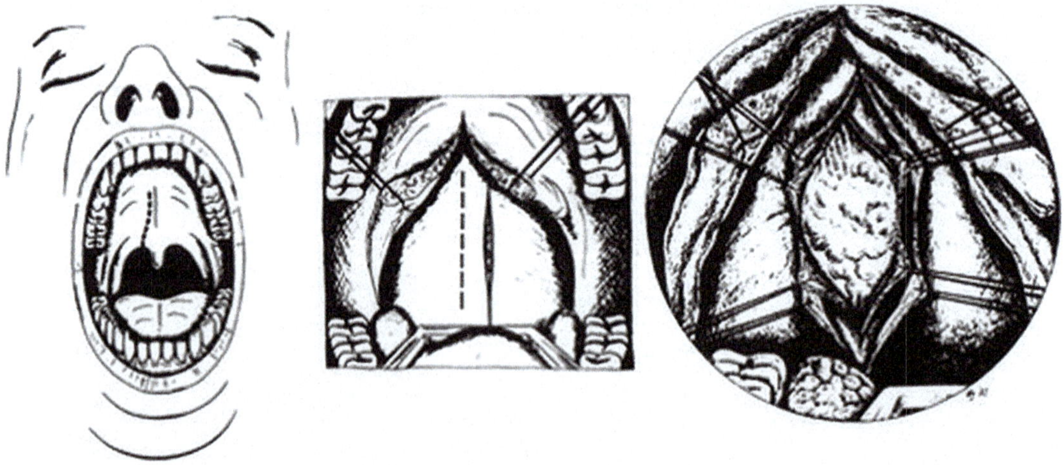

Fig. 2.3 Transoral surgical approach with midline soft palate incision. (Reproduced with permission from Pasztor et al. [4])

requiring extensive retraction. While the transoral approach is still utilized for the inferior extent of axis tumors and en bloc resections, it is more often used in conjunction with transnasal endoscopy or advanced retropharyngeal reconstruction techniques that obviate soft palate or mandible splitting approaches. This has led to significant decreases in long-term intubation and need for gastrostomy tube placements for this approach to the craniocervical junction.

Case Presentation

A 57-year-old male with a current history of multiple myeloma presented in outpatient consultation for a 6-month history of torticollis, neck pain with any upright posture, and sudden painful upper extremity paresthesias whenever he removed his hard cervical collar. He also noted being unable to maintain an upright head position out of his cervical collar for any length of time without severe pain and hand numbness. The patient had been on effective therapy for his myeloma and was declared prior to presentation to be in complete remission, without detectable markers. He had previously completed a course of focused beam radiation to lytic lesions of his C2 and C3 vertebral bodies over 8 months ago. At that time, he was advised to wear a rigid cervical collar to maintain spinal stability without a defined endpoint.

Recent imaging reveals largely unchanged lytic lesions of the C2 and C3 vertebra with new anterior C2 vertebral body cortical fractures and reversible associated cervical kyphosis. There is no evidence of bony regrowth into the previous lesions. The C2 lesion continued to show as metabolically active on recent PET scanning, but this was of unknown significance given the presence of fractures. The patient was considered to have a very good long-term life expectancy from an oncological perspective and was chiefly affected only by his neck pain.

On physical examination, the patient was fully ambulatory with full motor strength in both arms and lower extremities. He had no sensory deficits, no coordination difficulty, and no balance issues. The patient noted no history of swallowing difficulty but showed difficulty with chewing because of his collar and neck pain. Visually, the patient had a slight cock-robin neck turn, which cannot be modified without extreme pain. Removal of the cervical collar results in pain, with gradual head drop followed by arm paresthesias.

The patient is hesitant to consider operative options that would result in permanent loss of head motion. He is open to the possibility of needing gastric tube feeding if a surgery can be done to relieve his neck pain and concerning arm symptoms. After considering alternative nonoperative approaches to his condition, the patient would like to pursue surgery to improve his head position and neck pain symptoms.

Operative treatment was offered in the form of a posterior C1–C4 screw fixation and fusion with supplemental posterior sublaminar wiring followed by anterior combined retropharyngeal and transoral resection of tumor and expandable cage strut grafting. Posterior instrumentation and grafting were performed first. Surgery through the transoral exposure was done under transnasal endoscopic guidance requiring a minimal pharyngeal opening to resect tumor just inferior the C1 anterior arch. A standard retropharyngeal approach was undertaken to perform a C3 corpectomy and C2 partial inferior resection. A titanium expandable cage was then placed spanning the C4 superior endplate to the anterior ring of C1 under visual and mechanical guidance from the transoral approach. The pharyngeal soft tissues were approximated in two layers using interrupted Vicryl and Prolene sutures. An orogastric tube for possible short-term alimentation was placed prior to emergence from anesthesia. He was extubated without difficulty and transferred to the general ward.

The patient recovered normally without neurological deficits. He noticed immediate relief of previous neck pain symptoms as well. After a postoperative swallowing screen, he was allowed to begin soft foods on postoperative day 2 without difficulty. He was tolerating a regular diet by postoperative day 3 and was discharged home on the postoperative day 4 without needing home services.

Final pathology revealed small rests of viable myeloma tumor cells involving the C2 vertebra. He was re-started on appropriate systemic therapy within 2 weeks of surgery. The patient followed up for 3-month and 6-month appointments with stable postoperative radiographs and evidence of partial posterolateral bony union. He continued to have no difficulty with swallowing or recurrent neck pain. There was no recurrence of lytic lesions in any adjacent location.

Discussion

In the abovementioned case, surgical resection through a transoral approach was considered, given the patient's very good prognosis and functional status. It was believed that he would gain significant long-term benefit if his mechanical pain and functional kyphosis were treated surgically with appropriate stabilization. The patient's perceived Lhermitte's symptoms were considered to be ominous for future neurological deficit if the patient's head drop was not treated in the long term. In this case, indications for surgery would not be for curative resection or neurological compression but for deformity stabilization and fracture management while maintaining occipitocervical motion. An alternative dorsal-only approach could be conceived with occipitocervical fusion to the subaxial spine. This may provide adequate mechanical stability and would be highly dependent upon bony union in the long term as well as sacrificing head movement. In this case, bony union was not assured, given the previously irradiated field. A dorsal fusion to C1 without anterior strut reconstruction was not considered to be mechanically viable, given the lack of significant vertebral body support.

The elements of this patient's disease that would argue against using a transoral approach would be the presence of a previously irradiated field as well as significant subaxial disease. These factors went into designing a modified surgical approach that involved transnasal endoscopic visualization of a mini-open transoral resection in combination with a routine retropharyngeal approach to reconstruction. This allowed for proper clearance of the caudal margin of the anterior C1 ring from devitalized bone and tumor as well as proper guidance of the metallic graft. Furthermore, it allowed for minimizing of trauma to the posterior pharyngeal muscles by avoiding long-term retraction and decreasing incision size. Another advantage to this endoscopic mini-open approach is the avoidance of saliva pooling around the mucosal defect as the incision is made far more cranially without need for soft palate splitting. This allows for early resumption of diet and minimal soft-tissue reconstruction.

Conclusion

The transoral approach is a useful and technically expedient option for surgical resection of craniocervical junction tumors. This is especially true if dorsal surgical treatment options do not allow for proper access to the tumor or adequate reconstruction options. Modifications in techniques, especially those that allow for endoscopic visualization, may allow for decreased mucosal and pharyngeal disruption and retraction. This may decrease postoperative needs and complications. However, surgical methods should be tailored to the patient's tumor size, type, and comorbid conditions. The use of a team approach with oncologists, otorhinolaryngologists, and speech and nutrition staff is absolutely required to deal with variances in tumors types, intraoperative challenges, and postoperative complications.

References

1. Crockard HA. The transoral approach to the base of the brain and upper cervical cord. Ann R Coll Surg Eng. 1985;167:321–5.
2. Yadav YR, Madhariya SN, Parihar VS, Namdev H, Bhatele PR. Endoscopic transoral excision of odontoid process in irreducible atlantoaxial dislocation: our experience of 34 patients. J Neurol Surg A Cent Eur Neurosurg. 2013;74(3):162–7.
3. Lee JY, Lega B, Bhowmick D, Newman JG, O'Malley BW Jr, Weinstein GS, et al. Da Vinci robot-assisted transoral odontoidectomy for basilar invagination. ORL J Otorhinolaryngol Relat Spec. 2010;72(2):91–5.
4. Ponce-Gómez JA, Ortega-Porcayo LA, Soriano-Barón HE, Sotomayor-González A, Arriada-Mendicoa N,

Gómez-Amador JL, et al. Evolution from microscopic transoral to endoscopic endonasal odontoidectomy. Neurosurg Focus. 2014;37(4):E15.
5. Shriver MF, Kshettry VR, Sindwani R, Woodard T, Benzel EC, Recinos PF. Transoral and transnasal odontoidectomy complications: a systematic review and meta-analysis. Clin Neurol Neurosurg. 2016;148:121–9.
6. Mazzatenta D, Zoli M, Mascari C, Pasquini E, Frank G. Endoscopic endonasal odontoidectomy: clinical series. Spine (Phila Pa 1976). 2014;39(10):846–53.
7. Pasztor E, Vajda J, Piffkó P, Horváth M, Gádor I. Transoral surgery for craniocervical space-occupying processes. J Neurosurg. 1984;60:276–81.
8. Bettegowda C, Shajari M, Suk I, Simmons OP, Gokaslan ZL, Wolinsky JP. Sublabial approach for the treatment of symptomatic basilar impression in a patient with Klippel-Feil syndrome. Neurosurgery. 2011;69(1 Suppl Operative):ons77-82. discussion ons82.
9. Liu JK, Couldwell WT, Apfelbaum RI. Transoral approach and extended modifications for lesions of the ventral foramen magnum and craniovertebral junction. Skull Base. 2008;18(3):151–66.

3 Transmandibular Approach to Craniocervical Spine

Xun Li, Jared Fridley, Thomas Kosztowski, and Ziya L. Gokaslan

Background

Transoral surgery can trace its origin back to Dr. Wilfred Trotter, who in 1929 outlined a surgical approach to lesions of the epiglottis or glossoepiglottic fossa [1]. In 1947, Thomson and Nagus published a case report of the drainage of a retropharyngeal abscess by using a transoral approach. Over the ensuing decades, the indications for these approaches to the posterior pharynx were expanded to the treatment of various pathologies of the craniocervical junction (CCJ), such as tumor and trauma [2–4]. Although the approach was initially met with difficulties stemming from limited exposure, poor illumination, and the lack of appropriate surgical instruments, interest in the approach resurfaced in the 1960s, aided by the introduction of the operating microscope, customized instruments, and technological advancement [4, 5]. In 1980, Wood et al. published a series of two patients who underwent an expanded transoral approach in which he split the lip, mandible, and tongue for further caudal exposure, termed a median labiomandibular glossotomy, a subtype of the transmandibular approach [6].

Access to the CVJ can be obtained via anterior, anterolateral, posterior, and posterolateral surgical approaches. Anterior approaches are comprised of transoral approaches and their variations including the transmandibular approach. Anterolateral approaches include the high cervical retropharyngeal approach and the mandibular swing variation of the transmandibular approach. These anterior approaches provide access for direct ventral decompression of the spinal cord, although they can carry substantial morbidity. The midline posterior approach is utilized for posterior and lateral spinal cord decompression as well as instrumented stabilization across the CVJ. Ventral cord decompression via a posterior approach is limited due to the inability to manipulate the spinal cord without incurring significant neurologic morbidity and the proximity of important neurovascular structures. The far-lateral/extreme-lateral transcondylar approaches provide better visualization of the ventral spinal cord via a posterolateral corridor and can be useful for tumors adjacent to the foramen magnum and upper cervical spine.

The most common anterior approaches to the CCJ are the transoral approach and the high cervical retropharyngeal approach. The transoral approach permits access from the lower clivus down to C2, but the exposure can be severely narrowed by physical restrictions such as mouth-opening ability or limited neck extension. The extra-oral anterolateral

X. Li · J. Fridley · T. Kosztowski · Z. L. Gokaslan (✉)
Department of Neurosurgery, Rhode Island Hospital, Warren Alpert School of Medicine at Brown University, Providence, RI, USA
e-mail: ziya.gokaslan@lifespan.org

D. M. Sciubba (ed.), *Spinal Tumor Surgery*, https://doi.org/10.1007/978-3-319-98422-3_3

cervical approach, as described by Drs. Smith and Robinson, is usually limited to C3 rostrally due to the presence of the internal branch of the superior laryngeal nerve. The C2–C3 interspace can be accessed above the superior laryngeal nerve via the submandibular approach, which provides a small corridor that is in turn limited rostrally by the hypoglossal nerve; this provides access to approximately the mid body of C2 [7].

Like the transoral approach, the transmandibular approach necessitates dissection through the pharynx to access the CCJ. However, the transmandibular approach provides significantly improved CCJ exposure, from the lower one-third of the clivus down to C4. The transmandibular approach is most commonly used for resection of CCJ tumors, particularly primary tumors of the spine that necessitate en bloc resection, such as chordomas. Compared to the high cervical retropharyngeal approach, the transmandibular approach has several advantages: (1) access via a relatively avascular plane; (2) avoidance of critical structures such as the internal carotid arteries, lower cranial nerves, muscles of mastication, temporomandibular joints, and vestibulocochlear apparatus; and (3) improved visualization of ventral/ventrolateral CCJ pathology, particularly tumors, by allowing an off-midline pharyngeal incision to provide a more oblique angle to the lesion [8]. There are two variations of the transmandibular approach: (1) transmandibular circumglossal (also termed as the mandibular swing technique) and (2) median labiomandibular glossotomy [8].

Risks

Although the transmandibular approach is a very effective way of accessing pathology ventral to the spinal cord, it is a potentially morbid procedure with many inherent risks including dysphagia, airway compromise, infection, pharyngeal dehiscence, and jaw malocclusion. Dysphagia is commonly seen after undergoing a transmandibular approach. This is likely from a combination of the circumglossal incision, retropharyngeal dissection, and sectioning of the tensor and levator veli palatini muscles [9]. The risk is increased with prolonged overall length of surgery and the duration of retraction of the pharynx and tongue [10].

Infection is a significant risk of the transmandibular approach due to bacterial colonization of the oral cavity. Precautions are taken when prepping the operative field, including sterilization of the mouth and even nose to decrease the bacterial load. Reported rates of infection in the literature with a transmandibular approach vary from 6% up to 50% [11]. Infection types include parapharyngeal abscesses, soft tissue infection, and meningitis. Parapharyngeal space abscess or a chronic nonhealing pharyngeal dehiscence can potentially lead to orocutaneous fistula [10]. Bacterial meningitis, particularly with gram-negative bacteria, can be difficult to treat and is best avoided by not lacerating the dura, and if a durotomy is necessary, the dura is closed in a watertight fashion.

Tongue swelling is frequently encountered in the postoperative period, which can cause potentially life-threatening airway obstruction. For this reason, a tracheostomy is often placed prior to surgery [9]. Malocclusion of the teeth results from incorrectly aligning both halves of the mandible during mandible reconstruction. This can result in difficulty with chewing food and present a cosmetic defect. This can be avoided by predrilling screw holes in the mandible prior to performing the mandibulotomy. Injury to the lower cranial nerves, particularly the hypoglossal nerve, can occur during dissection beneath the mandible. Vertebral artery injury can occur during dissection lateral to the cervical spine while the vertebral artery travels within the transverse foramen. Tumors of the CCJ can cause distortion of the adjacent neurovascular structures, thereby increasing the potential for injury, particularly if encasing these structures [12]. Other less common risks that have been reported include serous otitis media from sectioning of the Eustachian tube as well as conductive hearing loss [9, 10].

Alternative Surgical Approaches

Standard Transoral Approach

The standard transoral approach, also known as the transoral transpharyngeal approach, provides the most direct access to a ventral spinal lesion from the lower one-third of the clivus rostrally to the body of C2 caudally. For tumors, rheumatoid arthritis pannus, or other C2 dens lesions, the transoral approach is an effective means of decompressing the ventral spinal cord. One of the significant downsides of the transoral approach is the narrow operative field through the oral cavity. This is primarily due to the front teeth rostrally and the mandible/tongue caudally. To increase exposure, the uvula can be retracted with a suture, and the soft palate can be retracted with a soft rubber tubing through the nose and under the palate. Specialized oral retractors can be utilized to retract the tongue out of the way. The overall working area can be limited if the patient's mouth opening is <2.5 cm or if the patient has restricted neck extension [3, 4, 13].

Transmaxillary Approaches

Transmaxillary exposures can expand the rostral limit of the CCJ by exposing the upper clivus. Most commonly, this is done via a Le Fort I osteotomy through the maxilla. The downside of this approach is the limited caudal exposure due to the down-fractured maxilla and hard palate complex obstructing the view of C2 [14]. To circumvent the caudal limit of exposure experienced in the Le Fort I approach, the transmaxillary palatal split approach creates a midline opening of the maxilla and hard palate complex, thereby allowing access from the upper clivus to C2. However, this approach poses the risk of velopharyngeal insufficiency consisting of dysphagia, nasal regurgitation, and hypernasal voice [14]. It is also associated with a higher risk of wound infection, swallowing dysfunction, and difficulty. Performing a unilateral Le Fort I osteotomy can aid in preservation of the soft palate and the other maxilla and thus result in more rapid recovery of oropalatal function.

Endoscopic Approaches

Advances in neuroendoscopy technology and techniques for the treatment of head and neck pathology over the past decade have been adopted by some spine surgeons for the treatment of CCJ pathology. The visualization afforded by endoscopes is not limited by the borders of the mouth and palate, making even those patients with limited mouth-opening ability or restricted neck range of motion candidates for an endoscopic CCJ approach. There are two different routes for an endoscopic approach to the CCJ: transoral or transnasal.

The transoral endoscopic approach allows access from the lower third of the clivus down to approximately the level of the C2–C3 disc space. It has the advantage of eliminating the need to split the soft palate, particularly because of the availability of angled endoscopes. By avoiding soft palate dissection, the risk of velopharyngeal insufficiency is reduced. The transnasal endoscopic approach allows access from the anterior skull base down to the odontoid process. Both routes can be combined for access to pathology that extends from the skull base down to the upper cervical spine. There are disadvantages to endoscopic CCJ approaches, including technical difficulty with pharyngeal wall closure and a steep learning curve to become facile with this technique. Closure of the posterior pharyngeal wall can be particularly difficult caudally in the region of the lower clivus, C1, and C2, where the prevertebral muscles insert [13].

Preoperative Assessment

The assessment of patients who may be candidates for a transmandibular approach necessitates careful clinical evaluation and interpretation of relevant imaging. A full neurological examination including cranial nerve and sensorimotor evaluation is necessary for each patient. In addition, assessment of cervical spine range of motion and an oral cavity examination should be performed. Preexisting jaw or dentition abnormalities should be noted. Imaging, including computed tomography (CT) and magnetic resonance imaging (MRI), of the head and neck should be performed for each patient.

Imaging

Conventional radiographs and CT of the cervical spine are helpful for examining relevant cervical spine bone anatomy, as it relates to the underlying pathology as well as planning for possible instrumented spinal stabilization. Attention should be paid to C1 and C2 anatomy, as this region tends to have more anatomic variations than the subaxial cervical spine. Flexion–extension cervical spine radiographs may be helpful if there is suspicion of dynamic instability, although in most cases instability is introduced iatrogenically by the surgery itself and therefore may ultimately be of limited utility [13].

MRI of the cervical spine with and without contrast is necessary to understand the relationship of the underlying pathology to the surrounding soft tissue and neural elements. In the case of primary tumors of the upper cervical spine, surgical planning is based on what part(s) of the spine is involved, what soft tissues are involved, and whether any neural element compression is present. If an en bloc resection is being considered, surgical planning may encompas multiple approaches based on the involved bony elements and paraspinal tissues, as well as the location of neural element compression if present.

If there is concern for involvement by tumor of vascular structures, such as the vertebral arteries, either conventional angiography or CT angiography of the neck can be helpful in delineating the relationship between relevant vasculature and the lesion of interest [13]. Conventional angiography should be performed if preoperative embolization of a hypervascular tumor is indicated or sacrifice of a vertebral artery is being contemplated. Prior to vertebral artery sacrifice, a balloon test occlusion is performed to determine if collateral vasculature is sufficient to supply blood flow to the brain and brain stem.

Tracheostomy/PEG

A tracheostomy and a percutaneous endoscopic gastrostomy (PEG) are often performed preoperatively or in the operating room immediately prior to a transmandibular approach, given the significant risk of postoperative dysphagia and airway obstruction. Tracheostomy has a number of advantages compared to the placement of an oral or nasal endotracheal tube: (1) improves intraoperative airway security by avoiding endotracheal tube manipulation, (2) allows an unobstructed surgical view of the oropharynx, (3) prevents mechanical pressure from being exerted by an endotracheal tube on the pharynx, possibly decreasing the potential for wound dehiscence, and (4) improves the ability to perform routine mouth care and improves the clearance of saliva, thereby decreasing risk of infection.

PEG tube placement prior to surgery offers many advantages and mitigates potential approach-related morbidity. Early postoperative nutrition is essential for wound healing, and PEG access allows enteral feeding to begin soon after surgery. Unlike nasal or oral enteral tubes that run adjacent to pharyngeal tissues, PEG tubes avoid the risk of mechanical pressure on the pharyngeal incision site after surgery and the risk of injuring the same tissues during tube placement. Barring any permanent dysphagia post surgery, the PEG tube is removed as soon as the pharyngeal wound is healed and after a formal swallowing evaluation.

Multidisciplinary Care

It is important for the spine surgeon to involve other surgical subspecialties that will be involved in performing the transmandibular approach itself and assist in caring for the patient postoperatively. Plastic surgery, oromaxillofacial surgery, and an otolaryngology are subspecialties that each play a key role in the management of patients undergoing this surgical approach. Otolaryngology helps perform the dissection of the oropharynx and can perform a tracheostomy preoperatively as well. The oromaxillofacial and plastic surgery teams are often involved in performing the mandibulotomy and reconstruction of the mandible, as well as wound closure. Postoperative services such as speech therapy, physical therapy, and nursing teams are critical to reduce the risk of perioperative morbidity.

Surgical Technique

Positioning

Patients are positioned supine on a standard operating table. If needed, Gardner-Wells tongs are applied to attempt reduction of any CCJ malalignment for patients, such as those with basilar invagination. The oropharynx, mouth, perioral region, jaw, and neck are thoroughly prepped with betadine wash. The nasopharynx is also prepped, as it is in communication with the oropharynx. The area from below the eyes down to the bottom of the neck is toweled off and draped.

Surgical Technique

The oromaxillofacial surgeon and otolaryngologist perform much of the initial exposure until the spine is encountered. Incision is made from the lower lip at the midline and carried caudally to the hyoid. The incision then is continued out laterally to the border of the sternocleidomastoid muscle and then curved up to the mastoid process (Fig. 3.1). Subperiosteal dissection along the mandible is performed starting at the midline, dissecting medial to lateral, to approximately 2 cm from midline. Care should be taken to avoid dissection too lateral, which risks injury to the mental nerve exiting from the mental foramen (Fig. 3.2). The mandibular osteotomy is sometimes marked in a zigzag or step-like pattern to allow easier reapproximation. Holes are predrilled on either side of the planned mandibulotomy site, and titanium mini-plates prefitted for later placement. Prefitting of plates and drilling of holes is important prior to performing osteotomies because it ensures that the mandible will be reapproximated perfectly later. Poor alignment of the jaw may not only result in poor cosmesis but also risk malocclusion. A tooth may need to be removed if it obstructs the path of the mandibulotomy.

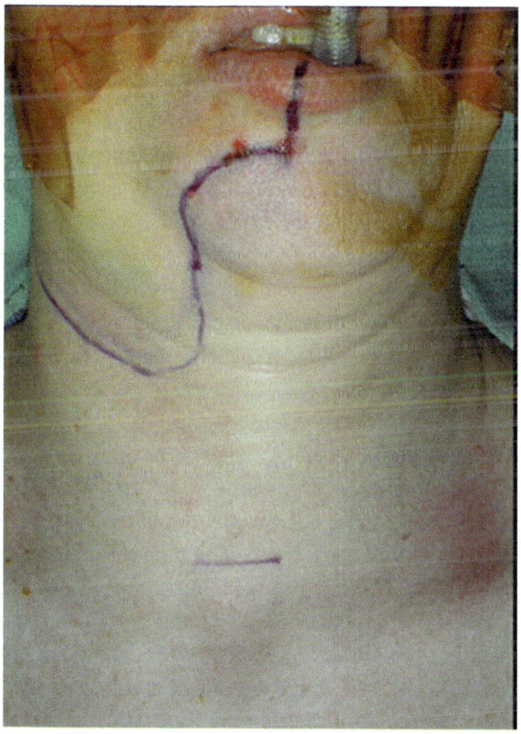

Fig. 3.1 Incision is marked from the lower lip down, rounding the chin, to the hyoid bone and curving up over the sternocleidomastoid muscle to the mastoid tip

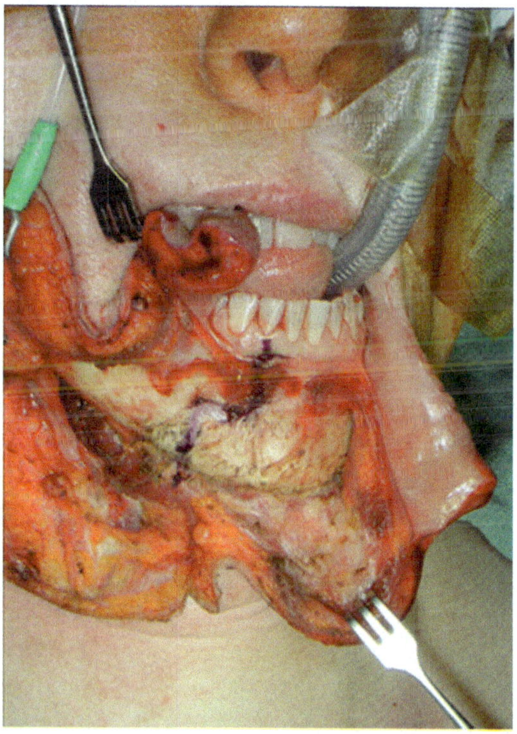

Fig. 3.2 Mandibular osteotomy is marked in a step-like fashion to prevent postoperative mandible slippage and malocclusion

If significant lateral exposure of the CCJ lesion is needed, the tissues below the neck can be dissected prior to performing the mandibulotomy. Subplatysmal dissection is performed, and dissection continues deep into the submandibular gland. The sternocleidomastoid muscle is retracted posteriorly, and the carotid sheath is identified and exposed. To facilitate the exposure below the level of the mandible, the digastric muscle is split. This is followed by dissecting the mylohyoid from the hyoid and dissecting the geniohyoid from the mandible.

The mandibulotomy is then performed, and the mandible is swung out laterally to open the mandibulopharyngeal space (Fig. 3.3). To mobilize the tongue, an incision is performed starting underneath the tongue at the midline where the osteotomy was made. This incision is extended around the tongue, terminating at the tonsillar pillar. As the mandible is opened laterally with the cervical myocutaneous flap, the tongue is retracted medially away from the operative field (Figs. 3.4 and 3.5). This space is further enlarged through the transection of the facial artery and the inner pterygoid muscle from the lateral pterygoid plate. To increase exposure, the muscles attached to the styloid process are detached: the stylohyoid, stylopharyngeal, and styloglossus muscles. The cranial nerve IX is identified to ensure that it is spared. If it is obstructive to the approach, the external carotid artery may need to be transected at the level of the facial artery or the occipital artery, thereby allowing entry into the retrostyloid space. This is done only when the vessels cannot be mobilized. Other maneuvers that increase the operative field include splitting the digastric muscle between the anterior and posterior bellies. The tensor veli palatini muscles, soft palate, and the Eustachian tube can also be divided to increase the exposure, but oftentimes, this is avoided as these maneuvers increase the potential morbidity of the procedure. In the exposure, the lower cranial nerves, primarily the hypoglossal nerve, need to be carefully identified and protected.

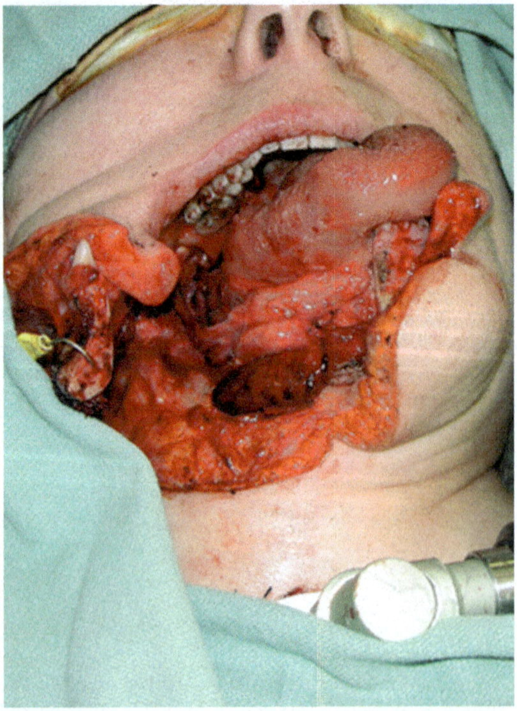

Fig. 3.3 The mandible is swung laterally to open the mandibulopharyngeal space

To expose the spine through the mouth, the posterior pharyngeal wall is divided. The clivus and upper cervical spine should now only be covered by the longus capitis muscles, which are detached. The prevertebral fascia is opened sharply, and the longus colli are undermined and dissected from medial to lateral. At this point, the anterior arch of C1 can be palpated. If the lesion is centered on the vertebral body and dens of C2, the anterior arch of C1 may need to be opened. The anterior longitudinal ligament is identified, and the anterior arch of C1 is drilled and rongeured until the odontoid process is visualized. If the surgical plan necessitates resection of the dens, the transverse ligament lateral attachments adjacent to the C1–C2 articular process need to be released. Alar and apical ligaments should be transected prior to bony removal of the dens to prevent upward retraction of the dens toward the clivus, which could then impinge into the spinal cord. If an en bloc resection for primary spinal tumor is planned, the posterior longitudinal ligament is exposed and cut rostral and caudal to the limits of the lesion.

If the lesion wraps around the thecal sac dorsally, further bony resection of the C2 ring can be done while being mindful of the ipsilateral vertebral artery. The upper cervical nerve roots can be sacrificed to gain access to the dorsal aspect of the thecal sac (Fig. 3.6). C1–C2 nerve root sacri-

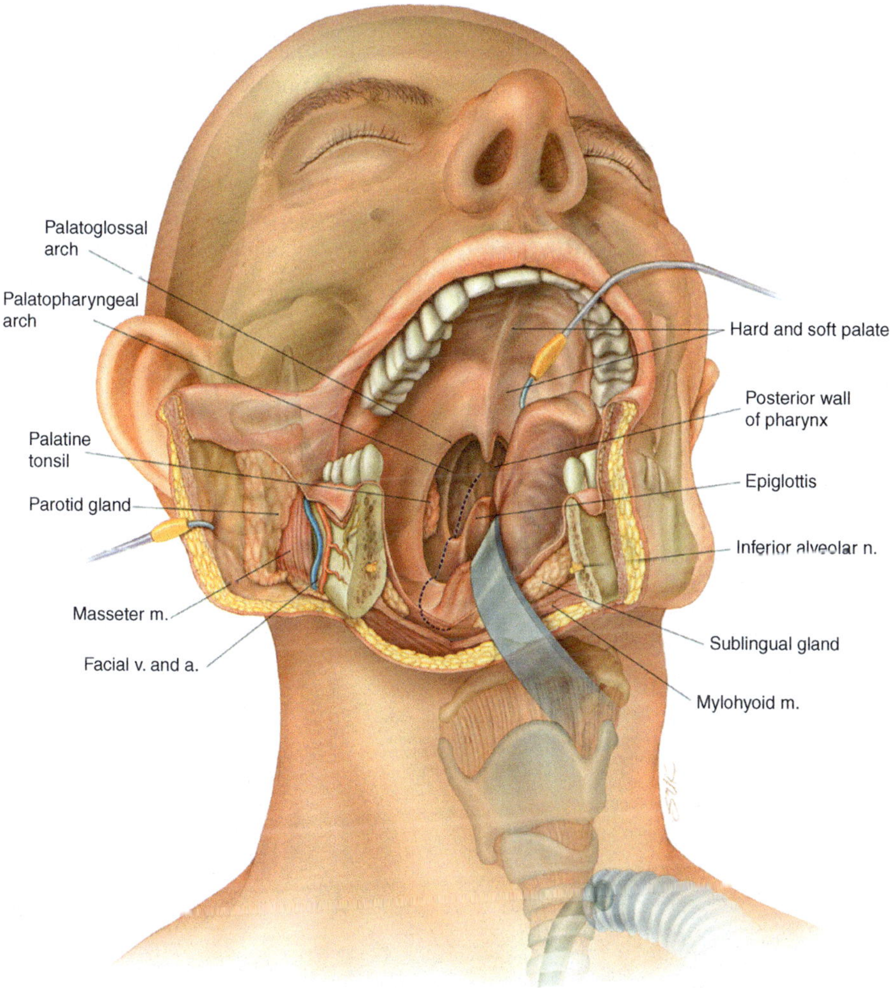

Fig. 3.4 Artist illustration of the transmandibular approach. (Reproduced with permission from Rhines et al. [16])

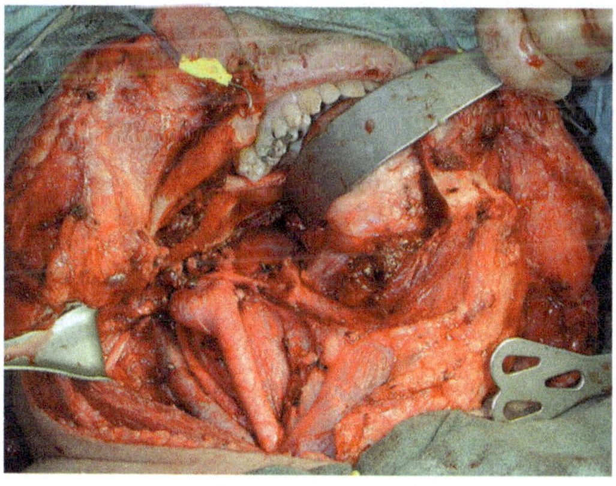

Fig. 3.5 Operative view following further lateral dissection, including exposure of the carotid artery. The tongue is retracted away from the posterior pharyngeal wall for better visualization

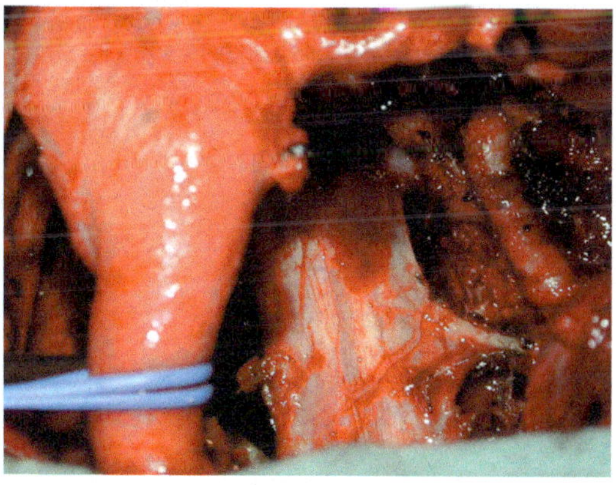

Fig. 3.6 Following CCJ bone resection, the thecal sac is visualized. An ipsilateral upper cervical nerve root is ligated and sacrificed

fice typically causes no significant clinical deficit other than dermatomal numbness. If the root is cut distal to the dorsal root ganglion, neuralgia may result. Sacrifice of the C3–C5 nerve roots can lead to diaphragmatic paresis/paralysis, and sacrificing C5–T1 nerve roots will result in sensorimotor deficits in the upper extremities.

If a durotomy is planned, or caused iatrogenically, primary repair of the dura is preferred to reduce the chance of a clinically significant cerebrospinal fluid (CSF) leak. Dural sealants, synthetic dural products, and fat/muscle/fascia grafts are useful adjuncts, particularly if primary repair is tenuous or unable to be directly performed. A Valsalva maneuver is performed to ensure there is a watertight closure. A lumbar drain should be placed if there is concern that dural closure is tenuous or a CSF leak occurs postoperatively.

If instability is introduced following resection of CCJ pathology, anterior reconstruction is performed (Fig. 3.7). A Harms cage or a similar construct is appropriately fitted to span the area of

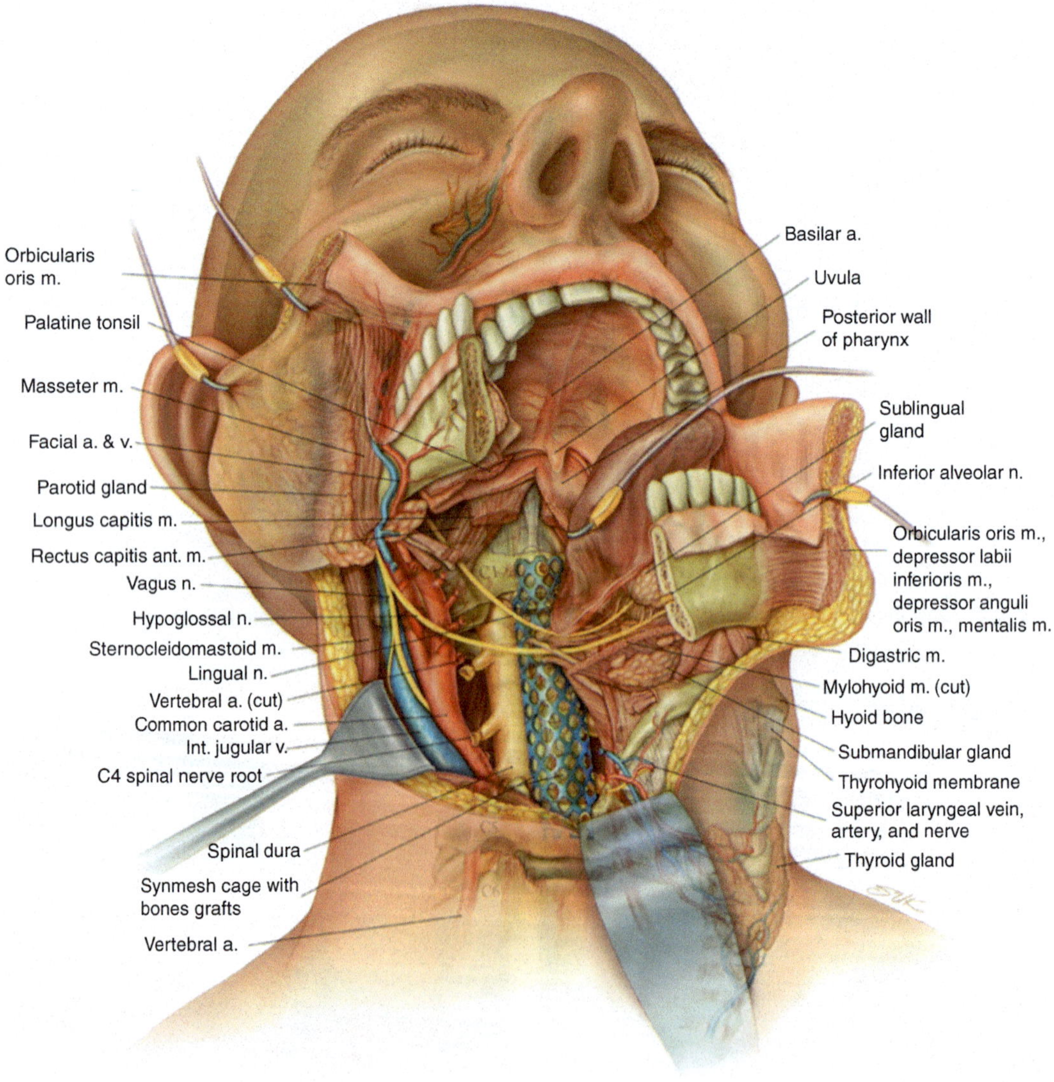

Fig. 3.7 Artist illustration demonstrating anterior column reconstruction following en bloc tumor resection. (Reproduced with permission from Rhines et al. [16])

the spine defect, ensuring that neither the rostral nor caudal ends impinge dorsally on the spinal cord. This is most important on the rostral end as the vertebral body cross-sectional area will be smaller than the caudal end. Sometimes, cages can be tailored such that the ends are flared out to provide a tab for the cage to be fixated to the vertebral bodies anteriorly. If this is not feasible, a plate can also be used.

For closure, plastic surgery has proven to be an invaluable service in addition to the presence of otolaryngology and maxillofacial surgery. The pharyngeal structures as well as the mylohyoid and digastric muscles are reattached. The split mandible is reapproximated with fixed plates with screws in the predrilled holes. This is followed by closure of the oral mucosa. Care must be taken to realign the vermillion border when suturing the lip. Likewise, the neck tissues and platysma are reapproximated in anatomic layers, with attention paid to not strangulate the tissue.

Postoperative Care

Postoperative transfer of the patient to an intensive care unit is essential following surgery. It is extremely important to frequently monitor these patients clinically as the neck soft tissues may become significantly edematous postoperatively. The tongue is likely to also swell significantly in the postoperative period, which may compromise both airway and swallowing. Topical corticosteroid application to the tongue immediately after surgical closure can reduce postoperative edema. Most of these patients will have had a tracheostomy placed prior to surgery, which, pending decreased edema and ventilator weaning, will ultimately be removed.

Prophylactic, targeted antibiotic coverage based on cultures taken preoperatively should be continued for 5 days postoperatively. The patient needs to be carefully monitored postoperatively for signs of infection. There should be a low threshold for imaging, as there are multiple sources of possible infection, including an injury to the pharyngeal tissues or esophagus.

The patient should have nothing by mouth initially until tongue and neck swelling subside. Nutritional support provided by a PEG tube in the interim is extremely important for nutrition and wound healing. Laryngoscopy and esophagoscopy usually are required in those undergoing a dysphagia workup, although some surgeons perform these routinely on postoperative day 7 [13].

Lumbar drain can be weaned when no cerebrospinal fluid leakage is observed in the drains. If there is any suspicion of there being a planned or unintentional durotomy during the surgery, care should be taken not to wean the lumbar drain too quickly. CSF diversion is important while the dura is healing and creating a watertight seal. Furthermore, if there is suspicion of CSF leakage into the wound, there should be a low threshold for wound re-exploration since the risk of meningitis is very high with this procedure.

Other commonly cited complications including localized infection in the acute to subacute period may need targeted intravenous antibiotics as guided by infectious disease specialists and, additionally, surgical drainage by otolaryngologists. Vigilance must be maintained for velopharyngeal insufficiency, as it usually presented 3–6 months postoperatively, especially in approaches that required a palatal incision [15].

Conclusion

The CCJ is a challenging area to approach surgically due to the complex bony anatomy and adjacent neurovascular structures. The median labiomandibular glossotomy represents an expanded transoral approach that provides direct access to the midline structures from the clivus to mid-cervical spine. This approach provides exceptional surgical freedom and visualization but carries significant risk for morbidity and mortality, both intraoperatively and postoperatively. As always, less invasive approaches should be employed whenever possible, but in patients with primary neoplasms requiring en bloc resection, this approach affords a relatively safe and effective avenue to resect, reduce, and stabilize pathology of the CCJ.

References

1. Trotter W. Purvis oration on the surgery of malignant disease of the pharynx. Br Med J. 1929; 1(3398):269–72.1.
2. Delgado TE, Garrido E, Harwick RD. Labiomandibular, transoral approach to chordomas in the clivus and upper cervical spine. Neurosurgery. 1981;8(6):675–9.
3. Balasingam V, Anderson GJ, Gross ND, Cheng CM, Noguchi A, Dogan A, et al. Anatomical analysis of transoral surgical approaches to the clivus. J Neurosurg. 2006;105(2):301–8.
4. Liu JK, Couldwell WT, Apfelbaum RI. Transoral approach and extended modifications for lesions of the ventral foramen magnum and craniovertebral junction. Skull Base. 2008;18(3):151–66.
5. Steinberger J, Skovrlj B, Lee NJ, Kothari P, Leven DM, Guzman JZ, et al. Surgical morbidity and mortality associated with transoral approach to the cervical spine. Spine. 2016;41(9):E535–40.
6. Wood BG, Sadar ES, Levine HL, Dohn DF, Tucker HM. Surgical problems of the base of the skull. An interdisciplinary approach. Arch Otolaryngol. 1980;106(1):1–5.
7. Russo A, Albanese E, Quiroga M, Ulm AJ. Submandibular approach to the C2-3 disc level: microsurgical anatomy with clinical application. J Neurosurg Spine. 2009;10(4):380–9.
8. Neo M, Asato R, Honda K, Kataoka K, Fujibayashi S, Nakamura T. Transmaxillary and transmandibular approach to a C1 chordoma. Spine. 2007;32(7):E236–9.
9. DeMonte F, Diaz E Jr, Callender D, Suk I. Transmandibular, circumglossal, retropharyngeal approach for chordomas of the clivus and upper cervical spine. Technical note. Neurosurg Focus. 2001;10(3):E10.
10. Krespi YP, Sisson GA. Transmandibular exposure of the skull base. Am J Surg. 1984;148(4):534–8.
11. Hodges SD, Humphreys SC, Brown TW Jr, Eck JC, Covington LA. Complications of the anterior retropharyngeal approach in cervical spine surgery: a technique and outcomes review. J South Orthop Assoc. 2000;9(3):169–74.
12. Choi D, Melcher R, Harms J, Crockard A. Outcome of 132 operations in 97 patients with chordomas of the craniocervical junction and upper cervical spine. Neurosurgery. 2010;66(1):59–65. discussion.
13. Konya D, Ozgen S, Gercek A, Celebiler O, Pamir MN. Transmandibular approach for upper cervical pathologies: report of 2 cases and review of the literature. Turk Neurosurg. 2008;18(3):271–5.
14. Youssef AS, Sloan AE. Extended transoral approaches: surgical technique and analysis. Neurosurgery. 2010;66(3 Suppl):126–34.
15. Dlouhy BJ, Dahdaleh NS, Menezes AH. Evolution of transoral approaches, endoscopic endonasal approaches, and reduction strategies for treatment of craniovertebral junction pathology: a treatment algorithm update. Neurosurg Focus. 2015;38(4):E8.
16. Rhines LD, Fourney DR, Siadati A, Suk I, Gokaslan ZL. En bloc resection of multilevel cervical chordoma with C2 involvement. J Neurosurg Spine. 2005;2:199–205.

4 Craniocervical Approach: Transcervical

Wataru Ishida, Kyle L. McCormick, and Sheng-fu Larry Lo

Overview

The ventral craniovertebral junction (CVJ) is difficult to safely access surgically due to its deep, anatomically complex location that can be affected by diverse pathologies, including basilar invagination, congenital skull base malformations, lower clival chordomas and chondrosarcomas, metastatic diseases, rheumatoid pannus, and the intradural pathologies of meningiomas and vascular malformations [1]. The most direct and widely used approach to reach the ventral CVJ has been the ventral transoral route, introduced by Fang and Ong in 1962 [2]. The approach has been successful in its ability to directly reach the region, offering the widest view of the anatomy and the options to combine it with transfacial and/or high cervical retropharyngeal approaches to improve the narrow and deep working channel [3–11].

Currently, the standard direct approach is a transoral-transpharyngeal approach with the option to add a transmandibular route [10, 12–16] or Le Fort osteotomy [3, 17–19] for increased visualization of lesions as well as the surgical bed. However, this approach comes with significant morbidities, including postoperative bacterial meningitis, especially in the setting of intraoperative dural tears, the need for tracheostomy, dysphasia, changes in phonation, airway impairment, pharyngeal wound dehiscence, and suboptimal esthetic outcomes [20]. In addition, the operative microscope, while allowing for direct illumination of the operative field, is not well suited to this type of approach, which requires a wide range of movement and visualization beyond a narrow cone of direct light [21]. Fortunately, the endoscope has been a major advancement for this type of surgery, as it offers direct illumination and a wider panoramic view of the field [22–24]. Because its illumination is at the end of a long rod, it allows light to penetrate deeper and closer to the surgical target. In addition, it offers a field of view of approximately 80° [21, 24], providing the surgeon with a panoramic perspective. In effect, the eyes of the surgeon are brought directly into the surgical field. Its shape can be used to gently retract structures, preventing retraction-associated morbidities [1, 20]. In addition, both the endoscope and its related technology are widely available in hospitals and operating rooms.

In 2002, Frempong-Boadu and Fessler used the endoscope for an endoscopically assisted transoral approach [2], followed in 2005 by Kassam at the University of Pittsburgh with the first fully transnasal endoscopic resection of the

W. Ishida
The Johns Hopkins Hospital, Department of Neurosurgery, Baltimore, MD, USA

K. L. McCormick
Neurosurgery Department, Columbia University Medical Center, New York, NY, USA

S.-f. L. Lo (✉)
Johns Hopkins University School of Medicine, Department of Neurosurgery, Baltimore, MD, USA
e-mail: larrylo@jhmi.edu

D. M. Sciubba (ed.), *Spinal Tumor Surgery*, https://doi.org/10.1007/978-3-319-98422-3_4

odontoid [23]. Finally, it was Wolinsky et al. who completed the first endoscopic transcervical odontoidectomy for basilar invagination [21]. It is our hope that this chapter may provide neurosurgeons with an additional method of an approach to the CVJ when indicated to increase safety and improve patient outcomes.

Indications, Contraindications, and Advantages

The principal indication for a transcervical approach to the cervical spine is basilar invagination of C2, with no need for clival resection [3, 22]. The use of the endoscope limits the degree of morbidities associated with retraction [20] and has been effective in all three approaches to the CVJ [1–4, 10, 22, 24–30]. The transcervical approach also offers the benefit of familiarity—the anatomy of the exposure is familiar to neurosurgeons, which, given the narrowness of the approaches to the CVJ, leads to a significant surgical advantage. This approach also adds a new trajectory (Fig. 4.1), allowing for the resection of more caudal vertebral bodies below the odontoid and for the decompression of deeper basilar invagination [3]. This allows surgeons to treat a wider range of pathologies than with just the transoral or transnasal approach [3, 31].

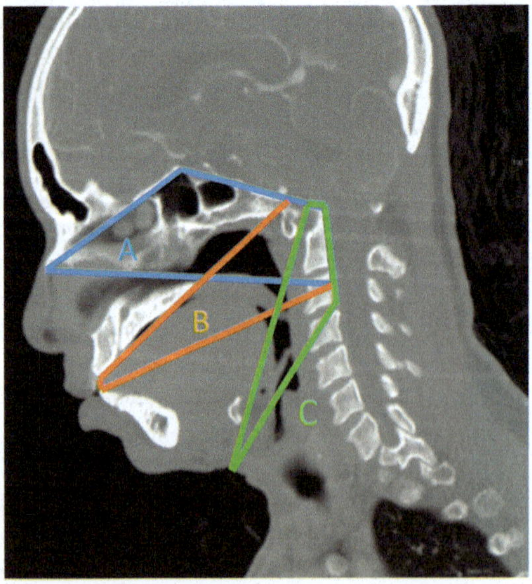

Fig. 4.1 Comparing the (A) transnasal and (B) transoral approaches to the CVJ with the (C) endoscopic transcervical approach

Another advantage of this approach is the preservation of a sterile surgical field to reduce the risk of postoperative complications [1, 3, 10, 20–22, 25]. The transoral and transnasal approaches violate the oropharyngeal and nasopharyngeal mucosa, respectively. This increases the chances of infection or wound dehiscence of the posterior pharyngeal wall secondary to the invasion of bacterial flora native to these regions [3, 6, 20, 30, 31]. The transoral approach also may require palate splitting and tongue retraction, which may require postoperative intubation for extended periods [2, 5, 6, 8, 14, 15, 20, 21, 31–36]. The transnasal approach, as mentioned, also requires crossing a cavity with bacteria, increasing the chance of postoperative meningitis in the setting of a cerebrospinal fluid (CSF) leak [20–22, 30, 31, 34, 37]. In addition, the anatomy encountered in the transoral and transnasal approaches may be less familiar to neurosurgeons and places the vidian nerves and Eustachian tubes at risk [20, 38]. The transcervical approach involves anatomy more familiar to neurosurgeons and does not violate the unsterile mucosal membranes, thereby decreasing the chance of postoperative meningitis in the case of an inadvertent or intentional breach of dura mater and subsequent CSF contamination [1, 3, 10, 20–22, 25].

In addition, patients treated with endoscopic-assisted transcervical approach were found able to ingest food orally after removal of the endotracheal tube, with a decreased need for tracheostomy and tube feeding [10, 22]. This approach also decreases the risk of postoperative phonation difficulty potentially present in the transoral approach because the soft palate is neither split nor retracted [3, 10, 20–22]. There is also no need to split the mandible or maxilla, thereby minimizing the risk of complications such as difficulty in mastication or suboptimal aesthetic outcomes [1–3, 10–12, 14, 20, 21, 25]. Although the risk of injury to the recurrent laryngeal nerve exists, it is not increased when compared with an anterior cervical approach [10].

Not all patients, however, are candidates for this approach. This trajectory may not be achieved in patients who are obese, barrel-chested, or severely kyphotic [1, 3, 10, 21]. Based on its trajectory, this approach should not be used to access the clivus and related pathologies, as accessing the lower clivus for resection requires undue retraction and is restricted by constraints of the chest on the angle of attack [3].

Clinical Materials and Methods

Surgical Preparation and Positioning

The surgical positioning for a transcervical anterior Craniocervical approach is similar to that of the anterior cervical discectomy and fusion (ACDF) but with nasotracheal intubation using a soft armored endotracheal tube rather than orotracheal intubation [1, 3, 10, 22]. The patient is positioned supine on a flat Jackson table with a shoulder roll placed behind the neck for gentle neck extension. The level of neck extension the patient can tolerate should be determined preoperatively [1]. Somatosensory evoked responses and motor evoked responses are monitored throughout the procedure. The head is fixed to the table via a halo ring attached to a Mayfield halo adaptor (Fig. 4.2a).

Two table-mounted arms are attached to the table contralateral to the surgeon: one to fix the retractor to the table and the other to hold the endoscope. They are both attached to the table caudal to the cervical spine such that they do not interfere with lateral fluoroscopy. The endoscopy monitor is contralateral to the surgeon, with the frameless stereotactic display just rostral to

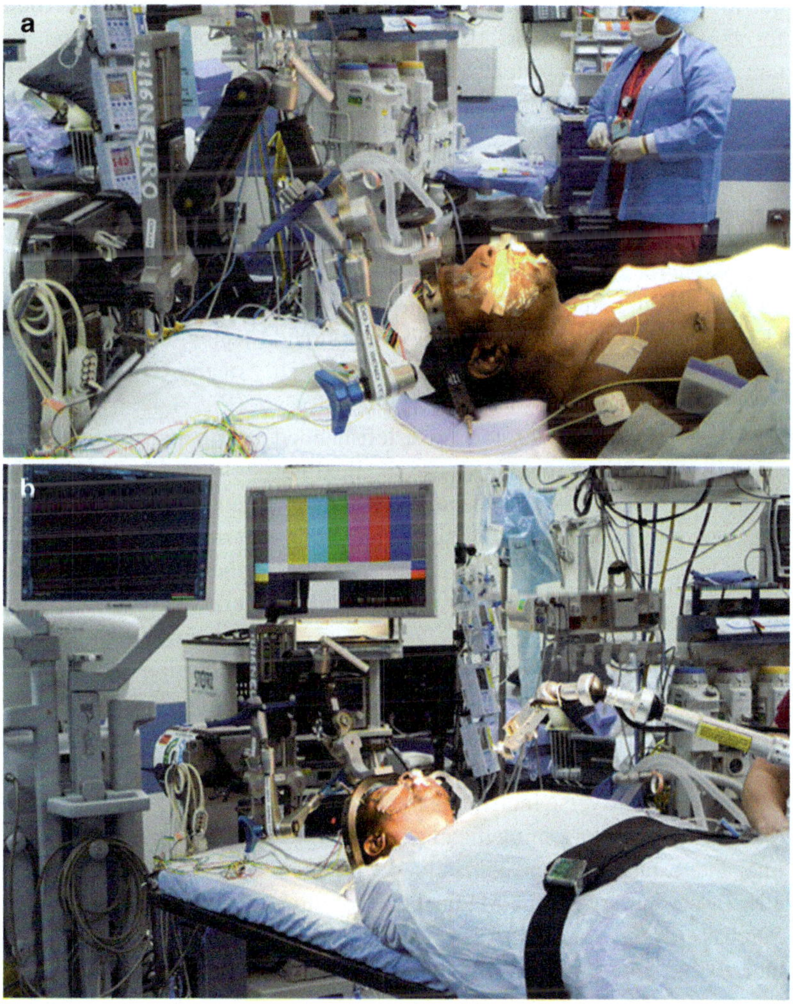

Fig. 4.2 (**a**) The head is fixed to the table using a halo ring attached to a Mayfield halo adaptor. (**b**) Final setup

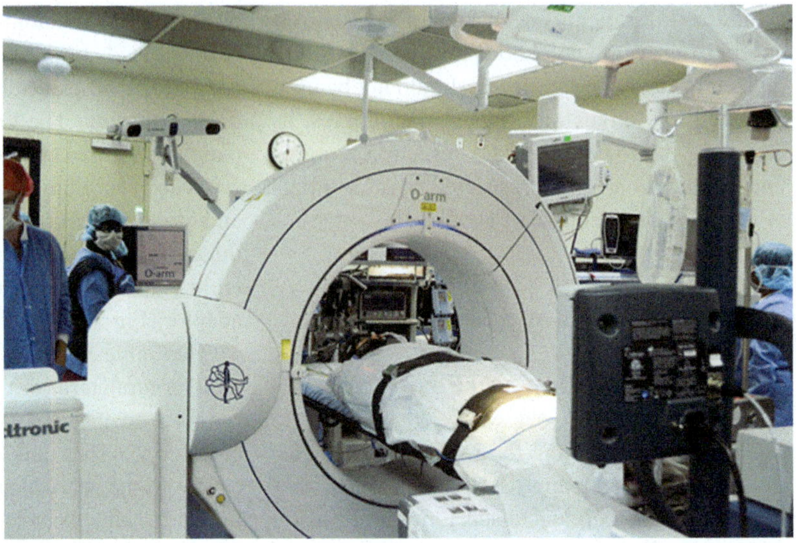

Fig. 4.3 Registration for neuronavigation using O-arm

the monitor and the fluoroscopy monitor caudal to the endoscopy monitor. Reference array for the frameless stereotactic navigation system is fixed to the patient via the halo ring (Fig. 4.2b). The patient is registered intraoperatively using the Medtronic O-arm intraoperative CT (Medtronic, Minneapolis, MN, USA) and Medtronic StealthStation S7 System for navigation (Medtronic, Minneapolis, MN, USA) (Fig. 4.3) [10, 22, 26]. The neck is then prepped and draped in a sterile fashion as for an ACDF [1, 3, 10, 22]. The side of approach is determined by the handedness of the surgeon: the approach is made from the right side of the patient for a right-handed surgeon and left for a left-handed surgeon [1]. Image guidance use is flexible: because the head is fixed in place, imaging guidance selection may be based on surgeons' preference [1, 3, 10, 22].

Surgical Techniques

The standard Smith-Robinson approach to the cervical spine is used for incision and initial exposure. A transverse incision is made near the C4–C5 level starting immediately off the midline and extending approximately 4 cm laterally. Bovie cautery (Bovie Medical Corporation, Purchase, New York, USA) is used to incise underlying cutaneous and platysma muscles. To access the cervical spine, dissection is done medial to the sternocleidomastoid muscle and carotid sheath and lateral to the strap muscles. Blunt dissection aimed superiorly between plane tissues is performed with the esophagus and trachea swept medially and sternocleidomastoid muscles swept laterally, allowing access to the anterior tubercle of C1. Retraction of the esophagus may be maintained using a handheld Cloward retractor. Kitner dissectors are used to sweep open loose areolar tissue anterior to the spine, exposing the spine rostrally to the level of the C1 tubercle. A beveled, tubular retractor (Fig. 4.4a, b) is positioned flat against the spine with its most rostral tip at the anterior tubercle of C1. The position of the retractor is then confirmed using the navigation system. A soft armored endotracheal tube is utilized to allow the retractor to push the trachea to the contralateral side with minimal resistance from the tube; the armor simultaneously prevents distortion or occlusion of the endotracheal tube.

The longus colli muscles are dissected through the retractor and moved laterally off the spine to expose the ventral aspect of C2.[1] A Misonix

[1] *Vertebral Arteries*. Following the dissection of the longus colli muscles through the retractor, the ventral aspect of C2 will become exposed. The vertebral arteries lie ventral to C2, especially just rostral to the C2–C3 disc space [38]. Great care should be taken to avoid injury to the vertebral arteries during this portion of the procedure.

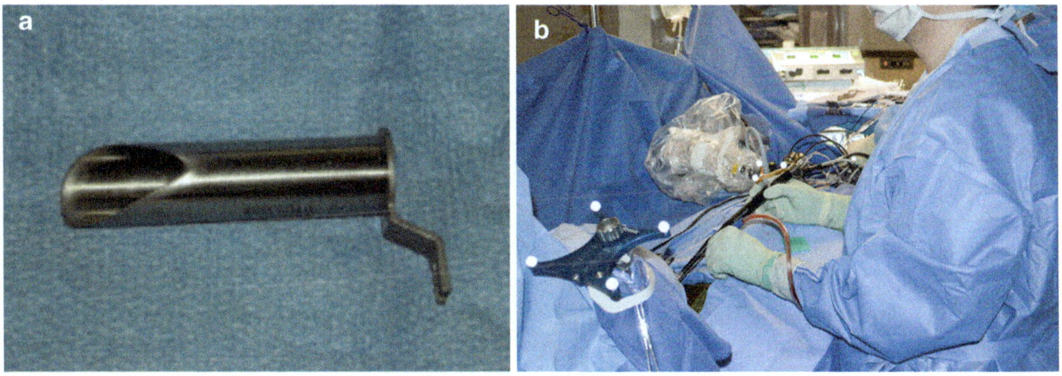

Fig. 4.4 (**a**, **b**) Beveled, tubular retractor and Medtronic Sofamor Danek METRx tubular retractor system. The retractor is modified such that the base of the tubular retractor is cut at a customizable angle, which allows the retractor to be directly attached to the spine in a stable fashion, providing an optimal view and trajectory for inserting the transodontoid screw through the base of C2 and the odontoid, while minimizing tissue retraction and offering 360° protection of the soft tissue surrounding the surgical area. In addition, if it is fixed to the table, it removes the need for an assistant to perform the retraction

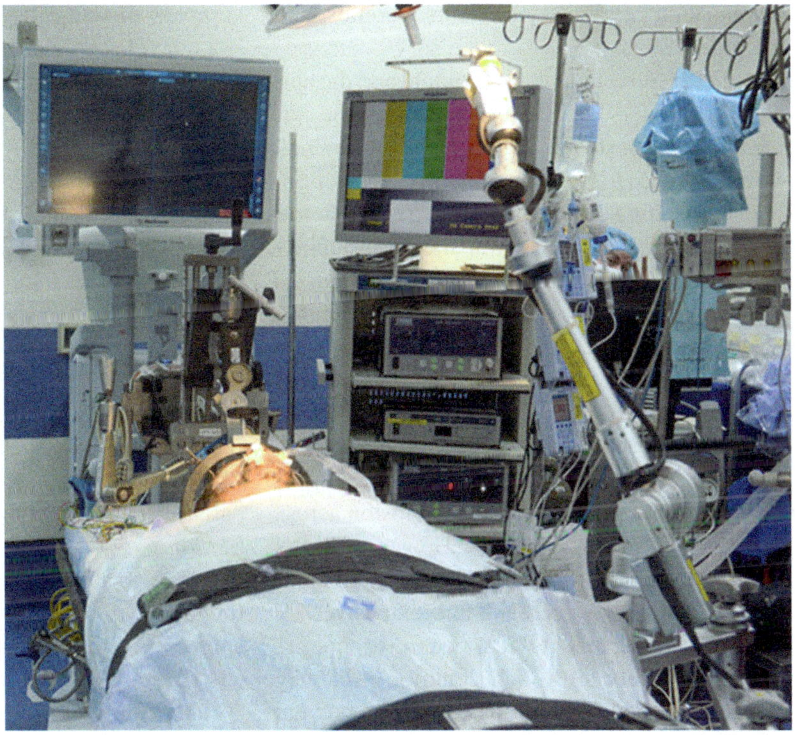

Fig. 4.5 Neuro-endoscope. An endoscope may be used free-hand or put into a holding system to let the surgeon use both hands during the procedure. A 30° 4-mm endoscope is described here, but 0, 30°-upviewing and 30-downviewing endoscopes are also available; the greater angle endoscopes may provide adequate visualization without corresponding ability to perform manual dissection [3]

BoneScalpel M.I.S. (Misonix, Farmingdale, New York, USA) is then calibrated and used in conjunction with the neuronavigation system, with the BoneScalpel recalibrating for each different drill bit and drill attachment. A 30° 4-mm neuro-endoscope is attached to the endoscope arm, where it will stay for the remainder of the operation to provide visualization down the retractor (Fig. 4.5). In order to capture a view of C2 from above, the neuro-endoscope is positioned within the retractor such that it lies flat against the retractor superior surface.

Resection begins between the posterior aspect of the anterior ring of C-1 and the odontoid. Drilling then proceeds rostrally until the tip of the odontoid is encountered. Progression of resection is continuously monitored via direct visualization through the endoscope as well as via the stereotactic neuronavigation. Once the tip of the odontoid is visualized, resection should proceed in a "top-down" fashion throughout the length of the odontoid until all bony structures are removed. A 3-mm diamond burr is then used to completely resect the remaining bone. Once the osseous resection is complete, the resection of the ligaments (transverse, alar, and apical) and any pannus, if present, should be performed, exposing the underlying dura.[2] Since the dens is completely mobile, it can be disconnected at its base and delivered in an en bloc fashion using a combination of pituitary rongeurs, curettes, and microdissectors.

Once the resection of the odontoid and the apical and transverse ligaments is complete, the cervical spine is unstable [10, 32, 33, 39, 40]. Great care is required for further transport or repositioning in the setting of a combined anterior-posterior approach. For the majority of patients, instability exists from the occiput through C2, although, in certain instances, especially those in which C1 has been assimilated into the occiput, the instability is between C1 and C2. For those patients with localized C1–C2 instability, an anterior arthrodesis is achieved using the same approach with bilateral anterior lateral mass/pedicle/transarticular screw instrumentation and fusion across the C1–C2 joints [10, 22, 41]. However, if it is not feasible due to anatomical considerations or if the instability is present more extensively, a second-stage occiput-cervical fusion is required. For further safety, a 1/8-inch Hemovac drain may be tunneled deep into the osteotomy to prevent a post-operative hematoma compressing the ventral brainstem.

The next steps depend on the nature of the procedure. The C1 ring can be left intact if only the odontoid was to be removed. However, in order to gain access to the lower clivus, the C1 ring must be removed, requiring the retractor to be angled more anteriorly to gain access to the lower clivus. Realistically, however, the angle of attack, depth of surgical field, and position of the retractor relative to the chest make this portion of the dissection difficult or impossible to achieve [3, 10, 21, 22, 34].

[2]*Apical and transverse ligaments*. These ligaments should not be resected during the odontoid resection, as they provide a protective barrier between the osseous resection and the dura mater.

Surgical Anatomy

Access Granted by Procedure and Surgical Corridors

The entry point is the midline of the skin at the C4–C5 cervical disc level [1, 3, 10, 22]. The approach theoretically permits access to the anterior tubercle of C1 superiorly and the lower cervical spine inferiorly [3]. Within the surgical field, the most superior access is the point in the middle at 1 cm above basion, and the most inferior access is the inferoposterior aspect of the body of C2, based on access using surgical trajectory through the retractor. However, this approach can technically access the cervical spine from C5 to the basion [3]. As noted by Syre and Lee, there is theoretically no lower limit because a wide cervical incision can expose the entire cervical spines through to the cervicothoracic junction (Figs. 4.6, 4.7, and 4.8) [1].

Cadaveric and image-based studies have compared the surgical corridors of the transcervical, transoral, and transnasal approaches. The actual distances to the surgical targets, however, were found to be 94 mm for the extended endonasal approach, 102 mm for the transoral approach, and 100 mm for the transcervical approach [3–11, 25]. The transcervical approach has the narrowest angle of attack, at 15°, compared to 30° for the transoral approach and 28° for the extended endonasal approach [3–11, 25]. Finally, the transoral approach offers the widest working area at 1402 mm^2, followed by the extended transnasal approach at 1305 mm^2, and the transcervical approach at 743 mm^2 [3–11, 25]. These findings are summarized in Table 4.1.

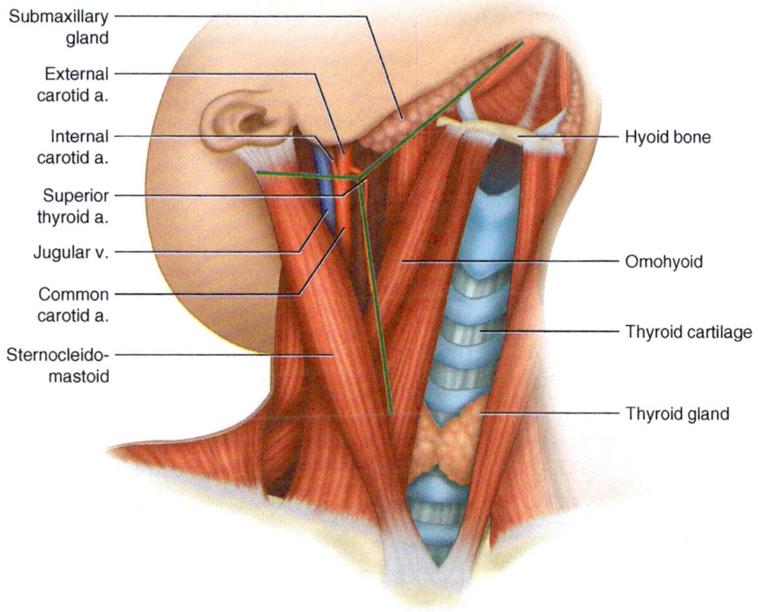

Fig. 4.6 Lateral rotation and head hyperextension for transcervical exposure. (Reproduced with permission from Stevenson et al. [49])

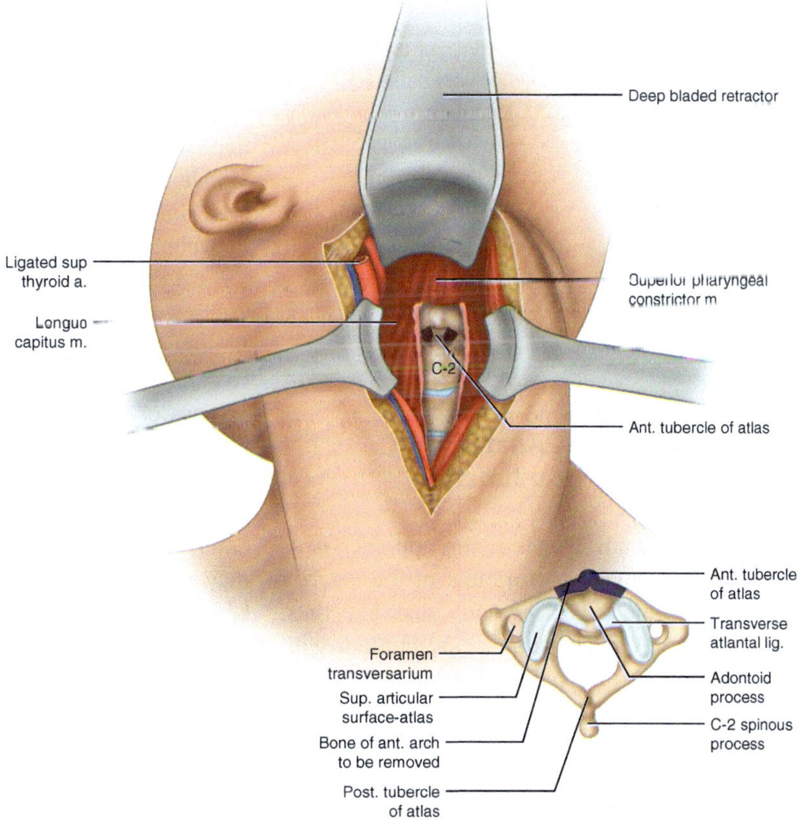

Fig. 4.7 Retraction and exposure of upper cervical spine. (Reproduced with permission from Stevenson et al. [49])

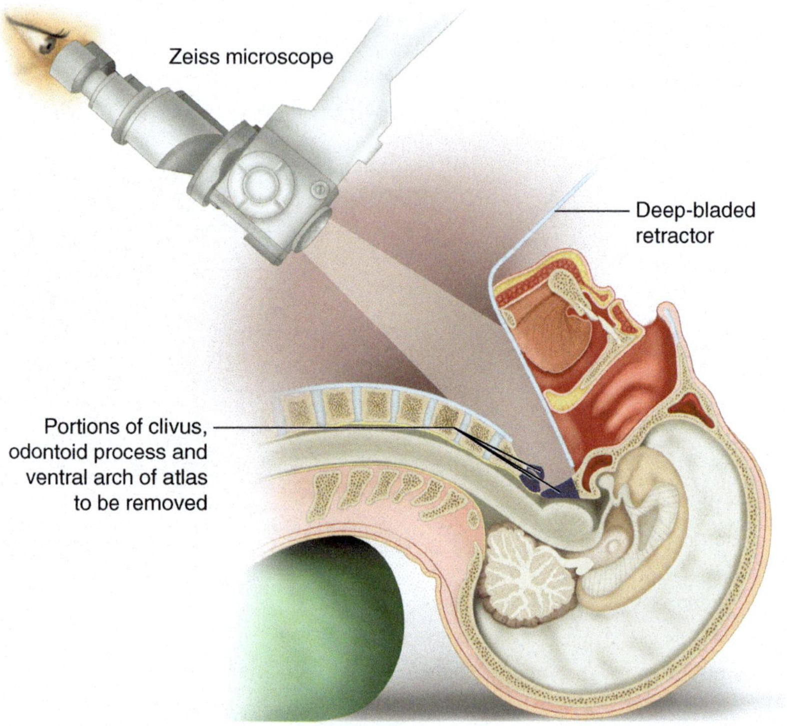

Fig. 4.8 Deep-blade retraction for visualization of the clival area with the transcervical approach. (Reproduced with permission from Stevenson et al. [49])

Table 4.1 Comparison of the features of the transcervical, transoral, and transnasal approaches to the CVJ

	Transcervical approach	Transoral approach	Transnasal approach
Distance to surgical target (mm)	100	102	94
Angle of attack (°)	15	30	28
Working area (mm^2)	743	1406	1305

Understanding the Anatomy of the Craniocervical Junction

One of the key advantages of this approach is its surgical anatomy: it mirrors that of the anterior approach to the lower cervical spine, and thus, the majority of spine surgeons are familiar with it. However, a thorough understanding of the anatomy of the CVJ adds an additional level of safety to the procedure. There are several considerations based on the anatomy of the CVJ, which will be discussed as follows:

Arteries

As mentioned in footnote 1, special attention should be paid to the vertebral arteries during this approach. The ventral aspect of C2 will become visible following the dissection of the longus colli muscles [1, 10, 42]. The vertebral arteries lie ventral to C2, especially just rostral to the C2–C3 disc space [1, 10, 38, 42]. The vertebral arteries that lie caudal to C3 lie in the transverse foramen of the cervical spine [1, 10, 22, 38, 42]. Eventually, these arteries enter the transverse process of C2, at which point the anatomy can be variable. The vertebral artery in this region may swing ventral to C2 prior to coursing laterally [10, 42]. This, in conjunction with possible craniocervical bone abnormalities of the region, may put the vertebral arteries at risk. Risk can be minimized with careful preoperative analysis using a 3D CT reconstruction in conjunction with MR imaging [10].

C1 and C2

The C1–C2 junction is intrinsically very mobile and has the potential to move even while the head is immobilized using the halo ring [10, 38]. This creates a unique challenge for both registration and accurate navigation of the three-dimensional relationship between intraoperative CT scan images and the actual surgical anatomy [3, 10, 21, 34, 38]. The patient's head should be secured to the table using the halo ring and Mayfield adaptor prior to image acquisition in order for us to minimize movement and thereby registration inaccuracy [10].

Ligaments

There are many anatomical layers between the osseous odontoid and the dura mater as well as between the dura mater and the brainstem. These include multiple ligaments providing protection to the brainstem and spinal cord; these ligaments create a boundary through which one should not drill [10, 22, 38, 43]. Immediately posterior to the dens, the transverse ligament inserts into the tubercles on the medial aspects of the lateral masses of C1 and surrounds the odontoid [10, 38]. The apical ligament lies rostrally, inserting into the tip of the dens and base of the clivus. The apical ligament is often associated with pathological conditions of the region, usually resulting in laxity (rather than destruction) of the ligaments [10]. During the approach, the apical and transverse ligaments should be resected only after completion of the odontoid resection to provide a protective barrier for the dura mater [10, 22, 43]. Finally, posterior to the apical and transverse ligaments are the vertical and horizontal ligaments and tectorial membrane; these exist as the final barrier before encountering the dura mater [10, 38]. In the case of an advanced disease, the ligaments stabilizing the dens can be thin or almost nonexistent [1, 10, 38].

Other Anatomical Structures

One of the caveats of this approach is the narrow workspace provided. Retraction, while integral to the procedure, can create potential risks [1, 3, 10, 20–22, 29]. The tubular retractor can help minimize overly aggressive retraction [10]. This may be especially useful in preventing traction injury to the digastric muscles and hypogastric nerves due to their proximity to the point of retraction [1, 38]. This, used in conjunction with a 30° endoscope placed at the superior portion of the tubular retraction, can look down on the anatomy, thus providing a familiar perspective of the head-on view of the ventral cervical spine [1, 10]. Notably, the tubular retractor does limit visualization of the surgical field through a narrow rigid corridor. Should more visualization be required, both the tubular retractor and endoscope must be repositioned [1, 3, 10, 22]. This removes the ability to visualize anatomic relationships of neighboring structures, obligating a fundamental knowledge of anatomy essential for successful surgery. As stated earlier, it is also advisable to use intraoperative frameless stereotactic navigation adjunctively to allow an appreciation of surface anatomy not seen through the endoscope and to provide feedback on the location of neural structures as they relate to the bone being resected [1, 10].

Complications

Dasenbrock et al. [22] described the outcomes of 15 patients who underwent endoscopic image-guided transcervical odontoidectomies. Of the 15 patients, 6 presented with postoperative complications, including upper airway swelling ($n = 2$), urinary tract infection ($n = 2$), dysphasia ($n = 2$), an asymptomatic pseudomeningocele ($n = 1$), and gastrostomy tube placement ($n = 1$). One patient required intubation for more than 48 h postoperatively. However, no patients presented with late neurological deterioration, bacterial meningitis, venous thromboembolic event, or need for tracheostomy. Meanwhile, McGirt et al. described the outcomes of four patients who also underwent surgery using an endoscopic transcervical approach and reported that one patient experienced subluxation in the halo vest [21, 43]. In a retrospective analysis of three patients, Wolinksy et al. found that one patient had the complication of an intraoperative CSF leak [10, 21]. Due to the limited number of clinical studies reported in the literature, further multicenter, prospective studies are warranted to better understand the benefits of this novel approach.

Discussion

When approaching the anterior cervical spine to reach the CVJ, there is no standardized approach; the transoral, transnasal, and transcervical approaches all have their own advantages and disadvantages. The transoral approach has several advantages: when combined with other approaches (e.g., Le Fort osteotomy or transmandibular-circumglossal approach), it provides a wide working area and allows for top-down drilling [2–19]. However, one of the greatest disadvantages is a contaminated surgical field, making CSF leak management significantly more difficult [21, 35, 36, 44–46]. Furthermore, it requires tongue retraction and palate splitting, which can cause several severe complications and the need for extensive postoperative intubation as elaborated earlier [2, 5, 6, 8, 14, 15, 20, 21, 31–36]. Finally, the anatomy is also less familiar to neurosurgeons in general and may require the expertise of an otolaryngologist.

The transnasal approach was developed in response to these disadvantages and also has its own set of advantages and disadvantages. It allows for top-down drilling, causes fewer retraction complications, and provides a wide working area [23, 30, 31, 37, 45, 47, 48]. However, it requires crossing a cavity with natural bacterial flora, increasing the risk of postoperative meningitis in the event of a CSF leak [20–22, 30, 31, 34, 37]. Both the transoral and transnasal approaches also place the vidian nerves and Eustachian tubes at risk, should exposure be made too wide [20, 38].

While these approaches remain ideal for treating tumors or rheumatoid disease involving the clivus through C2, the transcervical approach presents a new and potentially advantageous approach in the case of basilar invagination of C2 without clival resection [3, 22]. It proceeds through a sterile surgical field, presents familiar anatomy to spine surgeons, causes fewer retraction complications, and may decrease postoperative complications [1, 3, 10, 20–22, 25].

However, there are several drawbacks related to this technique, which includes its narrow working angles (15° compared to 30° in the transoral approach and 28° in the extended endonasal approach), long working distances (approximately 100 mm), and pharyngeal retraction, all while requiring the maintenance of a midline dissection trajectory [3–11, 21, 22, 25, 34]. It may also increase the likelihood of durotomy due to the need to pull the odontoid tip [22, 43]. However, the consequences of a CSF leak may be potentially neutralized by the sterile surgical field provided by the approach. The bony resection of the odontoid is more difficult than in the other approaches which allow the odontoid process to remain attached at the base to C2 earlier in the surgical dissection [3].

The endoscope provides surgeons with a technically feasible way to treat a wider array of pathology in the region with more flexibility and less morbidities [1, 20–24]. However, like the microscope, the endoscope only provides a two-dimensional image. This can be overcome by moving the scope and using manual palpation to provide secondary depth perception clues [1, 3, 10, 21, 22, 25, 29, 34]. Resolution of the endoscope is only as good as its attached camera and screen (in comparison to the microscope, which uses direct visualization by the human retina, with resolving power greater than the best high-definition video) [1, 3, 10, 21, 22, 24, 25, 29, 34]. Rapid improvements in video technology and the current phasing-in of three-dimensional endoscopes will hopefully solve this problem in the future.

Multiple approaches provide spine surgeons the opportunity to personalize their surgical approach in order to optimize the effectiveness of surgery and maximize patient safety. The appropriate surgical exposure varies and is based on the surgical pathology, operative objective, medical history, and the surgeon's experience. We hope to have provided insight into a new approach that may allow for easier, more sterile access to the ventral CVJ when pathology and its localization support it.

Conclusion

The endoscopic transcervical approach to the ventral CVJ can be a useful tool to safely decompress the brainstem and spinal cord while adding the extra safety feature of sterility of surgical field. It also offers the benefit of decreased recovery time by minimizing postoperative periods where patients are intubated and/or under nasogastric tubes for feeding. This procedure is contraindicated for those patients who present with pathologies predominantly at the clivus, or who are obese, barrel-chested, or kyphotic. However, in those for whom the approach is indicated, the anterior transcervical approach to the CVJ offers a useful tool in the arsenal that so far had only consisted of the transoral-transpharyngeal approach and the transnasal approach, by providing a more specific trajectory for treating pathologies of the CVJ and upper cervical spine.

References

1. Syre PLJ. Endoscopic approaches to the craniovertebral junction. In: Surgical anatomy and techniques to the spine E-book. Philadelphia: Elsevier Health Sciences; 2013. p. 60–8.
2. Frempong-Boadu AK, Faunce WA, Fessler RG. Endoscopically assisted transoral-transpharyngeal approach to the craniovertebral junction. Neurosurgery. 2002;51:S60–6.
3. Baird CJ, Conway JE, Sciubba DM, Prevedello DM, Quinones-Hinojosa A, Kassam AB. Radiographic and anatomic basis of endoscopic anterior craniocervical decompression: a comparison of endonasal, transoral, and transcervical approaches. Neurosurgery. 2009;65:158–63.; discussion 163-154. https://doi.org/10.1227/01.neu.0000345641.97181.ed.
4. Cavallo LM, Messina A, Cappabianca P, Esposito F, de Divitiis E, Gardner P, Tschabitscher M. Endoscopic endonasal surgery of the midline skull base: anatomical study and clinical considerations. Neurosurg Focus. 2005;19:E2.
5. Crockard HA. The transoral approach to the base of the brain and upper cervical cord. Ann R Coll Surg Engl. 1985;67:321–5
6. Crockard HA. Transoral surgery: some lessons learned. Br J Neurosurg. 1995,9:283–93.
7. Hadley MN, Spetzler RF, Sonntag VK. The transoral approach to the superior cervical spine. A review of 53 cases of extradural cervicomedullary compression. J Neurosurg. 1989;71:16–23. https://doi.org/10.3171/jns.1989.71.1.0016.
8. Mummaneni PV, Haid RW. Transoral odontoidectomy. Neurosurgery. 2005;56:1045–50. discussion 1045-1050
9. Spetzler RF, Hadley MN, Sonntag VK. The transoral approach to the anterior superior cervical spine. A review of 29 cases. Acta Neurochir Suppl. 1988;43:69–74.
10. Wolinsky JP, Sciubba DM, Suk I, Gokaslan ZL. Endoscopic image-guided odontoidectomy for decompression of basilar invagination via a standard anterior cervical approach. Technical note. J Neurosurg Spine. 2007;6:184–91. https://doi.org/10.3171/spi.2007.6.2.184.
11. Youssef AS, Guiot B, Black K, Sloan AE. Modifications of the transoral approach to the craniovertebral junction: anatomic study and clinical correlations. Neurosurgery. 2008;62:145–54.; discussion 154-145. https://doi.org/10.1227/01.neu.0000317386.99055.3f.
12. Arbit E, Patterson RH Jr. Combined transoral and median labiomandibular glossotomy approach to the upper cervical spine. Neurosurgery. 1981;8:672–4.
13. Bertrand J, Luc B, Philippe M, Philippe P. Anterior mandibular osteotomy for tumor extirpation: a critical evaluation. Head Neck. 2000;22:323–7.
14. Delgado TE, Garrido E, Harwick RD. Labiomandibular, transoral approach to chordomas in the clivus and upper cervical spine. Neurosurgery. 1981;8:675–9.
15. Kanamori Y, Miyamoto K, Hosoe H, Fujitsuka H, Tatematsu N, Shimizu K. Transoral approach using the mandibular osteotomy for atlantoaxial vertical subluxation in juvenile rheumatoid arthritis associated with mandibular micrognathia. J Spinal Disord Tech. 2003;16:221–4.
16. Menezes AH, VanGilder JC, Clark CR, el-Khoury G. Odontoid upward migration in rheumatoid arthritis. An analysis of 45 patients with "cranial settling". J Neurosurg. 1985;63:500–9. https://doi.org/10.3171/jns.1985.63.4.0500.
17. Anand VK, Harkey HL, Al-Mefty O. Open-Door Maxillotomy Approach for Lesions of the Clivus. Skull Base Surg. 1991;1:217–25.
18. Balasingam V, Anderson GJ, Gross ND, Cheng CM, Noguchi A, Dogan A, et al. Anatomical analysis of transoral surgical approaches to the clivus. J Neurosurg. 2006;105:301–8. https://doi.org/10.3171/jns.2006.105.2.301.
19. James D, Crockard HA. Surgical access to the base of skull and upper cervical spine by extended maxillotomy. Neurosurgery. 1991;29:411–6.
20. Shriver MF, Kshettry VR, Sindwani R, Woodard T, Benzel EC, Recinos PF. Transoral and transnasal odontoidectomy complications: A systematic review and meta-analysis. Clin Neurol Neurosurg. 2016;148:121–9. https://doi.org/10.1016/j.clineuro.2016.07.019.
21. Visocchi M, Di Martino A, Maugeri R, Gonzalez Valcarcel I, Grasso V, Paludetti G. Videoassisted anterior surgical approaches to the craniocervical junction: rationale and clinical results. Eur Spine J. 2015;24:2713–23. https://doi.org/10.1007/s00586-015-3873-6.
22. Dasenbrock HH, Clarke MJ, Bydon A, Sciubba DM, Witham TF, Gokaslan ZL, Wolinsky JP. Endoscopic image-guided transcervical odontoidectomy: outcomes of 15 patients with basilar invagination. Neurosurgery. 2012;70:351–9.; discussion 359-360. https://doi.org/10.1227/NEU.0b013e318230e59a.

23. Kassam AB, Snyderman C, Gardner P, Carrau R, Spiro R. The expanded endonasal approach: a fully endoscopic transnasal approach and resection of the odontoid process: technical case report. Neurosurgery. 2005;57:E213; discussion E213.
24. Pillai P, Baig MN, Karas CS, Ammirati M. Endoscopic image-guided transoral approach to the craniovertebral junction: an anatomic study comparing surgical exposure and surgical freedom obtained with the endoscope and the operating microscope. Neurosurgery. 2009; 64:437–42; discussion 442–34. https://doi.org/10.1227/01.neu.0000334050.45750.c9.
25. Hsu W, Kosztowski TA, Zaidi HA, Gokaslan ZL, Wolinsky JP. Image-guided, endoscopic, transcervical resection of cervical chordoma. J Neurosurg Spine. 2010;12:431–5. https://doi.org/10.3171/2009.10.spine09393.
26. Ma H, Lv G, Wang B, Kuang L, Wang X. Endoscopic transcervical anterior release and posterior fixation in the treatment of irreducible vertical atlantoaxial dislocation. Eur Spine J. 2014;23:1749–54. https://doi.org/10.1007/s00586-014-3352-5.
27. Singh H, Rote S, Jada A, Bander ED, Almodovar-Mercado GJ, Essayed WI, et al. Endoscopic endonasal odontoid resection with real-time intraoperative image-guided computed tomography: report of 4 cases. J Neurosurg. 2017;128:1–6. https://doi.org/10.3171/2017.1.jns162601.
28. Yadav YR, Madhariya SN, Parihar VS, Namdev H, Bhatele PR. Endoscopic transoral excision of odontoid process in irreducible atlantoaxial dislocation: our experience of 34 patients. J Neurol Surg A Cent Eur Neurosurg. 2013;74:162–7. https://doi.org/10.1055/s-0032-1327441.
29. Yadav YR, Ratre S, Parhihar V, Dubey A, Dubey NM. Endoscopic technique for single-stage anterior decompression and anterior fusion by transcervical approach in atlantoaxial dislocation. Neurol India. 2017;65:341–7. https://doi.org/10.4103/neuroindia.NI_1276_16.
30. Yu Y, Hu F, Zhang X, Sun C. Endoscopic transnasal odontoidectomy. Sports Med Arthroscop Rev. 2016;24:2–6. https://doi.org/10.1097/jsa.0000000000000081.
31. Choi D, Crockard HA. Evolution of transoral surgery three decades of change in patients, pathologies, and indications. Neurosurgery. 2013;73:296–304. https://doi.org/10.1227/01.neu.0000430324.24623.10.
32. Di Lorenzo N. Craniocervical junction malformation treated by transoral approach. A survey of 25 cases with emphasis on postoperative instability and outcome. Acta Neurochir. 1992;118:112–6.
33. Goel A. Progressive basilar invagination after transoral odontoidectomy: treatment by atlantoaxial facet distraction and craniovertebral realignment. Spine. 2005;30:E551–5.
34. Lin ZK, Chi YL, Wang XY, Yu Q, Fang BD, Wu LJ. The influence of cervical spine position on the three anterior endoscopic approaches to the craniovertebral junction: an imaging study. Spine J. 2014;14:80–6. https://doi.org/10.1016/j.spinee.2013.06.079.
35. Menezes AH. Surgical approaches: postoperative care and complications "transoral-transpalatopharyngeal approach to the craniocervical junction". Childs Nerv Syst. 2008;24:1187–93. https://doi.org/10.1007/s00381-008-0599-3.
36. Perrini P, Benedetto N, Guidi E, Di Lorenzo N. Transoral approach and its superior extensions to the craniovertebral junction malformations: surgical strategies and results. Neurosurgery. 2009;64:331–42.; discussion 342. https://doi.org/10.1227/01.neu.0000334430.25626.dc.
37. Lee A, Sommer D, Reddy K, Murty N, Gunnarsson T. (2010) Endoscopic transnasal approach to the craniocervical junction. Skull Base. 2010;20:199–205. https://doi.org/10.1055/s-0029-1246220.
38. Türe U, Kaya AH. Surgical anatomy of the craniocervical junction. In: Pathology and surgery around the vertebral artery. Paris: Springer Paris; 2011. p. 317–28.
39. Menezes AH, VanGilder JC. Transoral-transpharyngeal approach to the anterior craniocervical junction. Ten-year experience with 72 patients. J Neurosurg. 1988;69:895–903. https://doi.org/10.3171/jns.1988.69.6.0895.
40. Sakou T, Morizono Y, Morimoto N. Transoral atlantoaxial anterior decompression and fusion. Clin Orthop Relat Res. 1984;187:134–8.
41. Hwang SW, Heilman CB, Riesenburger RI, Kryzanski J. C1–C2 arthrodesis after transoral odontoidectomy and suboccipital craniectomy for ventral brain stem compression in Chiari I patients. Eur Spine J. 2008;17:1211–7. https://doi.org/10.1007/s00586-008-0706-x.
42. Vanek P, Bradac O, de Lacy P, Konopkova R, Lacman J, Benes V. Vertebral artery and osseous anomalies characteristic at the craniocervical junction diagnosed by CT and 3D CT angiography in normal Czech population: analysis of 511 consecutive patients. Neurosurg Rev. 2017;40:369–76. https://doi.org/10.1007/s10143-016-0784-x.
43. McGirt MJ, Attenello FJ, Sciubba DM, Gokaslan ZL, Wolinsky JP. Endoscopic transcervical odontoidectomy for pediatric basilar invagination and cranial settling. Report of 4 cases. J Neurosurg Pediatr. 2008;1:337–42. https://doi.org/10.3171/ped/2008/1/4/337.
44. Dhaliwal PP, Hurlbert RJ, Sutherland GS. Intraoperative magnetic resonance imaging and neuronavigation for transoral approaches to upper cervical pathology. World Neurosurg. 2012;78:164–9. https://doi.org/10.1016/j.wneu.2011.09.020.
45. El-Sayed IH, Wu JC, Ames CP, Balamurali G, Mummaneni PV. Combined transnasal and transoral endoscopic approaches to the craniovertebral junction. J Craniovertebr Junction Spine. 2010;1:44–8. https://doi.org/10.4103/0974-8237.65481.
46. Salunke P, Sharma M, Sodhi HB, Mukherjee KK, Khandelwal NK. Congenital atlantoaxial dislocation:

a dynamic process and role of facets in irreducibility. J Neurosurg Spine. 2011;15:678–85. https://doi.org/10.3171/2011.7.spine1152.

47. Gladi M, Iacoangeli M, Specchia N, Re M, Dobran M, Alvaro L, Moriconi E, Scerrati M. Endoscopic transnasal odontoid resection to decompress the bulbo-medullary junction: a reliable anterior minimally invasive technique without posterior fusion. Eur Spine J. 2012;21(Suppl 1):S55–60. https://doi.org/10.1007/s00586-012-2220-4.
48. Hickman ZL, McDowell MM, Barton SM, Sussman ES, Grunstein E, Anderson RCE. Transnasal endoscopic approach to the pediatric craniovertebral junction and rostral cervical spine: case series and literature review. Neurosurg Focus. 2013;35:E14. https://doi.org/10.3171/2013.5.focus13147.
49. Stevenson GC, Stoney RJ, Perkins RK, Adams JE. A transcervical transclival approach to the ventral surface of the brain stem for removal of a clivus chordoma. JNS Spine. 1996;24:544–51.

Anterior Subaxial Cervical Approach

5

George N. Rymarczuk, Courtney Pendleton, and James S. Harrop

Part I: General Considerations of the Anterior Cervical Approach

History of the Anterior Cervical Exposure

Detailed descriptions of anterior exposure of the subaxial cervical spine for treatment of ventral spinal pathology first appeared with descriptions written by Smith-Robinson [1], followed closely by Cloward [2] in the mid-twentieth century. Improvements in the comprehension of anatomy and biomechanical principles, advancements in the design of self-retaining retractor systems and intraoperative lighting, and widespread microscope availability have made the anterior approach to the cervical spine a common and safe technique.

General Considerations of the Anterior Cervical Approach Versus Posterior Approach

Although posterior decompressive laminectomy has been a mainstay of treatment, use of anterior (also referred to as "ventral") approaches for direct decompression in the setting of subaxial cervical spine tumors has become increasingly popular as techniques for spine stabilization and reconstruction have evolved.

Posterior laminectomy with or without instrumented fusion may potentially afford the opportunity for decreased operative time while simultaneously addressing compressive symptoms from tumors lying either dorsal or ventral to the spinal cord. It additionally provides a means for decompressing nerve roots at the level of the foramen, and complete access to tumors lying dorsal to the thecal sac. However, posterior-only approaches, even in the face of instrumentation, may carry a risk of progressive kyphotic deformity [3, 4], and furthermore may be ill-suited for obtaining oncologic control of ventrally-located tumors.

Anterior cervical approaches provide a route for direct decompression of neural elements as well as resection of ventral subaxial tumors, and allow for immediate reconstruction and stabilization of the spinal column. They offer the opportunity for tissue diagnosis, oncologic control, and carry lower risks of infection, lengthy hospital course, and pseudoarthrosis than the posterior approach alone. Patients with kyphosis, particularly those with fixed kyphotic deformities, may experience better correction of alignment through inclusion of an anterior or combined approach [5]. Anterior-alone approaches do, however, have limited utility in addressing tumors dorsal to the spinal cord, may have a longer operative time, and carry risks of dysphagia and injury to the recurrent laryngeal nerve [6, 7], carotid sheath, and mediastinal

G. N. Rymarczuk (✉) · C. Pendleton · J. S. Harrop
Department of Neurological Surgery, Thomas Jefferson University Hospital, Philadelphia, PA, USA
e-mail: george.n.rymarczuk.mil@mail.mil

D. M. Sciubba (ed.), *Spinal Tumor Surgery*, https://doi.org/10.1007/978-3-319-98422-3_5

structures. Anterior approaches requiring partial or complete corpectomies carry additional risk of injury to the vertebral artery as it passes through the transverse foramina, particularly if the tumor distorts the anatomy.

Pertinent Neural Anatomy

Symptoms from subaxial cervical spine tumors include intractable pain, which may be mechanical or radicular in nature, as well as myelopathic symptoms from compression of the spinal cord. The median cervical spinal cord diameter is 10 mm, and the median cervical canal diameter is 17 mm; symptoms may be more likely to develop when canal diameter is reduced to 10 mm or less [8, 9].

Pathology

The majority of tumors found in the subaxial cervical spine include primary mesenchymal neoplasms, meningothelial tumors, nerve sheath tumors, hematopoietic lesions, and metastases.

The cervical spine is also subject to spondylotic change, which when superimposed upon the neoplastic disease, must be taken into consideration when formulating a management algorithm. Changes such as degenerative disc disease, hypertrophy or ossification of the posterior longitudinal ligament (OPLL), facet arthropathy, and osteophyte formation may occur in isolation or as part of a syndromic constellation (diffuse idiopathic skeletal hyperostosis, ankylosing spondylitis, etc.). Reducible, non-ankylosed deformity may be corrected utilizing lordotic grafts, positioning techniques including extension and traction, convergent Caspar pin placement, and instrumentation. Non-reducible deformity requires more surgical techniques such as osteotomies, and may necessitate combined anterior/posterior approaches for adequate reduction of listhesis and correction of kyphosis [5]. Plans to correct alignment in the setting of oncologic burden should weigh the risk of morbidity associated with extensive deformity correction with the patient's oncologic prognosis, degree of systemic disease control, and medical comorbidity.

Anterior Cervical Exposure and Local Anatomy

Some literature supports a left-sided approach to the spine, as the recurrent laryngeal nerve (RLN) lies protected between the trachea and esophagus during exposure, compared to the relatively more vulnerable course of the right recurrent laryngeal nerve [6]. Subsequent studies have shown that surgeon handedness and preference, revision surgery, and tumor configuration may dictate a right-sided approach, which can be performed with no increased rate of transient of permanent dysphonia [7]. In patients with prior anterior cervical spine exposures or potential lower cranial nerve involvement by the neoplastic process, evaluation by otolaryngology is recommended to assess vocal cord function. In the presence of preexisting injury, surgical approach should be planned for the ipsilateral side to avoid a devastating bilateral RLN injury. Further, the anatomic location of the tumors should be evaluated and considered since its involvement with the neural or vascular structures may alter approach strategies. The surgeon should feel comfortable with both approaches (right versus left) such that they choose the approach with the least potential morbidity.

A horizontal incision within a skin crease is commonly used for short segment and degenerative fusions. However, when performing multilevel procedures or when approaching a ventral spine tumor, a wide exposure is often beneficial. This can be accomplished with a carotid-type incision to provide adequate exposure while minimizing retraction on soft tissue structures.

The operative exposure traverses a predictable anatomic course. After opening the initial skin incision, the platysma is divided either transversely or in parallel with the direction of its fibers. With adequate dissection of the pre- and postplatysmal planes, four or even five levels may be readily accessed through a single transverse incision. Passing medially to the SCM, the omohyoid is identified and circumferentially dissected; it may be divided without significant consequence, but often it is easily simply retracted out of the surgical corridor. An avascular plane is developed medial to the carotid sheath and lateral to the esophagus/trachea. The spine is palpated and the anatomic levels are identified and confirmed with radiography. The longus colli muscles, an important landmark identifying the midline, are reflected laterally with subperiosteal dissection and may serve as an anchor point for the self-retaining retractor system. Discectomy with or without corpectomy and tumor resection may be carried out. Spinal tumors typically do not invade the disc spaces, which should be preserved initially such that discectomies can be done above and below the tumor, leaving the en bloc removal of the lesion as the final portion of the procedure. If the tumor is vascular in nature, consideration of preoperative embolization is often beneficial. Once the surgeon enters the tumor, bleeding will decrease significantly once the lesion is circumferentially dissected and vascular supply is removed. It is our practice to remove the posterior longitudinal ligament, as we have found that it is often infiltrated with tumor cells.

Reconstruction and Stabilization: Options and Challenges

Unfortunately, with oncologic patients there is always the concern for pseudoarthrosis, particularly those with a history of tobacco or chronic steroid use, or patients who will require aggressive postoperative chemotherapy or radiation. In these patients, autologous bone such as iliac crest or even vascularized free-flap grafts should be strongly considered as the graft material. The patient should be positioned, prepped, and draped in a way that facilitates graft harvesting. The use of vascularized free grafts from long bones requires coordination between the surgical teams and should be planned well in advance. Additional alternatives to autograft include cadaveric tricortical graft as well as synthetic materials (i.e., PEEK, titanium, etc.). These minimize the donor site morbidity and allow for ease of sizing and choice of lordosis but may have an increased risk of nonunion. Various plating systems exist, and choice is dependent on surgeon preference, as well as institutional vendor availability. Placement of screws should be divergent in the sagittal plane and convergent in the axial plane to minimize the risk of pull-out. If there is concern for the bone purchase and/or construct stability, posterior augmentation should be considered (Figs. 5.1 and 5.2).

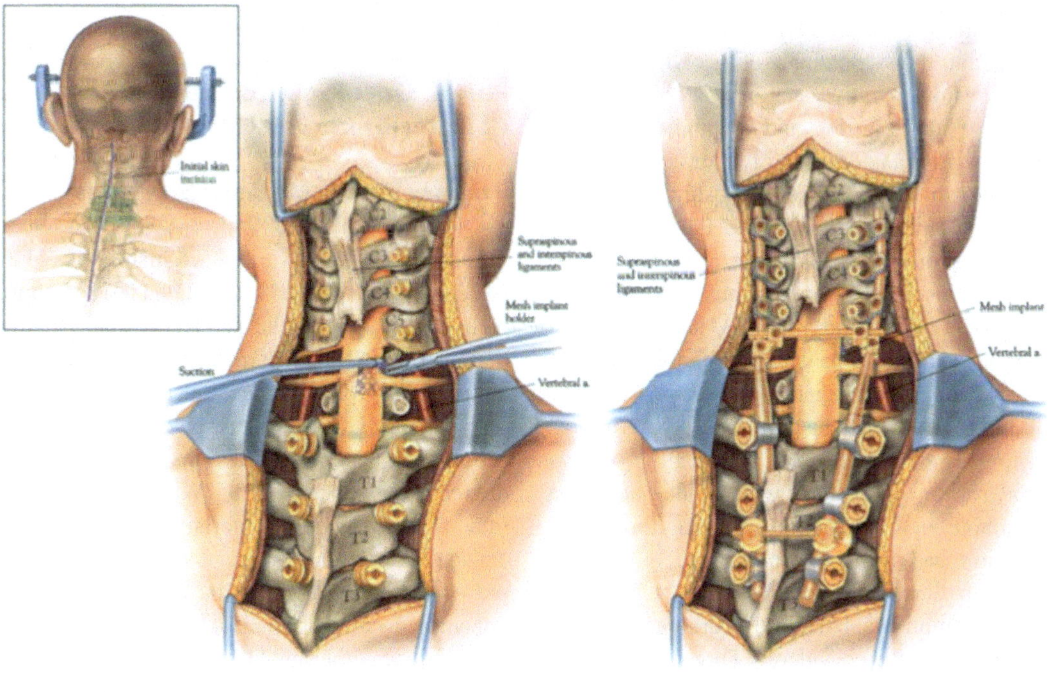

Fig. 5.1 Posterior stabilization for cervical spondylectomy to achieve oncologic margins for cervical osteogenic sarcoma. (Reprinted with permission from Cohen et al. [10])

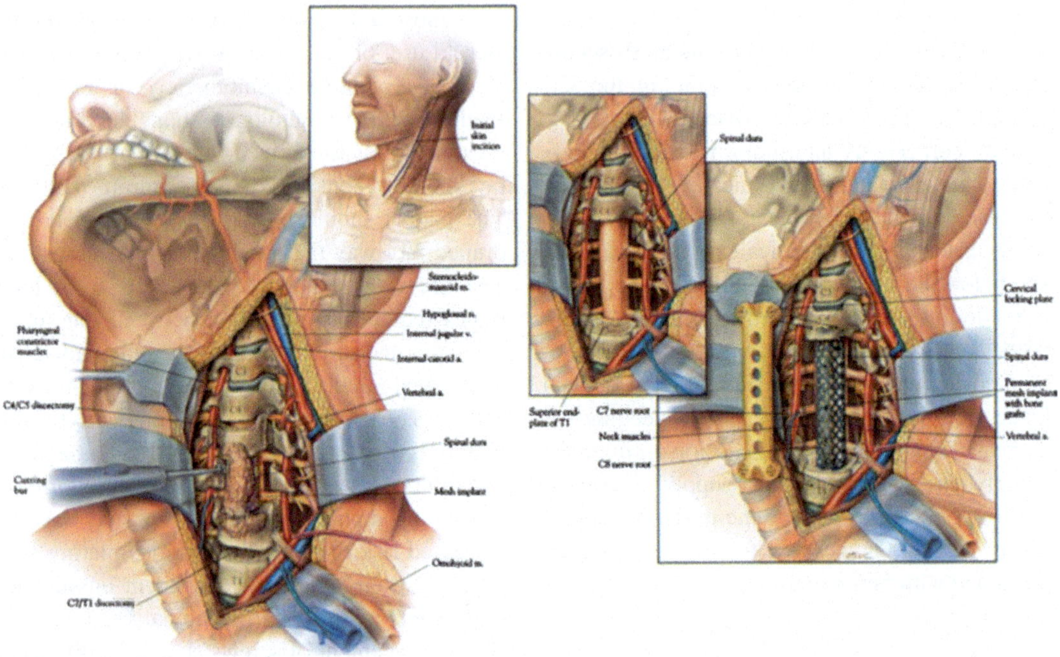

Fig. 5.2 Anterior subaxial cervical spondylectomy for osteogenic sarcoma. (Reprinted with permission from Cohen et al. [10])

Complications and Avoidance

The anterior cervical approach carries a risk of injury to the RLN, esophagus, thyroid, trachea, as well as the carotid or vertebral arteries, the vagus nerve, and the sympathetic chain. Knowledge of the relevant operative anatomy is paramount in avoiding such injuries, and the ability to recognize aberrant anatomy on preoperative imaging, or early in the operative exposure, will minimize intraoperative damage to these structures. Normal anatomical landmarks may be obscured by previous surgery or previous radiation, thus enlistment of a head-and-neck team for exposure should be considered. Although anterior cervical approaches generally carry a low risk of durotomy, in patients with underlying tumors, there may be calcification of the PLL or invasion/erosion of the dura, which make dural tear inevitable. In the event of a CSF leak, direct visualization and primary repair is recommended, although dural substitute or fibrin sealants, as well as lumbar subarachnoid drainage postoperatively, may be considered. Direct injury to the cord and nerve roots remains a risk and may be increased by tumor configuration, consistency, and invasion of neural structures. Long-term complications include the risk of pseudoarthrosis, graft displacement or migration, and instrumentation failure.

Part II: Oncologic Considerations of Anterior Cervical Surgery

Primary Versus Metastatic Lesions

Tumors of a wide variety of histologies may affect the subaxial cervical spine [11–18]. Tumor histology is one of the primary considerations that dictate treatment in a specific individual and can be broadly organized into two categories: primary spinal tumors and metastases. Both primary and metastatic lesions exhibit varying degrees of radiosensitivity. With the advent of image-guided radiation therapy techniques such as stereotactic radiosurgery (SRS), it is now possible to treat tumors that were traditionally considered radioresistant to conventional external beam radiotherapy [19, 20], as image-guided techniques have the capability to limit dosage received by the spinal cord and other critical nearby structures [21]. In light of this, nonsurgical options may have similar outcome in some instances of spinal metastasis [17, 18, 20, 22]. Conversely, many authors would advocate neurosurgical consultation for all primary tumors of the spine, as en bloc resection may be curative [19]. Therefore, surgeons should have an understanding of the histology, as it may alter the surgical approach and treatment. In isolated or unusual lesions, a biopsy should be considered in order to establish the diagnosis. For example, a cure can be effected in the case of a primary tumor treated with an en bloc resection, whereas an intra-lesional approach most likely will lead to recurrence. The potential morbidities of the more aggressive en bloc resection must be discussed with the patient so as to understand their goals and aims in terms of quality of life.

Primary Spinal Tumors

Primary spinal tumors are extradural lesions that are significantly less common than their metastatic counterparts. Primary lesions span the full spectrum of histological aggression. Furthermore, ultrastructurally benign lesions such as chordoma typically behave in a more locally destructive manner than their histology might belie. Primary neoplasms are most typically mesenchymal in origin and include benign lesions (chondroma, osteoma, hemangioma) as well as malignant tumors (sarcomas).

Primary tumors are often considered separately, as complete resection has the potential to be curative. With the ever-expanding role that SRS has been shown to occupy with metastatic disease, there is more leeway with the extent of resection that is necessary for metastatic lesions, and in many instances, a smaller and potentially less morbid procedure is indicated.

Metastatic Lesions

The great majority of extradural spinal cord tumors represent metastases. Among the most common primary spine tumors are breast, prostate, gastrointestinal, and lung cancers, as well as lymphoma and melanoma [19]. Metastases by definition are histologically aggressive; however, some lesions behave more indolently than others, and susceptibility to radiation therapy varies markedly. All of these attributes factor into the surgical decision-making process.

The NOMS Framework [19] is a multidisciplinary algorithm that has been developed at Memorial Sloan-Kettering Cancer Center to facilitate the decision-making process regarding metastatic disease of the spine. The algorithm assesses four aspects of the patient's clinical presentation: the patient's neurologic status ("N"), the oncologic behavior of the tumor ("O"), the mechanical stability of the spine ("M"), and the patient's systemic disease burden and degree of medical comorbidity ("S") [19].

For the assessment of the degree of spinal stability, the NOMS Framework draws on previous work done by the Spine Oncology Study Group. The Spine Oncology Study Group's Spinal Instability Neoplastic Score (SINS) is itself a tool that assigns a continuum of points based on seven of the patient's radiographic and clinical features [23]. According to the criteria set forth by the SINS algorithm, and with specific regard to the subaxial cervical spine, instability is more likely when junctional levels (occiput–C2, C7–T2) are involved as opposed to the relatively "mobile" subaxial region, if the patient experiences mechanical pain, if lesions appear lytic, if there is radiographic deformity present, if translation or subluxation is apparent on dynamic imaging, if vertebral body collapse is present, or if there is involvement of the posterior elements. These criteria are summarized in Table 5.1, which is adapted from Fisher et al. [23]. Overt instability is an indication for fixation that is independent of other features of the patient's presentation.

The neurologic assessment according to the NOMS Framework is predicated upon the degree of radiographic epidural involvement of the epidural space [19, 24]. The scale ranges from 0 to 3, with a score of 1 being further subdivided into 1a, 1b, and 1c. In general, a lower score would direct care toward radiation therapy. Radiation may still be the optimum therapy in light of more significant compression if a tumor were to be particularly radiosensitive. The scale for neurologic assessment is summarized in Figs. 5.1 and 5.2, which has been reprinted from Bilsky et al. [24].

The patient's oncological assessment is primarily concerned with the tumor's anticipated response to radiation therapy [19]. Gerszten [18] and Laufer [19] have provided excellent summarizations of the findings of multiple authors regarding the relative radiosensitivity of various metastatic malignancies to SRS. Hematologic and germinomatous malignancies are generally considered radiosensitive [18, 19], whereas other tumor histologies vary widely with regard to their sensitivity [11–17]. According to Laufer [19], who drew on earlier work from Gerszten [18], relatively radiosensitive solid tumors include breast and prostate tumors, whereas tumors that typically exhibit radioresistance include such histologies as sarcoma, melanoma, renal cell malignancy, and non-small-cell lung carcinoma.

Table 5.1 Criteria of the Spine Oncology Study Group's Spinal Instability Neoplastic Scale (SINS)[a]

Location	
Junctional (occiput–C2, C7–T2, T11–L1, L5–S1)	3
Mobile spine (C3–C6, L2–L4)	2
Semirigid (T3–T10)	1
Rigid (S2–S5)	0
Pain	
Yes	3
Occasional pain but not mechanical	1
Pain-free lesion	0
Bone lesion	
Lytic	2
Mixed (lytic/blastic)	1
Blastic	0
Radiographic spinal alignment	
Subluxation/translation present	4
De novo deformity (kyphosis/scoliosis)	2
Normal alignment	0
Vertebral body collapse	
˃50% collapse	3
˂50% collapse	2
No collapse with ˃50% body involved	1
None of the above	0
Posterolateral involvement of spinal elements	
Bilateral	3
Unilateral	1
None of the above	0
Total score	
Stable	0–6
Indeterminate	7–12
Unstable	13–18

[a]Adapted from Fisher et al. [23]

Finally, the patient's systemic disease burden and overall degree of medical comorbidity, suitability for surgery, and life expectancy must be assessed [19]. A thorough oncologic staging can have profound implications regarding the potential for prolonged palliation and therefore underscores the rationale for aggressive intervention. The major points of the NOMS Framework for the management of metastatic spinal disease are summarized in Fig. 5.3. However, tumor sensitivity and response to treatment are changing rapidly with the use of new chemotherapy agents and additional radiosurgery techniques such that surgeons need to coordinate care with the radiation oncology and medical oncology colleagues.

Diagnostic and Therapeutic Adjuncts to Surgery

Positron emission tomography ("PET scan") can be a useful adjunct to standard CT and MRI for evaluation of newly discovered spinal lesions. In

NOMS	Variable	1	2	3	4
Neurologic	No significant compression/deficit	X	X		
	Epidural compression + neurologic deficit			X	X
Oncologic	Radio-sensitive	X		X	
	Radio-resistant		X		X
Therapy		Conventional XRT	SRS	Conventional XRT	Separation surgery + SRS

Fig. 5.3 Summary of the NOMS Framework. (Adapted from Laufer et al. [19])

instances where the diagnosis is still unclear and tumor histology may influence the choice of surgical procedure, CT-guided needle biopsy can be invaluable. Considerations such as needle insertion point and trajectory must be kept in mind for locally aggressive or frankly malignant lesions, as this may risk seeding surrounding unaffected tissues, and histology may ultimately dictate that the biopsy tract itself should be resected.

Endovascular therapy is a relatively recent adjunct that has the potential to facilitate safe and complete resection in many instances. Some lesions affecting the cervical spine have the propensity to recruit a particularly robust vascular supply. Other lesions, such as metastatic renal cell carcinoma and hemangioma, are notorious for their vascular channels that may bleed profusely when dissected. Lesions of a vascular nature such as these may be embolized preoperatively in an effort to limit the bleeding that may be encountered intraoperatively.

In addition, locally aggressive lesions such as chordoma may grow to engulf or even invade the adventitia of the critical vascular structures of the neck. In these instances, a preoperative angiogram may be indicated for several reasons. Irregularities of the lumen of a critical vessel noted on angiography may indicate vessel invasion by the tumor, and based on this finding, a contingency plan may be formulated preoperatively, including ensuring that vascular clamps and blood products are readily available in the event of hemorrhage. In addition, assessment of collateral flow and even test balloon occlusion (TBO) can be performed during the preoperative evaluation of the newly diagnosed lesion, providing valuable information regarding possible downstream sequelae from vessel injury or sacrifice. Finally, endovascular techniques may facilitate vessel sacrifice peroperatively.

Goals of Surgery

The traditional goals of spinal surgery are (1) neural decompression, (2) restoration of alignment, (3) stabilization, and (4) arthrodesis. The decompression of neural elements serves ultimately to preserve existing function. In instances of neurologic deficit in the face of epidural compression, multiple studies have demonstrated that timely surgical decompression affords the best opportunity to preserve or regain ambulatory function and maintain control of bowel and bladder.

Additional concerns that are specific to spinal oncology also include obtaining a tissue diagnosis, and the possibility of a surgical cure must be entertained in appropriate situations of primary neoplasms. For this to be achieved, a complete en bloc resection with margins must be performed. In instances where en bloc resection is not possible or is ill-advised due to the potential for morbidity or mortality, a spectrum of debulking exists, which ranges from gross total resection to separation surgery only, depending on the tumor histology. For all procedures, adjuvant therapies such as radiation therapy or chemotherapy form an integral part of the patient's treatment algorithm. For metastatic disease, the goal is palliation care and maximization of the patient's quality of life.

With regard to the treatment of spinal metastases, recent data seem to indicate that the concept of "separation surgery" combined with postoperative image-guided radiation therapy may provide local control, which is as effective as a more complete resection, however, without the morbidity of the more involved surgical procedure [16, 20, 22]. In this technique, the surgeon approaches and decompresses the neural elements such that there is a minimum critical distance between the residual tumor and the spinal cord, and radiation can be employed postoperatively. The patient therefore does not undergo an aggressive resection of the tumor, which will limit the operative time, blood loss, and potential need for reconstruction.

Other Concerns

After tumor resection, wound-healing concerns must be addressed. Perioperative radiation therapy as well as systemic chemotherapy may increase the risk of wound breakdown, wound infection, and poor healing. Plastic surgery consultation may be warranted for consideration of flap rotation, particularly in instances of revision surgery.

Part III: Case Illustrations

Hemangioma of C4

A 70-year-old female patient presented with the onset of axial neck pain and features of early myelopathy. Intake magnetic resonance imaging revealed a pathologic fracture of the C4 vertebral body, with retropulsed material effacing the ventral aspect of her cervical cord, and abnormal T2 signal apparent within the cord parenchyma. On CT, the lesion was noted to be osteolytic in nature, with significant loss of height and anterior wedging of the vertebral body. This imaging can be seen in Fig. 5.4. The patient had no history of malignancy and underwent CT-guided biopsy of the lesion, which was consistent with vertebral hemangioma.

Given the propensity for vertebral hemangioma to hemorrhage, the patient was taken for angiography. Feeding tributaries from the left thyrocervical trunk were found to provide the dominant source of irrigation of the lesion. Microcatheter runs can be seen in Fig. 5.5. Figure 5.5a represents the early arterial phase

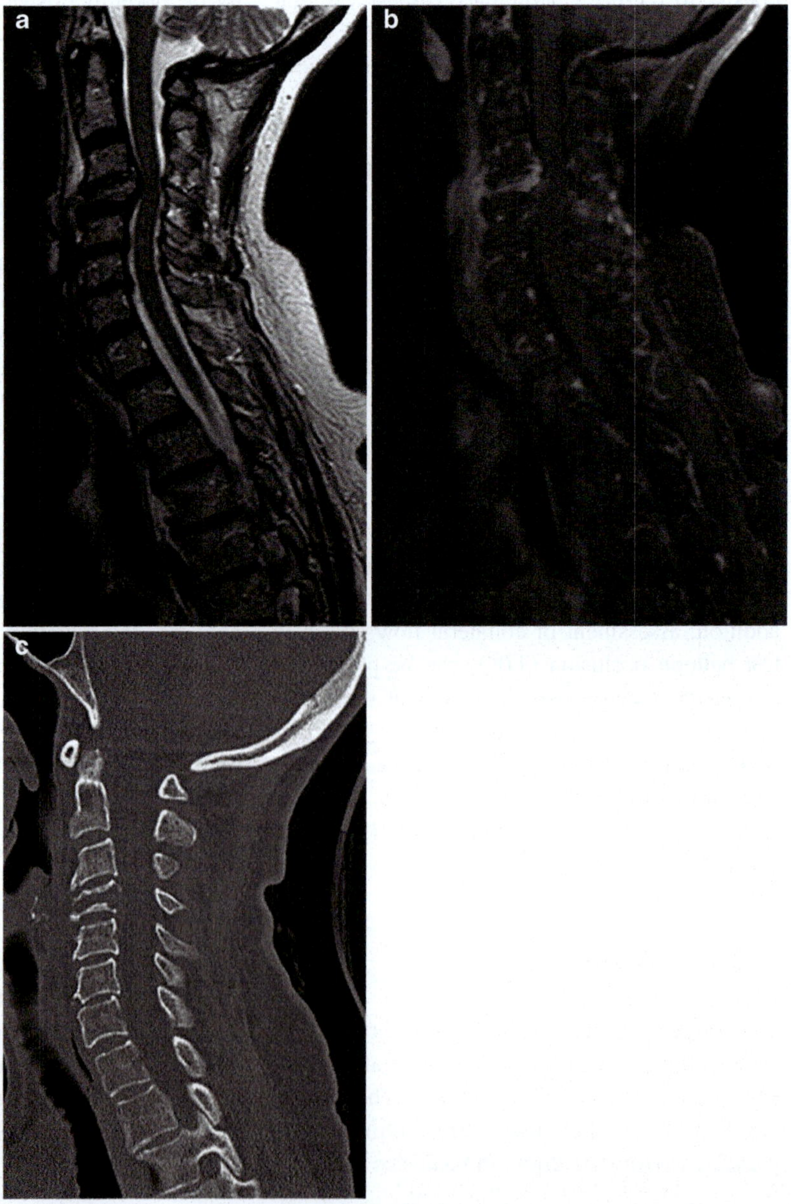

Fig. 5.4 (**a**) Preoperative imaging of a 70-year-old female with pathologic compression fracture of C4. Sagittal T2-weighted MRI. (**b**) Preoperative imaging of a 70-year-old female with pathologic compression fracture of C4. Sagittal T1-contrasted MRI. (**c**) Preoperative imaging of a 70-year-old female with pathologic compression fracture of C4. Sagittal CT

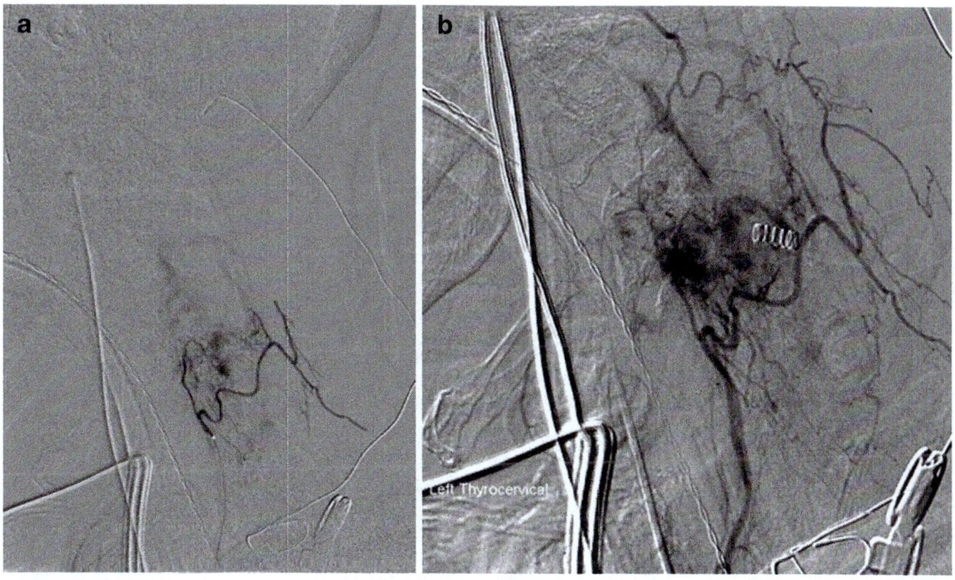

Fig. 5.5 (**a**) Angiography, early arterial phase, lateral projection, demonstrating arterial feeders from the thyrocervical trunk. (**b**) Angiography, late arterial and capillary phase, oblique working projection prior to embolization

on a lateral projection, whereas Fig. 5.5b represents a late arterial and capillary phase depicted on a more oblique working projection for pending embolization. Note the significant vascular blush of the tumor. The feeders were successfully embolized with Onyx® liquid embolic agent. The cast of embolic material can be seen on the lateral projection depicted in Fig. 5.6.

After angiography, the patient underwent a circumferential decompression and fusion, consisting of corpectomy of the C4 vertebral body followed by posterior arthrodesis from C3 to C5. Postoperative radiography is apparent in Fig. 5.7.

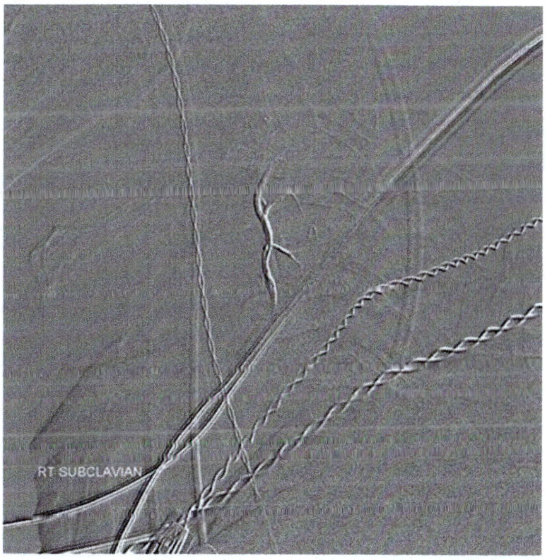

Fig. 5.6 Postembolization. Cast of the embolic material is apparent in the feeding artery, which originated from the thyrocervical trunk

Ventral Meningioma at C4–C5

A 55-year-old female initially presented with axial neck pain as well as radiculopathy of the right upper extremity. Imaging was notable for a calcified mass eccentric to the right side of the canal, dorsal to the C4 vertebral body, and spanning the C4–C5 disc space. A sagittal and axial computed tomography image is shown in Fig. 5.8. Given the ventral location of the lesion, the patient underwent a C4 corpectomy for exposure of the lesion. Intraoperatively, it was noted to be a partially calcified, dural-based mass. The lesion was resected along with its dural attachment. A patch duraplasty was performed, followed by insertion of an expandable corpectomy cage and anterior arthrodesis from C3 to C5. Finally, a lumbar drain was inserted. Final pathology was consistent with WHO grade I meningioma, psammomatous subtype. Postoperative lateral plain radiography is apparent in Fig. 5.9.

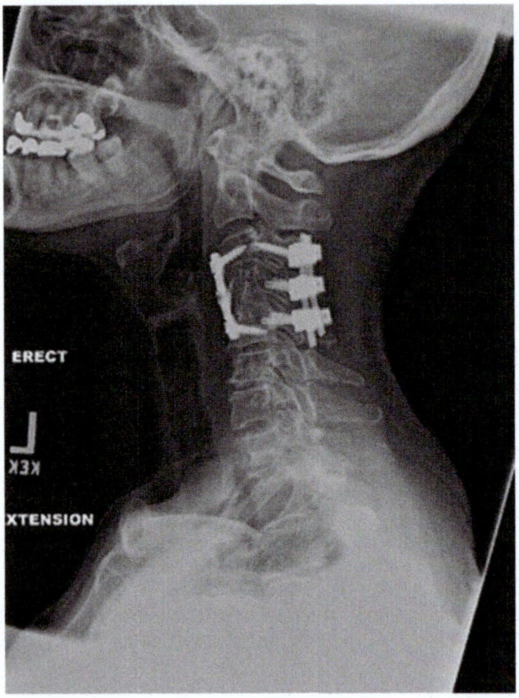

Fig. 5.7 The patient underwent C4 corpectomy with posterior augmentation. Pathology was consistent with vertebral hemangioma

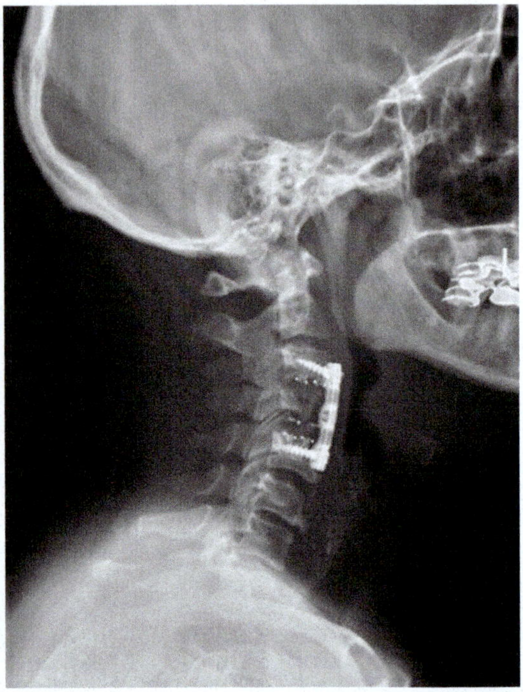

Fig. 5.9 The patient underwent C4 corpectomy; pathology was consistent with WHO grade I psammomatous meningioma

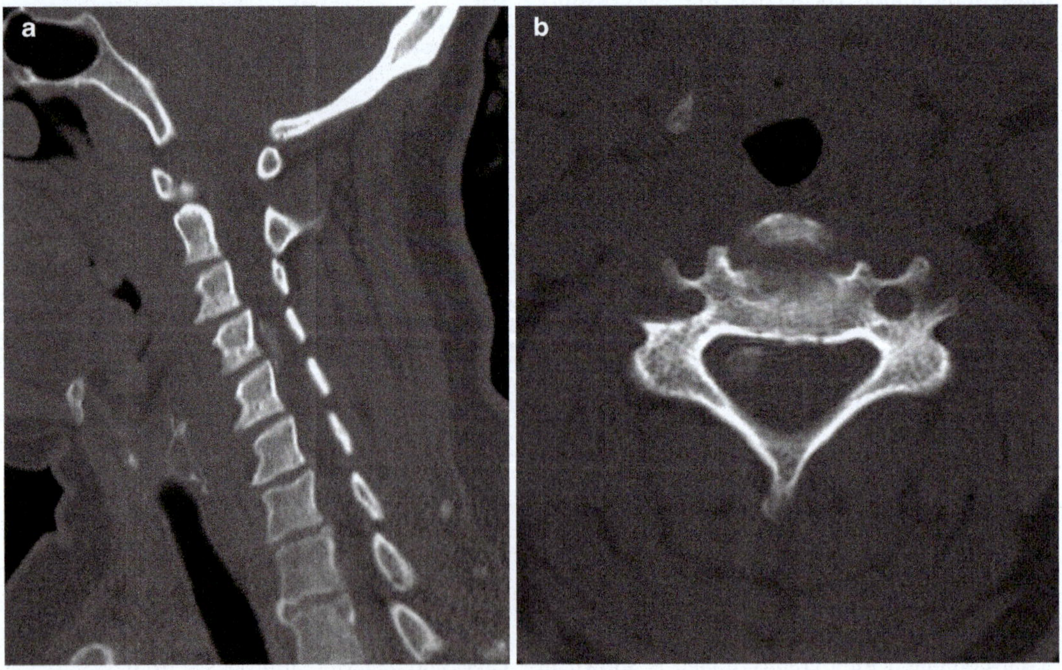

Fig. 5.8 (**a**) Sagittal CT demonstrating calcified mass dorsal to the C4 vertebral body. (**b**) Axial CT demonstrating calcified mass dorsal to the C4 vertebral body, eccentric to the right side

Cervical Chordoma

A 21-year-old female patient presented with progressive complaints of axial neck pain and right-hand clumsiness. Magnetic resonance imaging revealed a homogeneously enhancing, T2 intense epidural mass at the level of C3 through C5, exerting mass effect on the cervical spinal cord at these levels and extending out the right-sided neural foramina and into the anterior triangle of the neck. The lesion encased the right-sided vertebral artery. Figure 5.10 depicts the sagittal T2, sagittal T1 contrast-enhanced, and axial T1 contrast-enhanced MRI.

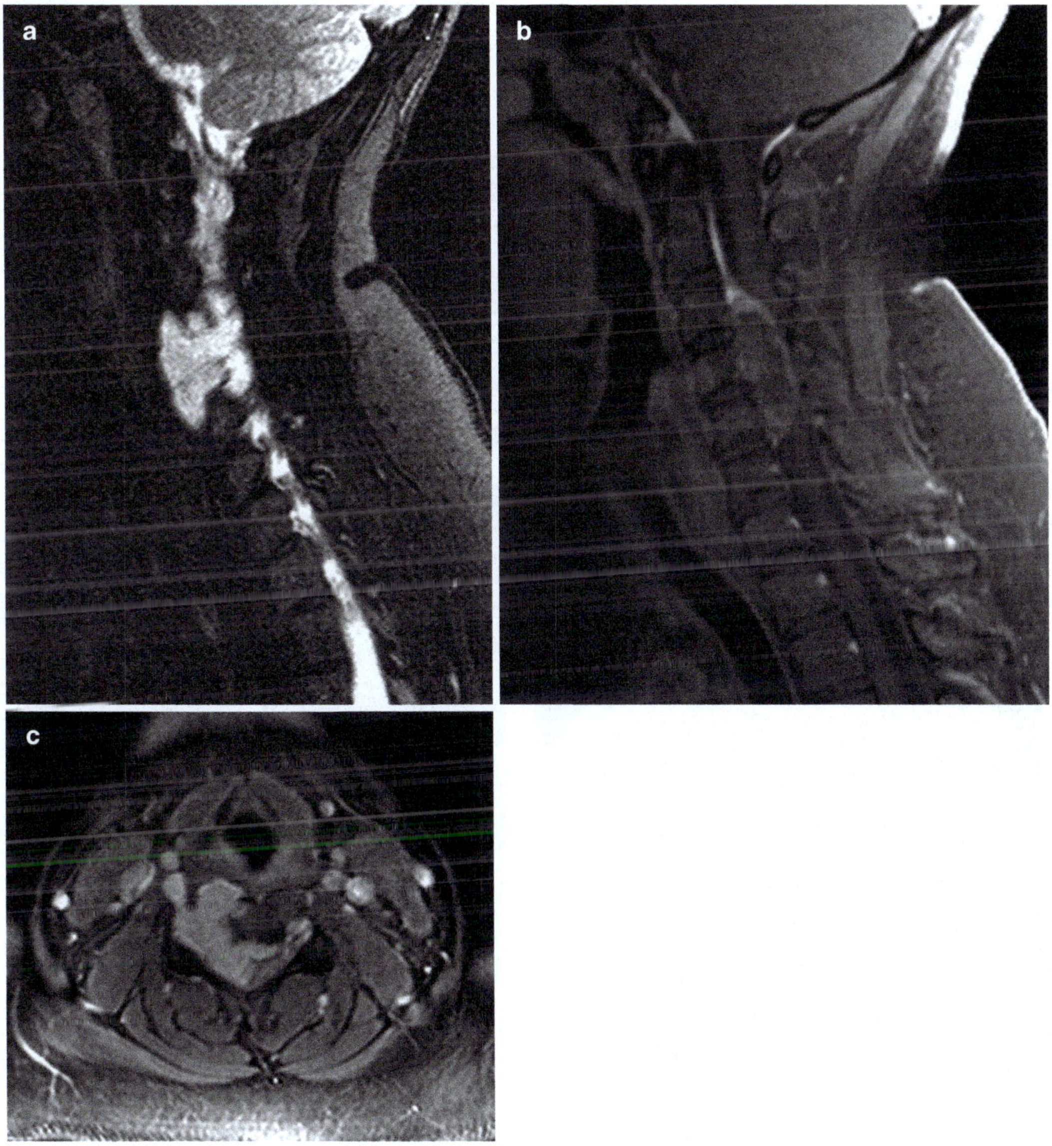

Fig. 5.10 (**a**) Anterior cervical epidural mass presenting in a 21-year-old female. Sagittal T2-weighted MRI. (**b**) Anterior cervical epidural mass presenting in a 21-year-old female. Sagittal T1-contrasted MRI. (**c**) Anterior cervical epidural mass presenting in a 21-year-old female. Axial T1-contrasted MRI

Computer tomography-guided biopsy was performed, and pathology returned consistent with chordoma. Given the encasement of her vertebral artery, the patient was taken for angiography and assessment of the collateral flow of her posterior cerebral circulation, along with test balloon occlusion of the right vertebral artery. She was found to have acceptable collateral flow, and the right vertebral artery was endovascularly sacrificed with Onyx® embolic material in order to facilitate en bloc resection of the chordoma. The postembolization Towne's projection of the left vertebral artery injection is shown in Fig. 5.11, which demonstrates the Onyx® cast within the right vertebral artery and appropriate collateral irrigation of the posterior circulation by the remaining left vertebral artery.

The patient next underwent a staged circumferential decompression, en bloc resection, and fusion procedure. The operation consisted of C3 through C5 corpectomy with anterior arthrodesis using a vascularized fibular free flap harvested and anastomosed in conjunction with plastic surgery, coupled with C3 through C7 laminectomy with right-sided C3 to C5 facetectomies, and C2 to T1 posterior arthrodesis. Postoperative CT is shown in Fig. 5.12. Figure 5.12a is a mid-sagittal

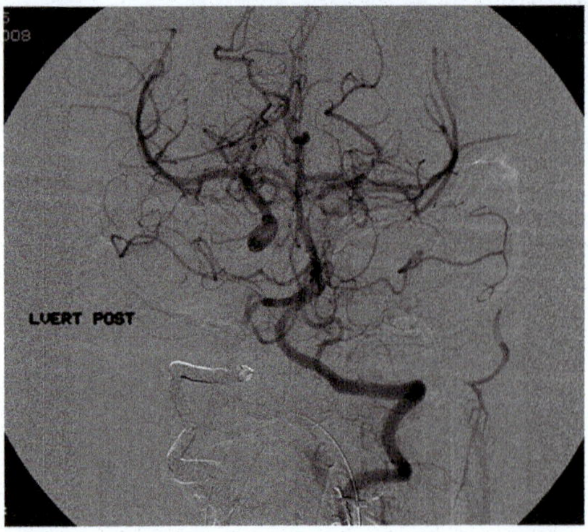

Fig. 5.11 Postembolization Towne's projection, left vertebral artery injection, demonstrating the Onyx® cast within the right vertebral artery and appropriate collateral irrigation of the posterior circulation by the remaining left vertebral artery

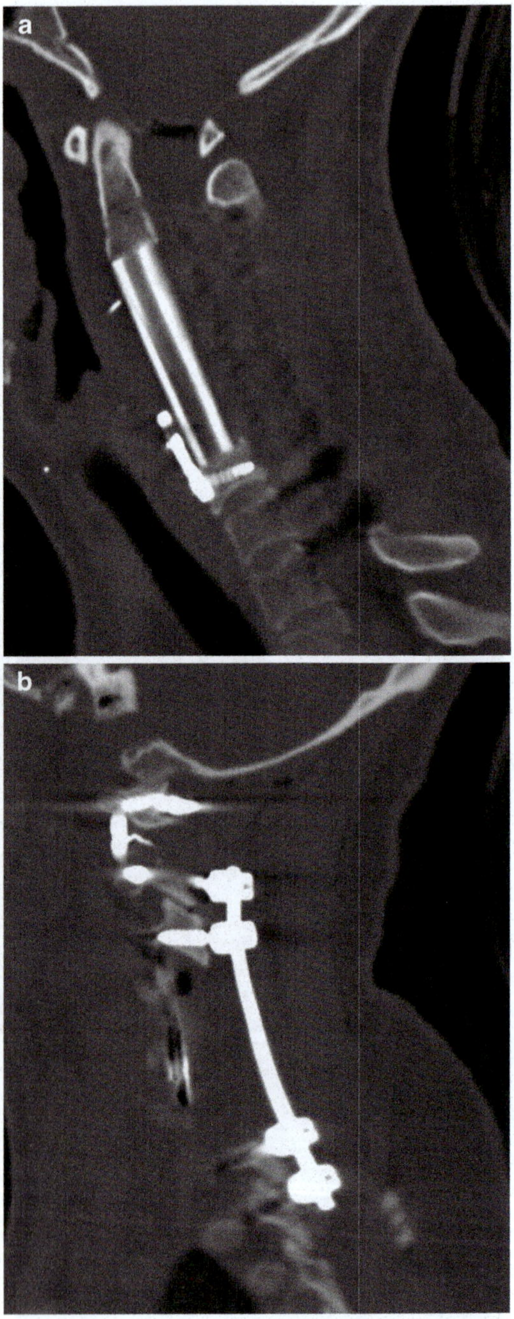

Fig. 5.12 (**a**) The patient underwent C3 through C5 corpectomy with anterior arthrodesis using a vascularized fibular free flap, coupled with C3 through C7 laminectomy with right-sided C3 to C5 facetectomies and C2 to T1 posterior arthrodesis. Sagittal postoperative CT. (**b**) The patient underwent C3 through C5 corpectomy with anterior arthrodesis using a vascularized fibular free-flap, coupled with C3 through C7 laminectomy with right-sided C3 to C5 facetectomies, and C2 to T1 posterior arthrodesis. Parasagittal postoperative CT

image demonstrating the position of the fibular graft. Figure 5.12b is a parasagittal image depicting the multi-level complete facetectomy. The patient tolerated the procedure well.

References

1. Smith GW, Robinson RA. The treatment of certain cervical-spine disorders by anterior removal of the intervertebral disc and interbody fusion. J Bone Joint Surg Am. 1958;40-A(3):607–24.
2. Cloward RB. The anterior approach for removal of ruptured cervical disks. J Neurosurg. 1958;15(6):602–17.
3. de Jonge T, Slullitel H, Dubousset J, Miladi L, Wicart P, Illés T. Late-onset spinal deformities in children treated by laminectomy and radiation therapy for malignant tumours. Eur Spine J. 2005;14(8):765–71.
4. Lonstein JE. Post-laminectomy kyphosis. Clin Orthop Relat Res. 1977;128:93–100.
5. O'Shaughnessy BA, Liu JC, Hsieh PC, Koski TR, Ganju A, Ondra SL. Surgical treatment of fixed cervical kyphosis with myelopathy. Spine. 2008;33(7):771–8.
6. Kriskovich MD, Apfelbaum RI, Haller JR. Vocal fold paralysis after anterior cervical spine surgery: incidence, mechanism, and prevention of injury. Laryngoscope. 2000;110(9):1467–73.
7. Shriver MF, Lewis DJ, Kshettry VR, Rosenbaum BP, Benzel EC, Mroz TE. Dysphagia rates after anterior cervical Diskectomy and fusion: a systematic review and meta-analysis. Global Spine J. 2017;7(1):95–103.
8. Pavlov H, Torg JS, Robie B, Jahre C. Cervical spinal stenosis: determination with vertebral body ratio method. Radiology. 1987;164(3):771–5.
9. Lim J-K, Wong H-K. Variation of the cervical spinal Torg ratio with gender and ethnicity. Spine J. 2004;4(4):396–401.
10. Cohen ZR, Fourney DR, Marco RA, Rhines LD, Gokaslan ZL. Total cervical spondylectomy for primary osteogenic sarcoma: case report and description of operative technique. JNS Spine. 2002;97:386–92.
11. Rades D, Fehlauer F, Stalpers LJA, Wildfang I, Zschenker O, Schild SE, et al. A prospective evaluation of two radiotherapy schedules with 10 versus 20 fractions for the treatment of metastatic spinal cord compression: final results of a multicenter study. Cancer. 2004;101(11):2687–92.
12. Rades D, Fehlauer F, Schulte R, Veninga T, Stalpers LJA, Basic H, et al. Prognostic factors for local control and survival after radiotherapy of metastatic spinal cord compression. J Clin Oncol. 2006;24(21):3388–93.
13. Rades D, Karstens JH, Alberti W. Role of radiotherapy in the treatment of motor dysfunction due to metastatic spinal cord compression: comparison of three different fractionation schedules. Int J Radiat Oncol Biol Phys. 2002;54(4):1160–4.
14. Gilbert RW, Kim JH, Posner JB. Epidural spinal cord compression from metastatic tumor: diagnosis and treatment. Ann Neurol. 1978;3(1):40–51.
15. Maranzano E, Latini P, Perrucci E, Beneventi S, Lupattelli M, Corgna E. Short-course radiotherapy (8 Gy x 2) in metastatic spinal cord compression: an effective and feasible treatment. Int J Radiat Oncol Biol Phys. 1997;38(5):1037–44.
16. Maranzano E, Bellavita R, Rossi R, De Angelis V, Frattegiani A, Bagnoli R, et al. Short-course versus split-course radiotherapy in metastatic spinal cord compression: results of a phase III, randomized, multicenter trial. J Clin Oncol. 2005;23(15):3358–65.
17. Katagiri H, Takahashi M, Inagaki J, Kobayashi H, Sugiura H, Yamamura S, et al. Clinical results of nonsurgical treatment for spinal metastases. Int J Radiat Oncol Biol Phys. 1998;42(5):1127–32.
18. Gerszten PC, Mendel E, Yamada Y. Radiotherapy and radiosurgery for metastatic spine disease: what are the options, indications, and outcomes? Spine. 2009;34(22 Suppl):S78–92.
19. Laufer I, Rubin DG, Lis E, Cox BW, Stubblefield MD, Yamada Y, et al. The NOMS framework: approach to the treatment of spinal metastatic tumors. Oncologist. 2013;18(6):744–51.
20. Laufer I, Iorgulescu JB, Chapman T, Lis E, Shi W, Zhang Z, et al. Local disease control for spinal metastases following "separation surgery" and adjuvant hypofractionated or high-dose single-fraction stereotactic radiosurgery: outcome analysis in 186 patients. J Neurosurg Spine. 2013;18(3):207–14.
21. Lovelock DM, Zhang Z, Jackson A, Keam J, Bekelman J, Bilsky M, et al. Correlation of local failure with measures of dose insufficiency in the high-dose single-fraction treatment of bony metastases. Int J Radiat Oncol Biol Phys. 2010;77(4):1282–7.
22. Bilsky MH, Laufer I, Burch S. Shifting paradigms in the treatment of metastatic spine disease. Spine. 2009;34(22 Suppl):S101–7.
23. Fisher CG, DiPaola CP, Ryken TC, Bilsky MH, Shaffrey CI, Berven SH, et al. A novel classification system for spinal instability in neoplastic disease: an evidence-based approach and expert consensus from the Spine Oncology Study Group. Spine. 2010;35(22):E1221–9.
24. Bilsky MH, Laufer I, Fourney DR, Groff M, Schmidt MH, Varga PP, et al. Reliability analysis of the epidural spinal cord compression scale. J Neurosurg Spine. 2010;13(3):324–8.

Cervicothoracic Approach: Manubriotomy and Sternotomy

6

Katherine Miller, Shanda H. Blackmon, and Rex A. W. Marco

Introduction

The anterior approach to the cervicothoracic junction (CTJ) is technically demanding, with exposure limited by the sternum, clavicle, and ribs, as well as neurovascular structures including the carotid sheath, trachea, esophagus, recurrent laryngeal nerves, great vessels, and sympathetic trunk. Recent experience at major spine centers suggests a trend toward posterior-only approaches to the cervicothoracic spine. Despite this trend, large extraosseous masses, primary malignant bone tumors, infections, unstable fractures, and tumors involving the chest wall or major vascular structures may necessitate the use of an anterior approach [1].

Tumors of the upper thoracic vertebrae (T1–T4) make up 15% of all spinal tumors and 10% of metastatic disease to the spine [2]. These lesions most commonly involve the anterior vertebral body with extension into the posterior elements. The CTJ, extending from C7 to T4, demonstrates unique biomechanics as the rigid, kyphotic thoracic spine transitions to a mobile, lordotic cervical spine. This in combination with a relatively small spinal canal makes neurologic involvement common in this region. Destruction of the vertebral body with progressive instability often leads to kyphosis and ventral spinal cord compression [3]. In this setting, disruption of the posterior elements through a posterior approach could further destabilize the area and an anterior approach may be preferable, thereby allowing direct decompression and sparing of the posterior elements. Extended constructs or circumferential fixation may also be required to provide adequate stability.

The appropriate anterior approach to the cervicothoracic spine is selected based on the level of the lesion, and selection requires careful review of preoperative imaging to determine accessibility of the level of interest. Imaging studies suggest that in approximately two-thirds of patients, a line drawn from the sternal notch to the thoracic spine intersects T3 or above. This suggests that a purely cervical approach without a sternal split may provide sufficient access to these levels in some patients [4, 5]. However, retraction of vital soft tissue structures often adds to bony constraints, limiting instrument maneuverability, especially in the setting of anterior stabilization and reconstruction of these upper thoracic segments [6]. Special attention should be given to the great vessels on review of preoperative imaging, as anatomic variation can result in their extension cranial to the sternal notch.

K. Miller (✉)
Houston Methodist, Department of Orthopedics and Sports Medicine, Houston, TX, USA
e-mail: kmiller@houstonmethodist.org

S. H. Blackmon
Mayo Clinic, Department of General Thoracic Surgery, Rochester, MN, USA

R. A. W. Marco
Musculoskeletal Oncology and Reconstructive Spine Surgery, Houston Methodist Hospital, Houston, TX, USA

D. M. Sciubba (ed.), *Spinal Tumor Surgery*, https://doi.org/10.1007/978-3-319-98422-3_6

Anterior approaches to the cervicothoracic junction include the following: (1) low anterior cervical approach, (2) modified anterior approach with medial claviculectomy, and (3) partial or complete sternotomy [2]. Low anterior approaches allow for access down to T2 (with limited applicability in patients with short necks), and modified anterior approaches allow for access as low as T4. If further exposure is necessary, a sternal splitting approach is usually required and allows for access from C3 to T5. The sternum comprises the manubrium, sternal body, and xiphoid process, which fuse during development, leaving a synostosis between the manubrium and the sternal body. This synostosis can be used to the surgeon's advantage in some sternal splitting approaches [7].

Approach Overview

The cervicothoracic junction falls between areas that can be approached without violating the sternum via a high lateral thoracotomy (T2–T5) or a purely cervical approach that allows access as far as T2. If exposure across this area is necessary, a sternal splitting approach may facilitate access to the CTJ. Traditional procedures designed provide this access while avoiding median sternotomy-involved disruption of the sternoclavicular joint. However, this was often found to result in unacceptable complication rates related to chronic pain and immobility of the upper extremity [1].

Median sternotomy in combination with a supraclavicular approach to the cervicothoracic junction was initially described by Cauchoix and Binet in 1957 [8]. Later, reports of high morbidity and mortality by Hodgson et al. led authors to recommend against this approach [9]. In the 1980s, Sundaresan et al. described a procedure that removed a rectangular portion of the manubrium along with one-third of the medial clavicle, repopularizing the trans-sternal approach [10]. Resection of the medial clavicle significantly improves exposure, and the resected clavicle can be used as a strut graft to reconstruct the anterior column [11]. Partial sternotomy has been described by several authors and involves a midline split of the manubrium with lateral division of the sternum, creating a reverse T- or Y-shaped osteotomy [3, 4, 12]. Alternatively, the lateral division can proceed through the synostosis between the manubrium and the body of the sternum as described by Darling et al. [7]. The manubrium can then be wired together so that neither the clavicle nor the manubrium is resected.

Authors advocating for a midline sternotomy believe this procedure has less morbidity associated with it compared to procedures involving resection of the medial clavicle or manubrium [9, 10, 13]. In most cases, a partial sternotomy is sufficient to allow access to upper thoracic vertebrae. Several authors report that partial sternotomy results in less blood loss and postoperative pain while providing the same exposure as complete sternotomy where the heart and great vessels impede more distal access [3, 4, 7, 12]. To facilitate resection of tumors with significant intrathoracic extension, Kraus et al. described a modification to the trans-sternal approach where the incision is continued laterally through the rib cage, resulting in a trapdoor, or clamshell, of the chest wall [14].

Surgical Technique

Patient Positioning

The patient is positioned supine on the table, with a bump placed transversely under the scapulae to allow for neck extension, to minimize thoracic kyphosis, and to allow the shoulders to fall away from the operative field. Usually, due to the more predictable course of the left recurrent laryngeal nerve running proximally in the tracheoesophageal groove, a left-sided cervical approach is preferable. Therefore, the neck is extended and tilted slightly to the right in a low anterior approach and hyperextended and turned 60 degrees to the right in modified anterior approaches and sternal splitting approaches. A nasogastric tube can be placed to facilitate palpation and identification of the esophagus intraoperatively [2, 15].

Low Anterior Approach

The low anterior approach, also known as the Smith-Robinson approach, is essentially the inferior extension of an ordinary anterior cervical approach and can be combined with a transsternal approach to provide extensile exposure to the anterior cervical spine. Used in isolation, a paramedian transverse skin incision can be utilized. For extensile exposure used in combination with a sternal splitting approach, a longitudinal skin incision medial to the sternocleidomastoid (SCM) muscle is employed. This incision can be extended caudally down the midline of the sternum toward the xiphoid process. Cauterization of the longus colli muscles allows for access as low as the T1–T2 disc space in some patients.

Modified Anterior Approach

A wider exposure at the cervicothoracic junction can be obtained via the modified anterior approach, which involves excision of the medial portion of the clavicle. Some argue that the wide anterolateral exposure afforded by medial clavicular excision is optimal for decompression but may be inadequate for tumor resection, reconstruction, and instrumentation due to limited cranial-caudal exposure, particularly in regard to the cranial angulation required for correct screw placement at caudal levels [4, 6]. Additionally, this resection is associated with complications related to disruption of the sternoclavicular joint and interclavicular ligament [11].

Kurz et al. describe a purely transclavicular approach in which a transverse skin incision is first made from the lateral border of the left SCM muscle to the midline, 1–2 cm above the left clavicle [13]. The medial end of the initial skin incision is then extended caudally to the junction of the sternum and the manubrium. The platysma and deep cervical fascia are incised. To expose the clavicle, sternal and clavicular heads of the SCM muscle and the inferior strap muscles must be elevated and retracted. Next, the medial third of the left clavicle is resected and disarticulated from the sternoclavicular joint with special attention to the subclavian vein, which lies posterior and inferior. By establishing a plane between the carotid sheath and the trachea and esophagus, the brachiocephalic vessels can be identified, which are then retracted caudally. These maneuvers allow for exposure from C4 to T4. This approach can be combined with manubriotomy in which a rectangular portion of manubrium is removed to facilitate caudal exposure as described by Sundaresan et al. [10]. Alternatively, the sternoclavicular joint can be kept intact, reflecting the manubrium and medial clavicle with the sternal head of the SCM.

Sternal Splitting Approach

The skin incision begins 4–8 cm cranial to the sternal notch at the anterior border of the sternocleidomastoid muscle. An oblique, longitudinal cut follows the medial border of the SCM to the sternal notch and continues midline over the sternum toward the xiphoid process. The platysma muscle and superficial cervical fascia are incised sharply, revealing the underlying strap muscles and SCM. Superficial branches of the cervical plexus supplying the skin of the anterior neck may cross the operative field at this time as well as the anterior jugular vein, which may be mobilized or sectioned. The investing layer of the deep cervical fascia can be seen encompassing the SCM; this is incised along with the pretracheal layer of deep cervical fascia which encompasses the strap muscles. This allows for blunt dissection, which mobilizes the SCM and creates a plane between the carotid sheath laterally and the trachea and esophagus medially.

The sternum is exposed subperiosteally, and retrosternal fat and residual thymus tissue are removed via digital dissection. A sternal saw is used to create the sternotomy according to surgeon preference. As discussed in the approach overview, several sternal splitting techniques can be used, including midline manubriotomy with unilateral or bilateral sectioning through the synostosis or partial sternotomy extending caudal to the synostosis with an inverted Y or T configuration. For improved access to intrathoracic structures, complete sternotomy or trapdoor approach with extension through the lateral thoracic wall can be used.

After completion of the sternotomy, hemostasis is achieved and bone wax is used to control bleeding from the sternum. A thoracic retractor is used to gently spread the rib cage. The sternohyoid and sternothyroid muscles connecting to the posterior aspect of the manubrium can be sectioned and retracted superiorly. Through the plane previously developed between the carotid sheath, trachea, and esophagus, the cauterization of the longus colli muscles allows access to the lower cervical levels. Deep to the underside of the manubrium, the left brachiocephalic vein can be identified. Blunt dissection can be used to follow the internal jugular vein as it enters the thorax beneath the SCM and joins the subclavian to form the brachiocephalic vein. Once identified, the left brachiocephalic vein can be gently retracted caudally. The inferior thyroid vein feeds into the brachiocephalic superiorly and can be ligated if necessary. Deep retractors are placed to protect the trachea and esophagus medially and the carotid sheath and left subclavian vessels laterally, creating a window to access the upper thoracic levels to T4 (Fig. 6.1).

Alternative Vascular Corridors

Access to the upper thoracic levels is achievable through gentle mobilization of vascular structures to create working windows. Traditionally, these windows are created superior to the left brachiocephalic vein. With this structure retracted caudally, windows medial and lateral to the brachiocephalic artery (BCA) can be utilized as described by Sattarov et al. [16]. A window medial to the BCA typically allows sufficient access to T3, which corresponds to the level of the left brachiocephalic vein. The lateral border of this window consists of the left common carotid artery, left internal jugular vein, and left vagus nerve. Alternatively, a window can be made lateral to the BCA allowing access to T4, which corresponds to the superior border of the confluence between the left and right brachiocephalic veins. The roof of this window is created by the right common carotid artery [16].

An interaortocaval subinnominate window has also been described by Cohen et al. and can provide access down to T5 [6]. In this approach, the left brachiocephalic vein is mobilized along its length to the superior vena cava (SVC). Mobilization of the proximal BCA is facilitated by incising the upper portion of the pericardial reflection covering the ascending aorta.

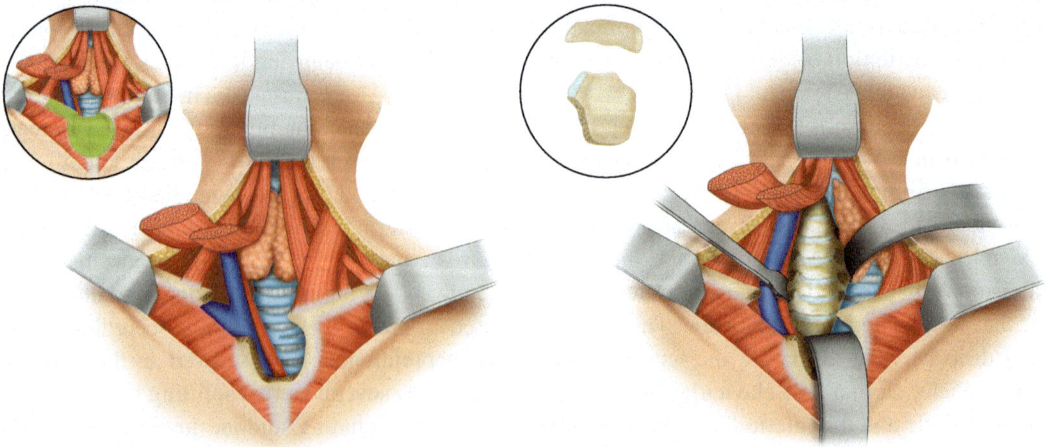

Fig. 6.1 Operative drawing of manubriotomy. (Reprinted with permission from Sundaresan et al. [10])

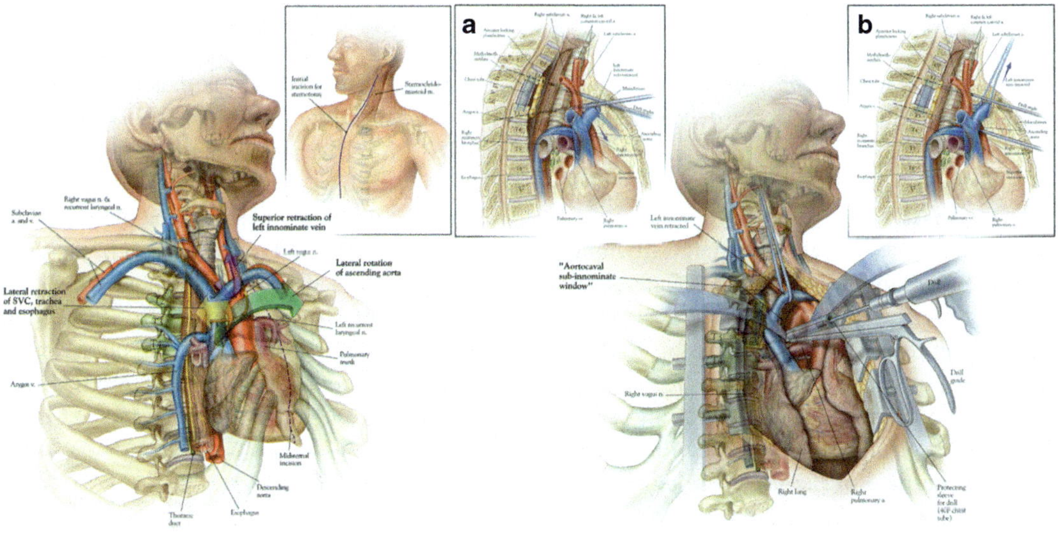

Fig. 6.2 Sternotomy to access the upper thoracic spine through the interaortocaval subinnominate window. (Reprinted with permission from Cohen et al. [6])

Retraction of the ascending aorta to the patient's left and the SVC, trachea, and esophagus to the patient's right then opens up a window inferior to the left brachiocephalic vein (Fig. 6.2).

Complications

Complications of anterior approaches to the cervicothoracic junction include risk of injury to the recurrent laryngeal nerve, the esophagus, the thoracic duct, the cervical sympathetic trunk, and the phrenic nerve. When a clavicle osteotomy is added, the possibility of vascular injury (subclavian vessels and brachiocephalic vessels) as well as nonunion of the clavicle is of importance.

Dangers

The Vagus and Recurrent Laryngeal Nerves

The vagus nerve descends within the carotid sheath between the common carotid artery medially and the internal jugular vein laterally. The left vagus nerve travels between the subclavian and common carotid arteries, traveling posterior to the left brachiocephalic vein to enter the thorax, descending on the left side of the aortic arch. The right vagus nerve crosses anterior to the right subclavian artery, traveling in the fat posterior to the brachiocephalic veins before coursing down the right side of the trachea.

The recurrent laryngeal nerve (RLN) is a branch of the vagus nerve supplying the laryngeal muscles; the course differs on the left and right, with the left considered to have less anatomic variation. The left recurrent laryngeal nerve descends within the carotid sheath and branches from the vagus at the level of the aortic arch, looping posterior to the arch distal to the ligamentum arteriosus. It courses proximally in the tracheoesophageal groove, its low origin giving it a more consistent and predictable course within the operative window for the anterior approach to the cervicothoracic spine. The right recurrent laryngeal nerve again descends within the carotid sheath, branching from the vagus as it crosses the right subclavian artery, usually occurring at the level of T3. It loops posterior to the subclavian artery and travels medially at an angle until reaching and ascending in the tracheoesophageal groove.

Damage to the recurrent laryngeal nerve leads to vocal cord paralysis and can result from vigorous retraction of the carotid sheath or trachea and esophagus. Dissection superficial to the longus colli puts the RLN and the esophagus at risk. Reduction of endotracheal cuff pressure after retractor placement can decrease the incidence of RLN palsy [17].

Thoracic Duct

The thoracic duct is the body's largest lymphatic vessel, providing drainage to the bilateral lower extremities, abdomen, left hemithorax and left upper limb, face, and neck. Crossing to the left of midline at around the level of T5, it ascends posterior to the aortic arch between the esophagus and left pleura to the left side of the thoracic inlet. At the base of the neck, the thoracic duct lies posterior to the left common carotid artery, vagus nerve, and internal jugular vein and is bordered by the esophagus medially, omohyoid muscle laterally, and vertebral bodies posteriorly. It rises 3–4 cm superior to the clavicle, passing anterior to the subclavian artery and forming an arch at C7 before draining into the angle created by the left subclavian and internal jugular veins.

Damage to the thoracic duct is an infrequent complication, with a recent retrospective review reporting an incidence of 0.02% for a total of 9591 patients undergoing an anterior approach to the cervical spine [18]. However, prolonged hospitalization and serious complications such as chylothorax, cervical chylous fistula, electrolyte disturbance, malnutrition, immunosuppression, and wound infection can result. If damage to the thoracic duct is suspected intraoperatively, a high-fat solution can be administered via nasogastric tube. In the presence of a chyle leak, milky fluid will appear at the operative site shortly after administration. Leaks identified intraoperatively should be repaired immediately. Conservative treatment for leaks identified postoperatively generally involves transition to a low-fat diet and management of fluid and electrolyte balance [19].

Cervical Sympathetic Trunk

The cervical sympathetic trunk (CST) courses posteriomedial to the carotid sheath, running on the anterior surface of the longus colli muscles (LCM). An anterior approach to the cervicothoracic spine puts this structure at risk for injury resulting in Horner's syndrome at the C6 level; the CST can be found approximately 1 cm lateral to the medial border of the LCM. To avoid risk to the CST, extensive anterolateral dissection over the lower cervical levels should proceed with caution, blunt retractors should be placed gently beneath the LCM, and transverse cut of the LCM should be avoided. In some patients, the CST can run within the posterior wall of the carotid sheath, therefore vigorous lateral retraction of this structure should also be avoided [20].

Case Report

History

A 60-year-old woman with a left-sided pancoast tumor measuring 8 × 8 × 6 cm arising from the upper lobe of the left lung and invading the T2 and T3 vertebral bodies presented with complaints of upper back pain as well as Horner's syndrome. She was a former smoker with a 20-pack-year smoking history. Of note, the patient originally presented to an outside facility with neck and arm pain that was thought to originate from a herniated disc at C5–C6. She was treated with an anterior decompression and fusion (ACDF) of C5–C6 6 weeks prior to referral to our center.

Examination and Imaging

On physical examination, the patient did not demonstrate any neurologic deficits or pathologic reflexes. The tumor was a solitary lesion, and outpatient workup for systemic disease was negative. Magnetic resonance imaging (MRI) revealed a large soft tissue mass involving the T2 and T3 vertebral bodies as well as multiple ribs. The mass appeared to extend into the foramen at T3 without evidence of spinal cord compression. The infiltrating tumor was found to partially encase the left subclavian artery and extend into the thoracic inlet with probable involvement of the brachial plexus (Fig. 6.3).

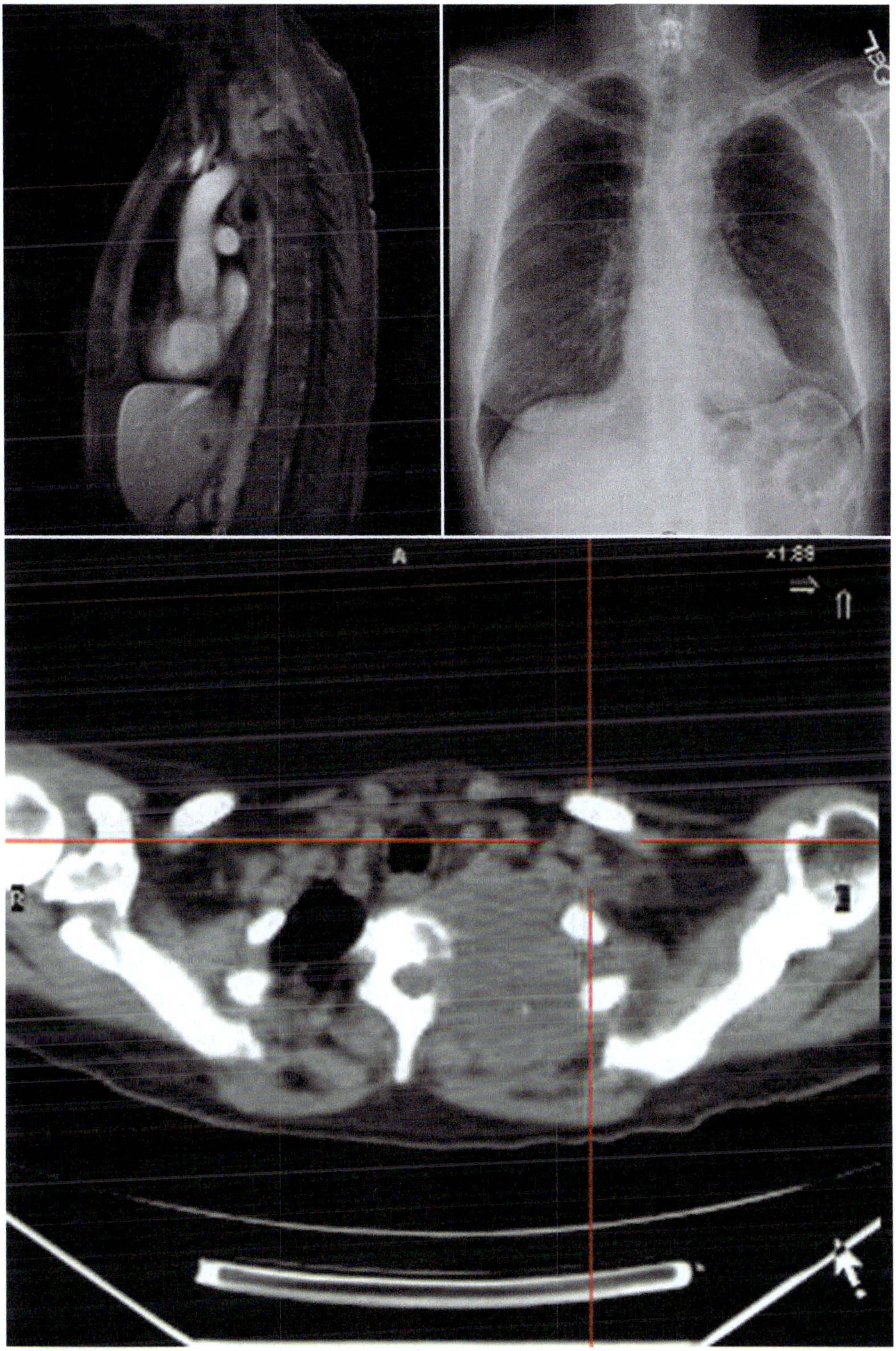

Fig. 6.3 Preoperative sagittal MRI postcontrast (upper left) showing involvement of the upper thoracic vertebrae. Preoperative AP chest radiograph (upper right) demonstrating a lesion in the left upper lobe. Preoperative axial CT (lower panel) demonstrating tumor extension into the T3 vertebra

Procedure

A staged procedure was decided upon, given the size and complexity of the tumor and intimate association with adjacent vital structures. In the first stage, bilateral posterior spinal instrumentation and fusion from C2 to T6 was carried out through a standard posterior midline approach, with the patient in the prone position (Fig. 6.4).

The second stage of the procedure consisted of an anterior corpectomy of T2 and T3 with removal of the tumor from the aorta, a wedge resection of the left upper lung lobe, and anterior spinal column reconstruction from T1 to T4. The patient was positioned supine on the table as previously described. The caudal extent of the tumor extended well below the sternal notch, with significant intrathoracic involvement necessitating a trans-sternal approach with extension through the rib cage to create a clamshell or trapdoor. A left trapdoor incision was created following the anterior border of the sternocleidomastoid muscle to the sternal notch, proceeding distally to bone in the midline of the sternum and continuing toward the left third intercostal space. This incision opened up a window to the sternum without division of the clavicle. The pectoral muscle was divided, and a small area of bleeding was noted in the soft tissue upon entry into the chest, which was subsequently found to lead directly to the internal mammary artery. The artery was ligated without complication. Median sternotomy was created with a sternal saw and extended laterally to the third intercostal space to allow for creation of the trapdoor. The left anterior chest wall was opened and held in place with a chest retractor. The left brachiocephalic vein and the left subclavian artery were identified via blunt dissection. After these structures were mobilized, dissection continued on the underside of the left first and second ribs to allow opening of the chest wall and create a plane anterior to the tumor. The tumor was noted to extend circumferentially around the left subclavian artery and superior to the aorta (Fig. 6.5).

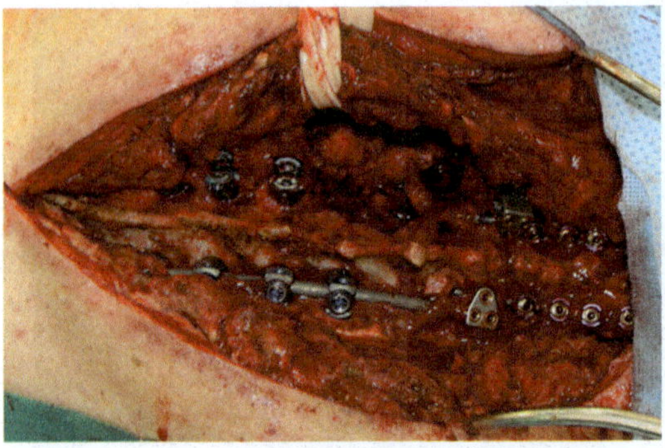

Fig. 6.4 Stage 1, standard posterior midline approach with spinal instrumentation and fusion C2–T6. Muscle-sparing high thoracotomy approach to remove the remaining tumor on the posterolateral aspect of the T1, T2, and T3 vertebra was performed during the third stage

Extensive dissection in this area was performed, specifically dissecting and identifying the phrenic

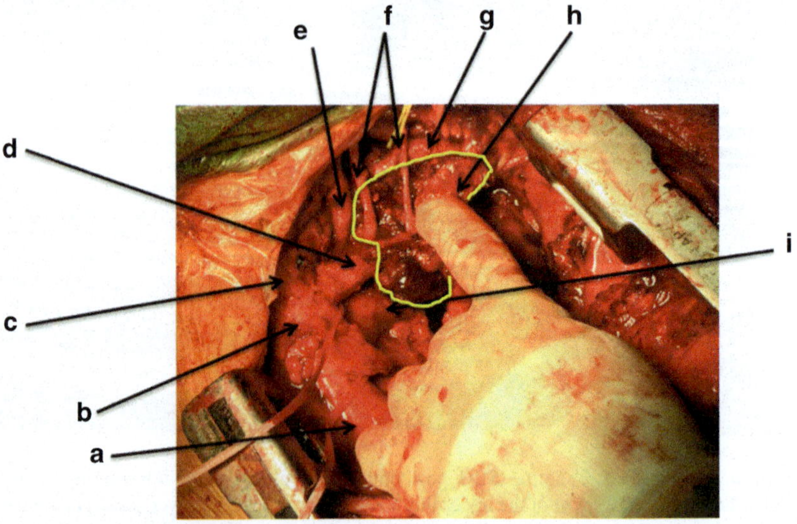

Fig. 6.5 Stage 2, cervicothoracic approach with trapdoor extension. Right atrium (A). Superior vena cava (B). Right innominate vein (C). Left innominate vein (D). Left common carotid artery (E). Inferior thyroid veins (F). Left subclavian artery (G). Tumor (H). Aorta (I)

nerve, vagus nerve, left recurrent laryngeal nerve, left subclavian artery, left common carotid artery, brachial plexus, thyrocervical trunk, and vertebral artery. After these structures were identified and tagged with vessel loops, the anterior and middle scalene muscles were divided to better expose the subclavian artery and brachial plexus. The tumor was mobilized from the adjacent soft tissue and peeled away from its medial attachment to the esophagus. The esophagus was air tested and noted to be intact. The aorta was noted to be directly adherent, and a small amount of tumor was left unresectable. Circumferential involvement of the left subclavian artery required a left carotid to subclavian bypass that was carried out by the thoracic surgeon. With the bulk of the tumor removed, corpectomy proceeded using Kerrison, Leksell, and pituitary rongeurs to excise all visible tumor from within the vertebral bodies of T2 and T3 (Fig. 6.6).

Anterior spinal column reconstruction proceeded using a mesh cage packed with calcium phosphate that was tamped into position. An anterior plate was placed at T1 through T4 and secured with screws. The sternum was reapproximated with sternal wires.

The third stage of the procedure involved a muscle-sparing, high thoracotomy with partial resection of the first, second, and third rib through which the tumor directly opposed to the posterolateral aspect of the spine was removed. The left T3 nerve root was ligated to facilitate removal of residual tumor.

Postoperative Course

The patient remained in the intensive care unit (ICU) between stages and was transferred to the surgical ICU postoperatively. Her estimated combined blood loss for the three procedures was 4 liters. Her hospital course was complicated by postoperative pneumonia, and she was discharged 16 days after the final procedure. Final pathology revealed positive margins, and the tumor

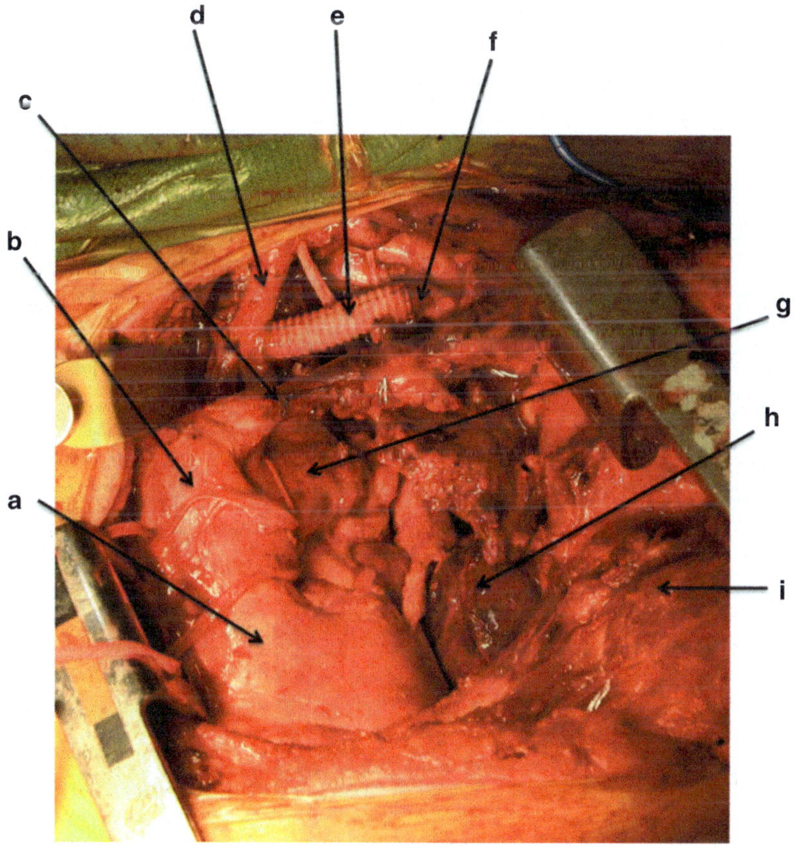

Fig. 6.6 Stage 2, posttumor resection. Right atrium (A). Superior vena cava (B). C. Left innominate vein (C). Left common carotid artery (D). Carotid artery to subclavian artery bypass graft (E). Left subclavian artery (F). Aorta (G)

was identified as undifferentiated carcinoma with sarcomatoid features. The patient received adjuvant chemotherapy and radiation and recovered well with surgery apart from two subsequent admissions for reactive bronchitis. A postoperative MRI at 2 years demonstrated no evidence of tumor recurrence, and she is currently living independently 9 years postoperatively (Fig. 6.7). Computed tomography (CT) at 4 and 8 years postoperatively revealed intact instrumentation without evidence of pseudarthrosis (Fig. 6.8). Plain films at her most recent follow-up demonstrated well-maintained alignment, without evidence of instrumentation failure or loosening (Fig. 6.9).

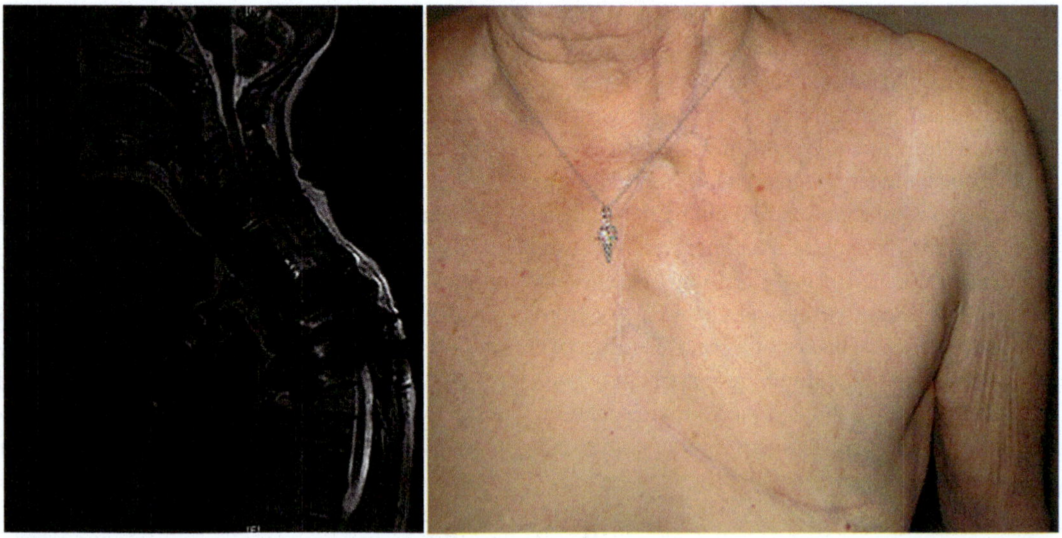

Fig. 6.7 Sagittal MRI 2 years postoperatively (left). Surgical scar following extended anterior cervical approach with median sternotomy and trapdoor extension (right)

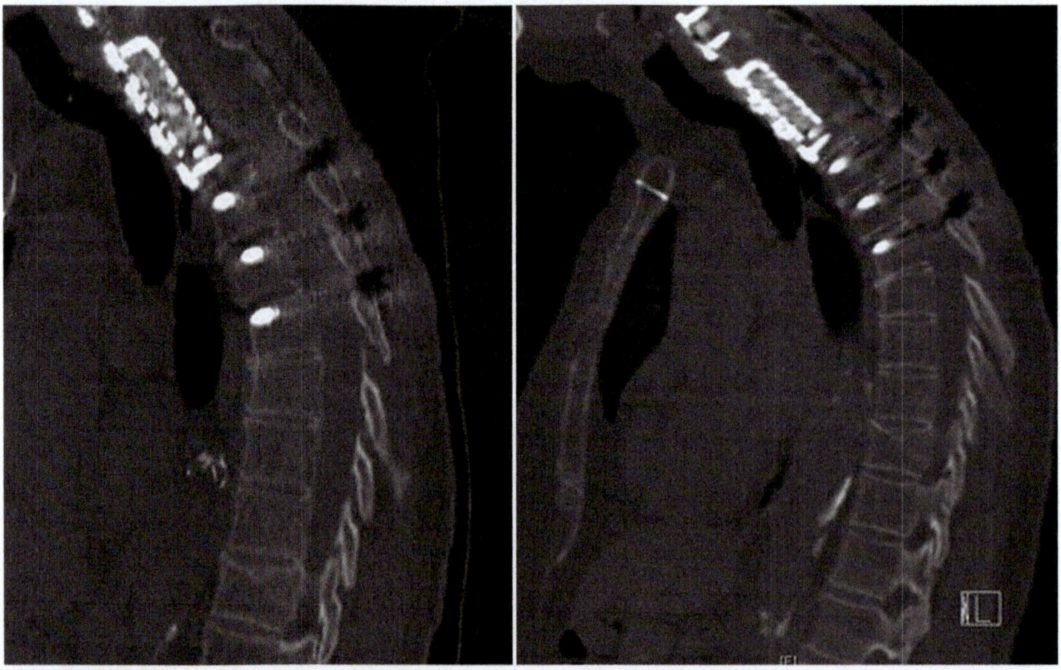

Fig. 6.8 Sagittal CT 4 years postoperatively (left) and 8 years postoperatively (right)

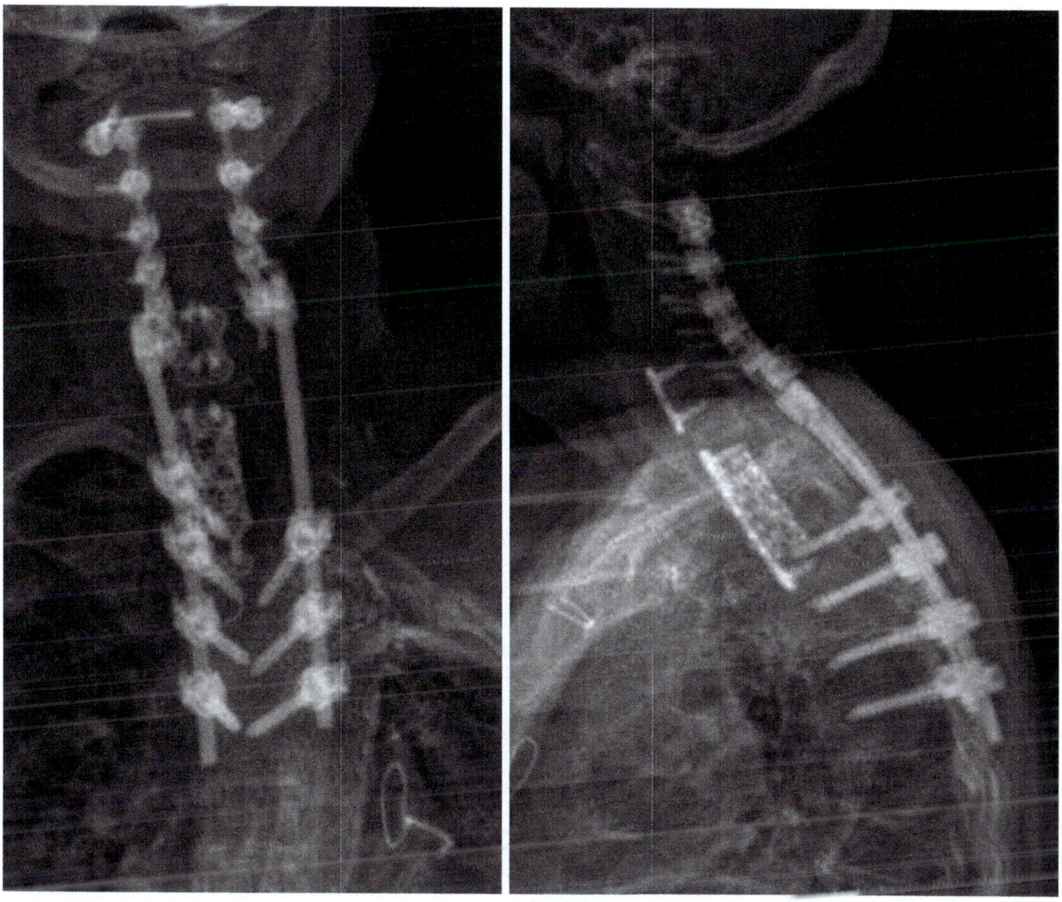

Fig. 6.9 AP (left) and lateral (right) radiographs 9 years postoperatively

References

1. Ames CP, Boriani S, Jandial R. Spine and spinal cord tumors: advanced management and operative techniques. Taylor and Francis Group, LLC: St. Louis; 2014.
2. Lam FC, Groff MW. An anterior approach to spinal pathology of the upper thoracic spine through a partial manubriotomy. J Neurosurg Spine. 2001;15(5):467–71.
3. Liu YL, Hao YJ, Li T, Song YM, Wang LM. Trans-upper-sternal approach to the cerivcothoracic junction. Clin Orthop Relat Res. 2009;467(8):2018–24.
4. Teng H, Hsiang J, Wu C, Wang M, Wei H, Yang X, Xiao J. Surgery in the cervicothoracic junction with an anterior low suprasternal approach alone or combined with manubriotomy and sternotomy: an approach selection method based on the cervicothoracic angle. J Neurosurg Spine. 2009;10:531–42.
5. Lakshmanan P, Lyons K, Davies PR, Howes JP, Ahuja S. Radiographic assessment of sternal notch level and its significance in approaching the upper thoracic spine. Am J Orthop. 2009;38(4):E71–4.
6. Cohen ZR, Fourney DR, Gokaslan AL, Walsh GW, Rhines L. Anterior stabilization of the upper thoracic spine via an interaortocaval subinnominate window: case report and description of operative technique. J Spinal Disord Tech. 2004;17:543–8.
7. Darling GE, McBroom R, Perrin R. Modified anterior approach to the cerivcothoracic junction. Spine (Phila Pa 1976). 1995;20(13):1519–21.
8. Cauchoix J, Binet JP. Anterior surgical approaches to the spine. Ann R Coll Surg Engl. 1957;21:234–43.
9. Hodgson AR, Stock FE, Fang HY, Ong GB. Anterior spinal fusion. The operative approach and pathological findings in 412 patients with Pott's disease of the spine. Br J Surg. 1960;48:172–8.
10. Sundaresan N, Shah J, Foley K, Rosen G. An anterior surgical approach to the upper thoracic vertebrae. J Neurosurg. 1984;61:686–90.
11. Sar C, Hamzaoglu A, Talu U, Domanic U. An anterior approach to the cerivcothoracic junction of the spine (modified osteotomy of manubrium sterni and clavicle). J Spinal Disord. 1999;12(2):102–6.

12. Shin D, Chae K, Shin D, Kim H. Modified manubriosternal approach to the cerivcothoracic junction. Kor J Spine. 2005;2(1):88–91.
13. Kurz LT, Pursel SE, Herkowitz HN. Modified anterior approach to the cerivcothoracic junction. Spine. 1991;16(10):542–7.
14. Kraus DH, Hua J, Burt M. Surgical access to tumors of the cerivcothoracic junction. Head Neck. 1995;17(2):131–6.
15. Schuchert MJ, McCormick KN, Abbas G, Pennathur A, Landreneau JP, Landreneau JR, et al. Anterior thoracic surgical approaches in the treatment of spinal infections and neoplasms. Ann Thorac Surg. 2014;97:1750–7.
16. Sattarov KV, Fard SA, Patel AS, Alkadhim M, Avila MJ, Walter CM, et al. Peribrachiocephalic approaches to the anterior cervicothoracic spine. J Clin Neurosci. 2015;22(11):1822–6.
17. Jung A, Schramm J. How to reduce recurrent laryngeal nerve palsy in anterior cervical spine surgery: a prospective observational study. Neruosurgery. 2010;67(1):10–5.
18. Derakhshan A, Lubelski D, Steinmetz MP, Corriveau M, Lee S, Pace JR, et al. Thoracic duct injury following cervical spine surgery: a multicenter retrospective review. Global Spine J. 2017;7(1):115S–9S.
19. Delaney SW, Shi H, Shokrani A, Sinha UK. Management of chyle leak after head and neck surgery: review of current treatment strategies. Int J Otolaryngol. 2017;2017:8362874. https://doi.org/10.1155/2017/8362874.
20. Civelek E, Karasu A, Cansever T, Hepgul T, Hepgul K, Sabanci A, et al. Surgical anatomy of the cervical sympathetic trunk during anterolateral approach to cervical spine. Eur Spine J. 2008;17(8):991–5.

7 Posterolateral Thoracotomy

Corinna C. Zygourakis and Dean Chou

Posterolateral thoracotomy is an excellent way to approach tumors in the ventral thoracic spine. It was first reported in the treatment of Pott's disease [1], but is now used not only for infections but also for conditions such as trauma, thoracic disc herniations, and spinal tumors. It provides a more direct visualization of the vertebral body and ventral dura than posterior approaches, and it may therefore be more effective for anterior pathology. It avoids damage to the posterior ligamentous complex, paraspinal muscles, and the majority of the posterior elements. The anterior approach also allows for minimal removal of uninvolved bone, efficient tumor removal, and effective reconstruction of the anterior weight-bearing column [2]. Thoracic surgeons often assist in order to perform this exposure because of the opening of the chest cavity, but it is nonetheless important for all spine surgeons to understand the anatomic nuances, limitations, complications, and consequences of this approach.

C. C. Zygourakis (✉)
Johns Hopkins Hospital, Department of Neurosurgery, Baltimore, MD, USA
e-mail: czygour1@jhmi.edu

D. Chou
University of California, San Francisco, Department of Neurosurgery, San Francisco, CA, USA

Anatomy

First, we review the anatomy of the rib cage, which is formed by the 12 thoracic vertebrae, sternum, costal cartilages, and usually 12 ribs on each side. One must be careful when localizing and assuming that every patient has 12 ribs; there are instances in which patients have 13 or 11 ribs, or the L1 transverse process can appear to be a rib when it really is an elongated transverse process. The intercostal muscles lie in the space between the ribs and are organized into three layers: the external intercostals (that run infero-anteriorly), the internal intercostals (that run infero-posteriorly), and the innermost intercostals. The neurovascular bundle runs along the inferior aspect of each rib, and includes, from top to bottom, the intercostal vein, artery, and nerve. Each rib head contains a superior facet that articulates with the vertebral body above and an inferior facet that articulates with the vertebra of the same number. The transverse process of each vertebra also articulates with the rib head of the same number.

For tumors that are located in the upper thoracic spine (T1–T4), a partial manubriotomy [3] or sternotomy may need to be performed in order to access the spine anteriorly, but this will be discussed further in another chapter. Here, we focus on the posterolateral thoracotomy approach.

D. M. Sciubba (ed.), *Spinal Tumor Surgery*, https://doi.org/10.1007/978-3-319-98422-3_7

Positioning

The patient is positioned in the lateral decubitus position with the back and legs gently bent to avoid tension on the peripheral nerves, similar to routine positioning for lateral spine approaches. Generally, for lesions in the upper thoracic spine, we approach from the patient's right side (i.e., left lateral decubitus) due to the obstruction of the spine on the left side by the aorta. In contrast, in the lower thoracic spine (T10–T12), a left-sided approach is preferred to avoid liver retraction, especially in patients with hepatomegaly. We are careful to pad the patient's knees and heels with gel bolsters and pillows. The dependent arm is outstretched on an arm-board, and the superior arm is placed at a right angle on a thoracotomy-specific arm holder. The arms are well-padded to prevent brachial plexus or shoulder injuries. Strips of tape are placed around the hips and the upper chest to secure the patient to the bed. Extreme care must be taken so as not to tape the patient too tightly to the bed in order to avoid nerve compression. Also, it is important to put tape on the skin itself since putting foam between the tape and the skin will allow the patient to rotate during the operation. We perform nearly all such cases with intraoperative neuromonitoring, including both motor and somatosensory evoked potentials (MEPs and SSEPs). We also request anesthesiologists to use a special endotracheal tube (with either a dual lumen tube or a bronchial blocker) so that they can perform single lung ventilation when necessary.

Procedure

Exposure

We begin with a curvilinear incision at the level of the anterior axillary line that runs posteriorly at the appropriate intercostal space. Because the ribs run in an inferior-anterior direction, we must typically enter an intercostal space two levels above the vertebral level we are trying to reach. For example, to perform a T7 vertebrectomy, we would place our incision at the fifth intercostal space. The latissimus dorsi muscle is opened by electrocautery. For the upper thoracic spine, we mobilize the scapula by dividing the trapezius and rhomboid muscles posteriorly. We try to spare the serratus anterior muscles, although these too may be divided if necessary. We are careful to avoid injury to the long thoracic nerve, which results in denervation of the serratus anterior muscle and a "winged scapula," by making our incision at least 6–7 cm anterior to the scapular tip [4]. Similarly, we avoid injury to the thoracodorsal nerve, which supplies the latissimus dorsi muscle. Even with such precautions, patients should be warned of possible postoperative shoulder dysfunction, which is an expected outcome from this thoracotomy.

We then open the intercostal space by taking the rib, although it is not necessary to take the rib if adequate visualization can be achieved through the intercostal space. We first perform a subperiosteal dissection of the rib (Fig. 7.1a), careful not to injure the neurovascular bundle that runs along its inferior surface. We use the rib cutter to divide the rib posteriorly (Fig. 7.1b) and anteriorly (Fig. 7.1c), and then remove it (Fig. 7.1d). We then ask the anesthesiologists to deflate the lung and switch to single lung ventilation. We place a large Finochietto-type retractor system to retract the ribs and scapula and keep the incision open (Fig. 7.2a). If necessary, large sponges are used to displace and pack the lung out of the field (Fig. 7.2b). On the right side, the azygos vein with its tributaries, the esophagus, and the thoracic duct should be noted in order to avoid injury. Generally, however, with standard lateral spine approaches, these structures are far enough away so that mobilization is not necessary.

Localization

At this point, we place a marker on the vertebral body of interest and obtain intraoperative AP X-rays in order to confirm that we are at the correct level. We usually count from rostral to caudal, using the typical broad and flat appearance to identify the first rib (T1) and the C7 vertebral body, which should not have a rib. Lateral X-rays are generally obscured in the upper thoracic spine because of the shoulders, so AP X-rays tend to be

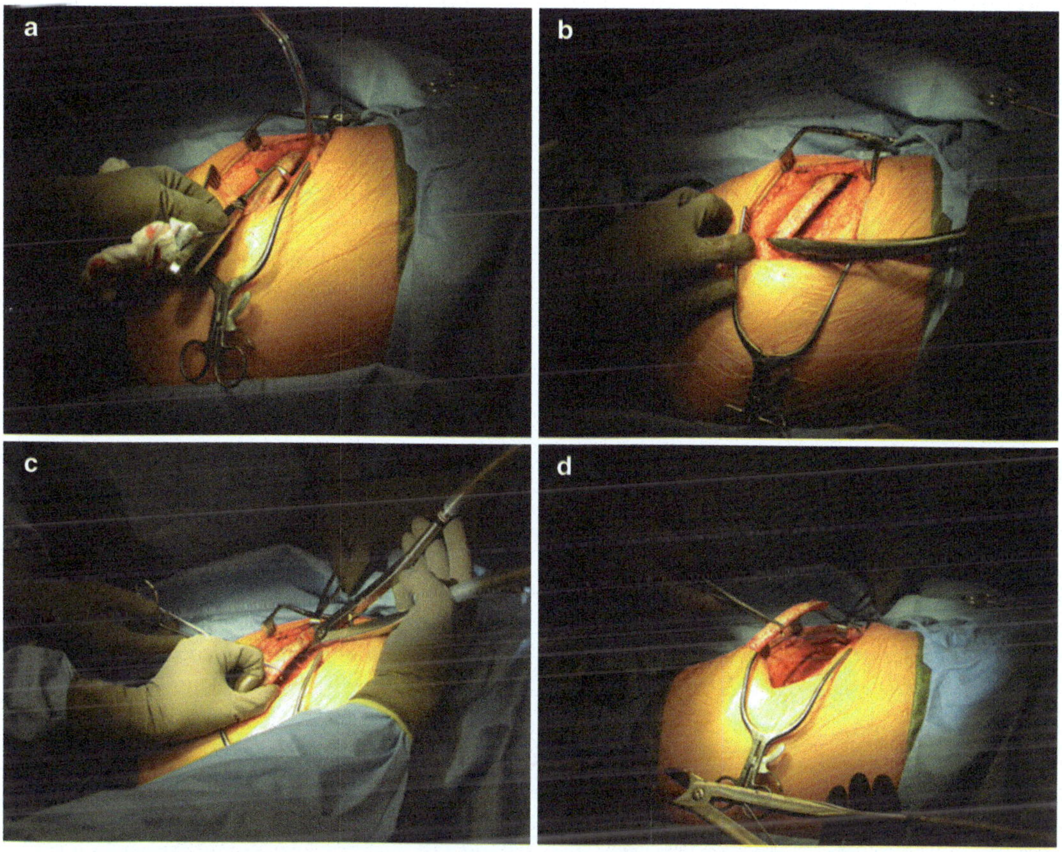

Fig. 7.1 Resection of the rib in thoracotomy procedure. (**a**) The periosteal dissection of the rib. (**b**) The posterior cut. (**c**) The anterior cut in the rib, which allows for rib removal (**d**)

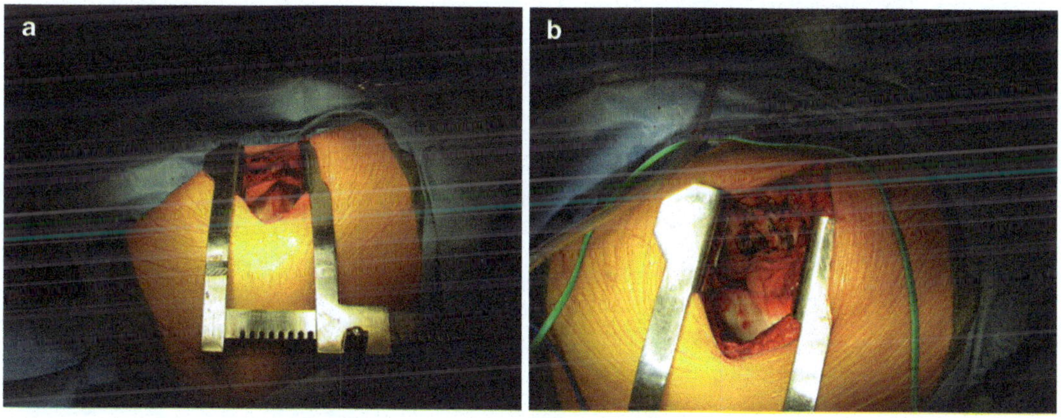

Fig. 7.2 Placement of the large Finochietto-type retractor system to retract the ribs and keep the thoracotomy open (**a**). Large sponges are often used to displace and pack the lung out of the field (**b**)

more useful. Correlation needs to be done with a preoperative X-ray to ensure that the patient has 12 ribs and does not have an anomalous cervical C7 rib. Once we have identified the correct level, we identify the intercostal artery and vein (also known as the segmental artery and vein) running along the vertebral body and use either a bipolar cautery or surgical clips to ligate the vessel.

If we are operating on the left side between T8 and T12, where the artery of Adamkiewicz usually arises, we will clip the segmental vessel first and wait 10 min to ensure that there are no changes in motor evoked potentials before ligating and sacrificing the vessel.

Corpectomy

We next turn our attention to the corpectomy and stabilization. We first identify and remove the rib head attached to the vertebral body of interest (Fig. 7.3a). We identify the pedicle and drill down the pedicle in order to identify the dura and spinal cord. We use a high-speed drill to perform the corpectomy (Fig. 7.3b) and then employ a combination of curettes and pituitary rongeurs to remove the discs above and below the vertebra of interest. After the vertebral body has been removed and the cord is adequately decompressed, we place a corpectomy cage (Fig. 7.3c) and lateral plate with screws (Fig. 7.3d) to achieve our spinal fixation. We may also consider additional posterior fixation (i.e., pedicle screws) if needed for long-segment spinal stabilization.

Closure

Prior to closure, we place a chest tube in the pleural space if the parietal pleura has been violated. The chest tube comes out through a small skin incision inferior to the surgical incision and aims toward the apex for a pneumothorax or to the dependent portion of the lung to assist with sucking up blood. Anesthesia re-inflates the lung under direct visualization. If there is any suspicion of air leak from the thoracotomy, large quantities of fibrin glue are applied over the lung and

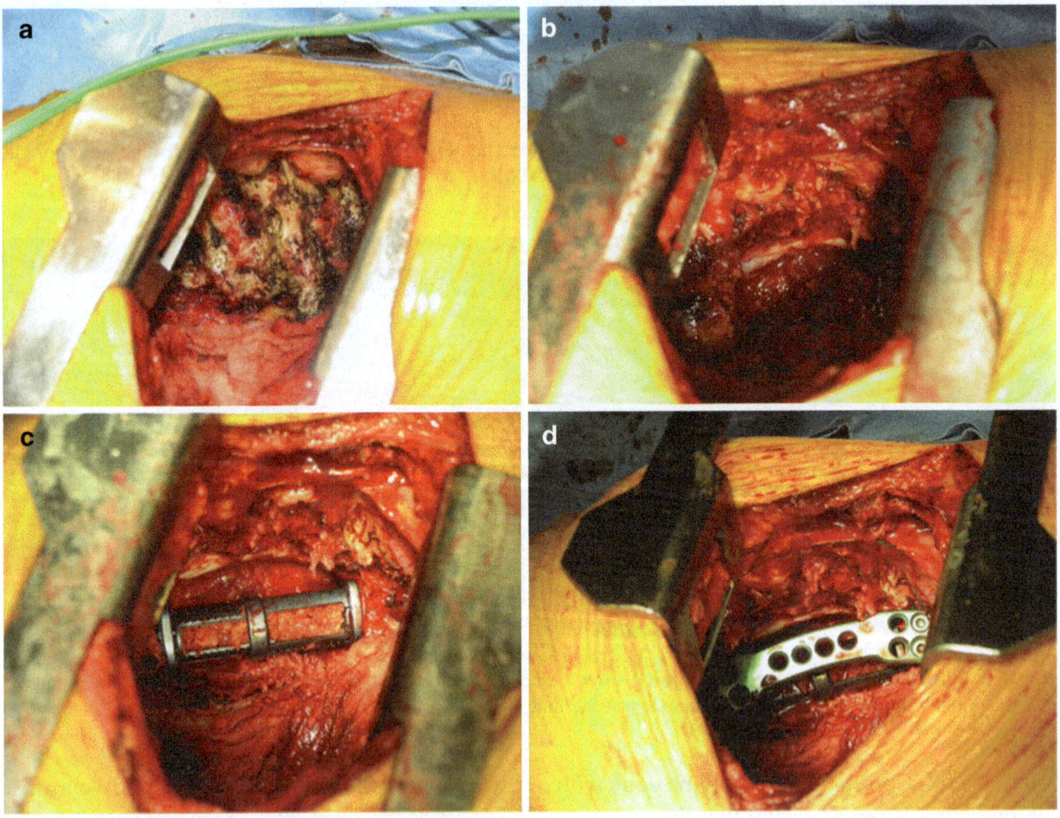

Fig. 7.3 The thoracic spine from the lateral view, before (**a**) and after (**b**) corpectomy is performed. (**c**) Corpectomy cage placement. (**d**) Lateral plate for stabilization

the area of suspected air leak. Larger air leaks will require thoracic surgery closure.

We bring together the ribs with a large figure of eight #2 Vicryl suture. We then use large Vicryl sutures to bring together first the serratus anterior muscle and then the latissimus dorsi muscle in two separate layers. The subcutaneous layer and the skin layer are then closed in succession. An air-tight closure is essential.

Postoperative Care

All patients have routine postoperative spinal care, including X-rays to evaluate implant placement, pain management, and physical therapy. The chest tube is initially placed to 20-mm H_2O suction, but is usually changed to water seal very quickly. We obtain daily chest X-rays to evaluate for pneumothorax or pleural effusion and remove the chest tube when the output is less than 250 cc for 24 h.

Complications

The most common complications of this procedure include chest wall pain, also known as post-thoracotomy pain syndrome, which may be seen in up to 50% of thoracotomy patients [5]. This phenomenon is not well understood but likely arises from compression of the intercostal nerve when spreading the thoracotomy with the retractor [5]. Aggressive multimodal pain regimens are an essential part of preventing and managing this pain.

Respiratory complications, such as atelectasis, pneumonia, and pneumothorax, may also occur in up to half of patients undergoing thoracotomies [6]. Preoperative pulmonary function testing should be considered in high-risk patients (such as those who smoke tobacco or have preexisting lung disease), and incentive spirometry and early mobilization are important in the immediate postoperative period. Ironically, many times atelectasis is seen in the contralateral (nonoperated) lung because of the dependent position during surgery. Other less common complications include wound infection, chylothorax, and shoulder girdle dysfunction, which result in decreased range of motion and pain in the shoulder joint [7]. Mortality rates are very low (<1%) [8, 9].

Taken together, these studies suggest that posterolateral thoracotomy is a safe and effective procedure for accessing ventral spinal tumors.

References

1. Hodgson AR, Stock FE. Anterior spinal fusion a preliminary communication on the radical treatment of Pott's disease and Pott's paraplegia. Br J Surg. 1956;44(185):266–75.
2. Gokaslan ZL, York JE, Walsh GL, McCutcheon IE, Lang FF, Putnam JB Jr, et al. Transthoracic vertebrectomy for metastatic spinal tumors. J Neurosurg. 1998;89(4):599–609.
3. Lam FC, Groff MW. An anterior approach to spinal pathology of the upper thoracic spine through a partial manubriotomy. J Neurosurg Spine. 2011;15(5):467–71.
4. Salazar JD, Doty JR, Tseng EE, Marin PC, Girotto JA, Rosebrough GS, et al. Relationship of the long thoracic nerve to the scapular tip: an aid to prevention of proximal nerve injury. J Thorac Cardiovasc Surg. 1998;116(6):960–4.
5. Karmakar MK, Ho AM. Postthoracotomy pain syndrome. Thorac Surg Clin. 2004;14(3):345–52.
6. Pettiford BL, Schuchert MJ, Jeyabalan G, Landreneau JR, Kilic A, Landreneau JP, et al. Technical challenges and utility of anterior exposure for thoracic spine pathology. Ann Thorac Surg. 2008;86(6):1762–8.
7. Miranda AP, de Souza HC, Santos BF, Abrã OJ, Cipriano FG, de Oliveira AS, et al. Bilateral shoulder dysfunction related to the lung resection area after thoracotomy. Medicine (Baltimore). 2015;94(44):e1927.
8. Burm W, Hübner F, Haffke T, Richter HP, Kast E, Rath SA. Approach-related complications of transthoracic spinal reconstruction procedures. Zentralbl Neurochir. 2004;65(1):1–6.
9. Ikard RW. Methods and complications of anterior exposure of the thoracic and lumbar spine. Arch Surg. 2006;141(10):1025–34.

Minimally Invasive Thoracoscopic Approach to the Anterior Thoracic Spine

8

Meic H. Schmidt

Introduction

Anterior approaches to the thoracic spine and the thoracolumbar junction have been progressively developing from traditional, open approaches to minimally invasive techniques. The use of endoscopic spine surgery has significantly expanded since its first description in the literature in the 1990s. Thoracoscopic surgeries have become safe and time efficient with comparable and better complication rates and outcomes than open approaches [1]. Common applications of thoracoscopy in spine surgery are anterior release for scoliosis, thoracic disc herniation, and corpectomy for traumatic fracture reconstruction. In this chapter, we discuss the role of thoracoscopic surgery in the management of metastatic spine disease.

Equipment for Thoracoscopic Surgery

Video Imaging System

One of the most important aspects for successful endoscopic surgery is to have high-quality images of the surgical field. The new high-definition video technology that is currently available has revolutionized image quality. A high-intensity xenon light source is typically connected to a 30-degree, 10-mm endoscope. This image is transmitted via a high-definition camera to two or three flat-screen monitors.

Endoscopic Tools

Tools for thoracoscopic surgery typically need to be long enough to allow for a three-point anchoring surgical technique. In addition, the tools should have depth markings and need to fit through 10-mm ports. Each port has a flexible black, threaded trocar with an inner diameter of 11 mm. It is important that the trocars are black to minimize light reflection from the camera. Similarly, all thoracoscopic tools should have nonreflective surfaces.

The harmonic scalpel is another invaluable tool for endoscopic surgery, although it is not commonly used in other spine surgeries. The harmonic scalpel cuts and coagulates by transferring mechanical energy to tissues. It therefore minimizes thermal injury and smoke that can interfere with visualization via an endoscope.

Endoscopic diaphragmatic retraction becomes necessary the closer one operates to the thoracolumbar junction. The diaphragm on the left side typically inserts along the lateral surface of the spine at the T12/L1 disc space. To create the working space, one must carefully retract

M. H. Schmidt
Brain and Spine Institute, Department of Neurosurgery, Westchester Medical Center at the New York Medical College, Valhalla, NY, USA
e-mail: meic.schmidt@wmchealth.org

D. M. Sciubba (ed.), *Spinal Tumor Surgery*, https://doi.org/10.1007/978-3-319-98422-3_8

the diaphragm, thereby expanding the costodiaphragmatic recess for surgery. Incising the diaphragm to expose the retroperitoneal space is necessary for placement of screws into the upper third of L1 or for L1 corpectomy with placement of screws into the top of L2.

For the corpectomy, it is recommended that one uses osteotomes with depth markings. Osteotomes allow for efficient vertebrectomies with minimal splattering of irrigation and blood, which can interfere with the optics on the endoscope. We do occasionally use an endoscopic drill (Midas Rex) to drill off the rib head or even out the endplates.

Endoscopic Spinal Reconstruction

Typically, either of two spinal implants can be placed for thoracoscopic spine surgery for metastatic disease: a vertebral body replacement (expandable cage) or an anterior lateral plating system. Expandable cages have become the preferred implant after corpectomy for metastasis. They are usually made from titanium alloy to minimize any postoperative imaging artifact. They can be placed via a small opening and expanded between the two endplates. Anterior lateral plates are commercially available from several companies. The MACS TL plate (Aesculap, Germany) is preferred for thoracoscopic surgery because it was designed for that purpose and has several features that make endoscopic implantation more efficient.

Preoperative Considerations

Patients are evaluated with standard spine imaging, including computed tomography (CT) and magnetic resonance imaging (MRI), and with anterior/posterior and lateral radiographs of the chest to evaluate for pleural effusion, fibrinous membranes, or dense adhesions in the pleural space.

Intravenous high-dose steroids are used in patients with symptomatic spinal cord compression or myelopathy. In addition, we routinely ask for endovascular embolization for most vascular metastasis.

Single-Lung Ventilation

Good single-lung ventilation is crucial for thoracoscopic spine surgery. It is best achieved with a double-lumen endotracheal tube. In smaller patients, an endobronchial blocker can be used. It is important to note that thoracoscopic spine surgery typically requires a longer time in the operating room than most other procedures performed with single-lung ventilation.

Indications and Contraindications

Indications for the thoracoscopic approach for metastatic spine disease are as follows:

- Pathological fractures
- Spinal cord compression
- Anterior column support after posterior surgery

Contraindications for the thoracoscopic approach are most commonly related to patient comorbidities that make single-lung ventilation difficult, such as cardiopulmonary disease, chronic obstructive pulmonary disease, extensive lung metastasis, and prior thoracic surgeries that create lung adhesions. In addition, patients should have acceptable bone quality and normal coagulation studies.

Patient Education and Informed Consent

The patient should be advised of the potential complications associated with anesthesia and surgery and give consent for the surgery. Risks associated with anterior thoracic spine surgery include the following:

- Spinal cord injury and nerve and sympathetic trunk injury
- Injury to the greater vessels
- Thoracic duct injury
- Injuries to the spleen, liver, and kidney
- Diaphragmatic hernia

Patients who agree to a thoracoscopic approach should also be advised of the possibility and give consent for possible conversion to a mini-open or open thoracotomy.

Operative Technique

The operative steps are illustrated in Fig. 8.1, which illustrates a patient treated with the thoracoscopic insertion of an expandable cage [2].

Patient Positioning

The approach side is selected based on the location of the great vessels (i.e., aorta and inferior vena cava) in relation to the spine. Most commonly, a left-sided approach is used to access the thoracolumbar junction (T11–L2). For the upper and mid-thoracic spine (T3–T10), a right-sided approach is preferred.

In the operating room, the patient is placed in the lateral decubitus position on a radiolucent table. We use three to four supports (sacrum, pubic bone, scapula, sternum) and a U-shaped cushion between the patient's legs to place the patient perpendicular to the floor. An axillary roll is placed, and the suspended arm is supported using a Krause armrest. Intraoperative fluoroscopy is used to verify patient's spine position, alignment, and level of pathology.

Thoracoscopic Access and Exposure

We use fluoroscopy to design our spine access. The skin surface is marked with the anatomical structures of interest—the vertebral bodies, the associated disc spaces, the anterior and posterior

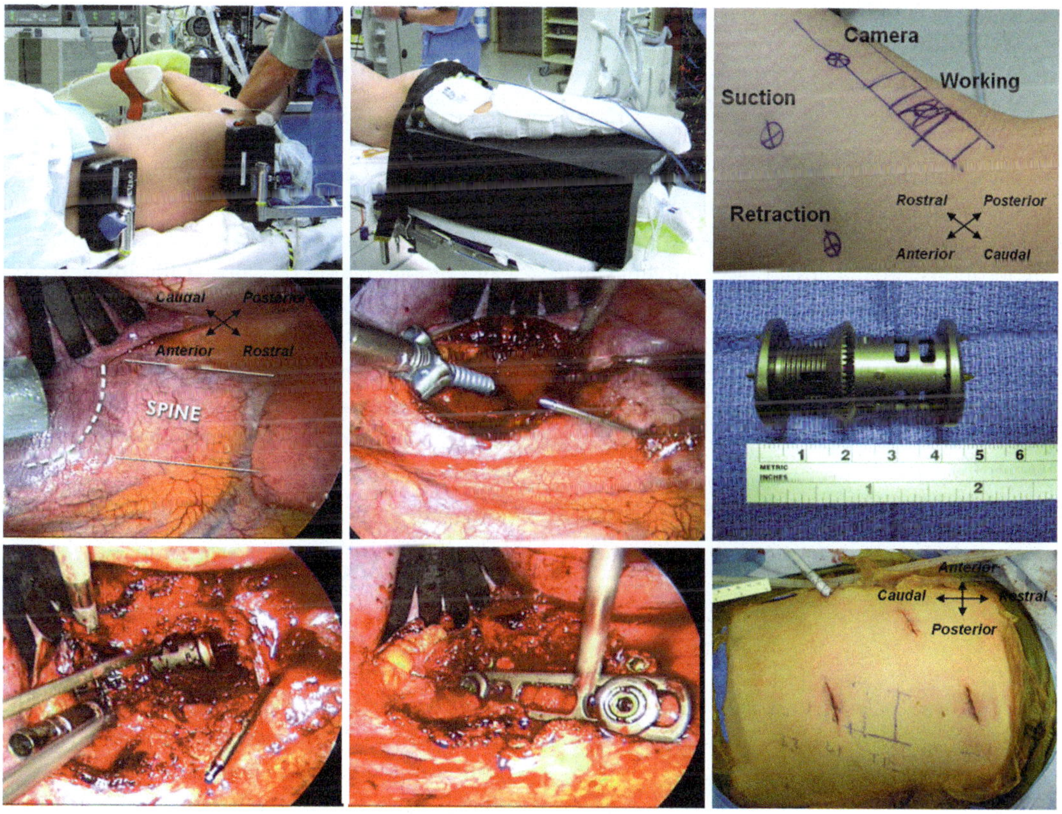

Fig. 8.1 Thoracoscopic decompression and fixation. (Reproduced from Ragel et al. [2], by permission of Oxford University Press)

spinal lines—as well as the surgical access sites (i.e., ports). For most thoracoscopic cases, a four-portal technique is sufficient for a corpectomy. In large patients, sometimes a fifth port is needed so that the targeted vertebra(e) can be reached more easily.

1. A *working portal* is placed directly over the vertebral body that is to be resected. It is typically larger than the other ports. This allows for access via two adjacent intercostal rib spaces and also allows for easier placement of an expandable cage through one incision.
2. An *endoscope portal* is placed two to three vertebral bodies above the working portal in line with the spine. For cases at the thoracolumbar junction, the endoscope is placed in a cranial direction relative to the working port. For upper thoracic cases, it is placed caudal to the working port.
3. The *retraction portal* is placed anterior to the working portal for safe retraction of the diaphragm and the lung.
4. A *suction irrigation portal* is placed between the retraction and the endoscope portals.

This configuration allows for all instruments to converge on the target vertebrae and avoids "fencing" of the endoscopic tools. After the portal locations are identified, we initiate single-lung ventilation to give the lung time to deflate (Fig. 8.2). The chest wall is then disinfected, and the area is sterilely draped to allow for possible conversion to an open technique if necessary.

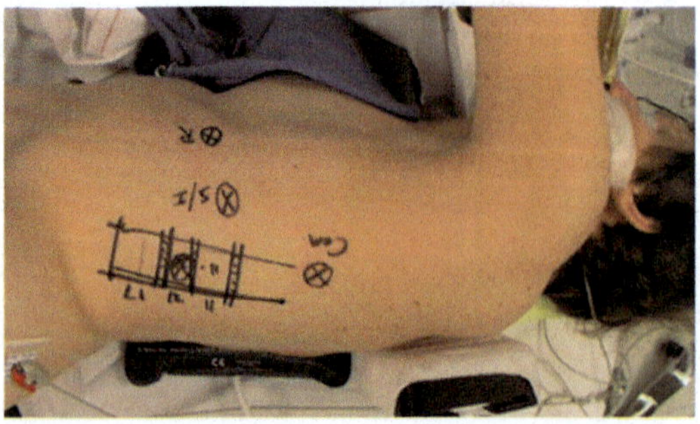

Fig. 8.2 Thoracoscopic patient positioning and working ports. (Reproduced with permission from Amini et al. [3])

To avoid iatrogenic injury to the underlying solid organs, the first port is placed at the location furthest away from the diaphragm. This incision is similar to the technique used to place a chest tube. After the skin incision, the rib is exposed. The thoracic cavity is entered carefully under direct vision with a blunt Kelly clamp. Once the pleural space is opened, manual palpation is performed to locate any pleural adhesions. Once it is determined that the pleural space is clear, the initial trocar is inserted and the 30-degree endoscope is introduced into the thoracic cavity. After a 360-degree survey has been performed, the remaining three trocar sites are placed under endoscopic visualization. Thus, no trocar is inserted "blindly." At this point, the key anatomical structures including the spine, diaphragm, aorta, and azygos vein, are identified. For orientation, we rotate the image on the monitor so that the spine is parallel to the lower edge of the video monitor.

Thoracolumbar Junction Access

The diaphragm typically inserts to the spine at the level of T12–L1 disc space. To gain access to the retroperitoneal portion of the upper lumbar spine, the diaphragm needs to be opened. This can be done endoscopically at the thinnest portion of the diaphragm with a harmonic scalpel. This allows for access to the L1–L2 levels. Once the diaphragm has been split, the retroperitoneal fat and peritoneum are bluntly dissected away from the fascia of the psoas muscle to expose the vertebral bodies.

Vertebral Body Exposure

Exposing the thoracic vertebral bodies and discs requires elevation of a pleural flap using the harmonic scalpel and identification of the segmental vessels, which lie transversely across the midportion of the vertebral body deep to the parietal pleura. These vessels are then ligated and divided, thus completing the exposure to the lateral vertebral body and discs.

Placement of Screws and Instrumentation

We use the MACS TL endoscopic anterolateral plate for anterior fixation in all cases. The system includes two clamps and four screws (two anterior stabilization screws and two posterior polyaxial vertebral body screws). One clamp and two screws are used at each vertebral body adjacent to the diseased vertebra. Using a short K-wire placed under fluoroscopic guidance as a guide, a cannulated awl is used to decorticate each screw entry point. The polyaxial screw clamp is assembled and inserted, and the K-wire is removed after the screw has engaged the cortical surface. To avoid the course of the segmental arteries along the midline of the vertebral bodies, the posterior polyaxial screw is inserted 10 mm anterior to the spinal canal in the upper or lower third of the vertebral body (for the screw above the diseased level and the screw below the diseased level, respectively). After the polyaxial posterior screws have been placed above and below the diseased body, the clamps are oriented perpendicular to the anterior aspect of the vertebral body with careful consideration to the surrounding great vessels.

Corpectomy and Spinal Canal Decompression

Discectomy and corpectomy are performed in a similar manner to an open procedure. The discs are incised using an elongated endoscopic scalpel and removed with rongeurs. The vertebral body in question is removed using a median corpectomy with straight and curved osteotomes. The ipsilateral rib head is traced to the ipsilateral pedicle and neural foramen located at its base so that the pedicle can be removed using a high-speed drill and endoscopic Kerrison punches. Free bone fragments and epidural tumor are maneuvered to the central corpectomy cavity and removed to avoid excessive manipulation of the spinal cord. These procedures allow for direct decompression and visualization of the anterior spinal cord.

Interbody Reconstruction and Endoscopic Stabilization

The thoracolumbar junction is reconstructed with an expandable cage inserted under direct fluoroscopic visualization after complete corpectomy. Once placed, the cage is expanded and distracted, and allograft is packed around the cage itself. The anterolateral plate is placed over the posterior polyaxial screws, the posterior screws are tightened, and the anterior stabilization screws are placed at each level. The screw plate construct is then locked and torqued. A final anterior/posterior and lateral fluoroscopic image is obtained prior to closure to verify hardware positioning.

Placement of Chest Tube and Closure

The diaphragm is sutured closed, and the operative field and the entire thoracic cavity are irrigated. A 24-Fr chest tube is placed through the inferolateral port or the lateral suction port under direct or thoracoscopic visualization, and the lung is reinflated. Before closure, the operative field is viewed to ensure proper lung reinflation and no bleeding from the surface. Port sites are closed in layers and the chest tube is secured in place.

Results

In a recent publication, we reviewed our experience in 12 patients who underwent a thoracoscopic spine surgery for metastatic disease [4]. The mean age of patients was 59 years, and the mean estimated blood loss was 613 ml. The mean duration of the operation was 234 minutes. The median length of stay in the hospital was 7.5 days (range 5–21 days). All 12 patients had improvement in their postoperative pain scores in comparison with their preoperative pain scores, and no patients suffered from worsening neurological function after surgery. Of the 7 patients who presented with neurological dysfunction, 6 (86%) had an improvement in their Frankel grade after surgery. No patients experienced delayed hardware failure requiring reoperation over a mean follow-up of 10 months (range 1–45 months).

Conclusion

Over the past two decades, endoscopic surgery has become a viable option for patients with metastatic spine disease. The retroperitoneal part of the thoracolumbar junction can be accessed with a small diaphragmatic incision. The results and outcomes of the thoracoscopic approach compare well with standard open surgery.

Acknowledgments This chapter is based on previous works by the authors Kalra RR, Schmidt MH, and Beisse R. Thoracoscopic decompression and fixation for thoracic and thoracolumbar junction lesions. In: Kim DH, Fessler RG, Regan JJ, editors. *Endoscopic Spine Surgery and Instrumentation*. New York: Thieme; 2016 and Ravindra VM, Brock A, Awad AW, Kalra R, Schmidt MH. The role of the mini-open thoracoscopic-assisted approach in the management of metastatic spine disease at the thoracolumbar junction. *Neurosurg Focus* 2016;41(2):E16.

References

1. Zuckerman SL, Laufer I, Sahgal A, Yamada YJ, Schmidt MH, Chou D, et al. When less is more: the indications for MIS techniques and separation surgery in metastatic spine disease. Spine (Phila Pa 1976). 2016;41(Suppl 20):S246–S53.
2. Ragel BT, Amini A, Schmidt MH. Thoracoscopic vertebral body replacement with an expandable cage after ventral spinal canal decompression. Neurosurgery. 2007;61(5 Suppl 2):317–22; discussion 22–3
3. Amini A, Beisse R and Schmidt MH. Thoracoscopic spine surgery for decompression and stabilization of the anterolateral thoracolumbar spine. Neurosurg Focus. 2005;19:E4.
4. Ravindra VM, Brock A, Awad AW, Kalra R, Schmidt MH. The role of the mini-open thoracoscopic-assisted approach in the management of metastatic spine disease at the thoracolumbar junction. Neurosurg Focus. 2016;41(2):E16.

9 Thoracoabdominal Approach for Tumors of the Thoracolumbar Spine

A. Karim Ahmed, Daniel M. Sciubba, and Feng Wei

Anatomic and Biomechanical Considerations

The thoracolumbar region (T11–L2) serves as an anatomic transition zone between the thorax and abdomen, a structural transition zone between the kyphotic thoracic and lordotic lumbar spine, and a dynamic transition zone between the semi-rigid thoracic and mobile lumbar spine.

The thoracolumbar spine, from T11 to L2, has unique structural and biomechanical challenges. Held in place by the ribs, the semirigid thoracic spine does not significantly contribute to mobility. This is in contrast to caudal lumbar segments which impart the majority of torso flexion and extension, particularly from L2 to L4.

Twelve paired ribs correspond to 12 thoracic vertebrae, containing superior and inferior costal facets for the articulation of the rib head, and an articular facet joint for articulation with the tubercle of the rib. The first seven paired ribs comprise the "true ribs," and the subsequent five comprise the "false ribs"—the latter two of which are known as "floating ribs" and lack costal articulation with the sternum.

With the exception of the T1 nerve root, responsible for finger abduction, the majority of thoracic motor nerves do not innervate critical muscles required for mobility or function, unlike in the cervical and lumbar spine. The anterior rami from T1 to T11 provide the intercostal nerves, which travel along the caudal aspect of the rib in the neurovascular bundle, located in between the internal intercostal muscle and innermost intercostal muscle, innervating skin and muscle of the chest and abdomen. Dermatomal innervation of the areola, umbilicus, and lower abdominal wall correspond to nerve roots from T4, T10, and T12 (subcostal), respectively. Hip flexion is mostly performed by the iliopsoas muscle, supplied in large part by the L2 nerve root. The upper lumbar segments from L1 to L3 innervate the psoas major muscle, via the lumbar plexus. Iliacus is innervated by the femoral nerve from L2 to L4.

The costal pleura, bordering the inner surface of the ribs, and parietal pleura represent the superficial boundary of the pleural space—bordered deeply by the visceral pleura. The diaphragmatic portion of the parietal pleura overlies the diaphragm, innervated by the phrenic nerve (C3–C5) and crucial for breathing function. Separating the thorax from the abdomen, the diaphragm is a sheet of muscle with two main components: the peripheral muscle and the central tendon. Including the opening for the inferior vena cava (~T8), the central tendon aponeurosis is an insertion point for respiratory muscles and essential to reduce pressure in the pleural space

A. Karim Ahmed · D. M. Sciubba
Department of Neurosurgery, The Johns Hopkins Hospital, Baltimore, MD, USA

F. Wei (✉)
Peking University Third Hospital, Department of Orthopedics, Beijing, China
e-mail: weifeng@bjmu.edu.cn

D. M. Sciubba (ed.), *Spinal Tumor Surgery*, https://doi.org/10.1007/978-3-319-98422-3_9

during inspiration. The peripheral muscles may be subdivided into the sternal, costal, and lumbar portions. The esophageal and aortic hiatus are formed by the peripheral muscle, at ~T10 and ~T12, respectively. The aortic hiatus allows for the passage of the aorta, azygos vein, hemiazygos vein, and thoracic duct. The psoas and quadratus lumborum muscles form the posterolateral border of the diaphragm, abutting the median and lateral arcuate ligaments. The paired tendinous crus of the diaphragm are tethered to the anterior longitudinal ligament of the lumbar vertebrae: the right (longer) crus attaches from L1 to L3 and the left attaches from L1 to L2 [1–7].

Operative Technique

Choosing Surgical Approach

The location of pathology and required exposure are critical to determine the best surgical approach. Anterior access to the thoracic spine, from T5 to T10, may be accomplished with a thoracotomy. For lesions of T5 or T6, the similarly numbered rib is removed (n). At T7 and T8, however, the rib of the suprajacent level is removed (n − 1). Removal of the rib two levels cranial to the lesion is required for exposure of T9 and T10 (n − 2). In the upper lumbar spine, however, anterior access may be performed via a retroperitoneal approach. As such, the thoracoabdominal approach is a combined thoracotomy and retroperitoneal exposure, with possible diaphragmatic detachment, for ventral access of the thoracolumbar junction, when either approach is not sufficient alone. The thoracoabdominal approach may be supplemented with a staged posterior approach for larger primary neoplasms requiring en bloc resection [8–11].

Patient Positioning

The patient is placed in the left lateral decubitus position. A left-sided thoracolumbar approach is favored due to large size and limited mobility of the liver on the right, compared with the contralateral spleen. Vascular injury to the left-sided thick-walled aorta is also considered to be easier to repair, compared to the right-sided vena cava; the former may be easier to mobilize, especially in the setting of radiation-induced retroperitoneal fibrosis [9].

Thoracoabdominal Exposure

An oblique flank skin incision is made from the 10th rib to the abdominal wall. Posterior retraction of the latissimus dorsi may be performed during muscle dissection. The rib is identified and subperiosteally dissected from its subcutaneous and muscular attachments (i.e., serratus anterior, latissimus dorsi, and intercostal muscles) on its superior border, thereby avoiding the neurovascular bundle. The rib may be resected for improved operative exposure, and the healthy bone is utilized for bone grafting. The rib is followed around to the costal margin, with careful dissection of the external and internal oblique muscles. Excessive dissection can result in abdominal flank bulging, pain, and weakness [8]. Division of the transversalis fascia, deep into the costal margin, exposes the peritoneum.

The peritoneum is dissected free from the bordering psoas, quadratus lumborum, and diaphragm to enter the retroperitoneal space. Ventral retraction of the peritoneum, posterior reflection of the psoas muscle, and detachment of the posterolateral diaphragm aid in exposure to the anterior spinal column. The diaphragm may be entered at its attachments with the median/lateral arcuate ligaments or crus. One must be mindful to preserve the distal muscular component of the diaphragm for repair and the central portion containing the phrenic nerve.

Detachment of the diaphragm, with gentle cranial retraction of the lung, exposes the diaphragmatic portion of the parietal pleura. Access to the lower thoracic spine and thoracolumbar junction may be accomplished by sharply incising the parietal pleura. Dissection of the segmental vessels allows for exposure of the anterior disk spaces and vertebral bodies but should be carefully performed due to the risk of hemorrhage. A preoperative angiogram of the artery of Adamkiewicz may be warranted if a large amount of lower thoracic segmental vessels will be sacrificed. In order to preserve collateral circulation nerve and/or spinal cord (i.e., radicular artery, anterior spinal artery), ligation of the segmental vessels should occur at the anterior vertebral body. Retroperitoneal lymphatics (i.e., thoracic duct, cisterna chyli) should also be approached with caution in order to avoid the development of postoperative lymphoceles. Bipolar electrocautery, cottonoids, and hemostatic agents are useful to maintain hemostasis throughout the case [9–11].

Decompression

With the anterior spinal column exposed, the annulus of the intervertebral disk spaces may be sharply incised in preparation for discectomy. During this process, the great vessels should be mobilized anteriorly to prevent vascular injury. A high-speed burr, Leksell rongeurs, and Kerrison punch are useful to remove the disks above and below the diseased level. Disk fragments are taken piecemeal with pituitary rongeurs, and the posterior longitudinal ligament is removed with a Kerrison punch. Corpectomy is performed by first removing the rib head and proximal pedicle. Removal of the proximal pedicle exposes the dura [9–11].

Reconstruction and Instrumentation

Anterior column support is accomplished with the placement of an expandable cage in the vertebral defect and may be packed with healthy autologous (i.e., resected rib) bone, or allograft. A lateral screw-rod system, or plate, stabilizes the segment above and below. Posterior transpedicular screw and rod instrumentation may be appropriate to obtain added stability following extensive resection [9–11].

Closure

Closure is initiated in a watertight fashion. If the diaphragm was taken down during the exposure, a large-bore chest tube is placed, and primary repair of the diaphragm is performed with non-absorbable sutures. The parietal pleura may be sutured, and rib-approximating sutures close the thoracic cavity. The intercostal muscles, abdominal wall, serratus anterior, and latissimus dorsi muscles are closed, in a layered fashion, with nonabsorbable sutures. The fascia is reapproximated with 0 Vicryl, with reapproximation of the subcutaneous layer. The subcuticular layer may be closed with 3–0 Vicryl sutures [9, 10].

Case Presentation

This 63-year-old female presented with a 3-year history of an enlarging mass in the left side of her back, accompanied by progressive ipsilateral thoracolumbar pain and abdominal numbness. She previously underwent a thoracotomy for a T10 paraspinal fibroma, 6.5 years prior. On examination, the patient endorsed tenderness to palpation of the left-sided thoracolumbar mass but was otherwise neurologically intact.

Imaging

CT revealed an irregularly shaped soft-tissue mass (61.0 × 47.7 × 77.4 mm, hyperdensity 38.4 HU) immediately left to the spine at T9–T11 (Fig. 9.1f). CT with contrast demonstrated heterogeneous enhancement, and areas of hypodense necrosis were identified. Lytic invasion of the left posterolateral T10 and T11 vertebral bodies was identified, with extension into the pedicles (Fig. 9.1g). The left paraspinal muscles from T9 to L2 were noted to be wider than the contralateral side. MRI similarly revealed a large soft-tissue mass (112.7 × 104.3 × 62.6 mm) with irregular margins from T9 to T11 (Fig. 9.1a). The lesion was T1 hypo-intense, T2 hyper-intense, and DWI hyper-intense. Soft-tissue infiltration was noted through the left T10/T11 neural foramen, resulting in epidural spinal cord compression. At the levels of T9–L2, an irregularly shaped, multi-lobular soft-tissue mass was found in the left paraspinal muscles (Fig. 9.1b, c).

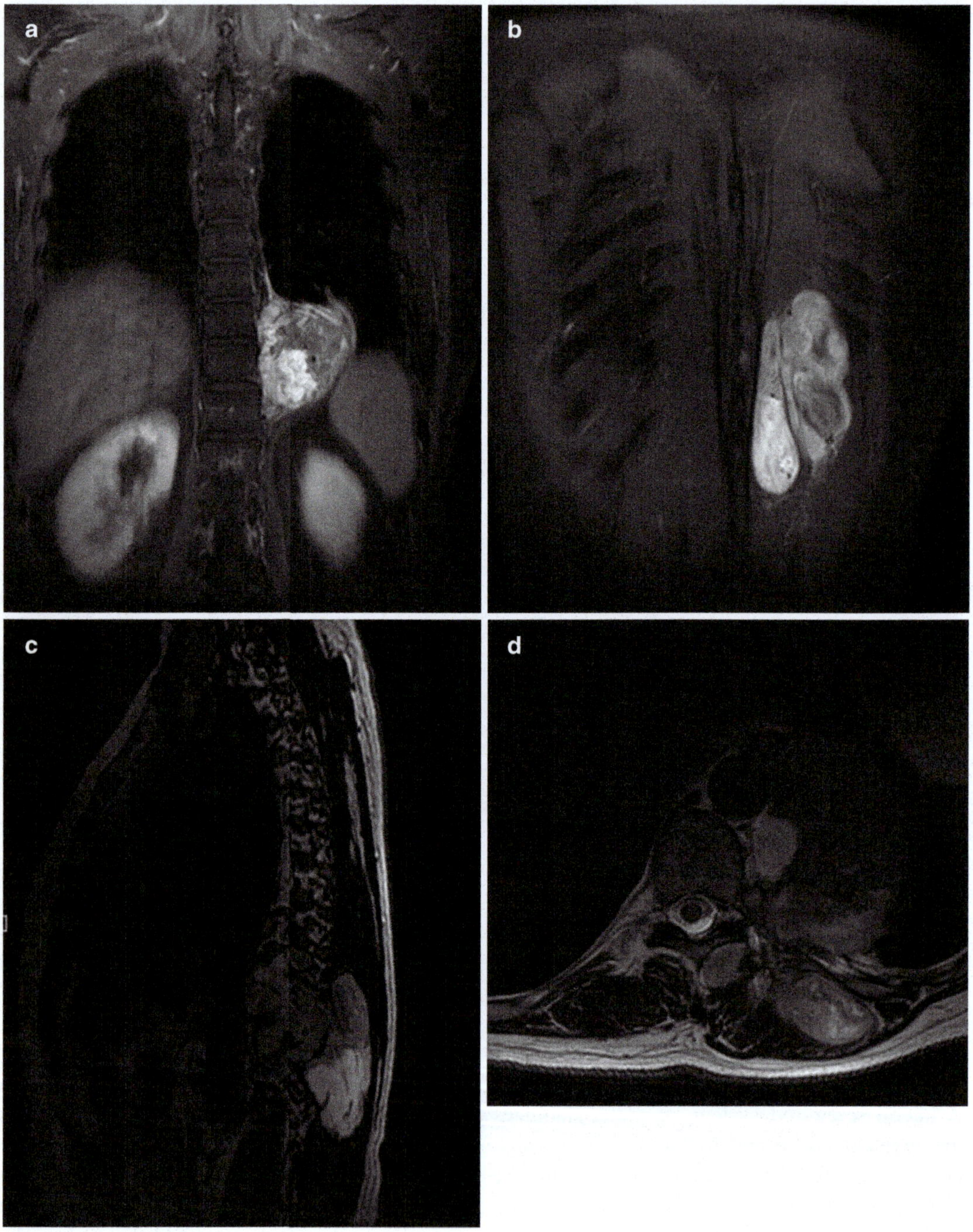

Fig. 9.1 Images of the patient on initial presentation, including magnetic resonance (**a–e**) computed tomography of the thoracic spine. (**a**) Image of magnetic resonance in the coronal plane shows the tumor on the left side of the vertebral body of T9 – T11. (**b**) Image of magnetic resonance in the coronal plane shows the tumor in the iliocostalis thoracis which reaches the level of L1 – L2. (**c**) Image of magnetic resonance in the sagittal plane shows the tumor in the iliocostalis thoracis, which reaches the level of L1 – L2. (**d**) Image of magnetic resonance in the axial plane of T9. (**e**) Image of magnetic resonance in the axial plane of T10 – T11. (**f**) Image of computed tomography in the axial plane of T9. (**g**) Image of computed tomography in the axial plane of T10 – T11. The black arrow shows the position of the diaphragm. (**h**) Image of computed tomography in the coronal plane shows the tumor on the left side of the vertebral body of T9 – T11. The white arrow shows the position of the diaphragm. (**i**) Image of computed tomography in the sagittal plane. The white arrow shows the position of the diaphragm, which reveals that the tumor is above the diaphragm

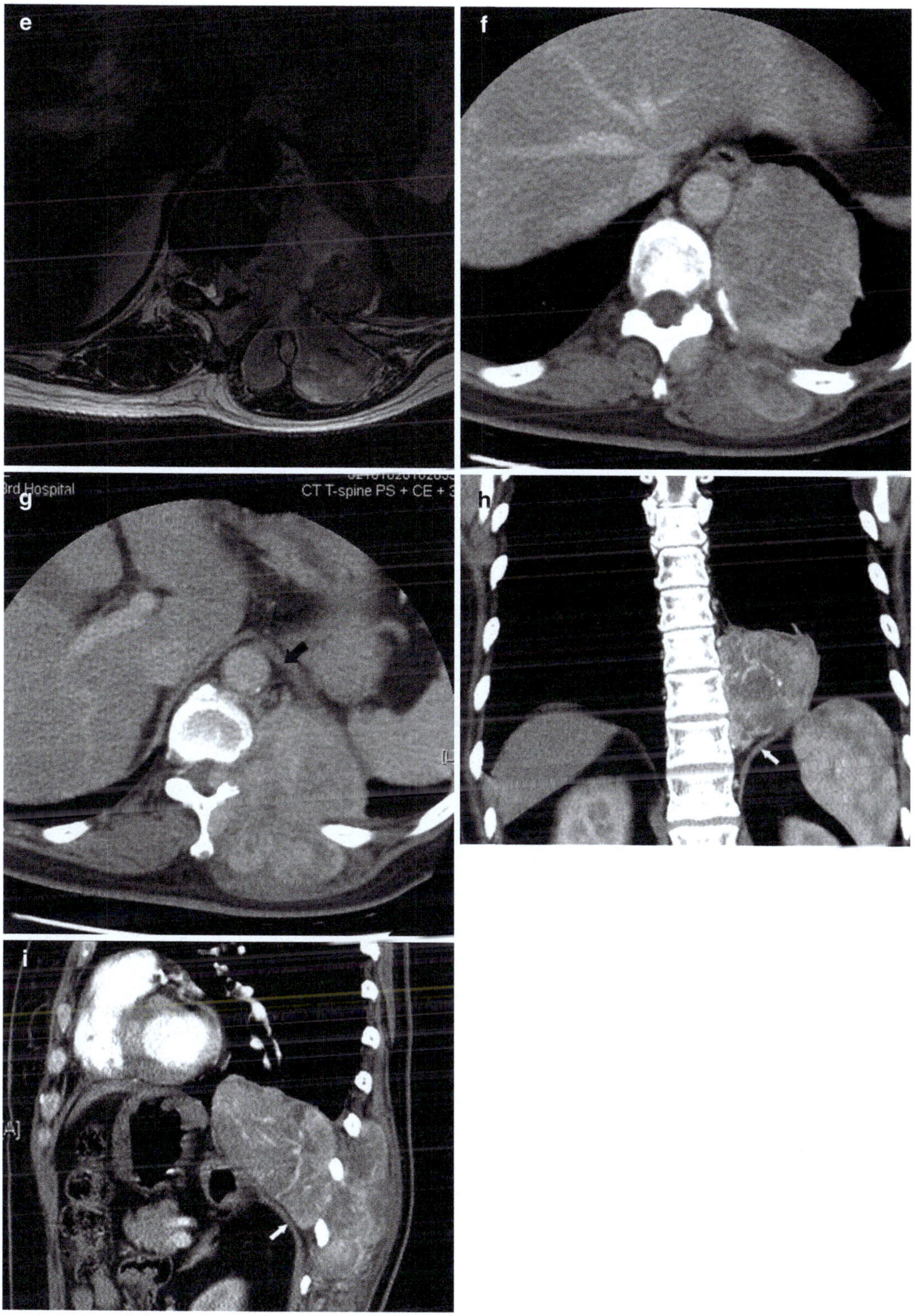

Fig. 9.1 (continued)

Pathologic Diagnosis

Pathology slides from the previous surgical resection were not available for review. A CT-guided biopsy was therefore performed, which revealed a spindle-cell mesenchymal tumor with profuse stromal vascularity, determined by the numerous branching vessels. There was no significant pleomorphism, and the extracellular matrix was collagenous. These characteristics suggested the diagnosis of a solitary fibroma. Even though the tumor cells were not highly mitotic (low Ki-67), large (>10 cm) extrapleural solitary fibromas are generally considered aggressive, and an intracapsular surgical resection with positive margins is associated with a sub-optimal prognosis. These tumors were called hemangiopericytomas because of their profuse stromal angiogenesis, and an intracapsular resection will likely lead to significant intraoperative blood loss. A plan for extracapsular en bloc resection was therefore determined as appropriate in order to reduce blood loss, prevent recurrence, and prolong tumor-free survival.

Tumor Staging and Surgical Planning

The tumor was Enneking S3 and WBB 1–6, A–D (Figs. 9.1d, e and 9.2a). In accordance with the WBB guidelines for resection of thoracolumbar

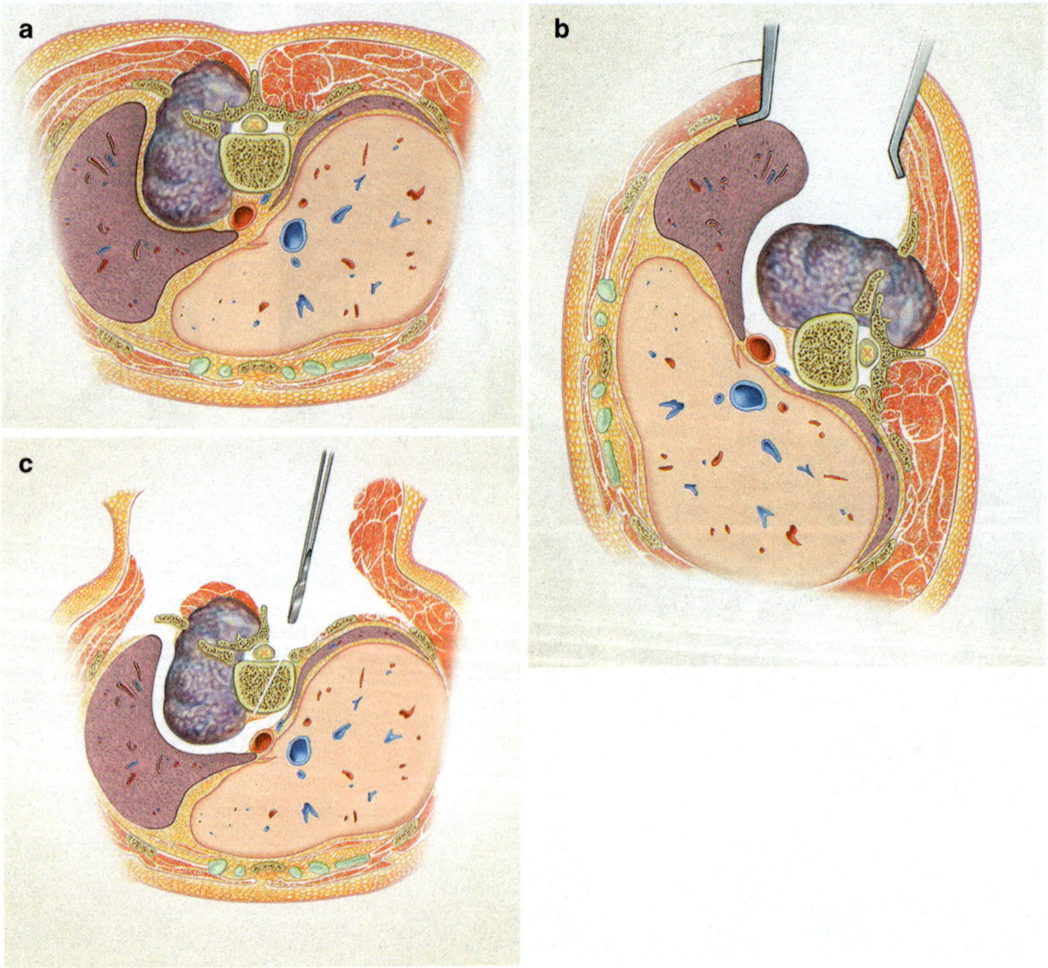

Fig. 9.2 Illustration of the tumor and stages of the surgery. (**a**) The illustration shows the tumor involving the wide areas of the lateral side of the vertebral body, appendix, and the intervertebral foramen. (**b**) Stage 1 operation involving left-sided thoracotomy and tumor released from the lung, aorta, diaphragm, and vertebral body. (**c**) Stage 2 operation involving the sagittal en bloc resection via posterior approach

tumors, a detailed surgical plan was adopted. In the first stage, an anterolateral approach was taken to separate the tumor from adjacent normal structures including the left lung, diaphragm, and aorta (Fig. 9.2b). In the second posterior stage, a plane was developed between the superficial and deep paraspinal muscles, advanced anterolaterally until the tumor was circumferentially released. The right posterior elements that were not involved by the tumor were removed in a piecemeal fashion to reveal the neural structures. The involved levels were separated from the normal spine by proximal and distal discectomies, and a sagittal osteotomy was performed diagonally from the right posterior to the left anterior in the involved vertebrae (Fig. 9.2c). The tumor mass was taken out en bloc from the posterior approach.

Preoperative Optimization

Feeding arteries to the tumor were selectively embolized by an interventional radiologist one day prior to the first stage. Angiography demonstrated a large tumor with proficient blood supply from the T9–T11 intercostal arteries, which were embolized using N-butyl cyanoacrylate (300–500 μm in size) and coils (Fig. 9.3).

Operative Technique

First stage: The patient was placed on right lateral decubitus and under general anesthesia with double-lumen endotracheal intubation. The T10 vertebra (where tumor diameter was the largest) was found to correspond to the level of the 8th rib on the mid-axillary line. A 15-cm incision through the skin, subcutaneous fascia, and the latissimus dorsi was made along the left 8th rib, centering on the mid-axillary line. The 8th rib was exposed and excised by about 12 cm. Following deflation of the left lung, the parietal pleura was opened to enter the thoracic cavity (Fig. 9.4). Electrocautery was used to dissect the adhesions between the tumor and the left lung. Manual palpation was utilized to identify the lower margin of the tumor, between the caudal aspect of the tumor and diaphragm. Because the aorta was dorsal to the tumor and not under direct visualization, blunt finger dissection helped separate the tumor

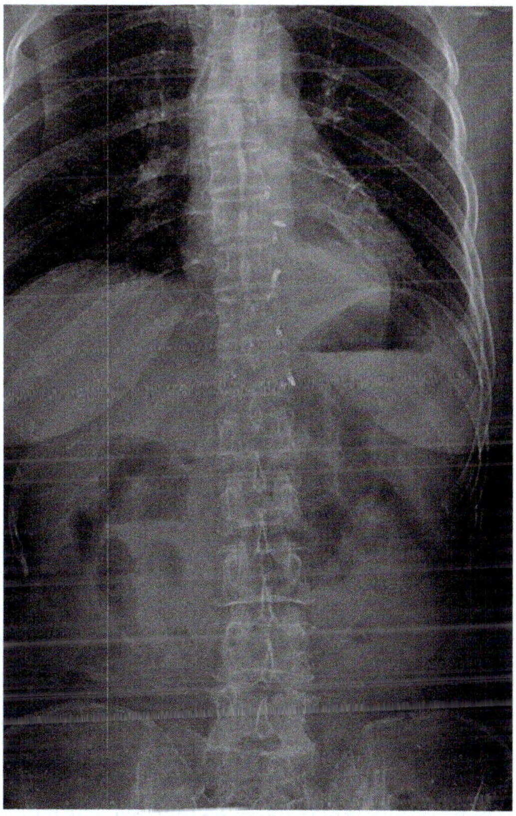

Fig. 9.3 Embolization of the segmental arteries of the left side

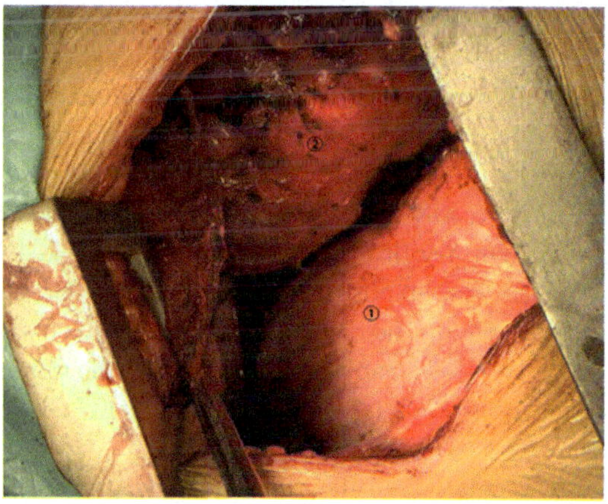

Fig. 9.4 Operative photograph of left-sided thoracotomy. ① diaphragm; ② tumor; and ③ lung

from the aorta and spine. Due to the preoperative embolization, only limited venous bleeding was encountered during the first-stage procedure. The parietal pleura and intercostal muscles were dissected, using electrocautery, with a 1-cm margin proximally and laterally. The 9th, 10th, and the 11th ribs were partially resected, with rib-cutting forceps. Proximally, the T9/T10 intervertebral disc was identified by fluoroscopy, and a lateral partial discectomy was performed. The left half of the anterior longitudinal ligament was also resected. The space formed between the aorta and the involved vertebrae was packed with large amounts of Gelfoam for both hemostasis and to prevent adhesions during the second stage. The wound was closed in a layered fashion, and a chest tube was placed.

Second stage: Seven days following the first surgery, the patient was placed prone on the table under general anesthesia with double-lumen endotracheal intubation. A mid-line incision was made from T7 to L2, followed by subperiosteal dissection. With fluoroscopic assistance, right-sided pedicles were placed from T7 to L1. The right-sided screws from T9 to T11 were removed temporarily to allow subsequent osteotomy. A left transverse incision down to the latissimus dorsi, perpendicular to the mid-line, was extended laterally into the previous incision. The thoracolumbar fascia was exposed by reflecting the latissimus dorsi and serratus muscles cranially. The rib cut ends from the first-stage procedure could be palpated. The thoracolumbar fascia was incised lateral to the longissimus thoracis, from T7 to L2. The uninvolved, more superficial longissimus thoracis was divided from the deeper iliocostalis thoracis. The tumor was palpable deep into the iliocostalis thoracis from T9 to T12. The iliocostalis thoracis was transected proximally and distally with 1-cm margins to the tumor. The left T7–T8 laminae were exposed, and two pedicles screws were inserted. The distal cut end of the iliocostalis thoracis was cranially reflected, with the tumor exposing the left facet joints of T11–L1. Pedicle screws were inserted at T12 and L1.

The cut ends of the 9th to 11th ribs from the first stage were palpated, and the lateral 3 cm of the cut ends was resected further to allow access to the left thoracic cavity. Once the left lung was deflated, blunt dissection was utilized to free the tumor anteriorly, releasing the loose connective tissues between the tumor and the adjacent lung, diaphragm, aorta, and spine. Gauze was placed temporarily between the tumor mass and adjacent structures. The intercostal muscles were transected along the upper edge of the 9th rib and the lower edge of the 11th rib down to the level of the facet joints of T8/T9 and T11/T12, respectively. The involved intercostal vessels and nerves were sacrificed. The tumor mass was now completely freed from adjacent organs, anteriorly, and uninvolved back muscles, posteriorly.

Subsequently, the spinous process, lower half laminae, inferior articular processes of T8, and superior articular processes of T9 were resected using an ultrasonic blade. The T11/T12 intervertebral level was similarly released. Right hemilaminectomies and facetectomies were performed from T9 to T11. The right T9–T11 nerve roots were ligated, and the dural sac was released from the posterior longitudinal ligament using a Penfield elevator. The proximal (T8/T9) and distal (T11/T12) intervertebral discs and posterior longitudinal ligament at the corresponding levels were resected. The proximal release was easier since part of the T8/T9 disc and the anterior longitudinal ligament was resected in the first stage. The T11/T12 disc was not accessible during the first stage, and the anterior longitudinal ligament at that level was resected from the posterior approach. In order to prevent injury to the aorta, an abdominal spatula was inserted along the cut ends of the ribs and placed between the aorta and the spine, before the anterior annulus fibrosus and longitudinal ligament were transected with an osteotome. The left half of T9–T11 vertebrae and their posterior elements were now ready to be removed en bloc with sagittal resection. According to CT-based preoperative planning, an osteotomy line from the medial wall of the pedicles to the left anterior part of the vertebral body with a 30° angle from the vertical axis of the patient body would allow sufficient distance from the tumor margin. An ultrasonic blade was used to perform osteotomies of the T9–T11 vertebral bodies, while the dura and aorta were protected with a nerve elevator and an abdominal spatula, respectively. Partial discectomies of T9/T10 and T10/T11 were performed using a No. 15 blade scalpel and a pituitary rongeur. The entire tumor mass, including the left half of T9–T11 vertebrae, posterior elements, and proximal ends of the corresponding ribs, was mobilized.

A ball-tip probe was used to palpate the medial wall of the right pedicle screw tracts within the bodies of T9 and T11. Both were intact and the two screws were re-inserted. A precontoured connecting rod was placed and locked in on the right side. The tumor mass was gently pushed laterally until the left margin of the thecal sac and left T9–T11 nerve roots were visible. The nerve roots were ligated. After carefully releasing the adhesion with the dura, near the T10/T11 neural foramen, the tumor mass was taken out en bloc (Figs. 9.5 and 9.6).

The inferior endplate of T8 and the superior endplate of T12 were decorticated using a curette, and a 15-mm titanium cage with allografted bone was placed between T8 and T12. The left connecting rod was placed and locked in, with compression between T8 and T12. Two cross-links were used to brace the construct. In order to repair the defect in the left thoracic wall from the 10-cm resection on the 9th, 10th, and 11th ribs, two titanium rods mimicking the contour of ribs were connected to the left rod using dominos (Fig. 9.7). A hernia repair film was sutured to the rib rods and a chest tube was placed (Fig. 9.8). Our plastic surgeon colleagues used a retrograde latissimus dorsi musculocutaneous flap to repair the large paraspinal soft-tissue defect (Fig. 9.9). One Jackson-Pratt drain was placed underneath the surgical wound and one under the donor site.

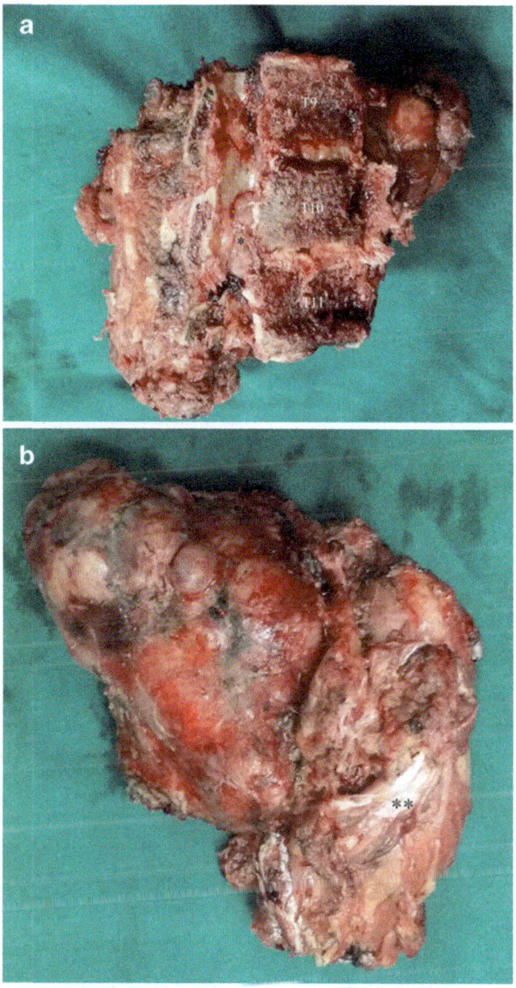

Fig. 9.5 Photographs of the removed specimen. (**a**) Sagittal view. The star (*) shows the tumor in T10 – T11 intervertebral foramen. (**b**) Lateral view. The double star (**) shows the iliocostalis thoracis embracing the tumor inside

Clinical Outcome

The patient was neurologically intact following the surgery. Within the first week, the chest tube and drains were discontinued and the patient began to ambulate. Postoperative X-ray and CT confirmed implant position (Fig. 9.10), and pathology review of the margins was negative for invasion of the tumor capsule. The patient was doing well 8 months postoperatively, with no signs of tumor recurrence or complication.

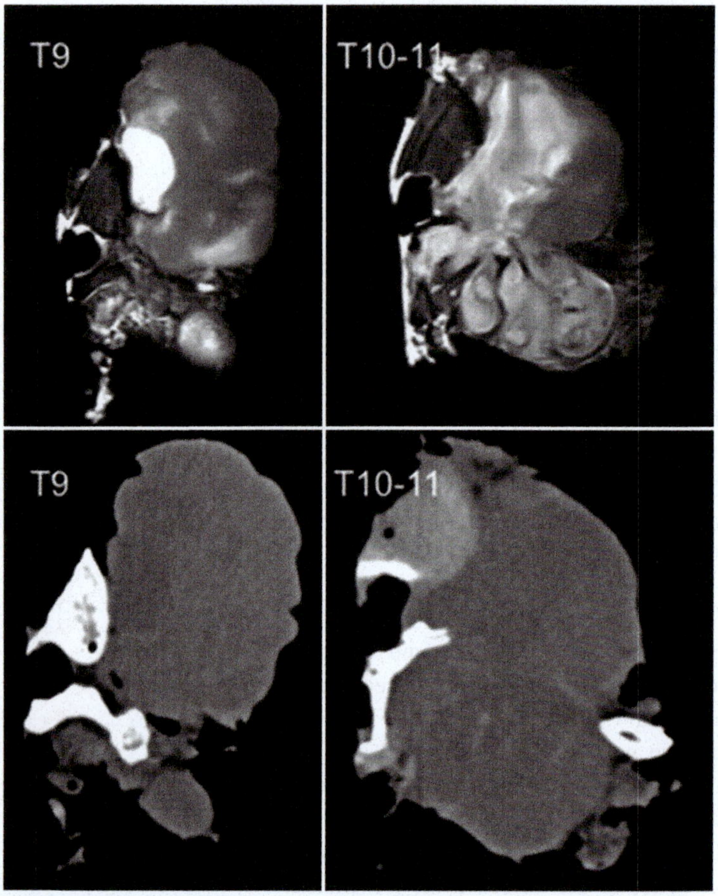

Fig. 9.6 Magnetic resonance of the removed specimen (the above two images) and computed tomography of the specimen (the below two images)

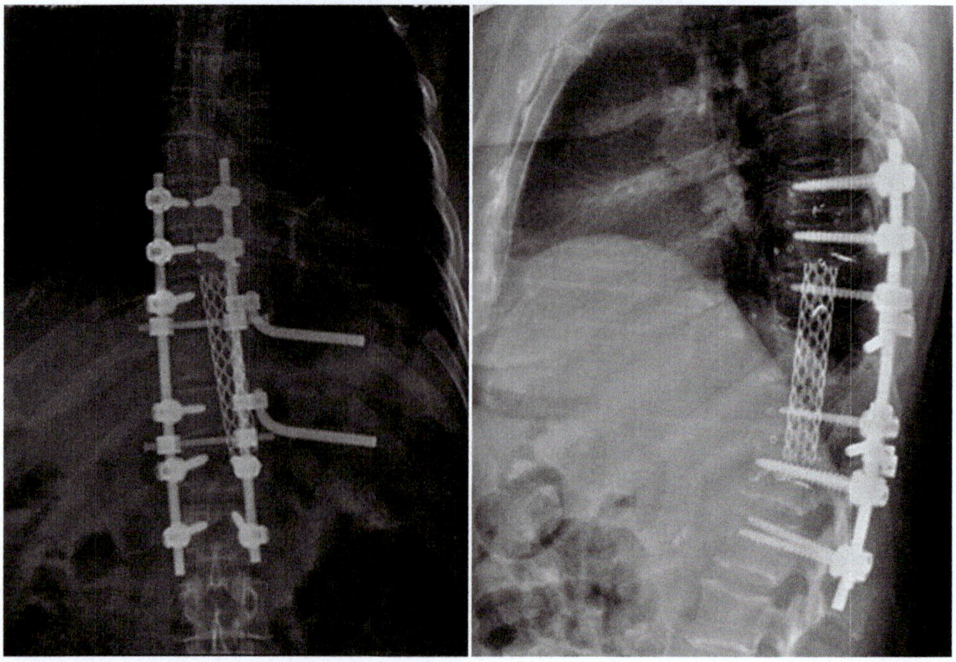

Fig. 9.7 The X-ray film of the final construct

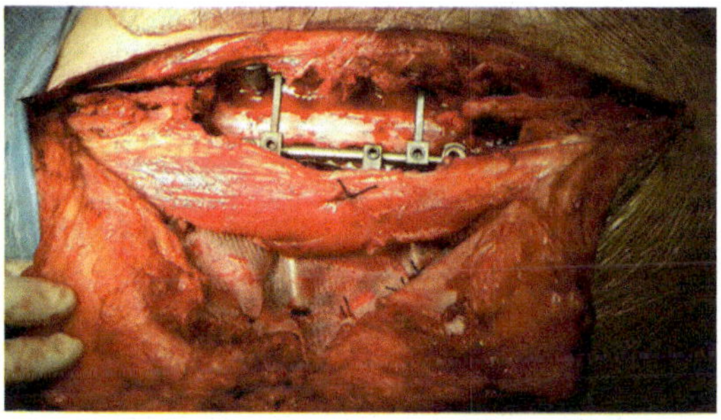

Fig. 9.8 Operative photograph of the surgery of the posterior approach

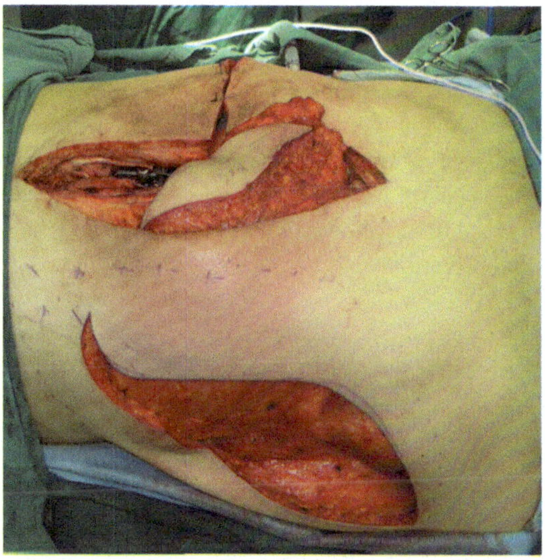

Fig. 9.9 Operative photograph of retrograde latissimus dorsi myocutaneous flap

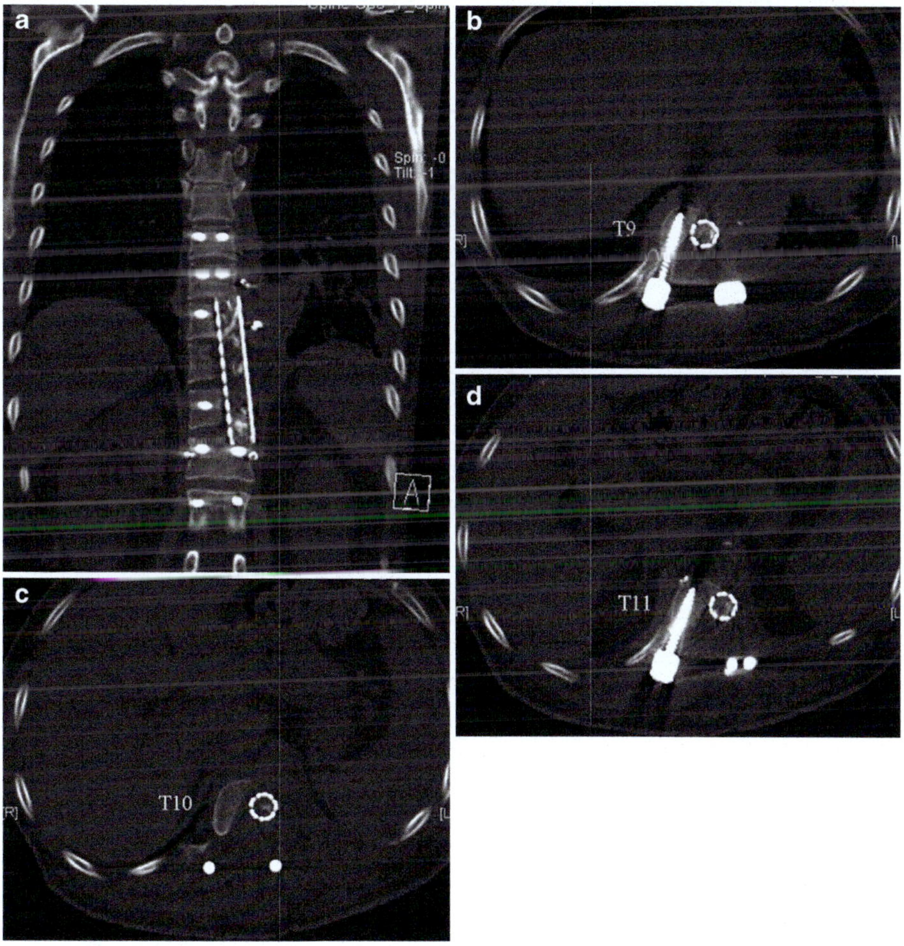

Fig. 9.10 The computed tomography of the final construct. (**a**) Coronal view. (**b**) Axial view of T9 level. (**c**) Axial view of T10 level. (**d**) Axial view of T11 level

Conclusion

Large thoracolumbar tumors involving at least three levels could be removed according to the WBB guidelines as staged procedures. An anterolateral trans-thoracic release could be performed first, followed by a posterior en bloc sagittal resection.

References

1. Vollmer DG, Banister WM. Thoracolumbar spinal anatomy. Neurosurg Clin N Am. 1997;8:443–53.
2. Willard FH, Vleeming A, Schuenke MD, Danneels L, Schleip R. The thoracolumbar fascia: anatomy, function and clinical considerations. J Anat. 2012;221:507–36.
3. Baaj AA, Papadimitriou K, Amin AG, Kretzer RM, Wolinsky JP, Gokaslan ZL. Surgical anatomy of the diaphragm in the anterolateral approach to the spine: a cadaveric study. J Spinal Disord Tech. 2014;27:220–3.
4. du Plessis M, Ramai D, Shah S, Holland JD, Tubbs RS, Loukas M. The clinical anatomy of the musculotendinous part of the diaphragm. Surg Radiol Anat. 2015;37(9):1013–20.
5. Lumsden AB, Colborn GL, Sreeram S, Skandalakis LJ. The surgical anatomy and technique of the thoracoabdominal incision. Surg Clin North Am. 1993;73:633–44.
6. Konig MA, Milz S, Bayley E, Boszczyk BM. The direct anterior approach to the thoracolumbar junction: an anatomical feasibility study. Eur Spine J. 2014;23:2265–71.
7. Dakwar E, Ahmadian A, Uribe JS. The anatomical relationship of the diaphragm to the thoracolumbar junction during the minimally invasive lateral extracoelomic (retropleural/retroperitoneal) approach. J Neurosurg Spine. 2012;16:359–64.
8. Fahim DK, Kim SD, Cho D, Lee S, Kim DH. Avoiding abdominal flank bulge after anterolateral approaches to the thoracolumbar spine: cadaveric study and electrophysiological investigation. J Neurosurg Spine. 2011;15:532–40.
9. Molina CA, Gokaslan ZL, Sciubba DM. Retroperitoneal approaches to the thoracolumbar spine. Neupsy key 2011. Available from: https://neupsykey.com/retroperitoneal-approaches-to-the-thoracolumbar-spine/
10. Fourney DR, Gokaslan ZL. Thoracolumbar spine: surgical treatment of metastatic disease. Curr Opin Orthop. 2003;14:144–52.
11. Walsh GL, Gokaslan ZL, McCutcheon IE, Mineo MT, Yasko AW, Swisher SG, et al. Anterior approaches to the thoracic spine in patients with cancer: indications and results. Ann Thorac Surg. 1997;64:1611–8.

10 Retroperitoneal Approach to the Lumbar Spine: A Case-Based Approach for Primary Tumor

Étienne Bourassa-Moreau, Joel Gagnon, and Charles G. Fisher

Introduction

Primary spinal tumors are rare, require precise oncological margins, and are associated with difficult anatomy, thus placing their surgical management at the highest level of complexity. Several validated classifications have been developed to help guide the spine surgeon in the management of these challenging tumors. The Enneking classification [1] uses histological grade, local extent, and the presence of distant metastasis to guide in selecting the appropriate oncological margin to be achieved. Applying Enneking's principles has shown the best outcomes with regard to local recurrence and survival [2]. Once the appropriate oncological margin is determined, the Weinstein-Boriani-Biagini (WBB) [1] classification is used to plan the technical aspect and feasibility of the surgical resection (Fig. 10.1).

Surgical planning for a primary lumbar spine tumor frequently requires anterior access. Therefore, the surgical team must have a deep understanding of the anatomy, surgical techniques, and pitfalls of the anterior retroperitoneal approach.

É. Bourassa-Moreau
Hôpital du Sacré-Coeur de Montréal, Department of Orthopaedic Surgery, Montreal, Canada

J. Gagnon
Vancouver General Hospital, Department of Vascular Surgery, Vancouver, BC, Canada

C. G. Fisher (✉)
Vancouver General Hospital, Department of Orthopaedics, Division of Spine, Vancouver, BC, Canada
e-mail: Charles.Fisher@vch.ca

Planning Principles

A precise common terminology for oncologic resection is key for appropriate surgical planning and communication among a multidisciplinary team. The resection strategy is based on the margins to be achieved as dictated by the Enneking classification. The potential margins are intralesional, marginal, and wide, with the latter two being the standard for aggressive benign or malignant primary spine tumors.

Intralesional resection means the tumor is removed within its margins. This resection strategy can be achieved by various techniques including curettage, piecemeal resection, gross total resection, or debulking. With intralesional resection, microscopic and possibly macroscopic tumors are left behind, and any chance of tumor-free margin is lost.

Wide or marginal margins are achieved through en bloc resection. This means the tumor is removed in one piece fully encased in a cuff of healthy tissue (wide margin) or along the tumor capsule (marginal margin). In the spine, the resection is often a combination of wide and marginal (marginal along critical structures such as the dura). Despite the surgeon's impression being important, the resection margins can only be confirmed by an experienced musculoskeletal pathologist (Fig. 10.2).

D. M. Sciubba (ed.), *Spinal Tumor Surgery*, https://doi.org/10.1007/978-3-319-98422-3_10

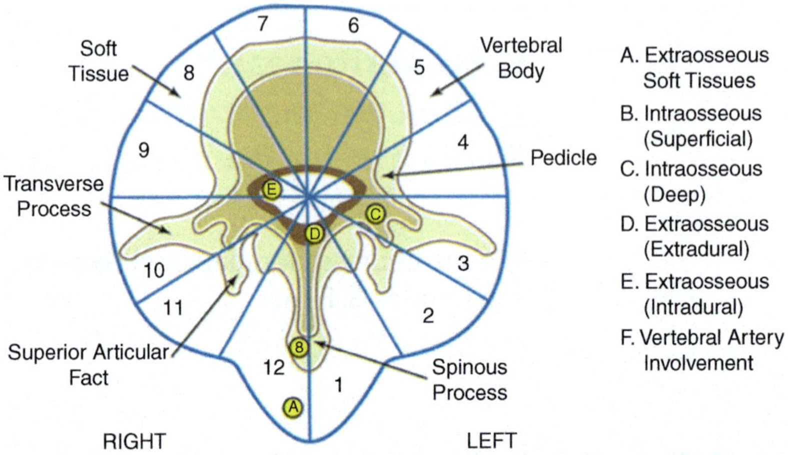

Fig. 10.1 Weinstein-Boriani-Biagini diagram. The vertebra is divided into 12 radiating sectors. These sectors are numbered going counter-clockwise from the left side of the spinous process (sector 1) to the right side of the spinous process (sector 12). The tumor is further divided into five concentric layers in an alphabetical order from the periphery to the center

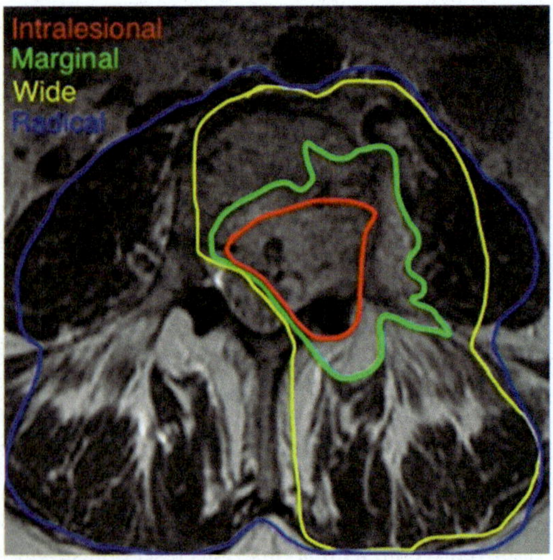

Fig. 10.2 Different types of resection based on margins. From the center to the periphery: intralesional—violates the tumor margin; marginal—along the pseudocapsule; wide—outside the pseudocapsule; radical—the whole compartment is excised

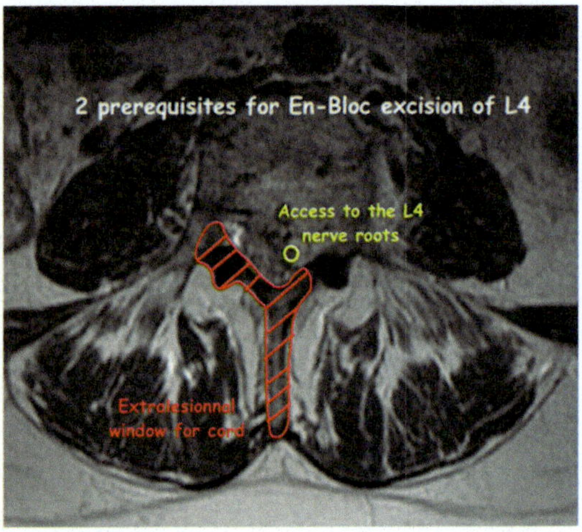

Fig. 10.3 In this case, the two prerequisites for en bloc resection of the L4 vertebra were met with the obligatory sacrifice of the L4 left nerve root

In the spine, the two prerequisites for en bloc delivery of a tumor are as follows:

1. Enough of the vertebral ring can be removed outside the tumor margins to create a window allowing safe delivery of the tumor without traction on the spinal cord/cauda.
2. Any nerve root involved with the tumor can be accessed outside the tumor margin to be tied off at the dura and cut.

Planning for en bloc resection requires careful analysis of three-dimensional imaging (CT and MRI scan) (Fig. 10.3). Pathologist, oncologist, radiologist, and surgeon together determine the appropriate margins of resection for each specific tumor. This decision is based on the Enneking grade but also on the location of the tumor and the functional consequences of the resection.

Indications for Anterior Lumbar Retroperitoneal Approach

Expertise in both posterior and anterior approaches to the spine is essential to treat primary spinal tumors. The most common indication for the anterior retroperitoneal approach is en bloc resection of a tumor growing eccentrically anteriorly through the bone into the soft tissues (through layer A of WBB). In that scenario, the anterior approach is necessary to provide adequate direct visual control of the surgical margins over the sectors 5 to 8. Another indication is a single anterior approach to enable en bloc resection of a small tumor in the vertebral body of the lumbar spine (sectors 5 to 8).

Surgical Anatomy of the Anterior Lumbar Retroperitoneal Approach

The patient is generally positioned supine for the anterior retroperitoneal approach for oncologic resections. Although a lazy lateral positioning can be used for thoracoabdominal exposure in other circumstances (trauma, deformity, and infection), it is generally not used in tumor because the lateral position renders the dissection of the contralateral side technically more demanding.

Lumbar lordosis makes approaching the upper lumbar vertebra (L1–L2–L3) easier. The amount of lordosis can be controlled with an inflatable bag positioned under the lumbar spine or by breaking the table in extension.

The side of the retroperitoneal anterior approach is dictated by the location of the tumor and the anticipated difficulty of the dissection. Sectors 4 to 6 are best approached from the left, whereas sectors 7 to 9 are best approached from the right.

The incision of the posterior sheet of the transversalis fascia gives access to the retroperitoneal space. During this dissection, the rectus is retracted medially to allow surgical access in line with the retroperitoneal plane (Fig. 10.4).

During the retroperitoneal dissection, the surgeon should routinely identify important structures including the psoas, the lateral femoral cutaneous nerve, the genitofemoral nerve (GFN), sympathetic trunk, the ureter, and the major vascular structures (aorta, inferior vena cava, iliac vessels, the segmental vessels, and the iliolumbar vein) [3] (Fig. 10.5).

Because psoas is palpated blindly with finger dissection, it is a key landmark early in the approach.

The lateral femoral cutaneous nerve (LFCN) pierces out of the psoas muscle at the L3–L4 levels and generally travels on the lateral margin of the psoas. The genitofemoral nerve should be identified on the anterior aspect of the psoas below the L2–L3 disc level where it exits. Its location relative to the psoas can vary, but the GFN is commonly found close to the medial margin of the psoas [4]. Stretching or laceration of the GFN and LFCN can cause postoperative numbness and anesthesia.

The sympathetic trunk can be identified at the medial margin of the psoas or slightly more medially over the lumbar spine (see Fig. 10.5). It runs under the iliac vessels below the L4–L5 level. However, the sympathetic trunk can be displaced further medially by osteophytes or tumor [5]. When the surgical resection allows, the surgeon should preserve the sympathetic trunk to avoid postoperative hypotension (bilateral injuries) or local vasodilation and dryness of the skin (unilateral injuries).

The ureter is a small translucent tubular structure that can easily be overlooked if not formally identified. Most often, the ureter remains adherent to the parietal peritoneum as it gets lifted away from the psoas, but adherences could alter this relationship. Therefore, ureter peristalsis (Kelly sign) is very helpful for identification. Ureteral injury is uncommon but a challenging condition to diagnose and treat [6, 7]. The absence of a urine leak cannot be used as a reliable sign to rule out injury. Therefore, if a ureteral injury is suspected intraoperatively, the spine surgeon should seek urology consultation immediately. Once peripheral nerves and ureter are identified, vascular structures can be mobilized.

Vascular structures should be swept away from the spine without any tension or resistance. Anticipating pathological and congenital anomalies of vascular anatomy is critical to execute the anterior retroperitoneal approach safely. Surgical planning routinely includes the review of the CT angiography. Vascular calcifications and osteophytes near vascular structures increase the risk of vascular injury during mobilization and are both common findings in elderly patients [8].

All segmental vessels in the surgical field should be identified in the mid-valleys of the

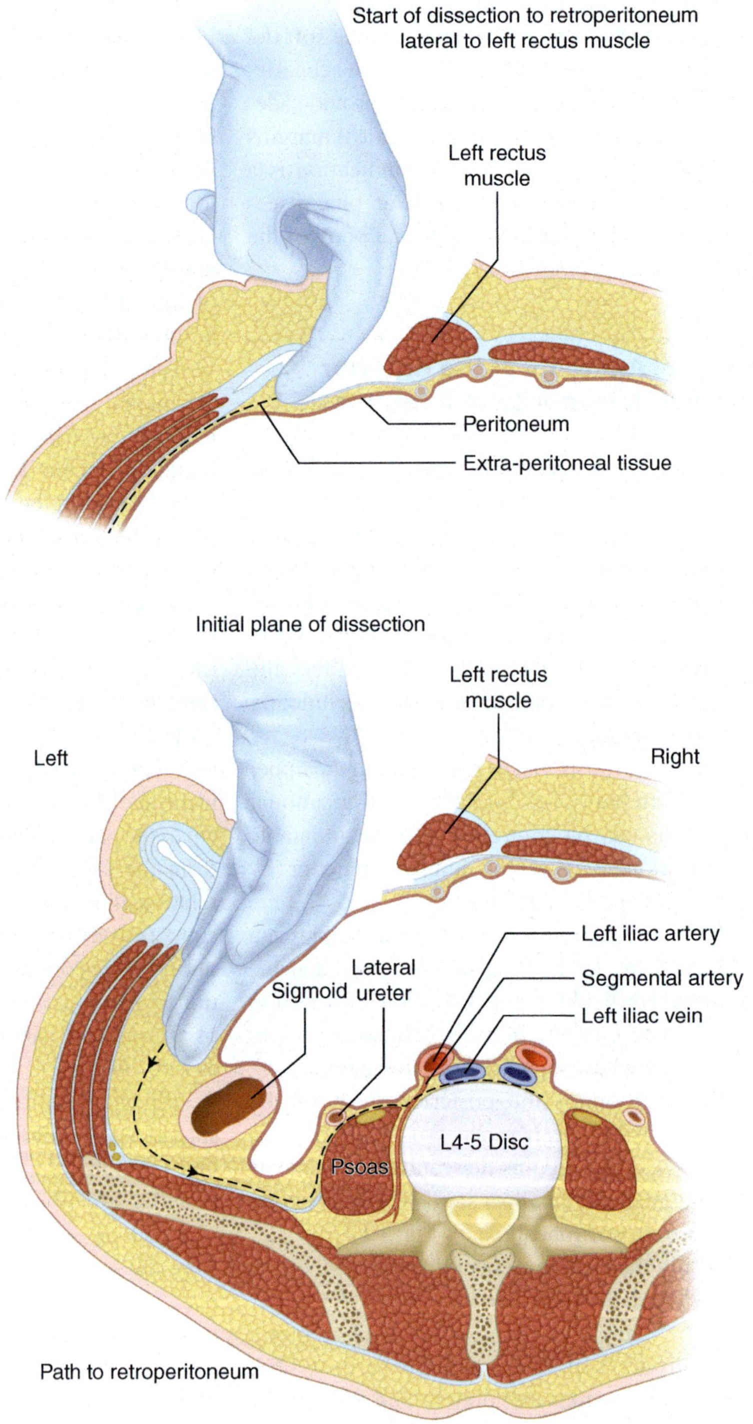

Fig. 10.4 The access to the retroperitoneal space is obtained after the incision of the posterior sheet of the transversalis. Note that the dissection is carried laterally to the rectus to avoid tension on it. (Reprinted from Brau [3], Copyright 2002, with permission from Elsevier)

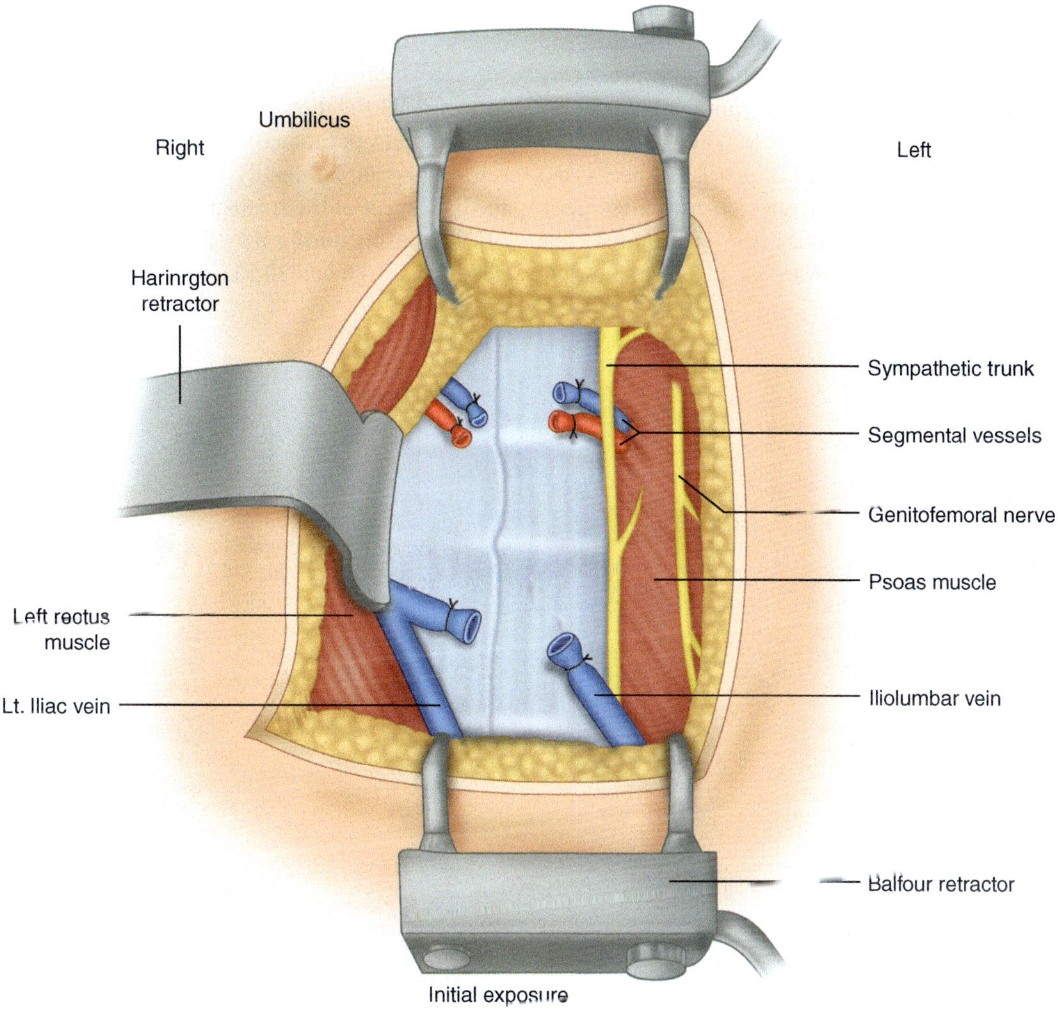

Fig. 10.5 Critical structures of the retroperitoneal space. Ilio-lumbar vein and segmental vessels are tied and sectioned. Note that this anatomy can be modified by congenital anomaly, degenerative process, and by the tumor itself. (Reprinted from Brau [3], Copyright 2002, with permission from Elsevier)

vertebral bodies and ligated using vascular clips. It is safe to get at least one fingerbreadth between the veins and the vertebra all the way in front of the vertebra and to the opposite side.

Specific Considerations by Level

The exposure of L5–S1 level requires dissection of the iliac bifurcation and ligation of the middle sacral artery. The iliac bifurcation lies in close proximity with the hypogastric plexus. In males, the hypogastric plexus should be protected to prevent retrograde ejaculation [3]. In addition, the spermatic cord in males should be mobilized carefully when approaching L5–S1 in order to prevent excessive traction that can cause thrombosis of artery.

Access to the L4–L5 disc involves the mobilization of the common iliac vessels and the ligation of ilio-lumbar vein. The ilio-lumbar vein drains the L5 vertebrae into the inferior vena cava (IVC). If not properly identified and ligated, the retraction of the ilio-lumbar vein can cause tear at the back of the IVC. Surgeons should be aware of common anatomical variation of the ilio-lumbar vein, with up to 25% of patients having multiple veins [9]. The plane between the vein and the artery needs to be dissected with great care because this plane can be quite inflamed and tedious.

When access to L1, L2, and L3 is necessary, mobilization of the pancreas, superior mesenteric arteries, and renal arteries is often required. The surgeon should be aware of possible multiple (polar) renal arteries or the left retroaortic renal artery [10]. If a polar artery needed to be ligated for access, this would inevitably engender some loss of renal function.

Once retroperitoneal dissection is completed, retractors can be finally re-positioned on the medial aspect of the rectus to release the tension off the muscle during the other steps of the surgery (Figs. 10.6 and 10.7).

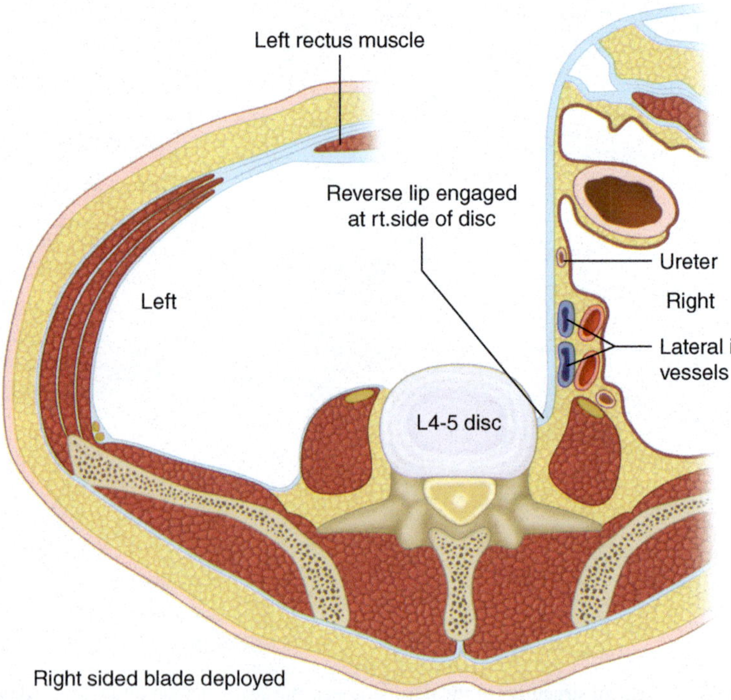

Fig. 10.6 Positioning of a retractor blade during the left retroperitoneal approach of a normal spine. Note that the blade of the retractor is re-positioned medial to the rectus muscle. Vascular structure needs to be mobilized safely to achieve this retraction. (Reprinted from Brau [3], Copyright 2002, with permission from Elsevier)

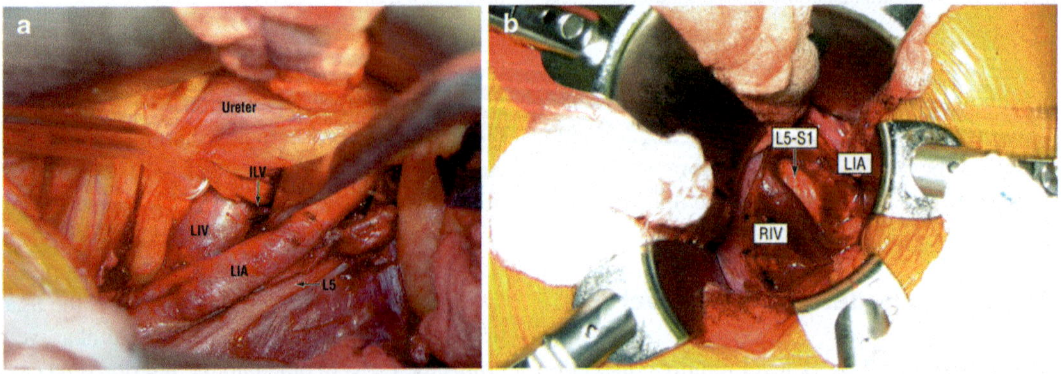

Fig. 10.7 Intraoperative images of the retroperitoneal exposure to the lumbar spine with the patient's head pointed to the upper left of the image. A. Lateral retraction of the left common iliac artery exposes the common iliac vein. B. The L5–S1 disc space is located between the left common iliac artery and right common iliac vein. LIV: left common iliac vein; LIA: left common iliac artery; ILV: ileolumbar vein; RIV: right common iliac vein. (Reproduced with permission from JAMA Surgery. 2005. 140(4): 339–343. Copyright©(2005) American Medical Association. All rights reserved)

Complications

Postoperative adverse events in oncologic spine surgery are extremely common, especially for en bloc resection [11, 12]. The surgeon performing the anterior retroperitoneal approach of the lumbar spine should be able to screen, identify, and manage the approach-specific postoperative complications.

Although rare, arterial thrombosis or dissection can be devastating, especially if the diagnosis is delayed [13]. During surgery, limb perfusion can be monitored with an oxy-meter usually secured on the great toe. Postoperative palpation of peripheral pulses is routinely performed, and any anomaly warrants immediate arterial Doppler or angiography. Urgent vascular surgery consultation is mandatory for possible thrombectomy or stent angioplasty.

Significant risk of developing deep vein thrombosis after spine surgery for tumor implies routine postoperative thromboprophylaxis to start once the surgeon feels it is safe. A high level of suspicion and aggressive screening are also necessary.

Rectus abdominis muscle paralysis can occur when wide exposure from lateral dissection occurs. This exposure could result in injury of multiple lateral terminal branches of the intercostal nerve. Therefore, wide lateral exposure of the rectus should be avoided and replaced by an approach medial to the muscle. Postoperative ileus tends to happen with intraperitoneal procedures, but rarely with retroperitoneal approaches. Therefore, when ileus is present, incisional herniation should be ruled out with a CT scan.

Case Description: History, Examination, and Radiological Diagnosis

A 38-year-old female sought medical attention after a 9-month history of progressive low back pain associated with a left L4 radiculopathy. She denied any night pain or weight loss.

Her physical exam demonstrated some tenderness in the left lower lumbar region and normal neurology.

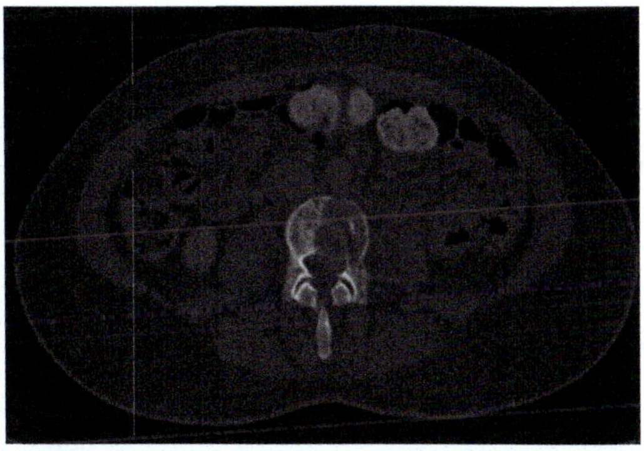

Fig. 10.8 Axial CT scan cut centered at the L4 pedicle level demonstrates the lytic lesion involving 50% of the vertebral body and expanding in the epidural space with obliteration of the left lateral recess

A CT scan showed a lytic lesion of the fourth lumbar vertebra involving over 50% of the vertebral body and sparing the disc spaces. The axial CT cut demonstrates stenosis of the left L4 lateral recess (Fig. 10.8).

The differential diagnosis included primary malignant or benign neoplastic lesion, lymphoma, multiple myeloma, and, less likely, metastasis.

Case Description: Staging

Local staging included a magnetic resonance imaging (MRI) that revealed a large L4 mass expanding through to the anterior soft tissue on the left side, left anterior epidural space, and obliterating the left L4–L5 foramen (Fig. 10.9). It was noted that the aorta was in close relation with the left anterior tumor expansion (Fig. 10.10). Systemic staging included bloodwork, bone scan, and chest and abdo-pelvis CT scan. Pancreatic tumor and benign intracranial and intramedullary tumors were found. Lastly, a percutaneous transpedicular CT-guided biopsy was performed using a posterolateral trajectory to enable subsequent removal of the biopsy tract during tumor resection (see Fig. 10.10).

The case was subjected to multidisciplinary tumor board. Final pathology report confirmed a clear cell chondrosarcoma grade 1/3. The incidental findings of a pancreatic tumor and benign

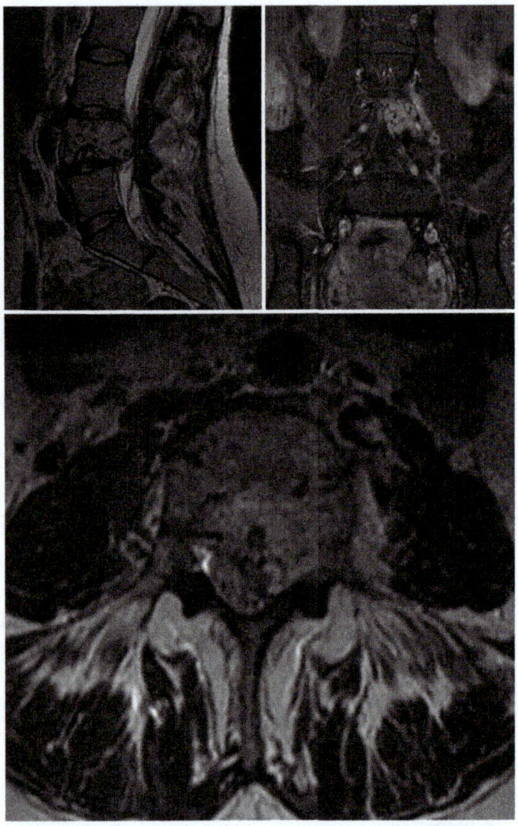

Fig. 10.9 Sagittal, coronal, and axial MRI cuts of T2 sequences centered on the lumbar spine. The left L4 nerve root is encased in the epidural and foraminal extension of the tumor. The axial cuts clearly demonstrate the expansion of the tumor is in close relation with the dura, the left psoas, and the aorta

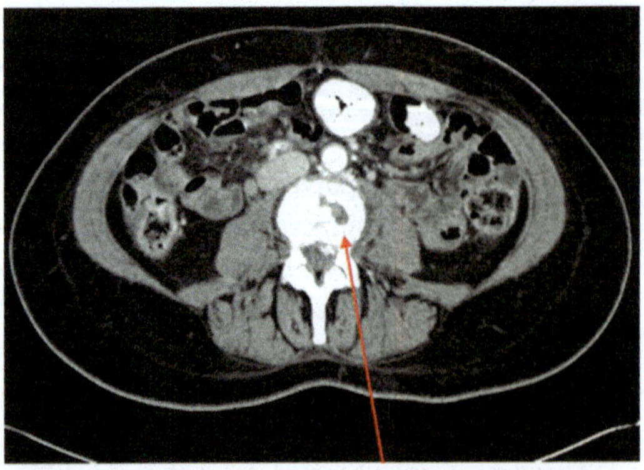

Fig. 10.10 Transpedicular CT-guided biopsy tract was planned to be excisable at the time of surgery

intracranial and intramedullary tumors were in keeping with the diagnosis of Von Hippel-Lindau syndrome [14]. The syndrome was considered as unrelated to the chondrosarcoma by the genetic and medicine teams. The case was categorized as Enneking IIB (low-grade extracompartmental with no local or distant metastasis). Accordingly, the consensus of the multidisciplinary team was for wide/marginal surgical resection of the tumor in an en bloc fashion and postoperative proton beam radiation (Fig. 10.11).

Case Description: Surgical Planning

The two prerequisites for en bloc resection were met. The tumor was confined within sectors 2 to 7 (layers A to D) of the L4 vertebra so that sectors 8 to 1 are disease free, providing an appropriate tumor-free window. The left L4 nerve root was encased in tumor at the level of the foramen (Fig. 10.12) and therefore needed to

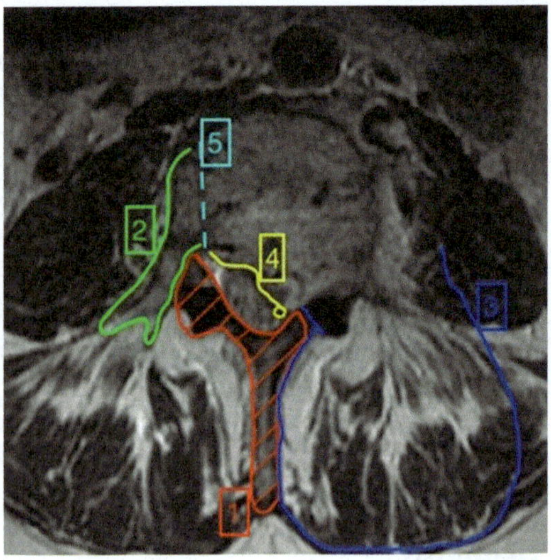

Fig. 10.11 Planning of the posterior approach; the dissection is divided into critical steps. (1) Piecemeal resection of the posterior arch sectors 11 to 1. (2) Sub-periosteal dissection of sectors 8 to 10. (3) Dissection through the posterior muscle of sectors 2 and 3. (4) Release of the dura from the tumor and section of the left L4 nerve root. (5) Sagittal osteotomy. (6) Cranial and caudal osteotomies (not shown)

be sacrificed. Access to tie off the L4 nerve root in the epidural space could be achieved without entering the tumor. The resection margins were in close proximity anteriorly with the aorta (sector 6, layer A) and medially with the dura (zones 3 to 7, layer D). Accordingly, the surgical team was prepared to include the dura and/or the aorta within the resection margins and, if needed, reconstruct these structures at the time of surgery.

The posterior approach was planned first with the following goals to achieve (Fig. 10.13):

1. Resection of the posterior arch not involved in the tumor (sectors 11 to 1).
2. Subperiosteal dissection of sectors 8 to 10.
3. Wide (layer a) dissection through the posterior muscle covering the tumor (sectors 2 and 3).
4. Release of the dura from the tumor and section of the L4 nerve root crossing the tumor.
5. Perform a sagittal osteotomy of the right fourth of the vertebral body.
6. Define the upper and lower margins with osteotomies through the lower L3 endplate and upper L5 endplate (not shown in Fig. 10.12).

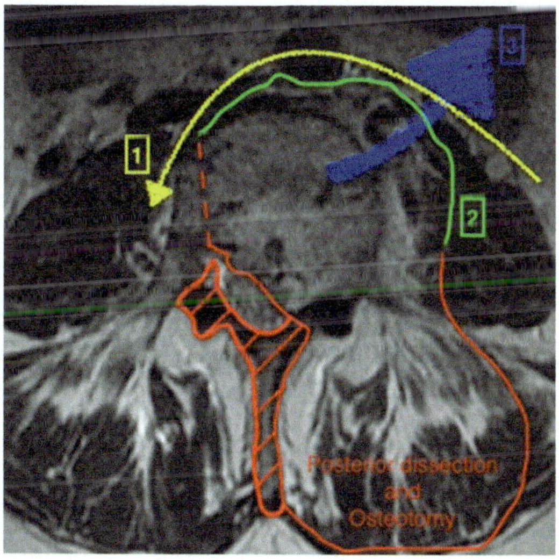

Fig. 10.12 Planning of the anterior approach. (1) Anterior retroperitoneal approach. (2) Wide margin dissection over the sectors 3 to 7 (through psoas, the possibility of resection of the aorta to obtain a disease-free margin was anticipated) with surgical section of the left L4 nerve root lateral to the tumor. (3) En bloc removal of the tumor. (4) Reconstruction of the anterior column (not shown)

The second stage of the case included a left-sided anterior lumbar retroperitoneal approach with the following goals to achieve (Fig. 10.14):

1. Identification and protection of critical retroperitoneal structures adjacent to the spine.
2. Appropriate wide margin over the tumor through the left psoas, possibly through the aorta and sacrifice of L4 root lateral to tumor.
3. Removal of the tumor in an en bloc fashion.
4. Reconstruction of the anterior column.

Case Description: Procedure

The en bloc resection was planned for 2 days, with the patient staying intubated for observation in the

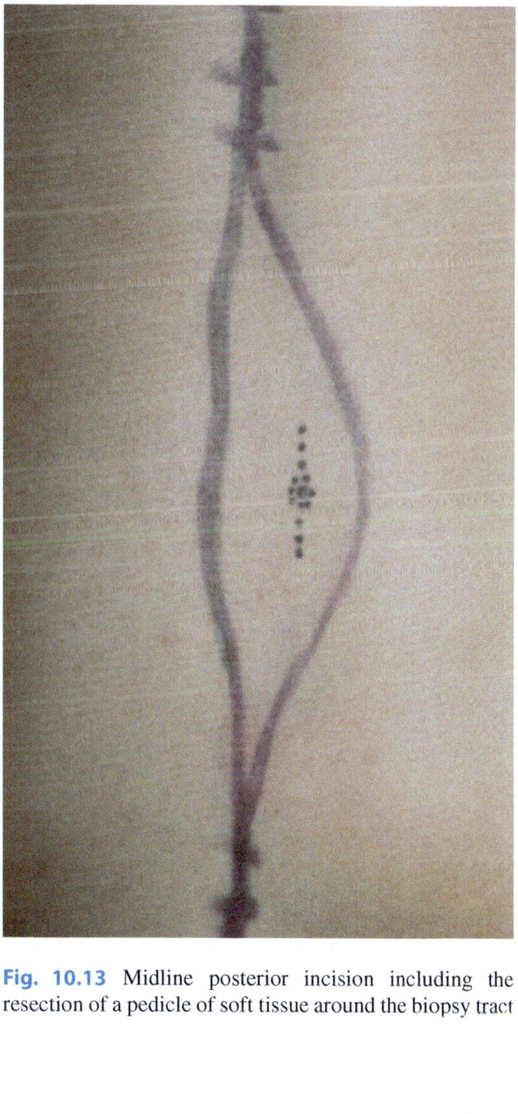

Fig. 10.13 Midline posterior incision including the resection of a pedicle of soft tissue around the biopsy tract

recovery room overnight. The posterior approach was carried out on day 1 and the anterior approach on day 2. The surgical team included two oncological spinal surgeons, one plastic surgeon, and one vascular surgeon.

Case Description: Posterior Approach

First, a tri-corticated iliac crest bone graft was harvested through a separate incision over the iliac crest. The graft was stored and the wound closed. The midline incision was then planned so that musculocutaneous tissues around the biopsy tract could be resected (see Fig. 10.14). The exposure was planned to give access to the pedicle entry points of L2–S1, and pedicle screws were inserted at all these levels except for L4. Importantly, posterior dissection of L4 on the left side (sectors 2 and 3) was carried out through a large cuff of healthy-looking multifidus and longissimus (layer A).

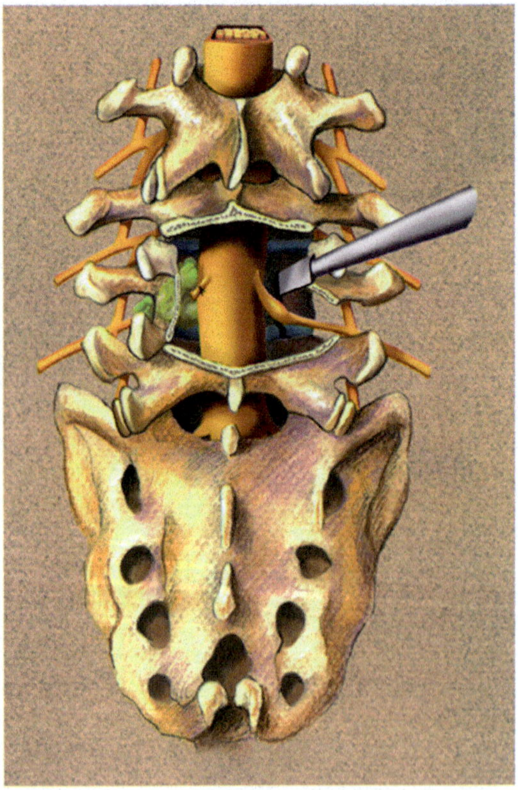

Fig. 10.14 Artistic representation of the extent of posterior piecemeal resection, posterior dissection, identification of nerve roots, and sagittal osteotomy. Note that the left L4 nerve root is tied and sectioned. The L3 and L5 posterior elements are disconnected of L4, but the left L4–L5 joint was left intact to resect the tumor's margin. (Figure courtesy of Charles G. Fisher, MD)

The right side of the L4 posterior elements was resected in a piecemeal fashion, away from the tumor (sectors 11 to 1). This resection also involved L3 pars osteotomies and disconnection of the L4–L5 facet joints to fully release L4 from the posterior elements. (see Fig. 10.14) Following the piecemeal resection, the right side of the L4 vertebral body (sectors 8 to 10) was bluntly dissected using a Penfield 1 and cautery. Gauzes were placed and left and would be recovered during the anterior approach.

Careful circumferential dissection of the epidural plane was done from L3 to L5. Although in close relation to the tumor (sectors 3 to 9, layer D), the epidural plane was easily developed outside the tumor margin. The L3, L4, and L5 nerve roots were all identified and followed laterally to the psoas, mobilized, and tagged with vessel loops with the exception of the left L4 nerve root. The left L4 nerve root was tied off and sectioned proximal to entering the foramen, in the epidural space.

Using straight osteotomes, three sagittal osteotomies were performed to isolate the tumor. The first sagittal osteotomy was performed just medial to the right pedicle through the L4 vertebral body (see Fig. 10.13).

Second, the L4 vertebral body was disconnected cranially and caudally by dissection through the inferior endplate of the L3 disc and the superior endplate of the L5 disc (Fig. 10.15).

Third, the posterior release of the L4 vertebral body from the ventral aspect of the dura was completed. This release is often difficult with several planes. All the Hoffman ligaments must be released to ensure a smooth en bloc delivery during the second anterior approach. Pedicle screws were connected to rods, and the wound was irrigated and closed with the help of the plastic surgery team. Drains were left in place and secured under the sterile dressing.

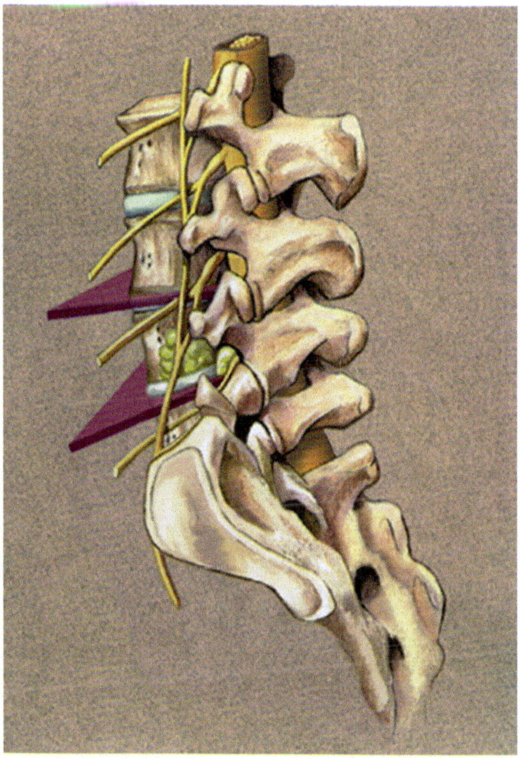

Fig. 10.15 Artistic representation of the osteotomy planes above and below the L4 vertebral compartment. (Figure courtesy of Charles G. Fisher, MD)

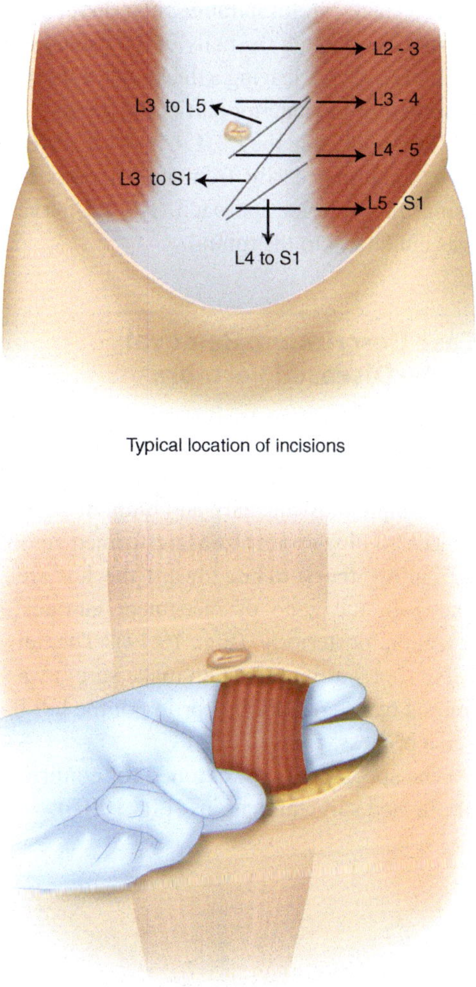

Fig. 10.16 Landmarks for cutaneous skin incision and circumferential mobilization of the rectus early during the exposure allow for manipulating it. (Reprinted from Brau [3], Copyright 2002, with permission from Elsevier)

Case Description: Anterior Retroperitoneal Approach

Between the first and the second stage of the surgery, the patient remained intubated and sedated in the recovery room. The patient was positioned supine on a radiolucent table. The operating surgeon stood on the left side of the patient (side of the retroperitoneal approach), and the assisting surgeon stood on the right side. A pulse oxymeter was placed on the left great toe.

In this case, a left oblique incision was used running from the midline (at the level of L5–S1) to the lateral edge of the left rectus (at the level of L2–L3) (Fig. 10.16). The incision was carried down, and the rectus sheet was incised obliquely. The rectus was mobilized from this sheet circumferentially. Dissection was performed carefully not to injure the epigastric vessels that run against the posterior aspect of the rectus.

The retroperitoneal space was bluntly dissected down to the psoas. Critical neural structures were identified. Localizing X-ray with a radio-opaque marker in a normal vertebral body confirmed the levels. Surgical section of L3, L4, and L5 segmental vessels and the ilio-lumbar vein allowed to analyze the plane between major vessels and the vertebra. The surgical dissection was performed carefully, starting from the normal tissue cranially and caudally to the tumor (L3 and L5) and moving carefully toward L4. There was a clear plane between the aorta, IVC, and common iliac vessels, precluding the need for vascular resection (sectors 6 and 7, layer A). The gauzes packed during the posterior approach were recovered under the right psoas. Then, careful intramuscular dissection was carried out through the belly of the psoas (sectors 5 and 4, layer A), leaving a thick cuff of the normal muscle over the anterior part of the tumor.

On the left side the L3, L4, and L5 nerve roots were identified easily from the markers placed using the posterior approach. The L4 nerve root was cut lateral to the tumor.

Case Description: Removal of the Diseased Vertebra

The cuts of the posterior osteotomies (sagittal, cranial, and caudal osteotomies) were identified and completed with sharp and blunt dissection.

The en bloc removal was performed smoothly by pulling the vertebra toward the left side, in line with the zone of piecemeal laminectomy resection posteriorly (Fig. 10.17). The left L3 nerve root was mobilized to make sure it was not injured by the remaining portion of the left transverse process.

The specimen was examined for confirmation of planned surgical margins (Fig. 10.18).

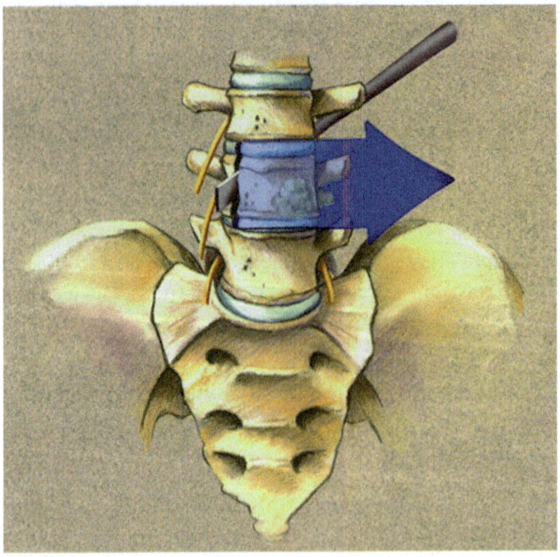

Fig. 10.17 Artistic representation of the direction of the en bloc delivery of the L4 vertebra. Note that the left L3 nerve root was mobilized posteriorly to the left transverse process to avoid excessive traction. The direction pull toward the left is in line with the extralesional window to avoid traction on the thecal sac. (Figure courtesy of Charles G. Fisher, MD)

The anterior column support was restored with a titanium cage filled with iliac crest bone graft (Figs. 10.19 and 10.20). The anterior dura was separated from the cage and bone graft by a piece of Gelfoam. Anteroposterior (AP) and lateral

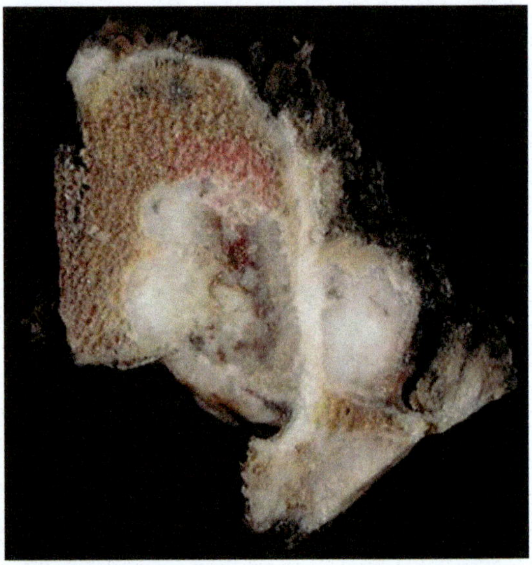

Fig. 10.18 Picture of the axial cut of the pathology specimen showing grayish-white, lobulated mass with focal calcification and necrosis of a chondrosarcoma. Note that the dissection in the left soft tissues (sectors 3 to 7) and the shape of the specimen correspond with the surgical planning in Fig. 10.8

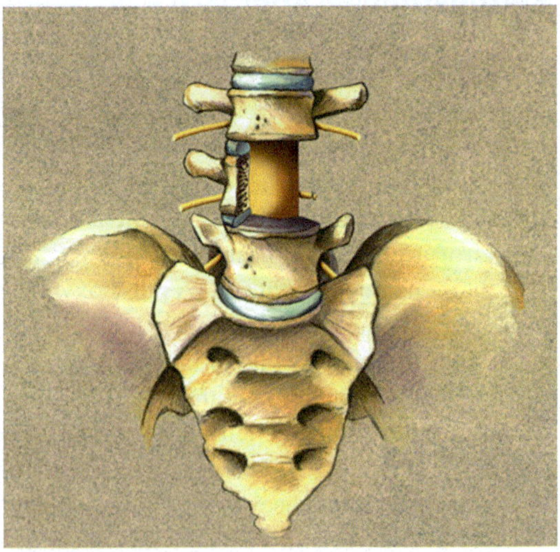

Fig. 10.19 Artistic representation of void created after the resection of the L4 vertebra. Note the left L4 nerve root tied proximally. (Figure courtesy of Charles G. Fisher, MD)

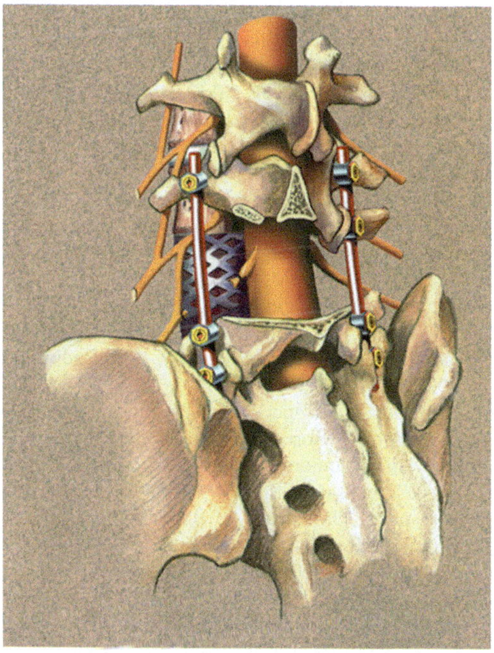

Fig. 10.20 Artistic representation of the reconstruction of the anterior column with a cage filled with bone graft and posterior pedicle instrumentation. (Figure courtesy of Charles G. Fisher, MD)

X-rays were obtained to confirm the appropriate position of the cage (Fig. 10.21). The wound was irrigated with free water and betadine before it was closed in layers.

Currently, an expandable PEEK cage would be used to facilitate placement and reduce imaging artifact.

Case Description: Postoperative Course

Postoperatively, the patient surprisingly had a right L4 neuropathy with an incomplete foot drop that fully recovered after 3 months. The patient had no significant impairment as a result of her left L4 nerve root sacrifice. The patient returned to all activities after 6 months.

The patient had a Whipple's procedure for her pancreatic tumor, without complication. The patient had 6-month imaging surveillance for 3 years and then yearly out to 10 years. There was no evidence of local recurrence or systemic disease.

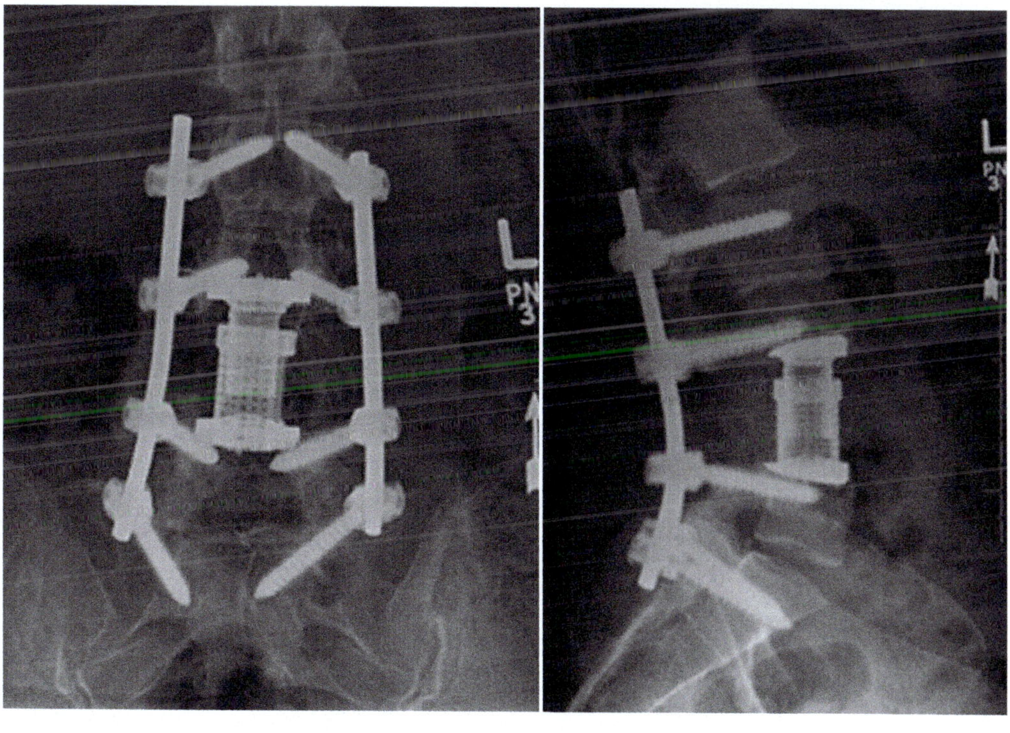

Fig. 10.21 Standing AP and lateral lumbar X-ray at the 8-year follow-up. The surgical instrumentation and posterior fusion were revised once because of nonunion. She otherwise had no local or systemic recurrence of her disease at the 8-year follow-up

References

1. Enneking WF, Spanier SS, Goodman MA. A system for the surgical staging of musculoskeletal sarcoma. Clin Orthop Relat Res. 1980;153:106–20.
2. Fisher CG, Saravanja DD, Dvorak MF, Rampersaud YR, Clarkson PW, Hurlbert J, et al. Surgical management of primary bone tumors of the spine: validation of an approach to enhance cure and reduce local recurrence. Spine (Phila Pa 1976). 2011;36(10):830–6.
3. Brau SA. Mini-open approach to the spine for anterior lumbar interbody fusion: description of the procedure, results and complications. Spine J. 2002;2(3):216–23.
4. Feigl GC, Dreu M, Ulz H, Breschan C, Maier C, Likar R. Susceptibility of the genitofemoral and lateral femoral cutaneous nerves to complications from lumbar sympathetic blocks: is there a morphological reason? Br J Anaesth. 2014;112(6):1098–104.
5. Feigl GC, Kastner M, Ulz H, Breschan C, Dreu M, Likar R. Topography of the lumbar sympathetic trunk in normal lumbar spines and spines with spondylophytes. Br J Anaesth. 2011;106(2):260–5.
6. Bjurlin MA, Rousseau LA, Vidal PP, Hollowell CM. Iatrogenic ureteral injury secondary to a thoracolumbar lateral revision instrumentation and fusion. Spine J. 2009;9(6):e13–5.
7. Isiklar ZU, Lindsey RW, Coburn M. Ureteral injury after anterior lumbar interbody fusion. A case report. Spine (Phila Pa 1976). 1996;21(20):2379–82.
8. Rothenfluh DA, Koenig M, Stokes OM, Behrbalk E, Boszczyk BM. Access-related complications in anterior lumbar surgery in patients over 60 years of age. Eur Spine J. 2014;23(Suppl 1):S86–92.
9. Nalbandian MM, Hoashi JS, Errico TJ. Variations in the iliolumbar vein during the anterior approach for spinal procedures. Spine (Phila Pa 1976). 2013;38(8):E445–50.
10. Satyapal KS, Haffejee AA, Singh B, Ramsaroop L, Robbs JV, Kalideen JM. Additional renal arteries: incidence and morphometry. Surg Radiol Anat. 2001;23(1):33–8.
11. Amendola L, Cappuccio M, De Iure F, Bandiera S, Gasbarrini A, Boriani S. En bloc resections for primary spinal tumors in 20 years of experience: effectiveness and safety. Spine J. 2014;14(11):2608–17.
12. Boriani S, Gasbarrini A, Bandiera S, Ghermandi R, Lador R. En bloc resections in the spine: the experience of 220 patients during 25 years. World Neurosurg. 2017;98:217–29.
13. Brau SA, Delamarter RB, Schiffman ML, Williams LA, Watkins RG. Vascular injury during anterior lumbar surgery. Spine J. 2004;4(4):409–12.
14. Maher ER, Yates JR, Harries R, Benjamin C, Harris R, Moore AT, et al. Clinical features and natural history of von Hippel-Lindau disease. Q J Med. 1990;77(283):1151–63.

Anterior Lumbar and Lumbosacral Approach: Transperitoneal

11

Cecilia L. Dalle Ore, Darryl Lau, and Christopher Pearson Ames

Case Presentation

A 57-year-old male presented with progressive low back pain resistant to nonsteroidal anti-inflammatory medications. Computed tomography (CT) and magnetic resonance imaging (MRI) demonstrated an expansile lesion involving the L2 vertebral body, epidural space, and the psoas muscle that was causing severe spinal canal stenosis (Figs. 11.1 and 11.2). On CT angiography, it was evident that the lesion was impinging upon the inferior vena cava as well. A CT-guided biopsy was performed, which showed the lesion to be a leiomyosarcoma. At this point, it was decided that a two-stage procedure was required for en bloc tumor resection. In addition, the patient would undergo phosphorus-32 (P-32) intraoperative implantation for radiation.

In the first stage, a posterior approach was used. Pedicle screws were placed from T12 to L4 (skipping L2), and osteotomies of the L1–L2 and L2–L3 facets were performed to allow for en bloc resection of the posterior elements of L2 (en bloc laminectomy and pediculectomy) and laminectomy of L1 and L3. The L1 and L2 nerve roots were resected proximal to the dorsal root ganglion, and a plane between the dura and the epidural tumor was developed in preparation for the second-stage anterior approach. Discectomies and resection of the posterior longitudinal ligament were carried out at the L1–L2 and L2–L3 levels. Rods were then contoured and secured to the pedicle screws, with additional satellite rods placed and locked to screws with locking caps. Posterolateral fusion from T12 to L4 was accomplished by decortication and placement of allograft, and the wound was closed.

The patient was then returned to the operating room for the planned second-stage anterior transperitoneal approach 2 days later. A vascular co-surgeon was involved for assistance in gaining anterior exposure to the lumbar spine. The abdomen was entered via a bilateral subcostal incision, and the retroperitoneum was exposed via a right visceral rotation, mobilizing the right colon, hepatic flexure, transverse colon, and duodenum superior to the left of the midline. The retroperitoneum was entered and the right kidney was mobilized posteriorly. The inferior vena cava (IVC) was isolated from the infrahepatic portion distal to nearly the caval bifurcation (Video 11.1), along with the left and right venal veins. The

Electronic Supplementary Material The online version of this chapter (https://doi.org/10.1007/978-3-319-98422-3_11) contains supplementary material, which is available to authorized users.

C. L. Dalle Ore · D. Lau · C. P. Ames (✉)
Department of Neurological Surgery, University of California, San Francisco, San Francisco, CA, USA
e-mail: christopher.ames@ucsf.edu

D. M. Sciubba (ed.), *Spinal Tumor Surgery*, https://doi.org/10.1007/978-3-319-98422-3_11

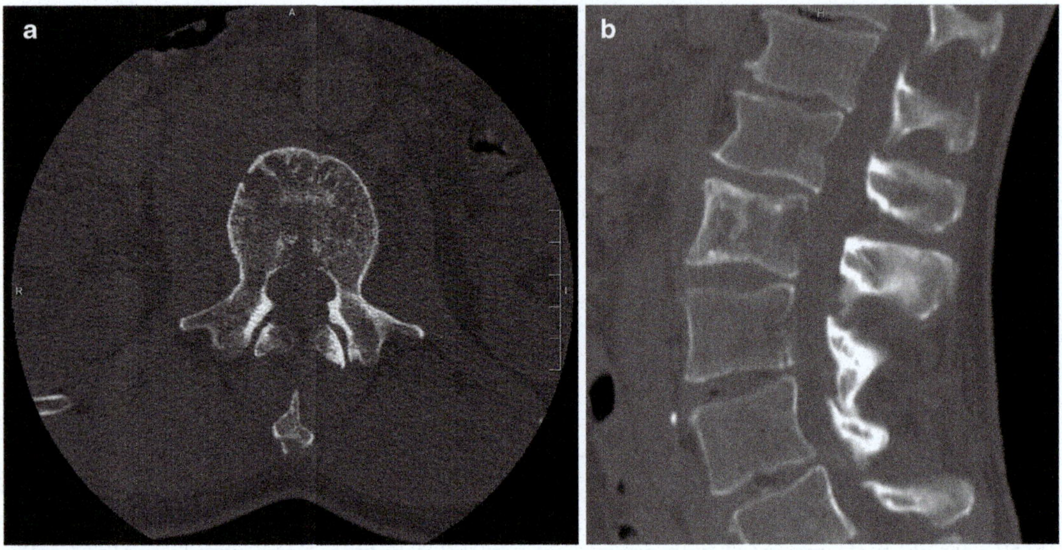

Fig. 11.1 Preoperative computed tomography of the lumbar spine demonstrating a destructive lesion of the L2 vertebral body. Axial lumbar CT demonstrating a destructive L2 vertebral body lesion with a right anterolateral prevertebral soft tissue component (**a**). Sagittal CT of the lumbar spine showing the same lytic lesion (**b**)

vena cava was separated from the tumor and mobilized away from the tumor. The lumbar arteries and the draining veins of the tumor were divided. The right renal artery and the aorta were then isolated to allow for complete exposure of the tumor (Video 11.2).

Localizing images were obtained to ensure we were in fact at the L2 vertebra. The anterior longitudinal ligament was resected, and the discectomy and osteotomy were completed at L1–L2 and L2–L3 levels. The right psoas muscle was divided in a transverse fashion to allow for clean distal and proximal margins. Following complete release, the L2 vertebral body and the tumor mass were carefully rolled out from underneath the inferior vena cava (Videos 11.3 and 11.4).

P-32 brachytherapy and a corresponding "dummy" source were prepared in a sterile fashion. The dummy source was used to test and verify placement on the dura and the IVC psoas muscle surgical margin. Following determination of the appropriate placement using the dummy source, the "live" source was placed in the same location for 14.25 min per site, corresponding to 10 Gy to 1-mm depth. The dural location was treated first, followed by the IVC and psoas muscle margin. During this time, the surgical bed was flooded with warm saline for shielding, and the source was held in place using wet gauze. Following the conclusion of the brachytherapy treatment portion, the saline was suctioned off, the wet gauze removed, and the source stored appropriately per radiation safety rules and regulations.

The appropriate interbody expandable cage was selected and filled with bone graft and was placed between L1 and L3. Intraoperative imaging confirmed appropriate placement. Following placement of the interbody graft, it was secured using an anterior plate and the wound was closed (Fig. 11.3).

The patient's postoperative course was complicated by MSSA (methicillin-sensitive *Staphylococcus aureus*) bacteremia and a fluid collection requiring drainage and an extended course of antibiotics. At 6-month follow-up, the patient had diminished sensation in the right L2 and L3 dermatomes and endorsed intermittent severe back pain but had normal strength in the bilateral lower extremities.

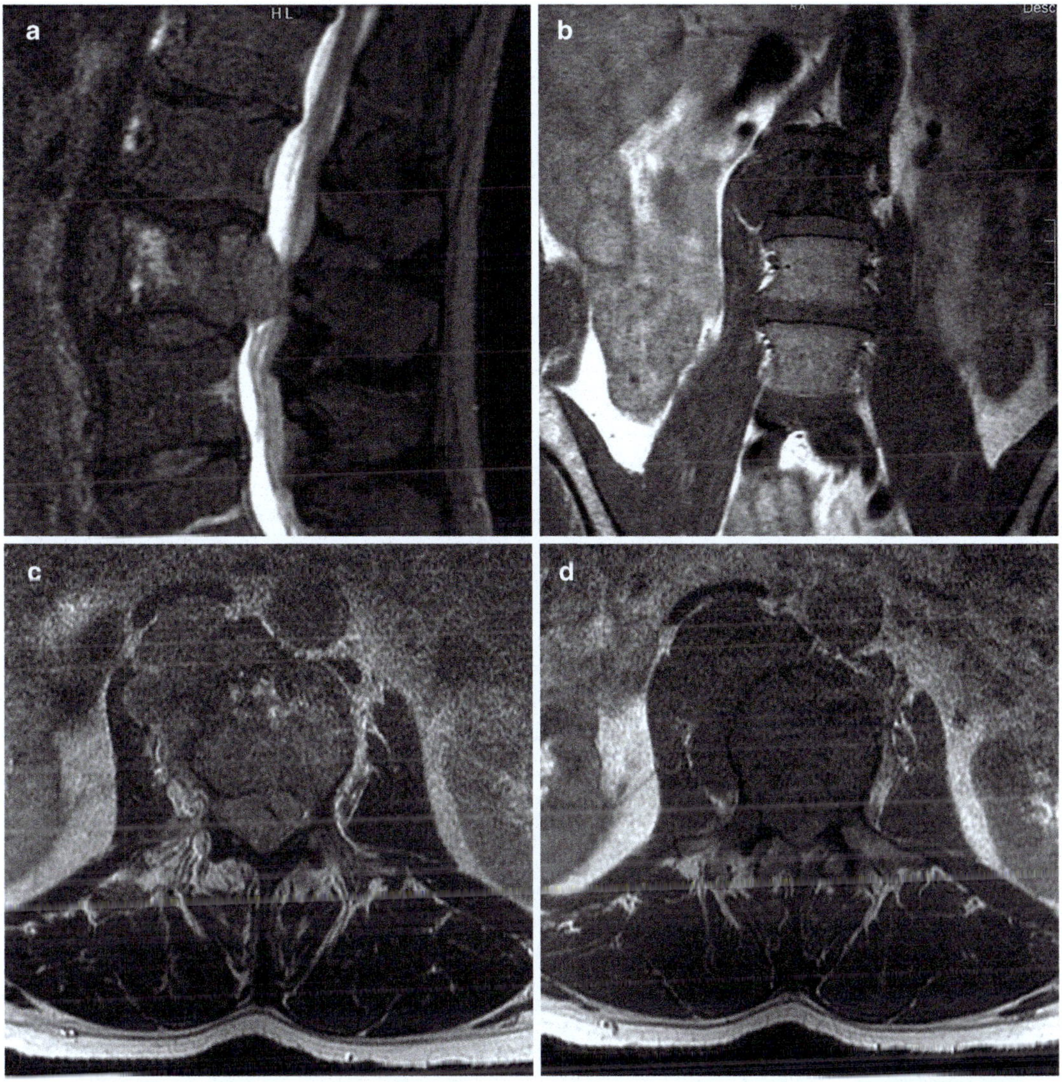

Fig. 11.2 Preoperative magnetic resonance imaging of the lumbar spine demonstrating a destructive lesion of the L2 vertebral body and prevertebral soft tissue. (**a**) T2 sagittal MRI showing a heterogeneously enhancing destructive lesion at L2. The lesion impinges upon the spinal canal causing severe spinal canal stenosis and obliteration of the CSF space. On coronal T1 (**b**), the anterolateral prevertebral soft tissue component of the lesion is evident within the right psoas muscle. Axial MRI cuts at the level of L2 (**c** is T2, **d** is T1) showing the destructive lesion with significant anterolateral expansion into the right psoas muscle. Severe canal stenosis with obliteration of the CSF space is again evident

Introduction

Primary tumors of the mobile spine were historically thought to be incurable due to chemotherapy and the radiation-resistant nature of these specific lesions, and the technical challenges posed in complete surgical resection further complicated by local anatomy. Tomita et al. transformed the treatment of primary spine lesions with the description of the posterior en bloc spondylectomy [1, 2]. While the posterior approach is the preferred intervention for many lesions, large lesions with significant ventral paravertebral extension or involvement of retroperitoneal vas-

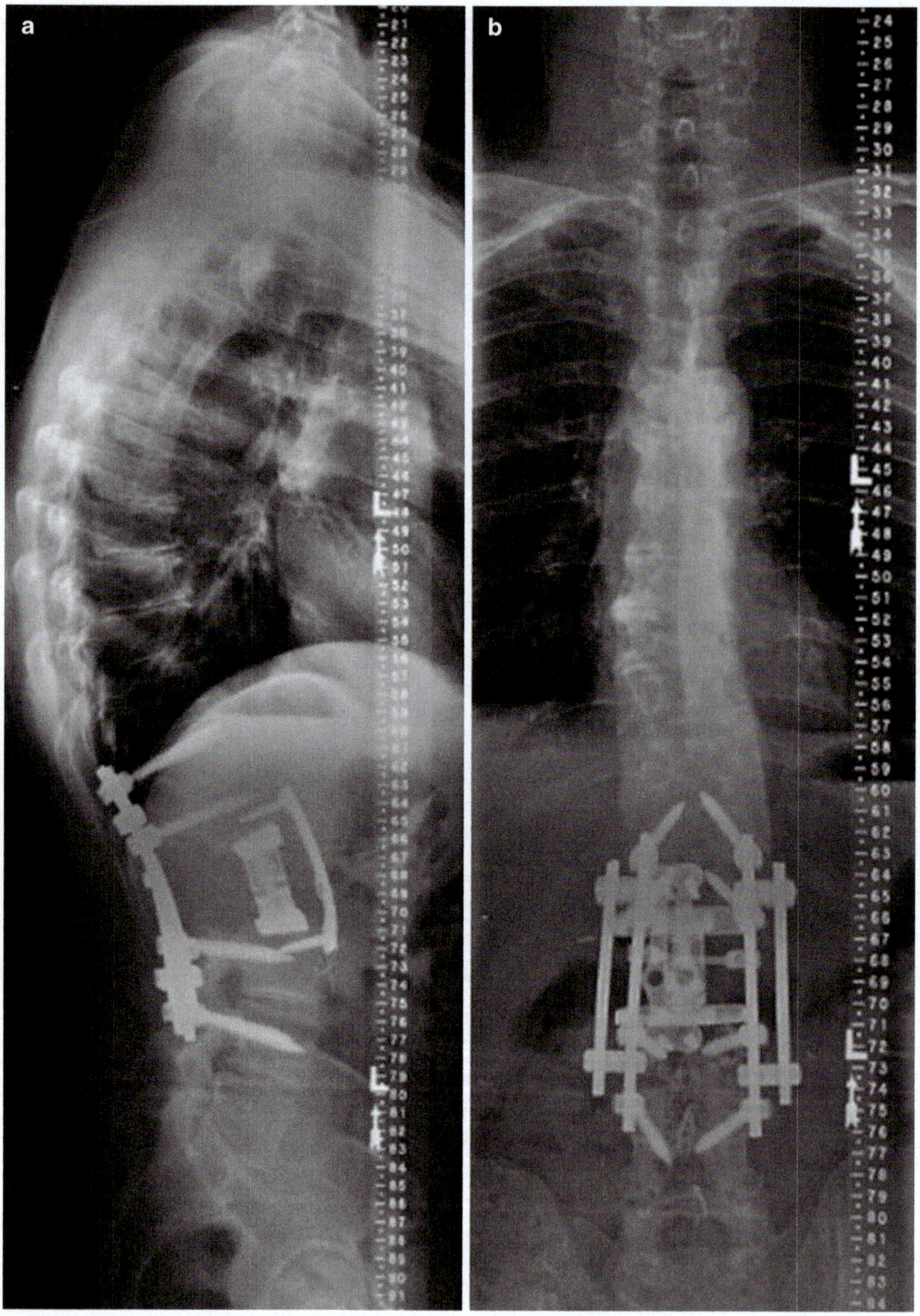

Fig. 11.3 Postoperative X-rays demonstrating final spinal construct from T12 to L4. Postoperative standing 3-foot lateral and anteroposterior X-rays (**a,b**). X-rays demonstrate normal regional and global spinal alignments. More importantly, the films demonstrate an intact construct consisting of the corpectomy cage and the new fusion construct consisting of T12–L4 bilateral pedicle screws secured with double bilateral rods (four total)

cular structures may not be amenable to posterior en bloc spondylectomy. The transperitoneal anterior lumbar and lumbosacral approach allows for direct visualization and access to the lumbar spine and associated structures such as the great vessels.

In contrast to intralesional surgical approaches, including curettage and piecemeal resection, en bloc resection consists of the removal of the lesion and affected portion(s) of the vertebra as a single piece [3, 4]. En bloc resection may be used in the treatment of solitary spinal metastases, locally invasive primary benign lesions, and malignant focal tumors [5]. The primary objective of en bloc spondylectomies is to remove the entirety of the tumor and the diseased vertebrae in one piece with an appropriate surrounding margin [3, 4]. Histologic examination of surgical specimens is necessary in order to determine whether en bloc resection was intralesional, marginal (entailing dissection along the pseudocapsule surrounding the tumor), or wide (in which the tumor and a continuous shell of healthy tissue are removed) [3, 6]. En bloc resection with appropriate margins for specific lesions has been demonstrated to minimize the chances of local recurrence and maximize patient survival and health-related quality of life (HRQoL) [5, 7–10].

Staging and Surgical Planning

Patients presenting with a suspected spine neoplasm must first undergo preoperative staging via X-rays, CT, and MRI, followed by biopsy [4]. Biopsy is essential in deciding whether an en bloc approach should be performed and whether neoadjuvant chemotherapy or radiation is warranted. Additional imaging modalities that may assist in the staging process include positron emission tomography (PET) scanning, CT scans of the chest and the abdomen (to look for metastatic disease), and bone scans [4].

The recommended biopsy approach is trocar biopsy under CT guidance [3, 4, 6], as open biopsy is associated with an increase in the risk of local spread and recurrence [3, 4]. Given that the biopsy tract may need to be excised during the definitive surgical intervention, it is recommended that the biopsy be performed at experienced centers with multidisciplinary teams to ensure adequate coordination with the surgeon [3, 4]. As biopsies do confer a risk of seeding, biopsies may be deferred in some cases, including certain cases of metastatic disease with known primary, recurrent disease, and some suspected chondrosarcomas, in which breaching of the pseudocapsule during a biopsy risks spread [6]. Following biopsy and imaging, patients should be staged at a multidisciplinary conference that includes surgeons, medical and radiation oncologists, radiologists, and pathologists [4].

The Enneking staging system allows for the application of oncologic principles initially developed in the long bones to the spine, based on grade (G), local extent (T), and metastasis (M) [3, 11]. Based on these features, the Enneking system prescribes appropriate margins [3, 12]. Margins consistent with the Enneking grade (i.e., Enneking appropriate (EA) margins) are associated with decreased local recurrence and improved survival in malignant spine tumors [3, 9, 13, 14]. The Enneking system recommends wide en bloc resection of stage 3 benign lesions (rapidly growing lesions with a thin, incomplete, or absent capsule) and of stage IA, IB, IIA, and IIB malignant lesions (i.e., all nonmetastatic malignant lesions, regardless of grade and local extension), with adjuvant therapy recommended for higher grade lesions [6].

Classification of staged lesions using Weinstein-Boriani-Biagnini (WBB) criteria may be useful in surgical planning, as WBB classification often suggests successful resection strategy [3, 6, 15]. In the WBB system, the vertebra is divided into 12 radiating zones and five layers [6]. Based on the zones involved, different techniques for en bloc spondylectomy are more likely to be feasible. In a meta-analysis of 89 articles, WBB classification was able to predict attainment of marginal or wide versus intralesional margins in 88% of cases [4].

Appropriate staging, surgical planning, and techniques are critical as multiple series have demonstrated that the first surgical treatment most strongly affects patient prognosis [4, 16,

17]. Intralesional and marginal surgical margins have been identified as impendent risk factors for local recurrence [16, 18], which in turn is strongly associated with survival [3]. Recurrent disease is also associated with significant reductions in patient quality of life (QoL) [4].

Adjuvant Therapy

Potential adjuvants to surgical treatment for primary spinal tumors include chemotherapy, percutaneous techniques, and radiation therapy [3]. Management in experienced centers by multidisciplinary teams capable of offering diverse treatment modalities is associated with improved outcomes [3, 4, 19].

Chemotherapy

The majority of primary spine tumors respond poorly to chemotherapy; however, adjuvant and neoadjuvant chemotherapy protocols exist for select lesions, including osteosarcoma, Ewing's Sarcoma, and giant-cell tumor [3, 20]. The use of denosumab neoadjuvant therapy for giant-cell tumor has been shown to improve disease control and allow for less morbid surgery [3, 20]. One series described the use of intraoperative chemotherapy using distilled water and cisplatin chemotherapy in cases where an intralesional T-saw cut of the pedicle was necessary to preserve the nerve roots in a series of patients with aggressive benign tumors and single metastatic lesions [21]. However, evidence regarding intraoperative chemotherapy for spinal tumors is very limited. An example of a malignant tumor that may warrant neoadjuvant chemotherapy prior to en bloc resection is Ewing's sarcoma.

Percutaneous Techniques

Percutaneous techniques such as selective arterial embolization (SAE) and thermal ablation may be appropriate for select lesions. Preoperative SAE is the standard treatment for aneurysmal bone cysts [22], and preliminary data indicate that multiple treatments of standalone SAE may be sufficient for treatment of select cases of aneurysmal bone cysts without extensive neural involvement or high-risk fractures [3]. SAE is also used preoperatively for the treatment of giant-cell tumors and vascular metastatic tumors, such as renal cell carcinoma, thyroid carcinoma, or hepatocellular carcinoma [23, 24], and may be of use prior to en bloc spondylectomy for recurrent low-grade osteosarcoma [25]. Percutaneous thermal ablation of osteoid osteoma has been shown to be highly efficacious [26].

Radiation Therapy

The majority of spinal lesions are radioresistant. However, select lesions are radiosensitive [24], and radiation therapy of an adequate dose (at least 60–65 Gy) can confer a survival advantage for patients with malignant spine tumors [3]. Radiation therapy is a useful adjuvant therapy in the treatment of chordomas and chondrosarcomas, particularly in lesions in which en bloc resection is not feasible [3, 27]. Multiple modalities have been demonstrated to be effective, including photon-based intensity-modulated radiation therapy, proton beam therapy, carbon ion, and high-dose single-fraction radiosurgery, all of which have been demonstrated to produce similarly high rates of 5-year local control when adequately dosed (typically, over 70 Gy) and combined with surgery for primary spine tumors [3, 28]. Some have advocated for both pre- and postoperative radiotherapy to reduce the rate of intraoperative seeding. The addition of preoperative radiation therapy has been shown to improve local control as compared to surgery and postoperative radiation therapy [3]; however, preoperative radiation therapy is associated with a significant increase in perioperative complications due to impaired wound healing and increased technical challenges intraoperatively due to scarring [3, 29, 30].

The use of Phosphorus-32 (P-32) brachytherapy in neurosurgery, as in this case, is relatively novel. Series regarding intracavitary P-32 brachytherapy for craniopharyngioma suggest that intracystic P-32 can be an effective treatment for craniopharyngioma, with limited morbidity related to the brachytherapy [31, 32], and a case report has described the use of P-32 brachytherapy plaque for the treatment of recurrent spinal neuroblastoma with good local control at 11 months [33].

Surgical Approaches

En bloc resection of spinal lesions poses a significant technical challenge and risk of morbidity due to the proximity of vital neural and vascular structures [3, 6]. Spondylectomies are also inherently destabilizing procedures and require reconstruction and instrumentation in order to allow for appropriate patient mobility. However, successful en bloc spondylectomy can confer a significant survival advantage. There are thus three key objectives in en bloc spondylectomy: successful resection of the lesion with acceptable margins to maximize local control and survival, limiting damage to the surrounding structures to limit morbidity and mortality and maximize functional outcomes, and reconstruction to restore stability and function [34]. Three major methods exist for en bloc spondylectomy: vertebrectomy, sagittal resection, and resection of the posterior arch [6]. Operative approach is selected based on the location, size, and local extent of the tumor.

Vertebrectomy

Vertebrectomies are defined as the en bloc removal of the body and lamina following detachment from the posterior elements via a transpedicular osteotomy [35] and are the preferred approach for centrally located lesions of the vertebral body with at least one pedicle free from disease (i.e., tumors involving WBB zones 4–8 or 5–9) [4]. This may be achieved via an anterior and/or posterior approach and may be accomplished in one or two stages [6].

Posterior Vertebrectomy

Posterior vertebrectomy is the most commonly utilized approach for resection of vertebral body lesions [5, 7, 21, 36–41]. The posterior approach allows for direct control of epidural venous plexus bleeding and posterior instrumentation [6]. Nerve roots may be sacrificed in the thoracic region to allow for sufficient space for resection of the vertebral body and anterior reconstruction when a posterior approach is taken [42, 43]; however, sacrifice of a nerve root in the thoracolumbar and lumbar spine is avoided when possible, and caution needs to be taken when operating near the artery of Adamkiewicz. Injury to the artery of Adamkiewicz leads to anterior spinal cord ischemia and loss of lower extremity function [5]. The single-stage posterior approach is associated with less morbidity for appropriate lesions and may be preferred, particularly for one- or two-segment en bloc resections [25].

Anterior Vertebrectomy

However, large lesions and lesions with significant ventral expansion may require a direct anterior approach [6]. Anterior vertebrectomies allow for easier ligation of the segmental vessels and may enable achievement of better margins in tumors with anterior paravertebral expansion or in recurrent disease where resection is complicated by adhesions and scar tissue [6, 25]. The anterior approach may be of particular utility for lesions in close proximity to major vessels; in cases in which the tumor is adherent to or involving major blood vessels, the assistance of a vascular surgeon may be of use, especially if repair of a vessel is warranted. The transperitoneal approach may also be necessary in L5 lesions with significant ventral extension, as the iliac crest may limit access via the sagittal approach [21].

Anterior vertebrectomies are often combined with a posterior laminectomy and instrumentation prior to anterior en bloc resection and instrumentation in a two-stage approach [5, 21, 34]. This allows for mobilization of the thecal sac and separation of the dural surface from the posterior longitudinal ligament or tumor capsule under direct visualization prior to anterior en bloc resection [21].

Sagittal Resection

Lesions located eccentrically in the body, pedicle, or transverse process (i.e., in zones 3–5 or 8–10) may be resected via sagittal resection [4]. This approach may be utilized for the en bloc resection of one or more levels [6, 44]. The patient is positioned in the lateral decubitus position, and the spine is accessed via the retroperitoneal approach [6]. Sagittal resection entails the removal of posterior structures, including the pedicle, to allow for dural displacement, followed by en bloc resection of anterior structures [6]. The sagittal approach may be combined with posterior approaches for instrumentation or to allow for anterior release prior to posterior resection of primary spinal tumors of posterior elements [6, 24, 44–46].

Resection of the Posterior Arch

Lesions restricted to zones 10–3 can be resected via an isolated posterior approach. Resection of posterior arch lesions entails a wide laminectomy above and below the lesion, exposing the dural sac above and below. Lateral dissection at the level of the lesion allows for exposure of the pedicles, which are then sectioned in order to achieve en bloc resection of the involved posterior elements [6]. Resection of tumors isolated to the posterior elements may not require resection of the vertebral body or anterior reconstruction [47].

Surgical Technique: Transperitoneal Vertebrectomy

Preoperatively, placement of a radiopaque localizing implant may aid in the intraoperative localization of lesions [48]. The patient should be positioned prone on a fluoroscopy-compatible table [48]. The use of intraoperative motor evoked potentials and somatosensory evoked potentials is recommended, and baseline measurements should be obtained prior to case initiation and before and after positioning changes [48].

En bloc spondylectomies are associated with substantial blood loss, and multiple units of packed red blood cells (PRBCs) should be available [48]. If available, use of a cell saver with leukocyte filter may reduce the transfusion burden [48].

Posterior laminectomy, pediculectomy, and instrumentation and fusion may precede anterior en bloc resection. The location of the pedicle cut should be informed by the degree of tumor extension, with the cut placed in a way to avoid intralesional margins. In the described case, the lack of tumor extension into the pedicles allowed for a posterior-based pediculectomy prior to anterior vertebrectomy.

Approach

Collaboration with general or vascular surgeon is recommended, particularly for patients with tumor compression or involvement of the major vessels. Pfannenstiel, horizontal, or vertical incisions may all be appropriate; the decision as to which incision to use is primarily cosmetic; however, for L4–L5 lesions, a vertical incision may allow for superior exposure [49]. Following incision, use electrocautery to dissect to the anterior rectus sheath. Open the rectus sheath using electrocautery and expose the paired rectus muscles. Retract the rectus muscles laterally to expose the transversalis fascia. Sharply dissect through the fascia to expose the peritoneum. Incise the peritoneum, taking care to avoid bowel [49].

Retract the small bowel and mesentery superiorly and to the left and pack with moist sponges [49]. Retract the sigmoid colon inferiorly and to the left to expose the posterior peritoneum. Visualize and palpate the aorta, vena cava, and sacral promontory. Following localization of retroperitoneal structures, elevate the posterior peritoneum with forceps and enter sharply [49].

Within the posterior peritoneum, avoid the use of electrocautery due to the risk for retrograde ejaculation due to hypogastric plexus injury [49].

Blunt dissect within the retroperitoneum using a Kittner swab to identify the disc space and vertebral bodies [49]. Intraoperative fluoroscopy may be used to confirm appropriate vertebral body level. Mobilize the ipsilateral kidney posteriorly. Prior to the mobilization of the great vessels, identify and ligate the iliolumbar vein and middle sacral artery [49]. Then, mobilize the great vessels. At the L5–S1 levels, it may be possible to pass between the great vessels; however, above L4–L5, mobilizing and sweeping the iliac vessels laterally is necessary for access [49]. Generally, a left-sided approach is preferred in order to limit injury to the IVC. However, a right-sided approach (as in this case) may be necessary if that is the side of maximal tumor extension [5].

En Bloc Corpectomy

Following exposure of the appropriate vertebral body and disc spaces and mobilization of great vessels, the en bloc corpectomy can be performed. Excise the discs distal and proximal to the affected vertebral body [5, 21]. Osteotomies through the vertebral body are not recommended due to the increased risk for graft subsidence into the cancellous bone of the vertebral body postoperatively [5, 50, 51]. Transect the annulus and the anterior longitudinal ligaments and then use a T-saw to divide the pedicle, if it has not been previously resected during an initial posterior stage [5, 21]. Paraspinal structures such as the psoas muscle may also require division around the tumor lesion depending on the extent of lesion extension. Following complete release of the vertebral body and the tumor, the involved vertebral body and the tumor can then be rolled out en bloc. Histopathological examination of the specimen is necessary in order to determine resection margins.

Reconstruction

En bloc spondylectomies are inherently highly destabilizing and require reconstruction. Options for anterior reconstruction include titanium mesh cages or carbon cages, filled with autograft material, or wide-diameter whole-shaft femur or tibia allografts [5, 25, 40]. Cages or allografts may be secured and the spine instrumented anteriorly using rods, plates, or cables [5, 24]. Anterior instrumentation may be augmented with posterior instrumentation, such as pedicle screw and rod constructs, in a staged approach [25, 52]. Pedicle screws provide superior support as compared to anterolateral plate fixation during flexion, extension, and axial rotation, and stability following en bloc spondylectomy is primarily a function of the number of screws in posterior instrumentation [5].

Complications

En bloc spondylectomies confer a substantial risk of morbidity. Series have reported rates of complications ranging from 13% to 65%, with 0 to 7.7% rates of mortality [4, 16, 17, 40, 53]. Reported rates of complications are slightly higher in resections for recurrent disease or following radiation therapy due to abnormal anatomy, adhesions, and fibrosis [4, 17, 25, 53]. Posterior-only approaches are associated with a lower rate of complications as compared to anterior or combined anterior/posterior approaches, although this may reflect the more complex lesions that typically require an anterior approach [17]. Similarly, multilevel en bloc spondylectomies are associated with increased morbidity due to the increased complexity [40]. Reported complications include surgical complications such as vascular injury, ureteral injury, hemorrhage, hematomas, wound necrosis, hardware failure, CSF leaks, deep wound infections, paraplegia, and local recurrence as well as medical complications such as pulmonary emboli, respiratory failure, myocardial infarctions, and acute kidney injuries [4, 17, 24, 39, 40]. The most common complications are wound complications and intraoperative blood loss [4, 54]. Of note, however, the majority of patients recover from their complications and are able to achieve good outcomes in the long term [40].

Surgical adjuncts are available to reduce the risk of perioperative complications. The use of intraoperative navigation may allow for tumor-free osteotomy cuts, improving surgical margins and the rate of Enneking appropriate resection while decreasing the risk of injury to surrounding structures [3, 55]. Strategies reported to reduce the rate of infections in en bloc spondylectomies include the use of intraoperative vancomycin powder [56], negative-pressure wound vacuums [57], and the assistance of a plastic surgery service in closing large wounds or areas with significant soft tissue deficits [58].

Conclusion

The resection of spinal tumors is technically challenging due to the proximity of vital structures. En bloc spondylectomies are associated with a relatively high risk of complications but have been shown to produce significant improvements in survival for patients with spinal tumors. Preoperatively, patients should be staged by multidisciplinary teams using MRI, CT, and additional imaging as necessary. CT-guided biopsies are strongly recommended for histopathological diagnosis of the lesion and should be performed at the same institution as the definitive surgical treatment in order to allow for communication with the spine surgeon and excision of the biopsy tract if necessary. Adjuvant therapeutic options may be appropriate for select patients. The surgical approach selected for resection is dependent upon the anatomy of the lesion within the vertebra. WBB classification of the tumor location may help guide surgical decision making, and the Enneking grade of the lesion prescribes appropriate margins. Enneking appropriate resection is associated with increased survival and HRQoL. Patients with lesions with significant anterior extension or that compress or involve the major vessels may require an anterior transperitoneal approach. Collaboration with vascular surgery may also be necessary. Anterior approaches may also be combined with posterior approaches in a two-stage procedure to allow for posterior decompression, dissection, and instrumentation prior to the anterior approach. Large lesions with significant anterior paraspinal involvement can be successfully resected en bloc via the anterior approach.

References

1. Tomita K, Kawahara N, Baba H, Tsuchiya H, Fujita T, Toribatake Y. Total en bloc spondylectomy. A new surgical technique for primary malignant vertebral tumors. Spine (Phila Pa 1976). 1997;22(3):324–33.
2. Tomita K, Kawahara N, Baba H, Tsuchiya H, Nagata S, Toribatake Y. Total en bloc spondylectomy for solitary spinal metastases. Int Orthop. 1994;18(5):291–8.
3. Dea N, Gokaslan Z, Choi D, Fisher C. Spine oncology – primary spine tumors. Neurosurgery. 2017;80(3S):S124–S30.
4. Yamazaki T, McLoughlin GS, Patel S, Rhines LD, Fourney DR. Feasibility and safety of en bloc resection for primary spine tumors: a systematic review by the spine oncology study group. Spine (Phila Pa 1976). 2009;34(22 Suppl):S31–8.
5. Zaidi HA, Awad AW, Dickman CA. Complete Spondylectomy using orthogonal spinal fixation and combined anterior and posterior approaches for thoracolumbar spinal reconstruction: technical nuances and clinical results. Clin Spine Surg. 2017;30(4):E466–E74.
6. Boriani S, Weinstein JN, Biagini R. Primary bone tumors of the spine. Terminology and surgical staging. Spine (Phila Pa 1976). 1997;22(9):1036–44.
7. Matsumoto M, Tsuji T, Iwanami A, Watanabe K, Hosogane N, Ishii K, et al. Total en bloc spondylectomy for spinal metastasis of differentiated thyroid cancers: a long-term follow-up. J Spinal Disord Tech. 2013;26(4):E137–42.
8. Boriani S, Bandiera S, Casadei R, Boriani L, Donthineni R, Gasbarrini A, et al. Giant cell tumor of the mobile spine: a review of 49 cases. Spine (Phila Pa 1976). 2012;37(1):E37–45.
9. Weinstein JN, McLain RF. Primary tumors of the spine. Spine (Phila Pa 1976). 1987;12(9):843–51.
10. Stener B. Complete removal of vertebrae for extirpation of tumors. A 20-year experience. Clin Orthop Relat Res. 1989;245:72–82.
11. Enneking WF. A system of staging musculoskeletal neoplasms. Clin Orthop Relat Res. 1986;204:9–24.
12. Chan P, Boriani S, Fourney DR, Biagini R, Dekutoski MB, Fehlings MG, et al. An assessment of the reliability of the Enneking and Weinstein-Boriani-Biagini classifications for staging of primary spinal tumors by the spine oncology study group. Spine (Phila Pa 1976). 2009;34(4):384–91.
13. Spanier SS, Shuster JJ, Vander Griend RA. The effect of local extent of the tumor on prognosis in osteosarcoma. J Bone Joint Surg Am. 1990;72(5):643–53.
14. Dekutoski MB, Clarke MJ, Rose P, Luzzati A, Rhines LD, Varga PP, et al. Osteosarcoma of the spine: prognostic variables for local recurrence and overall survival, a multicenter ambispective study. J Neurosurg Spine. 2016;25(1):59–68.
15. Boriani S, Biagini R, De Iure F, Bertoni F, Malaguti MC, Di Fiore M, et al. En bloc resections of bone tumors of the thoracolumbar spine. A preliminary

report on 29 patients. Spine (Phila Pa 1976). 1996;21(16):1927–31.
16. Lador R, Bandiera S, Gasbarrini A, Ghermandi R, Boriani S. Treatment of spinal tumors in a high volume center has direct impact on local recurrence, morbidity, and mortality. Clin Spine Surg. 2017 Oct;30(8):E1074–81.
17. Bandiera S, Boriani S, Donthineni R, Amendola L, Cappuccio M, Gasbarrini A. Complications of en bloc resections in the spine. Orthop Clin North Am. 2009;40(1):125–31. vii
18. Amendola L, Cappuccio M, De Iure F, Bandiera S, Gasbarrini A, Boriani S. En bloc resections for primary spinal tumors in 20 years of experience: effectiveness and safety. Spine J. 2014;14(11):2608–17.
19. Goldschlager T, Dea N, Boyd M, Reynolds J, Patel S, Rhines LD, et al. Giant cell tumors of the spine: has denosumab changed the treatment paradigm? J Neurosurg SpineJ Neurosurg Spine. 2015;22(5):526–33.
20. Thomas D, Henshaw R, Skubitz K, Chawla S, Staddon A, Blay JY, et al. Denosumab in patients with giant cell tumour of bone: an open-label, phase 2 study. Lancet Oncol. 2010;11(3):275–80.
21. Kawahara N, Tomita K, Murakami H, Demura S, Yoshioka K, Kato S. Total en bloc spondylectomy of the lower lumbar spine: a surgical techniques of combined posterior-anterior approach. Spine (Phila Pa 1976). 2011;36(1):74–82.
22. Vergel De Dios AM, Bond JR, Shives TC, McLeod RA, Unni KK. Aneurysmal bone cyst. A clinicopathologic study of 238 cases. Cancer. 1992;69(12):2921–31.
23. Mesfin A, El Dafrawy MH, Jain A, Hassanzadeh H, Kebaish KM. Total En bloc Spondylectomy for primary and metastatic spine tumors. Orthopedics. 2015;38(11):e995–e1000.
24. Santiago-Dieppa DR, Hwang LS, Bydon A, Gokaslan ZL, McCarthy EF, Witham TF. L4 and L5 spondylectomy for en bloc resection of giant cell tumor and review of the literature. Evid Based Spine Care J. 2014;5(2):151–7.
25. Druschel C, Disch AC, Melcher I, Engelhardt T, Luzzati A, Haas NP, et al. Surgical management of recurrent thoracolumbar spinal sarcoma with 4-level total en bloc spondylectomy: description of technique and report of two cases. Eur Spine J. 2012;21(1):1–9.
26. Tsoumakidou G, Thenint MA, Garnon J, Buy X, Steib JP, Gangi A. Percutaneous image guided laser photocoagulation of spinal osteoid osteoma: a single-institution series. Radiology. 2016;278(3):936–43.
27. Boriani S, Bandiera S, Biagini R, Bacchini P, Boriani L, Cappuccio M, et al. Chordoma of the mobile spine: fifty years of experience. Spine (Phila Pa 1976). 2006;31(4):493–503.
28. Imai R, Kamada T, Tsuji H, Sugawara S, Serizawa I, Tsujii H, et al. Effect of carbon ion radiotherapy for sacral chordoma: results of phase I-II and phase II clinical trials. Int J Radiat Oncol Biol Phys. 2010;77(5):1470–6.
29. Yokogawa N, Murakami H, Demura S, Kato S, Yoshioka K, Hayashi H, et al. Perioperative complications of total en bloc spondylectomy: adverse effects of preoperative irradiation. PLoS One. 2014;9(6):e98797.
30. Demura S, Kawahara N, Murakami H, Nambu K, Kato S, Yoshioka K, et al. Surgical site infection in spinal metastasis: risk factors and countermeasures. Spine (Phila Pa 1976). 2009;34(6):635–9.
31. Maarouf M, El Majdoub F, Fuetsch M, Hoevels M, Lehrke R, Berthold F, et al. Stereotactic intracavitary brachytherapy with P-32 for cystic craniopharyngiomas in children. Strahlenther Onkol. 2016;192(3):157–65.
32. Barriger RB, Chang A, Lo SS, Timmerman RD, DesRosiers C, Boaz JC, et al. Phosphorus-32 therapy for cystic craniopharyngiomas. Radiother Oncol. 2011;98(2):207–12.
33. Tong WY, Folkert MR, Greenfield JP, Yamada Y, Wolden SL. Intraoperative phosphorus-32 brachytherapy plaque for multiply recurrent high-risk epidural neuroblastoma. J Neurosurg Pediatr. 2014;13(4):388–92.
34. Clarke MJ, Hsu W, Suk I, McCarthy E, Black JH 3rd, Sciubba DM, et al. Three-level en bloc spondylectomy for chordoma. Neurosurgery. 2011;68(2 Suppl Operative):325–33. discussion 33
35. Kato S, Murakami H, Demura S, Yoshioka K, Kawahara N, Tomita K, et al. More than 10-year follow-up after total en bloc spondylectomy for spinal tumors. Ann Surg Oncol. 2014;21(4):1330–6.
36. Hsieh PC, Li KW, Sciubba DM, Suk I, Wolinsky JP, Gokaslan ZL. Posterior-only approach for total en bloc spondylectomy for malignant primary spinal neoplasms: anatomic considerations and operative nuances. Neurosurgery. 2009;65(6 Suppl):173–81. discussion 81
37. Tomita K, Kawahara N, Murakami H, Demura S. Total en bloc spondylectomy for spinal tumors: improvement of the technique and its associated basic background. J Orthop Sci. 2006;11(1):3–12.
38. Huang L, Chen K, Ye JC, Tang Y, Yang R, Wang P, et al. Modified total en bloc spondylectomy for thoracolumbar spinal tumors via a single posterior approach. Eur Spine J. 2013;22(3):556–64.
39. Neves RP, Oliveira VC, Costa LM, Soares DF, Cardoso PF, Costa PG, et al. Major complications following total en bloc spondylectomy for giant-cell tumor. J Surg Case Rep. 2014:1–4.
40. Luzzati AD, Shah S, Gagliano F, Perrucchini G, Scotto G, Alloisio M. Multilevel en bloc spondylectomy for tumors of the thoracic and lumbar spine is challenging but rewarding. Clin Orthop Relat Res. 2015;473(3):858–67.
41. Fang T, Dong J, Zhou X, McGuire RA Jr, Li X. Comparison of mini-open anterior corpectomy and posterior total en bloc spondylectomy for solitary metastases of the thoracolumbar spine. J Neurosurg Spine. 2012;17(4):271–9.

42. Abe E, Sato K, Tazawa H, Murai H, Okada K, Shimada Y, et al. Total spondylectomy for primary tumor of the thoracolumbar spine. Spinal Cord. 2000;38(3):146–52.
43. Melcher I, Disch AC, Khodadadyan-Klostermann C, Tohtz S, Smolny M, Stockle U, et al. Primary malignant bone tumors and solitary metastases of the thoracolumbar spine: results by management with total en bloc spondylectomy. Eur Spine J. 2007;16(8):1193–202.
44. Kato S, Kawahara N, Murakami H, Demura S, Shirai T, Tsuchiya H, et al. Multi-level total en bloc spondylectomy for solitary lumbar metastasis of myxoid liposarcoma. Orthopedics. 2010;33(6):446.
45. Oike N, Kawashima H, Ogose A, Hotta T, Hirano T, Ariizumi T, et al. A malignant solitary fibrous tumour arising from the first lumbar vertebra and mimicking an osteosarcoma: a case report. World J Surg Oncol. 2017;15(1):100.
46. Boriani S, Biagini R, De Iure F, Di Fiore M, Gamberini G, Zanoni A. Lumbar vertebrectomy for the treatment of bone tumors: surgical technique. Chir Organi Mov. 1994;79(2):163–73.
47. Vasudeva VS, Ropper AE, Rodriguez S, Wu KC, Chi JH. Contralateral osteotomy of the pedicle and posterolateral elements for en bloc resection: a technique for oncological resection of posterolateral spinal tumors. J Neurosurg Spine. 2017;26(3):275–81.
48. Jenkins AL III. Anterior surgery for metastatic spinal tumors. In: Connolly Jr ES, McKhann II GM, Huang J, Choudhri TF, Komotar RJ, Mocco J, editors. Fundamentals of operative techniques in neurosurgery. New York: Thieme; 2010. p. 587–92.
49. Steinmetz MP, Patel R, Resnick DK. Anterior transperitoneal lumbar approach. Fundamentals of Operative Techniques in neurosurgery. 2nd ed. New York: Thieme; 2010. p. 502–5.
50. Eswaran SK, Gupta A, Adams MF, Keaveny TM. Cortical and trabecular load sharing in the human vertebral body. J Bone Miner Res. 2006;21(2):307–14.
51. Rockoff SD, Sweet E, Bleustein J. The relative contribution of trabecular and cortical bone to the strength of human lumbar vertebrae. Calcif Tissue Res. 1969;3(2):163–75.
52. Disch AC, Schaser KD, Melcher I, Luzzati A, Feraboli F, Schmoelz W. En bloc spondylectomy reconstructions in a biomechanical in-vitro study. Eur Spine J. 2008;17(5):715–25.
53. Boriani S, Bandiera S, Donthineni R, Amendola L, Cappuccio M, De Iure F, et al. Morbidity of en bloc resections in the spine. Eur Spine J. 2010;19(2):231–41.
54. Liljenqvist U, Lerner T, Halm H, Buerger H, Gosheger G, Winkelmann W. En bloc spondylectomy in malignant tumors of the spine. Eur Spine J. 2008;17(4):600–9.
55. Dasenbrock HH, Clarke MJ, Bydon A, McGirt MJ, Witham TF, Sciubba DM, et al. En bloc resection of sacral chordomas aided by frameless stereotactic image guidance: a technical note. Neurosurgery. 2012;70(1 Suppl Operative):82–7. discussion 7-8
56. Ghobrial GM, Cadotte DW, Williams K Jr, Fehlings MG, Harrop JS. Complications from the use of intrawound vancomycin in lumbar spinal surgery: a systematic review. Neurosurg Focus. 2015;39(4):E11.
57. Adogwa O, Fatemi P, Perez E, Moreno J, Gazcon GC, Gokaslan ZL, et al. Negative pressure wound therapy reduces incidence of postoperative wound infection and dehiscence after long-segment thoracolumbar spinal fusion: a single institutional experience. Spine J. 2014;14(12):2911–7.
58. Garvey PB, Rhines LD, Dong W, Chang DW. Immediate soft-tissue reconstruction for complex defects of the spine following surgery for spinal neoplasms. Plast Reconstr Surg. 2010;125(5):1460–6.

Part II

Posterior Approaches

12 Occipital-Cervical Approach and Stabilization

A. Karim Ahmed, Ian Suk, Ali Bydon, and Nicholas Theodore

Anatomy

The occipital bone forms the foramen magnum, for which the basion and opisthion serve as the anterior and posterior midline landmarks. The skull base articulates with the atlas (C1) at the paired occipital condyles, accounting for the majority of head flexion and extension. Paired anterior and posterior arches of C1 form the anterior and posterior tubercles, respectively. The sulcus for vertebral artery can be appreciated as a smooth groove on the superior surface of the posterior arches. The ring of C1 is completed laterally, with the lateral masses and transverse foramen. Inferiorly, the C1 lateral mass joins C2 to form the atlanto-axial joint, responsible for the majority of head rotation. The fibrous apical ligament of C2 extends from the tip of the dens to the basion. The alar ligaments of the dens oppose excessive rotation, joining the occipital condyles, superolaterally. The cruciate ligament covers the posterior surface of the dens, attaching laterally to the C1 lateral masses, cranially to the foramen magnum, and caudally to the axis. Finally, the tectorial membrane forms the posterior longitudinal ligament (PLL), comprising the anterior surface of the central canal.

Originating from the subclavian arteries, the vertebral arteries are best characterized by anatomical location: preforaminal, from the subclavian artery to C6 (V1); foraminal, from the transverse foramen of C6 to C2 (V2); extradural, from C2 to the dura (V3); and intradural, forming the basilar artery (V4). The anterior spinal artery, formed from the vertebral arteries, and posterior spinal arteries, most commonly formed from the posterior inferior cerebellar arteries (PICA), supply the majority of the cervical spinal cord. Segmental arteries, arising from spinal branches of the vertebral artery, of the cervical artery, and of the deep cervical artery function to reinforce the anterior and posterior spinal arteries, as well as supply radicular arteries of nerve roots.

Adequate understanding of motor innervation and sensory dermatomes of cervical nerve roots is pivotal, especially if nerves are operatively sacrificed or injured. Sensory innervation to the posterior aspect of the occiput is provided by C2; C3 and C4 provide sensation to the neck and medial shoulders, respectively; C5 extends from the shoulder to the outer arm; C6 provides the lateral forearm and thumb; C7 for the middle digit; and C8 for the fifth digit. Motor innervation to the diaphragm is by the phrenic nerve (C3–C5). Motor innervation to the brachial plexus is from C5 to T1 [1–5].

A. Karim Ahmed · I. Suk · A. Bydon · N. Theodore (✉)
Department of Neurosurgery, The Johns Hopkins Hospital, Baltimore, MD, USA
e-mail: theodore@jhmi.edu

D. M. Sciubba (ed.), *Spinal Tumor Surgery*, https://doi.org/10.1007/978-3-319-98422-3_12

Diagnosis and Decision-Making

Occipito-cervical (OC) fusion may be indicated to address instability resulting from an infiltrating process or iatrogenic instability. The most common underlying etiologies include rheumatoid arthritis (41%), tumor (16%), trauma (15%), congenital abnormality (14%), metabolic conditions (6%), inflammatory conditions (6), and infection (2%) [6]. The accurate diagnosis of cervical spinal tumors has considerable implications for surgical management.

Metastatic spine disease is more common than benign primary spinal tumors, which is more common than malignant primary spinal tumors. Unlike primary spinal tumors, surgery for metastatic spine disease is generally palliative [7]. The spinal column is the most common site for skeletal metastases but involves the cervical spine in only 8–20% of cases [8]. Primary tumors arising at the anterior aspect of the craniovertebral junction may include chordoma, meningioma, schwannoma, chondrosarcoma, osteoblastoma, giant cell tumor, and plasmacytoma [9, 10].

For decision-making in metastatic spine disease, clinicians should rely on the NOMS Framework—an algorithm that consists of the patient's neurologic status (N), oncologic behavior of the tumor (O), spinal mechanical instability (M), and systemic burden of disease (S) [11]. As concluded by the Spinal Oncology Study Group's Spinal Instability Neoplastic Score (SINS), instability is more likely in pathologies involving junctional levels such as occiput–C2, as compared to the mobile subaxial spine. Instability is also more common if the patient complains of mechanical pain, the lesion is lytic, there is a radiographic deformity, there is translation or subluxation, there is vertebral body collapse, or there is involvement of the posterior elements [12]. Due to the risk of instability and wide diameter of the central canal from O to C2, patients most commonly present with mechanical instability and refractory neck pain, as opposed to neurologic deficits [13–15].

Operative Techniques

Approach

In the setting of cervical spine or craniovertebral junction tumors, the treatment goals for patients undergoing occipital-cervical stabilization are to decompress neural elements, realign the cervical spine, and stabilize the spinal column [16–18]. Nonoperative measures, including hard collar and external beam radiation, are recommended for patients with "normal alignment and minimal subluxation" [16].

Following a systematic review of the literature and modified Delphi method, the Spinal Oncology Study Group recommended posterior approaches for the majority of surgical cases involving metastatic disease in the craniovertebral junction (O–C2) [13]. Imaging criteria for instability, requiring posterior stabilization in this region, were described as "fracture subluxation of >5 mm, 70% unilateral condylar destruction, or >50% bilateral destruction" [13].

Positioning

Nasal intubation results in the least amount of cervical spine displacement, compared to other traditional methods, and may be preferred in the setting of cervical spine instability [19]. Arterial lines are placed and the patient is positioned prone on a Jackson table, on chest bolsters. A three-point mounted clamp, such as the Mayfield® Cranial Stabilization System (Integra LifeSciences Corporation, Plainsboro, NJ, USA), is used to immobilize the cervical spine and craniovertebral junction. Positioning during cranial stabilization is critical, because misalignment of the craniovertebral junction following rigid fixation can have a significant impact on sagittal alignment, swallowing function, and quality of life [20]. Moreover, OC fusions performed with an excessive posterior Occipito-cervical angle (POCA) face increased biomechanical stress and are associated with a higher incidence of dysphagia—potentially requiring reoperation [21].

Neuromonitoring

Due to the vital structures in the craniovertebral junction, it is necessary to have neuromonitoring. Ideally, this would consist of somatosensory evoked potentials (SSEP), transcranial motor evoked potentials (TcMEP), and neuromuscular junction testing (NMJ).

Somatosensory evoked potential monitoring, which can reduce postoperative paraplegia by 50–60% [22] and can be performed via bilateral median nerve stimulation at the wrist and posterior tibial nerve stimulation at the popliteal fossa. Waveforms should be carefully monitored for any deviation from the baseline. Of note, excessive neuromuscular blockade may reduce the sensitivity for detection of nerve root irritation during portions of the procedure.

Exposure

The Occipito-cervical area is shaved, prepped, and draped in sterile fashion. A midline incision is made from the occiput to the desired cervical level. This is deepened to the level of the spinous processes and the occipital bone. Subperiosteal dissection, using monopolar cautery, can be performed at the spinous processes and occipital bone. During the exposure it is necessary to not only identify structures directly visible but also remain cognizant of vital structures that may not be seen. This includes bony structures of the spinal column and occiput, the path and location of the vertebral arteries, and location of exiting nerve roots [17, 18, 23].

Decompression

Laminectomy, with or without foraminotomy, is useful in decompressing the central spinal canal. With exposure taken to the medial aspect of the facet complexes, a high-speed drill with a cutting bit is utilized to perform bilateral trough laminectomy. The spinous process and lamina can safely be removed in one piece and adjacent intraspinous ligaments divided with a Leksell rongeur. A Kocher or penetrating towel clamp is used to apply dorsal traction to lift the lamina and associated ligamentum flavum from the dura. An angled Kerrison punch can be used to divide the ligamentum flavum and lift residual lamina. Hemostasis of the epidural space is achieved by careful electrocautery and thrombin-soaked oxidized cellulose. Piecemeal laminectomy may also be performed with a Leksell rongeur [23, 24].

Instrumentation

Instrumentation of the occiput is achieved with a midline plate and bicortical keel screws. The plate is placed in close proximity, but caudal, to the external occipital protuberance (EOP). Plating directly at the EOP increases the risk for skin erosion. Due to the thickness of the skull base at the internal occipital crest, it is necessary to plate in the midline. The EOP and superior nuchal line can be utilized as anatomic landmarks. Preoperative CT scans should be used to plan the desired screw length. It is notable that screws placed laterally will be smaller due to the thinner bone, relative to the midline.

Instrumentation at C1 consists of lateral mass screws, with the entry point inferior to the posterior arch of C1 and superior to the C2 nerve root. Special attention should be paid to identify the C2 nerve root and remain medial to the vertebral artery. The arch of C1 may be utilized to guide screw trajectory, resulting in bicortical fixation with a long shank screw. The long shank screw includes an unthreaded portion due to the anterior location of the C1 lateral mass. Careful hemostasis should be maintained during instrumentation of C1, due to the propensity for venous bleeding. In order to minimize joint violation at O–C1 or C1–C2, the ideal screw trajectory should be between 0 and 15 degrees medial, with the screw tip lying from 20 to 40% of the anterior arch height, measured from the caudal border [25].

Instrumentation options at C2 include pars, pedicle, and intralaminar screws. Due to the lateral trajectory required for pedicle screw, the pars screw is often preferred in this location. The entry point for the C2 pars screw is 3–4 mm cranial relative to the C2–C3 facet joint and in the midpoint of the pars. The length of the unicortical C2 pars screw should end before reaching the transverse foramen, to minimize vertebral artery injury.

When possible, the surgeon should aim for two points of distal fixation. Notably, postoperative radiation, poor bone quality, osteoporosis, or multiple subaxial sites of disease may favor longer constructs [15]. Lateral mass screws are the instrumentation of choice for the subaxial cervical spine. The entry point is located 1 mm caudal and 1 mm medial to the midpoint of the lateral mass [26]. In order to minimize facet joint violation, screws are directed 30 degrees cranially and 20 degrees laterally. Screw length is planned from preoperative CT scans, typically ranging from 13 to 15 mm [27]. Decortication of the lamina, facet joints, and bone grafting at those decorticated sites allows for bony fusion. Additional axial stability may be achieved with transverse rod connectors (Fig. 12.1).

Closure

Closure may be initiated in a typical fashion, and flush placement of the occipital plate reduces the risk of skin erosion. Reapproximation of the fascial layer is performed with 0 Vicryl, followed by reapproximation of the subcutaneous layer. For reapproximation of the subcuticular layer skin edges, 3–0 Vicryl may be used.

Complications

Complications following Occipito-cervical fusion include dysphagia, dural venous sinus injury, CSF leak, pseudoarthrosis, wound infection, and wound dehiscence [6, 28, 29]. Additionally, anterior hip graft harvesting has a risk of injury to the lateral femoral cutaneous or ilioinguinal nerves, and long-term hip pain is reported to occur in 2.5% of cases [30, 31]. Risk factors for dural tear include old age, thin dura from chronic compression, synovial cysts, and scarring from previous surgery [31].

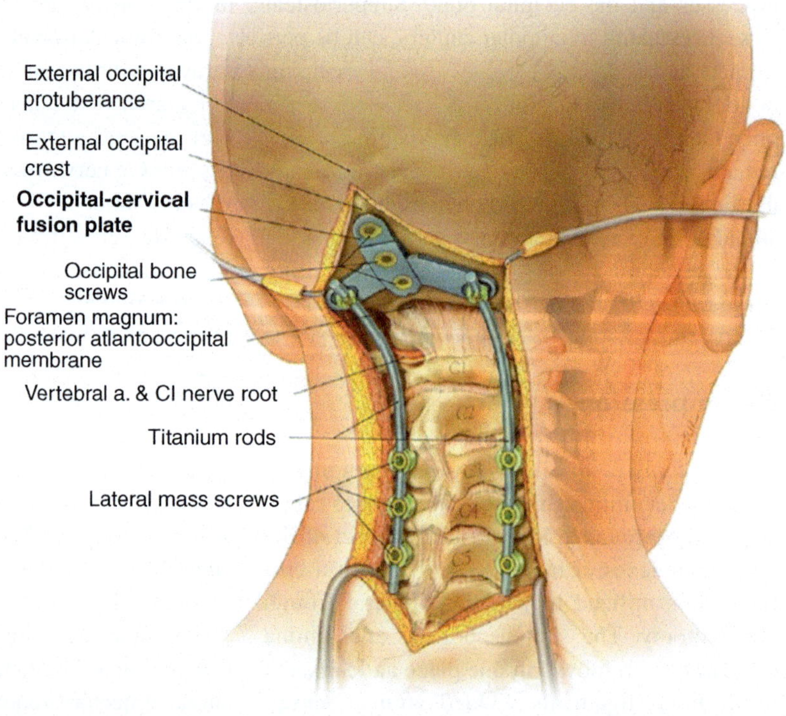

Fig. 12.1 Artist illustration of Occipito-cervical fixation. (Reprinted with permission from: Xu R, Sciubba DM, Gokaslan ZL, Bydon A. Metastasis to the Occipito-cervical junction: A case report and review of the literature. Surgical Neurology International;1:16, 2010. © 2010 Bydon A This is an open-access article distributed under the terms of the Creative Commons Attribution License, which permits unrestricted use, distribution, and reproduction in any medium, provided the original work is properly cited)

Case Presentation 1

A 67-year-old female with multiple medical comorbidities presented to the neurosurgical spine service with mechanical neck pain. She had a history of metastatic non-small-cell lung cancer (NSCLC) to her bone. She was worked up and found to have tumor infiltration on the right C1 lateral mass and right occipital condyle, resulting in destruction of the joint and occipito-atlantal instability. On physical examination, she was neurologically intact. She was placed in a Miami J collar with mild improvement in her pain, which was felt to be primarily due to mechanical instability.

Following an extensive discussion about the risks and benefits of surgery, the patient elected to proceed with surgery, consisting of a fusion from the occiput to C4. She was nasally intubated with a collar in place, placed prone, and her head was secured in a Mayfield head holder. A midline incision was fashioned from the occiput down to C5. Subperiosteal dissection was performed, with monopolar electrocautery, to the level of the spinous processes and the occipital bone. Anatomic landmarks were identified, including the occipital bone, posterior arch of C1, bilateral C2 lamina, and lateral masses of C3, C4, and C5.

The lateral masses of C3 and C4 were cannulated, bilaterally, followed by insertion of bicortical 16-mm Mountaineer screws. However, the thin right C4 lateral mass was noted to fracture laterally and could not be salvaged. In an effort to incorporate at least two points of distal fixation, the C5 lateral masses were cannulated for the placement of 16-mm lateral mass screws. Lateral mass screws were aimed ~20° superiorly and laterally. Bicortical purchase was achieved for every screw for C3 bilaterally, the left C4, and bilateral C5 lateral masses. Attention was then turned to placement of a midline plate on the occipital bone and secured with three bicortical keel screws. Two rods were bent to the cervical alignment, connected from the plate to the lateral mass screws and tightened.

Decortication with a cutting burr proceeded from the occipital bone, C1 lateral masses, bilateral laminae, and lateral masses of C2, C3, C4, and C5. The C2–C3, C3–C4, and C3–C4 joints were also decorticated, bilaterally. Irrigation was then performed with 1 liter of normal saline with antibiotics. Approximately 20 cc of Optium putty, mixed with bone croutons/chips, was placed on the decorticated lateral masses, lateral gutters, and medially over the spinous processes and the occipital bone. A drain was left in place and neuromonitoring was stable throughout the case. Closure was completed in typical neurosurgical fashion (Fig. 12.2).

Case Presentation 2

This is a 78-year-old gentleman who presented with a 7-week history of upper neck pain and lower extremity weakness, which was mechanical in nature. MRI demonstrated a lytic lesion present in the C2 vertebral body and dens, resulting in spinal cord compression at that level. The patient had a known history of colon cancer, resected 11 years prior, and bladder cancer, resected 5 years prior. Intraoral biopsy demonstrated metastatic urothelial carcinoma. Due to the mechanical neck pain, cord compression, and progressive lower extremity weakness, a posterior cervical decompression and Occipito-cervical stabilization were recommended. Due to the anterior location of the tumor, resection of the mass was not attempted. Rather, the goal of treatment was palliative in order to stabilize the region, improve pain, and preserve neurologic function.

The patient was placed prone on a Wilson frame with the head secured in a Mayfield frame. The posterior Occipito-cervical area was shaved, prepped, and draped in a sterile fashion. A midline incision was fashioned from the occiput to C4, and subperiosteal dissection was performed. Laminectomy decompression was performed at C1, C2, and C3. Meticulous hemostasis was maintained with bipolar electrocautery.

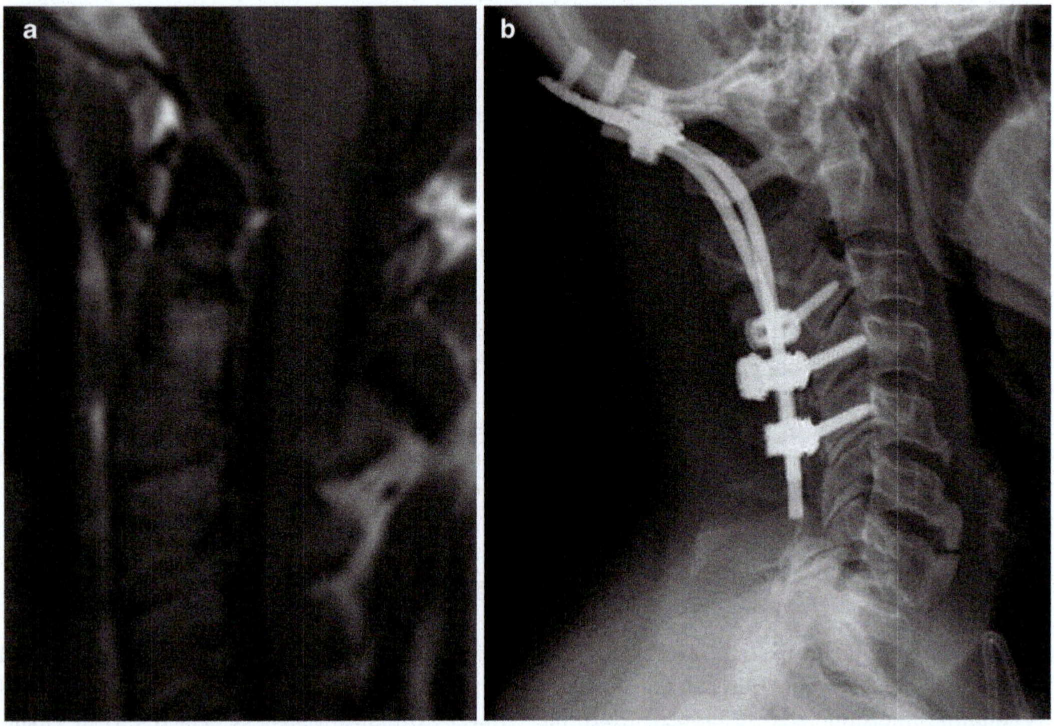

Fig. 12.2 Lytic metastatic non-small-cell lung cancer affecting the right occipital condyle and C1 facet joint. (**a**) Preoperative T1-weighted MRI. (**b**) Postoperative lateral radiograph demonstrating Occipito-cervical fusion from occiput down to C5

The bilateral laminectomies were performed by drilling troughs around them and removing them in one piece. Due to tumor extension in the posterior elements at these levels, this bone was not used as part of the autologous graft. The C2 pedicle was cannulated on the left side, and tissue was obtained for biopsy. A midline plate was secured on the occiput, with 8-mm keel screws. This was followed by placement of C3 lateral mass screws and C4 lateral mass screws. Decortication was performed at the occiput, the occiput–C1 joint, the C1–C2 joint, C2–C3 joint, and C3–C4 joint, using a high-speed cutting burr. Following decortication, two rods were fashioned to the patient's alignment and tightened. To optimize the strength of the construct, two cross-links were connected to the rods.

Copious irrigation was performed with normal saline and antibiotics. A drain was tunneled intramuscularly followed by the placement of 10 cc of optimum DBM putty, placed over the decorticated sites and lateral gutters. Closure was performed in the typical neurosurgical fashion, using 0 Vicryl for the fascial layer and 0 Vicryl for the subcutaneous layer. Skin edges were approximated with 3–0 stitches in the subcuticular layer, followed by skin staples. Neuromonitoring was utilized throughout the procedure and was stable for the entirety of the case (Fig. 12.3).

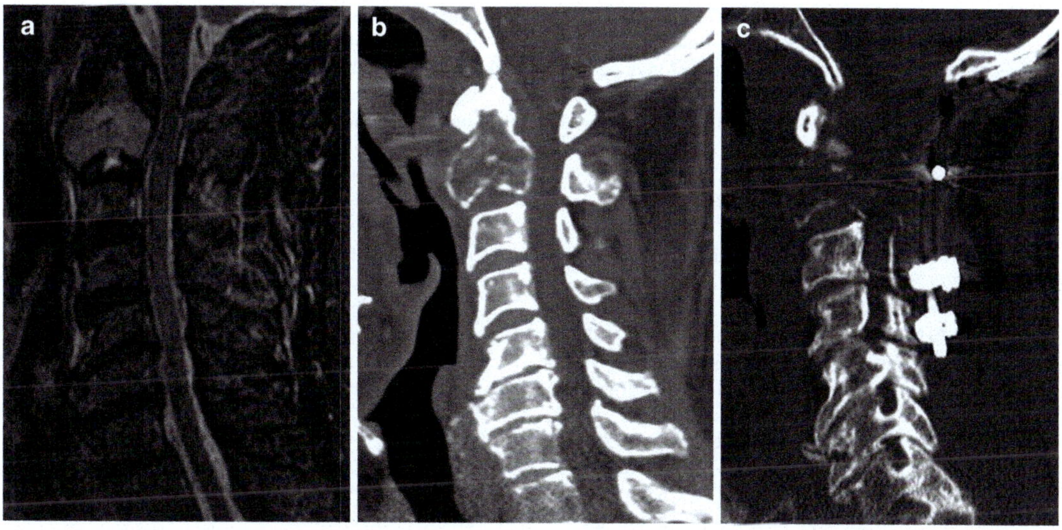

Fig. 12.3 Urothelial carcinoma metastatic to the C2 vertebral body and dens. (**a**) Preoperative sagittal T2-weighted MRI. (**b**) Preoperative sagittal CT. (**c**) Postoperative Occipito-cervical stabilization from occiput to C4

References

1. Smoker WR. Craniovertebral junction: normal anatomy, craniometry, and congenital anomalies. Radiographics. 1994;14(2):255–77.
2. Offiah CE, Day E. The craniocervical junction: embryology, anatomy, biomechanics and imaging in blunt trauma. Insights Imaging. 2017;8(1):29–47.
3. Schweitzer ME, Hodler J, Cervilla V, Resnick D. Craniovertebral junction: normal anatomy with MR correlation. AJR Am J Roentgenol. 1992;158(5):1087–90.
4. Lopez AJ, Scheer JK, Ke L, Smith ZA, Dlouhy BJ, Dahdaleh NS. Anatomy and biomechanics of the craniovertebral junction. Neurosurg Focus. 2015;38(4):E2.
5. Milligram MA, Rand N. Cervical spine anatomy. Spine State of the Art Rev. 2000;14(3):521–32.
6. Bhatia R, Desouza RM, Bull J, Casey AT. Rigid occipitocervical fixation: indications, outcomes, and complications in the modern era. J Neurosurg Spine. 2013;18(4):333–9.
7. Ciftdemir M, Kaya M, Selcuk E, Yalniz E. Tumors of the spine. World J Orthop. 2016;7(2):109–16.
8. Jenis IG, Dunn EJ, An HS. Metastatic disease of the cervical spine. A review. Clin Orthop Relat Res. 1999;359:89–103.
9. Guidetti B, Spallone A. Benign extramedullary tumors of the foramen magnum. Adv Tech Stand Neurosurg. 1988;16:83–120.
10. Shin H, Barrenechea IJ, Lesser J, Sen C, Perin NI. Occipitocervical fusion after resection of craniovertebral junction tumors. J Neurosurg Spine. 2006;4(2):137–44.
11. Laufer I, Rubin DG, Lis E, Cox BW, Stufflefield MD, Yamada Y, et al. The NOMS fraeworks: approach to the treatment of spinal metastatic tumors. Oncologist. 2013;18(6):744–51.
12. Fisher CG, DiPaola CP, Ryken TC, Bilsky MH, Shaffrey CI, Berven SH, et al. A novel classification system for spinal instability in neoplastic disease: an evidence-based approach and expert consensus from the spinal oncology study group. Spine. 2010;35(22):E1221–9.
13. Fehlings MG, David KS, Vialle L, Vialle E, Setzer M, Vrionis FD. Decision making in the surgical treatment of cervical spine metastases. Spine (Phila Pa 1976). 2009;34(22 suppl):S108–17.
14. Phillips E, Levine AM. Metastatic lesions of the upper cervical spine. Spine (Phila Pa 1976). 1989;14(10):1071–7.
15. Zuckerman SL, Kreines F, Powers A, Iorgulescu JB, Elder B, Bilsky MH, et al. Stabilization of tumor-associated craniovertebral junction instability: indications, operative variables, and outcomes. Neurosurgery. 2017;81(2):251–8.
16. Bilsky MH, Shannon FJ, Sheppard S, Prabhu V, Boland PJ. Diagnosis and management of a metastatic tumor in the atlantoaxial spine. Spine (Phila Pa). 2002;29:246–53.
17. Kukreja S, Ambekar S, Sin AH, Nanda A. Occipitocervical fusion surgery: review of operative techniques and results. J Neurol Surg B Skull Base. 2015;76(5):331–9.
18. Zou J, Yuan C, Zhu R, Zhang Z, Jiang W, Yang H. Effect of occipitocervical fusion with screw-rod system for upper cervical spine tumor. BMC Surg. 2014;14:30.
19. Austin N, Krishnamoorthy V, Dagal A. Airway management in cervical spine injury. Int J Crit Illn Sci. 2014;4(1):50–6.

20. Mazur MD, Sivakumar W, Riva-Cambrin J, Jones J, Brockmeyer DL. Avoiding early complications and reoperation during occipitocervical fusion in pediatric patients. J Neurosurg Pediatr. 2014;14(5):465–75.
21. Maulucci CM, Ghobrial GM, Sharan AD, Harrop JS, Jallo JI, Vaccaro AR, Prasad SK. Correlation of posterior occipitocervical angle and surgical outcomes for occipitocervical fusion. Evid Based Spine Care J. 2014;5(2):163–5.
22. Nuwer MR. Spinal cord monitoring. Muscle Nerve. 1999;22(12):1620–30.
23. Luksanapruksa P, Buchowski JM, Wright NM, Valone FH 3rd, Peters C, Bumpass DB. Outcomes and effectiveness of posterior occipital fusion for suboccipital spinal metastases. J Neurosurg Spine. 2017;26(5):554–9.
24. Lu JJ. Cervical laminectomy: technique. Neurosurgery. 2007;60(1 Suppl 1):S149–53.
25. Yeom JS, Buchowski JM, Park JW, Chang BS, Lee CK, Riew KD. Lateral fluoroscopic guide to prevent occipitocervical and atlantoaxial joint violation during C1 lateral mass screw placement. Spine J. 2009;9(7):574–9.
26. Eldin MM, Hassan ASA. Free hand technique of cervical lateral mass screw fixation. J Craniovertebr Junction Spine. 2017;8(2):113–8.
27. Mohamed E, Ihab Z, Moaz A, Ayman N, Haitham AE. Lateral mass fixation in subaxial cervical spine: anatomic review. Global Spine J. 2012;2(1):39–46.
28. Hwang SW, Gressot LV, Chern JJ, Relyea K, Jea A. Complications of occipital screw placement for occipitocervical fusion in children. J Neurosurg Pediatr. 2012;9(6):586–93.
29. Deutsch H, Haid RW Jr, Rodts GE Jr, Mummaneni PV. Occipitocervical fixation: long-term results. Spine (Phila Pa 1976). 2005;30(5):530–5.
30. Younger EM, Chapman MW. Morbidity at bone graft donor sites. J Orthop Trauma. 1989;3(3):192–5.
31. Cheung JP, Luk KD. Complications of anterior and posterior cervical spine surgery. Asian Spine J. 2016;10(2):385–400.

13 Posterior Subaxial Cervical Approach and Stabilization

Daniel L. Shepherd and Michelle J. Clarke

Introduction

The cervical spine can harbor many types of tumors, including primary bone malignancies and metastatic lesions (Table 13.1). Metastatic spinal cancers are far more prevalent than primary neoplasms. The spine is the most common site of skeletal metastases [1, 2] with an estimated 10% of cancer patients developing symptomatic metastases to the spine column [3]. Cervical spine metastases, though less prevalent than the thoracic and lumbar spine lesions, have been reported in up to 25% of patients with metastatic spinal tumors [1, 2, 4]. Approximately 85% of metastatic cervical tumors involve the subaxial spinal column [2, 5, 6]. Concomitant tumor involvement of the thoracolumbar spine is common [2, 6]. In contrast, primary tumors are rare and comprise less than 5% of all spinal column tumors [2].

Many tumors are discovered incidentally on radiographic studies or by physical examination findings. Symptoms may range from subtle stiffness or axial neck pain to more profound neurological deficits [2, 7]. Given the relatively wide spinal canal in the cervical spine, the incidence of neurological compromise is low, approximately 5% [2, 6, 8]. Neurological symptoms are typically due to extension of tumor into the spinal canal rather than deformity [2]. Severe night pain is a classic symptom that is often associated with cancerous neoplasms. Furthermore, a history of malignancy should raise clinical suspicion for potential recurrent or metastatic disease in patients with worsening or persistent neck pain. The etiology of axial neck pain may be a result of focal osseous destruction from the neoplasm or expansion of the periosteum. Osseous destruction can also lead to spinal instability resulting in pain on movement and increases the risk of a progressive kyphotic cervical deformity. Lesions that cause direct spinal cord or nerve root compression can also cause radiculomyelopathic symptoms. In severely stenotic cases, the spinal cord compression may result in quadriparesis.

The management of cervical spinal tumors depends not only on clinical presentation but also on histology, stage, and grade of the tumor. Although rare, primary tumors must be specifically addressed. Primary benign tumors are usually a focal problem but can be locally aggressive. Primary malignant tumors are always considered aggressive neoplasms. Because many primary lesions metastasize late, a radical en bloc tumor resection has potential to completely eradicate the disease [9–11]. If a primary lesion is suspected, a fine-needle biopsy can be performed to confirm the pathology. En bloc resections are technically challenging and are associated with

D. L. Shepherd
Mayo Clinic, Department of Neurosurgery, Rochester, MN, USA

M. J. Clarke (✉)
Mayo Clinic, Department of Neurologic Surgery, Rochester, MN, USA
e-mail: clarke.michelle@mayo.edu

D. M. Sciubba (ed.), *Spinal Tumor Surgery*, https://doi.org/10.1007/978-3-319-98422-3_13

Table 13.1 Classification of common tumors involving the spine

Benign primary tumors	Malignant primary tumors	Common metastatic tumors
Osteoid osteoma	Osteosarcoma	Lung
Osteoblastoma	Chondrosarcoma	Breast
Chondroblastoma	Hemangioendothelioma	GI tract
Hemangioma	Hemangiopericytoma	Prostate
Lymphangioma	Plasmacytoma, multiple myeloma	Melanoma
Giant-cell tumor	Lymphoma	Kidney
–	Leukemia	–
–	Chordoma	–
–	Ewing's sarcoma	–

significant morbidity and mortality. Conversely, aggressive en bloc resection of metastatic neoplasms is typically not indicated.

Nonoperative treatments with chemotherapy and/or radiotherapy may be effective in the initial stages of symptomatic cervical metastatic tumors [6], but surgery should be considered in patients who have failed nonoperative treatment or in patients who exhibit instability or neurological symptoms. Surgery is typically considered palliative in metastatic cancer patients. Surgery for metastatic spinal tumors does not alter the system disease, but local tumor control can improve the quality of the patient's remaining life with acceptably low mortality and morbidity rates [1, 4, 12–14]. The benefits of surgical intervention must be carefully weighed against the patient's estimated survival, their disease burden, their functional status, and the morbidity and recovery associated with the surgery. Together with adjuvant therapy, surgical intervention has the potential to provide symptomatic pain relief, reestablish spinal stability, and improve neurological status [1, 4, 12, 15].

Spinal tumors present complex surgical scenarios. In select cases a decompression alone may be sufficient, but in many instances a segmental fusion is required. Instability or prevention of iatrogenic instability is one of the major driving forces in adding a fusion construct to a tumor resection. In some circumstances instability can be noted preoperatively on flexion-extension lateral radiographs or if there is evidence of anterolisthesis of the vertebral bodies on computed tomography (CT) or magnetic resonance imaging (MRI). Patients who have lytic bony lesions, greater than 50% of vertebral body tumor involvement, evidence of vertebral body collapse, and destruction of the posterior facet joints have higher incidences of cervical instability. Finally, mechanical neck pain can also be a clinical indicator of dynamic spinal instability. Prophylactic fusion procedures are also performed in patients where postoperative instability or progressive deformity is anticipated. Situations that may predispose patients to worsening iatrogenic instability include combined anterior-posterior decompressions, extensive removal of ligamentous and bony structures, and multiple-level cervical laminectomies. An anterior decompression and reconstruction is useful in patients with extensive vertebral body tumor involvement or in patients who need support with axial loading of the spinal column. Posterior stabilization gives additional support to the posterior tension band and is best in tumors predominantly involving the posterior elements or dorsal epidural space. It is not uncommon for some cases to require a combined anterior and posterior approach to achieve appropriate tumor resection and fixation [16]. In these circumstances, posterior fixation provides additional stability to large anterior column resections. The use of lateral mass screw and rod constructs has become the gold standard method of providing posterior subaxial cervical spine fixation and stabilization.

Clinical Evaluation

Clinical evaluation of patients with a suspected spinal neoplasm should begin with a thorough history and physical examination. Diagnostic radiographic studies play a key role in investigation as they identify tumor anatomy and help narrow the differential tumor diagnosis. Appropriate studies for local assessment include plain radiographs, cervical computed tomographic (CT) scan, and magnetic resonance imaging (MRI). If a metastatic process is suspected, a chest radiographic as well as a CT scan of the chest abdomen and pelvis is indicated to evaluate for the primary lesion and to provide clinical oncological staging. A whole-body evaluation with positron emission tomography (PET) or bone scan should also be performed in patients with metastatic pathology to assess the overall extent of disease. The cervical MRI scan is helpful in determining the extent of local tumor involvement, differentiating tumor pathology, and assessing preoperative anatomy [2, 17]. Flexion and extension radiographs can be obtained to assess for dynamic instability. A cervical CT scan assesses bony integrity and shows viable screw options for cervical fusion constructs, if required.

Clinical Scenario

The patient is a 21-year-old Caucasian male who presents with a 3-week history of weakness and numbness of his bilateral upper extremities and a 3-day history of gait imbalance. His weakness is asymmetric with his left arm being more severely affected. He endorses constipation attributable to his current pain medicine regimen, but denies overt bowel and bladder incontinence. He has a history of osteosarcoma involving the distal right femur 5 years prior and has subsequently undergone tumor resection and endoprosthetic knee replacement. Since the time of his initial diagnosis, he developed a right-sided pulmonary nodule that was resected, and the pathology was consistent with metastatic osteosarcoma. On examination, he also has evidence of hyperreflexia in his lower extremities. An MRI evaluation revealed an enhancing epidural mass extending from C4 down to C7 that resulted in cervical spinal cord and nerve root compression (Fig. 13.1).

Positioning

Patient induction and surgical positioning warrant special consideration as many patients with cervical spine pathology have significant spinal canal stenosis [18]. Excessive neck flexion, extension, or rotation in this patient population has a potential risk for serious neurological complications. The head should be maintained in a neutral alignment until the head can be further secured. Similarly, fiberoptic intubation may reduce the amount of cervical extension required to place the endotracheal tube. The patient's blood pressure should be maintained at normotensive values, ideally with the systolic blood pressure being higher than 120 mmHg. Hypotension should be avoided in patients with spinal cord compression. Preoperative steroids can be considered if desired by the primary surgeon [19].

Neurological complications in the cervical spine can be potentially devastating, so preventative strategies such as intraoperative neurophysiological monitoring may be utilized to assess the psychological integrity of the spinal cord tracts. Monitoring the spinal column has potential to alert the surgeon prior to any irreversible neurological deterioration both during the positioning and the procedure [18, 20]. Combined motor evoked potential (MEP) and (somatosensory evoked potential (SSEP) monitoring can be used. The head should be kept in neutral alignment throughout the procedure and is secured to the bed frame with a Mayfield head holder.

Surgical Approach

Posterior cervical approaches begin with a midline incision over the intended levels of operation. The prominent C2 and C7 spinous processes can often be palpated to help with incisional planning, but fluoroscopy can be beneficial in smaller cases. The skin is incised sharply and the dissection is continued with electrocautery. The nuchal fascia is carefully dissected in line with

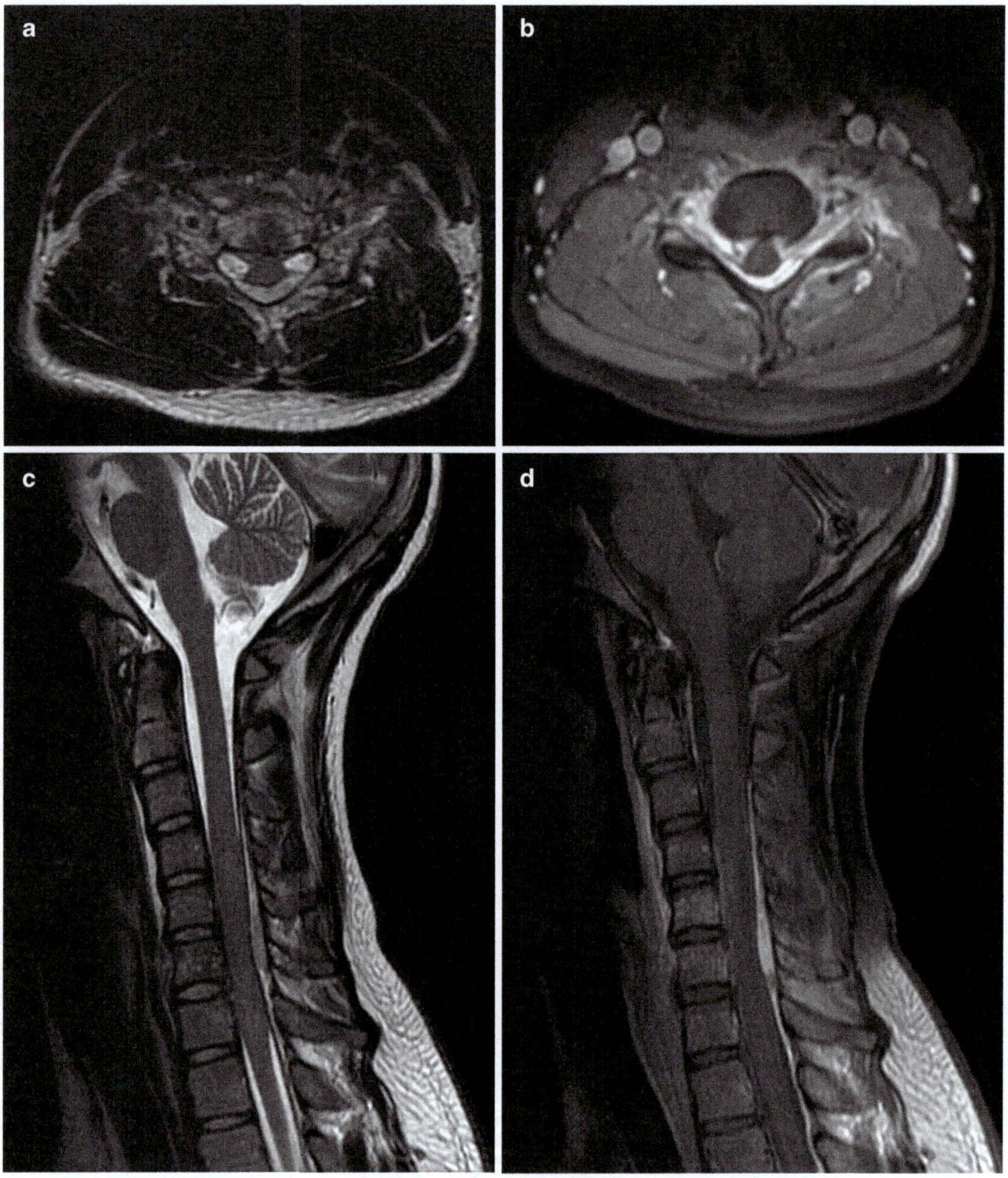

Fig. 13.1 MRI revealing an axial T2 (**a**), axial T1 with contrast (**b**), sagittal T2 (**c**), and sagittal T1 with contrast (**d**). There is evidence of epidural tumor involvement from C4 down to C7 resulting in moderate central spinal stenosis

the incision. The paraspinal musculature is then separated by identifying the relatively avascular midline raphe. Next, a subperiosteal dissection of the spinous processes, laminae, facet joints, and lateral masses is performed. The interspinous ligaments should be left intact when possible to help maintain stability. The intended levels of operation should be confirmed prior to any bone removal or instrumentation placement. Of note, the cervical facet capsules should not be violated until level localization has been verified radiographically to avoid unnecessary instability or autofusion of joints outside of the intended fusion construct.

Decompression and Tumor Resection

Resection of spinal tumors can be challenging. Surgical tenets such as adequate exposure, gentle tissue manipulation, continuous hemostasis, and approaching the lesion from normal to abnormal anatomy are vital. Goals of surgery vary widely depending on tumor pathology, extent of systemic disease, and patient health. If the lesion is a primary bony neoplasm, an aggressive en bloc resection with margins is desirable. Metastatic lesions are most often resected piecemeal, and surgery is considered palliative in this population. Regardless, the first priority is decompression of the neural elements, and this goal is often best achieved with a laminectomy. Multiple cervical laminectomy techniques have been described in the literature. One method involves drilling bilateral troughs along the laminar facet interface and removing the spinous processes and lamina in an en bloc fashion. Alternatively, the high-speed drill can be used to drill away the lamina while leaving an eggshell of thin cortical bone on top of the canal, which can then be removed with rongeurs. To ensure adequate decompression, the laminectomy should extend superior and inferior to the compressing lesion. Most operative patients with metastatic spinal tumors have some degree of spinal canal compromise, placing the patients at higher operative risks. In these circumstances, expedient tumor debulking can prevent any prolonged spinal cord compression during the procedure. Early decompression is especially important if monitoring changes occur. However, if spinal impingement is not a concern, performing screw placement prior to the decompression is reasonable.

The major limitations that can hinder tumor resection include involvement of the spinal dura, nerve roots, and vertebral arteries. Unlike spinal surgeries for degenerative pathology, oncological surgery often requires extensive bony removal of the posterior elements to adequately resect tumor and decompress neural elements. This enhances visualization of the spinal canal and exiting nerves and provides a corridor for tumor resection. However, excessive removal of the lateral mass and facet joints impairs axial loading, and in extreme cases, lateral mass reconstruction can be considered using a fibular strut or cage if there is competent bone above and below the defect to support the reconstruction [21].

Intraoperative bleeding can be excessive in patients with hypervascular spinal column tumors. Certain tumor pathologies such as renal cell carcinoma have a higher propensity for hemorrhage. Preoperative embolization of the feeding arteries can be helpful in reducing blood loss [2, 22–25]. However, embolization is rarely sufficient to stop bleeding altogether. Continued bleeding is often a result of residual tumor, especially in piecemeal resections, and the bleeding often slows upon completion of the tumor resection. Hemorrhagic areas can often be controlled with manual tamponade techniques using a cottonoid and gentle pressure from a suction device or the use of hemostatic agents.

In the provided scenario, the tumor predominantly involved the epidural space posteriorly. Laminectomies were performed from C4 to C7, exposing the underlying tumor. The lateral mass and facet joints were preserved. A surgical plane between the tumor capsule and spinal dura was identified and teased apart. The tumor was then resected in a piecemeal fashion until no remaining tumor was visible and all neural structures were adequately decompressed.

Fusion

Fusion procedures are often performed concurrently with tumor resections to prevent progressive deformity in the setting of pathologic or iatrogenic spinal instability. Having a firm knowledge of cervical anatomy and any pathological changes secondary to tumor displacement is pivotal in reducing fusion complication rates (Fig. 13.2).

While there have been many stabilization methods described in the literature, lateral mass screw constructs have become the gold standard for posterior cervical spine fixation (Fig. 13.3) [18, 26–28]. Three common lateral mass screw techniques have been described, the Magerl, the

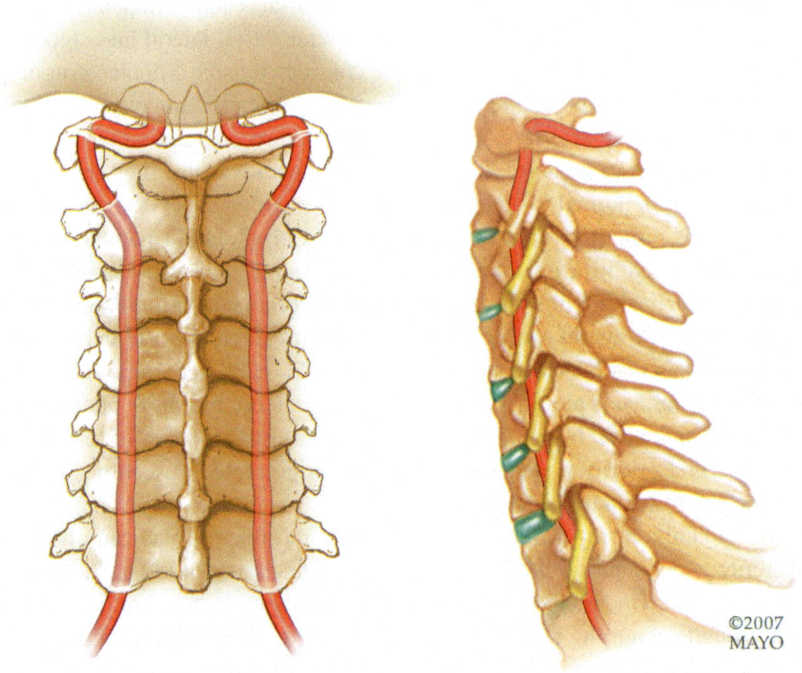

Fig. 13.2 AP and lateral views of the cervical spinal column referencing typical vascular and nerve anatomy. (Used with permission of Mayo Foundation for Medical Education and Research. All rights reserved)

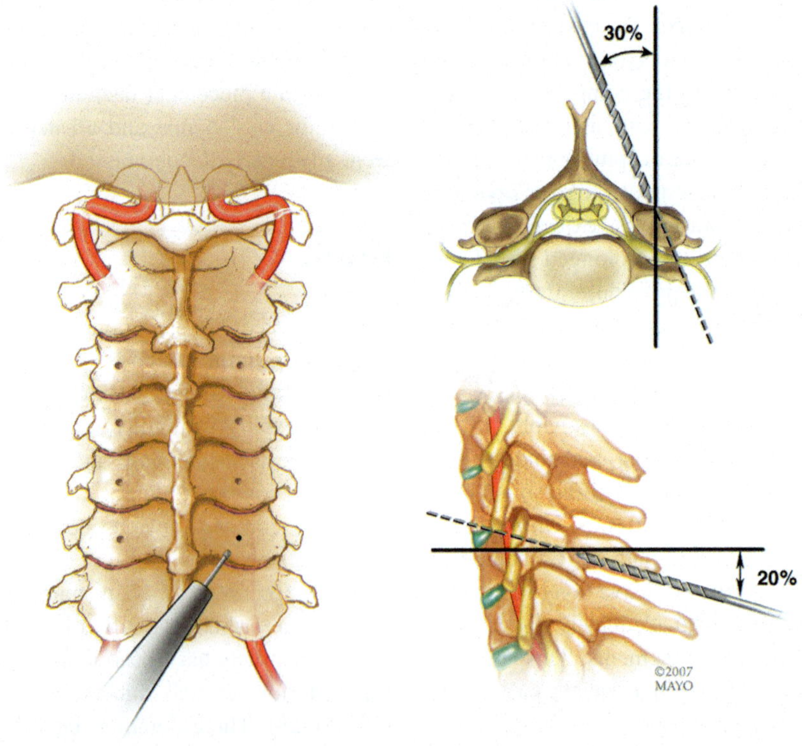

Fig. 13.3 Standard entry point location and lateral mass screw trajectory. (Used with permission of Mayo Foundation for Medical Education and Research. All rights reserved)

An, and the Anderson techniques. These techniques vary slightly on entry point and screw angulation, but are all similar in that they aim laterally to avoid injury to the vertebral artery and cephalad to avoid the exiting nerve root [18, 27].

Once the lateral mass landmarks are well visualized, the entry point is identified and a pilot hole is created. Using a high-speed drill, lateral mass tracts are cannulated utilizing a superior and lateral trajectory until the lateral mass floor can no longer be palpated with a ball probe. The tract is under-tapped. The depth is often between 12 and 16 mm depending on the presence of osteophytes, patient's body habitus, and the exact surgical trajectory that was taken.

Ending instrumentation at the C7 vertebral level is somewhat controversial as it creates long-arm vector forces between the cervical fusion and the physiological stiff thoracic spine, increasing the likelihood of adjacent segment disease. Longer cervical constructs are often extended to the upper thoracic spine to bridge the cervicothoracic junction to increase stability and avoid this complication (Fig. 13.4).

In patients with poor life expectancy, spinal stabilization alone may be appropriate, but if patients have a more indolent pathology or have a longer life expectancy, obtaining a solid fusion is preferred (Fig. 13.5). The facet joints and lamina should be exposed and decorticated with a cutting bit. Fusion preparation should be performed prior to lateral mass screw insertion as the screws can often inhibit visualization and drill access to the subaxial facet joints

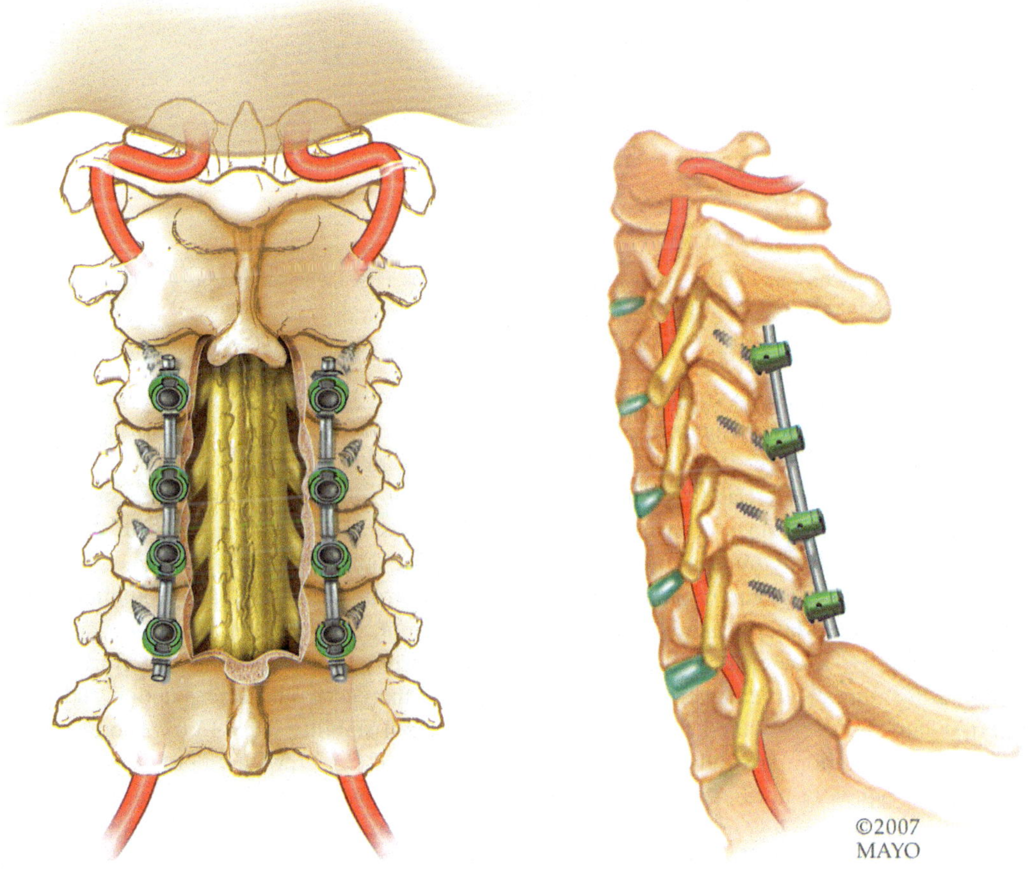

Fig. 13.4 AP and lateral view of subaxial laminectomies and fixation from C3 to C6. (Used with permission of Mayo Foundation for Medical Education and Research. All rights reserved)

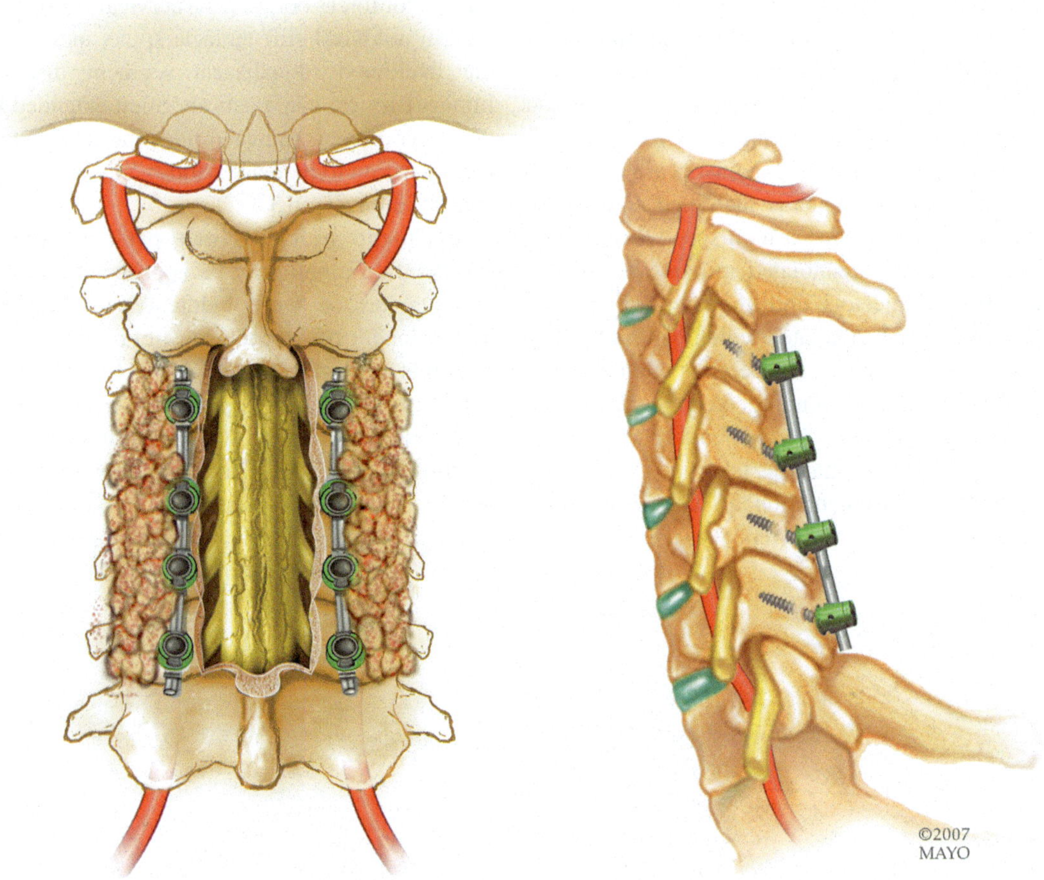

Fig. 13.5 AP and lateral view of subaxial fusion following arthrodesis. (Used with permission of Mayo Foundation for Medical Education and Research. All rights reserved)

[18]. The wound should be copiously irrigated prior to placement of graft materials. Polyaxial lateral mass screws are inserted. Excessive torque should be avoided as this can result in fracture of the lateral mass or strip the screw tract, reducing the bony purchase of the screw. Cervical alignment and screw position should be confirmed with a lateral radiograph or fluoroscopy. Finally, iliac crest autograft (if not involved by tumor) or cadaveric allograft is inserted into the decorticated facet joints and fusion bed to promote arthrodesis. Local bone autograft is typically not harvested in patients with active neoplastic lesions as the bone fragments could be seeded with cancerous cells, increasing the likelihood of local tumor recurrence or spread during arthrodesis. There should not be any free bone fragments in the spinal canal as this is a potential source of nerve compression.

Purely subaxial fixation is acceptable in certain cases. However, our clinical scenario had extensive epidural tumor involvement from C4 to C7 requiring multilevel laminectomies to resect the tumor. Therefore, the fusion captured C2 superiorly and was extended inferiorly to T2 to bridge the cervicothoracic junction and provide additional stability (Fig. 13.6). Thoracic pedicle screws and C2 screws are both outside the scope of this chapter. See Chaps. 12 and 17 for additional information on these techniques. It is also notable that the fusion construct in this case extends beyond the area of anticipated postoperative radiation treatment.

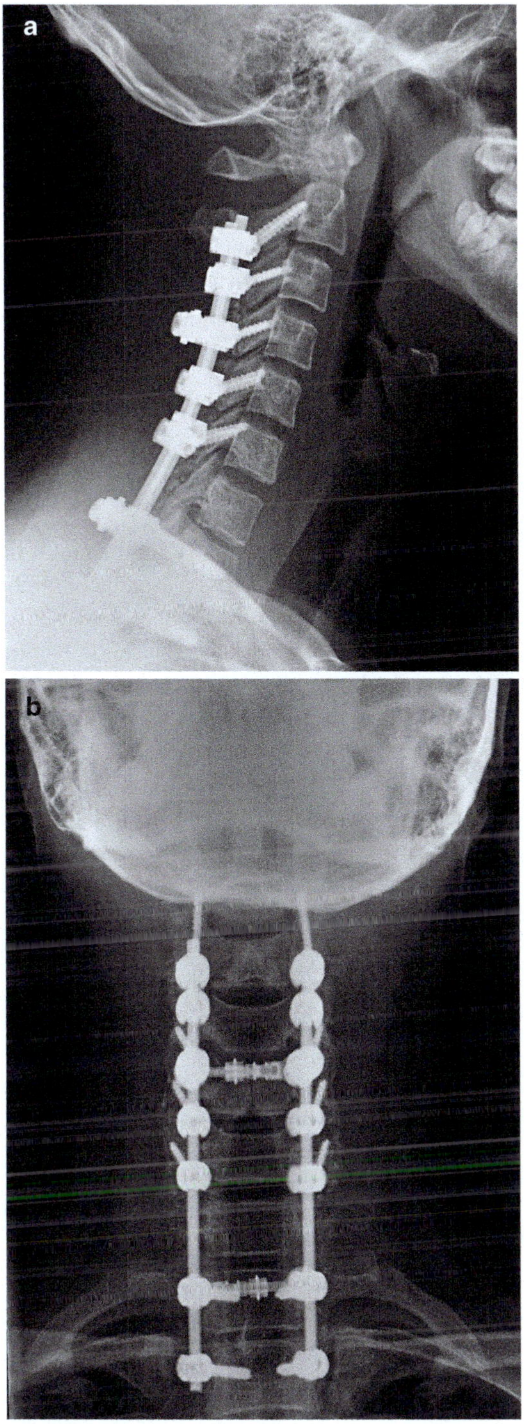

Fig. 13.6 Postoperative AP (**a**) and lateral (**b**) views of a C2–T2 posterior instrumented fusion with cross-links

Closure

A meticulous closure technique is important to minimize wound complication. Excellent hemostasis should be achieved prior to closing the wound. The extensive osseous decortication performed for arthrodesis often results in ongoing postoperative blood loss; therefore, subfascial and suprafascial drains are often placed.

Complications

The literature has shown that patients with spinal cancers have higher rates of surgical morbidity and mortality [3, 10, 29]. Optimizing outcomes in spinal tumor patients focuses on preservation of function and prevention of complications that can delay life-prolonging adjuvant treatments. Surgical site infections and wound complications are prevalent. Risk factors for wound complications include preoperative radiation and poor nutritional status [3]. Wound infections are highly problematic for cancer patients as this often requires additional surgery for irrigation and debridement, which temporarily suspends ongoing systemic chemotherapy and radiation treatments [3, 30]. Some studies have suggested that intraoperative vancomycin powder can reduce wound infection rates [31–33], but there is little evidence available to support this practice in cancer patients. Surgery is frequently followed by postoperative radiation, which can further impair wound healing and spinal fusion rates [3, 30]. Radiotherapy should be delayed for at least 2 weeks or more to minimize wound-related complications [34]. Furthermore, poor bone quality associated with the lesion or preexisting osteopenia or osteoporosis has been associated with higher rates of instrumentation failure in spinal tumor patients [30]. Finally, cancer patients are often hypercoagulable and are predisposed to deep venous thromboses, pulmonary emboli, or even disseminated intravascular coagulation [30]. Sequential compression devices and early mobilization are key to reducing the incidence of thrombotic complications in cancer patients.

There are inherent risks associated with posterior cervical lateral mass screw instrumentation as well. The structures most at risk during screw placement are the vertebral artery and the exiting nerve root. The screws should be directed laterally to avoid vascular injury to the vertebral artery, which typically lies ventral to the medial half of the lateral mass. If a vascular injury occurs during drilling, a short screw can be inserted along the tract to tamponade the arterial bleeding. Alternatively, the tract can be plugged with bone wax for hemostasis. Additional drilling of bone for visualization or any attempt to directly repair the vascular injury is not recommended as this may result in uncontrollable bleeding. If there is suspicion of vertebral artery injury, it is essential to avoid additional maneuvers that might put the contralateral vertebral artery at risk. Immediately following the procedure, the patient should undergo a diagnostic cerebral angiography for vascular assessment. If any ongoing bleeding or vascular dissection is identified, it can be further addressed in the angiography suite. Delayed cervical palsies are also a common complication following posterior cervical decompressions and most often occur in the C5 dermatome [35, 36]. Most patients make a full neurological recovery; however, it often takes up to 6 months or more to see maximal improvement [18]. Any patient who has radicular symptoms postoperatively should have advanced imaging performed to assess screw positioning and nerve root integrity.

If electrophysiological monitoring is being utilized, surgeons must know how to interpret and correct persistent monitoring changes. If a focal monitoring change is present, extremity repositioning can improve monitoring signals. Monitoring checks should be performed before and after any cervical deformity correction maneuvers are performed. If a monitoring change occurs following a correction in spinal alignment, it is recommended to reverse or lessen the degree of deformity correction.

Uncontrollable intraoperative hemorrhage from spinal tumors is a rare but potentially devastating intraoperative complication. Patients with metastatic cancer often have intrinsic coagulation dysfunction due to their systemic disease, and some lesions also have extensive involvement of local vascular anatomy. Certain tumor histologies, such as renal cell carcinoma, follicular thyroid carcinoma, and neuroendocrine tumors, have a higher propensity for intraoperative hemorrhage. If intraoperative bleeding is a concern, angiographic embolization can be performed to reduce intraoperative blood loss and provide better intraoperative visualization [2–25, 30]. Of note, intraoperative blood salvage is often avoided due to the risk of metastatic tumor contamination.

Clinical Pearls

Preoperative radiographic anatomy should be extensively reviewed to assess the extent of tumor involvement and to evaluate for aberrant vascular anatomy. Notify anesthesia prior to induction about cervical stenosis and implement standard positioning precautions of the cervical spine. Primary bony neoplasms require an aggressive en bloc surgical resection for surgical cure. Conversely, surgery for patients with metastatic spinal disease is palliative and is reserved for patients with intractable pain or neurological compromise. Lateral mass screws are recommended for posterior cervical constructs, and they should be directed laterally and superiorly (parallel to the facet joints) to avoid injury to the exiting nerve roots and vertebral artery.

References

1. Quan GM, Vital J-M, Pointillart V. Outcomes of palliative surgery in metastatic disease of the cervical and cervicothoracic spine. J Neurosurg Spine. 2011;14(5):612–8.
2. Abdu WA, Provencher M. Primary bone and metastatic tumors of the cervical spine. Spine. 1998;23(24):2767–77.
3. Mesfin A, Sciubba DM, Dea N, Nater A, Bird JE, Quraishi NA, et al. Changing the adverse event profile in metastatic spine surgery: an evidence-based approach to target wound complications and instrumentation failure. Spine. 2016;41(Suppl 20):S262–70.
4. Ibrahim A, Crockard A, Antonietti P, Boriani S, Bünger C, Gasbarrini A, et al. Does spinal surgery improve the quality of life for those with extradural

(spinal) osseous metastases? An international multicenter prospective observational study of 223 patients. Invited submission from the Joint Section Meeting on Disorders of the Spine and Peripheral Nerves, March 2007. J Neurosurg Spine. 2008;8(3):271–8.
5. Di Lorenzo N, Delfini R, Ciappetta P, Cantore G, Fortuna A. Primary tumors of the cervical spine: surgical experience with 38 cases. Surg Neurol. 1992;38(1):12–8.
6. Rao S, Badani K, Schildhauer T, Borges M. Metastatic malignancy of the cervical spine. A nonoperative history. Spine. 1992;17(10 Suppl):S407–12.
7. Arutyunyan GG, Clarke MJ. Management of primary and metastatic spinal tumors. J Neurosurg Sci. 2015;59(2):181–93.
8. Schiff D, O'Neill BP, Suman VJ. Spinal epidural metastasis as the initial manifestation of malignancy: clinical features and diagnostic approach. Neurology. 1997;49(2):452–6.
9. Boriani S, Gasbarrini A, Bandiera S, Ghermandi R, Lador R. En bloc resections in the spine: the experience of 220 patients during 25 years. World Neurosurg. 2017;98:217–29.
10. Clarke MJ, Mendel E, Vrionis FD. Primary spine tumors: diagnosis and treatment. Cancer Control. 2014;21(2):114–23.
11. Tomita K, Kawahara N, Murakami H, Demura S. Total en bloc spondylectomy for spinal tumors: improvement of the technique and its associated basic background. J Orthop Sci. 2006;11(1):3–12.
12. Davarski AN, Kitov BD, Zhelyazkov CB, Raykov SD, Kehayov II, Koev IG, et al. Surgical management of metastatic tumors of the cervical spine. Folia Med. 2013;55(3–4):39–45.
13. Laufer I, Sciubba DM, Madera M, Bydon A, Witham TJ, Gokaslan ZL, et al. Surgical management of metastatic spinal tumors. Cancer Control. 2012;19(2):122–8.
14. Fehlings MG, David KS, Vialle L, Vialle E, Setzer M, Vrionis FD. Decision making in the surgical treatment of cervical spine metastases. Spine. 2009;34(22 Suppl):S108–17.
15. Patchell RA, Tibbs PA, Regine WF, Payne R, Saris S, Kryscio RJ, et al. Direct decompressive surgical resection in the treatment of spinal cord compression caused by metastatic cancer: a randomised trial. Lancet. 2005;366(9486):643–8.
16. Sundaresan N, Steinberger AA, Moore F, Sachdev VP, Krol G, Hough L, et al. Indications and results of combined anterior-posterior approaches for spine tumor surgery. J Neurosurg. 1996;85(3):438–46.
17. Rupp RE, Ebraheim NA, Coombs RJ. Magnetic resonance imaging differentiation of compression spine fractures or vertebral lesions caused by osteoporosis or tumor. Spine. 1995;20(23):2499–503; discussion 2504.
18. Kurd MF, Millhouse PW, Schroeder GD, Kepler CK, Vaccaro AR. Lateral mass fixation in the subaxial cervical spine. J Spinal Disord Tech. 2015;28(7):259–63.
19. Kumar A, Weber MH, Gokaslan Z, Wolinsky J-P, Schmidt M, Rhines L, et al. Metastatic spinal cord compression and steroid treatment: a systematic review. Clin Spine Surg. 2017;30(4):156–63.
20. Kelleher MO, Tan G, Sarjeant R, Fehlings MG. Predictive value of intraoperative neurophysiological monitoring during cervical spine surgery: a prospective analysis of 1055 consecutive patients. J Neurosurg Spine. 2008;8(3):215–21.
21. Clarke MJ, Zadnik PL, Groves ML, Sciubba DM, Witham TF, Bydon A, et al. Fusion following lateral mass reconstruction in the cervical spine. J Neurosurg Spine. 2015;22(2):139–50.
22. Breslau J, Eskridge JM. Preoperative embolization of spinal tumors. J Vasc Interv Radiol. 1995;6(6):871–5.
23. Broaddus WC, Grady MS, Delashaw JB Jr, Ferguson RD, Jane JA. Preoperative superselective arteriolar embolization: a new approach to enhance resectability of spinal tumors. Neurosurgery. 1990;27(5):755–9.
24. Gellad FE, Sadato N, Numaguchi Y, Levine AM. Vascular metastatic lesions of the spine: preoperative embolization. Radiology. 1990;176(3):683–6.
25. Smith TP, Gray L, Weinstein JN, Richardson WJ, Payne CS. Preoperative transarterial embolization of spinal column neoplasms. J Vasc Interv Radiol. 1995;6(6):863–9.
26. Eldin MM, Hassan ASA. Free hand technique of cervical lateral mass screw fixation. J Craniovertebr Junction Spine. 2017;8(2):113–8.
27. Ebraheim NA, Klausner T, Xu R, Yeasting RA. Safe lateral-mass screw lengths in the Roy-Camille and Magerl techniques. An anatomic study. Spine. 1998;23(16):1739–42.
28. Coe JD, Vaccaro AR, Dailey AT, Skolasky RL Jr, Sasso RC, Ludwig SC, et al. Lateral mass screw fixation in the cervical spine: a systematic literature review. J Bone Joint Surg Am. 2013;95(23):2136–43.
29. Yang W, Jiang L, Liu X, Wei F, Yu M, Wu F, et al. Surgical complications of extraspinal tumors in the cervical spine: a report of 110 cases and literature review. Eur Spine J [Internet]. 2017. Available from: https://doi.org/10.1007/s00586-017-5259-4.
30. Clarke MJ, Vrionis FD. Spinal tumor surgery: management and the avoidance of complications. Cancer Control. 2014;21(2):124–32.
31. O'Neill KR, Smith JG, Abtahi AM, Archer KR, Spengler DM, McGirt MJ, et al. Reduced surgical site infections in patients undergoing posterior spinal stabilization of traumatic injuries using vancomycin powder. Spine J. 2011;11(7):641–6.
32. Theologis AA, Demirkiran G, Callahan M, Pekmezci M, Ames C, Deviren V. Local intrawound vancomycin powder decreases the risk of surgical site infections in complex adult deformity reconstruction: a cost analysis. Spine. 2014;39(22):1875–80.
33. Sweet FA, Roh M, Sliva C. Intrawound application of vancomycin for prophylaxis in instrumented thoracolumbar fusions: efficacy, drug levels, and patient outcomes. Spine. 2011;36(24):2084–8.

34. Itshayek E, Yamada J, Bilsky M, Schmidt M, Shaffrey C, Gerszten P, et al. Timing of surgery and radiotherapy in the management of metastatic spine disease: a systematic review. Int J Oncol. 2010;36(3):533–44.
35. Planchard RF, Maloney PR, Mallory GW, Puffer RC, Spinner RJ, Nassr A, et al. Postoperative delayed cervical palsies: understanding the etiology. Global Spine J. 2016;6(6):571–83.
36. Thompson SE, Smith ZA, Hsu WK, Nassr A, Mroz TE, Fish DE, et al. C5 palsy after cervical spine surgery: a multicenter retrospective review of 59 cases. Global Spine J. 2017;7(1 Suppl):64S–70S.

Anterior/Anterolateral Thoracic Access and Stabilization from Posterior Approach: Transpedicular, Costotransversectomy, Lateral Extracavitary Approaches: Standard Intralesional Resection

14

James G. Malcolm, Michael K. Moore, and Daniel Refai

Introduction

Surgical approaches to the anterior thoracic spine have evolved over the last century. As early as 1894, Menard developed the costotransversectomy (CT) for the treatment of Pott's disease [1]. Until 1976, when Larson popularized the lateral extracavitary approach (LECA), the most commonly performed procedure for ventral lesions remained a laminectomy. With the advent of the LECA, greater access to ventral lesions led to less morbidity and improved outcomes in ventral thoracic spine lesions [2]. Today surgeons have improved and expanded on surgical methods enabling virtually complete access to the ventral thoracic spine through dorsal approaches.

In consideration of dorsal versus ventral approaches to the anterior thoracic spine, the goal of surgery is paramount. Most tumors of the spine are metastases; therefore, debulking through intralesional (piecemeal) resection of the tumor, not en bloc resection, is the primary goal with gross total resection when possible. Resection of the tumor mass enables us to achieve three aims. First, it allows for stabilization of the spine. The compressive load carried by the vertebral body increases from 9% of total body weight at T1 to 47% of body weight at T12 [3]. Removal and replacement of a weakened anterior column restores biomechanical stability. This at minimum prevents progressive collapse in patients with pathologic fractures and can be used to correct kyphotic deformity. Cages or allograft struts are often used to achieve anterior column support. Second, the removal of the lesion reduces tumor burden creating a corridor between the neural structures and tumor. Third, to halt or reverse neurologic deterioration from compression of neural structures. In selecting a corridor, the surgeon must weigh surgical morbidity versus attainable outcomes.

While surgical decompression with radiotherapy is superior to radiotherapy alone in maintaining function [4], the decision to operate can be guided by the NOMS framework [5, 6]. Neurologic (N) considerations include the degree of myelopathy, functional radiculopathy, and epidural spinal cord compression [7]. When

J. G. Malcolm (✉) · M. K. Moore
Emory University, Department of Neurosurgery, Atlanta, GA, USA
e-mail: james.malcolm@emory.edu

D. Refai
Emory University, Department of Neurosurgery and Orthopaedics, Atlanta, GA, USA

D. M. Sciubba (ed.), *Spinal Tumor Surgery*, https://doi.org/10.1007/978-3-319-98422-3_14

possible, pain should be separated into biological and mechanical sources. Oncologic (O) considerations center primarily on the radiologic sensitivity of the tumor. For example, myeloma and lymphoma are considered radiosensitive; breast as moderately sensitive; colon and non-small-cell lung cancer as moderately resistant; and thyroid, renal, sarcoma, and melanoma as resistant [8]. Assessment of mechanical (M) instability includes movement-related pain and involved levels. Systemic (S) disease burden encompasses the extent of disease throughout the body as well as associated co-morbidities. With this framework in mind, resection is often recommended when there is high-grade epidural compression, radioresistance, mechanical radiculopathy or back pain, and instability and when the patient is able to tolerate surgery [5]. In cases with significant canal involvement for a tumor otherwise suitable for radiotherapy, surgery may be performed to separate the spinal cord from the tumor for subsequent stereotactic radiosurgery without damage to the cord [9]. This "separation surgery" enables the administration of adjuvant radiation therapy. In most institutions, the radiation oncologists request between 1 and 3 mm of cerebrospinal fluid (CSF) signal between the spinal cord and tumor margin to enable them to deliver complete lesional coverage with radiotherapy [7].

Access to the ventral thoracic spine has been historically accomplished through a variety of approaches with the main approaches being transthoracic or some combination of laminectomy (L) plus transpedicular (TP), costotransversectomy (CT) , or lateral extracavitary (LECA). Of these four approaches, the last three are posterior and can be thought of as in continuity with each other, and each extends upon a standard laminectomy (L) (Fig. 14.1). As the surgeon requires more anterior exposure, the dissection progresses from removal of the lamina (L), to pars and pedicle (TP), to removal of the transverse process and proximal rib (less than 4–6 cm) (CT), to a LECA in which extensive rib (beyond 6 cm) dissection is employed to enable contralateral access to ventral pathology from a unilateral posterior exposure (Figs. 14.2, 14.3, and 14.4) [10]. This may be accomplished in a traditional open or mini-open manner (Fig. 14.5).

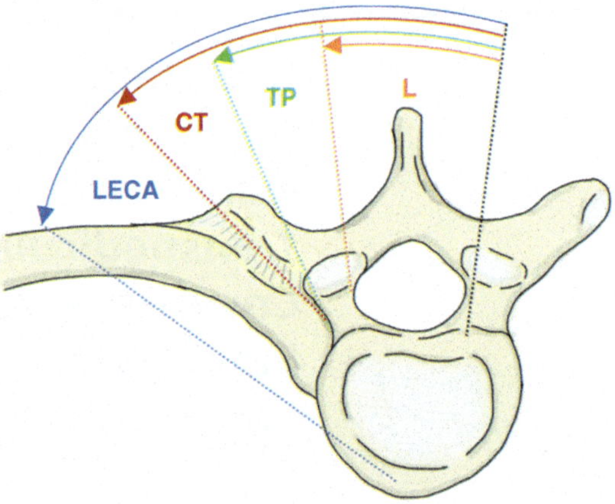

Fig. 14.1 Axial illustration of thoracic vertebral body and rib with various posterior approaches overlaid: lateral extracavitary approach (LECA), transpedicular (TP), and costotransversectomy (CT). Each of these extends the standard laminectomy (L). LECA provides greater access to the ventral aspect of the vertebral body, while TP and CT may be sufficient for more limited lesions

Case Description

For illustration, we present a 30-year-old female with a history of breast cancer who presented to clinic with progressive thoracic back pain radiating down her left flank through the T7 dermatome. Imaging revealed a lesion at T6–T7 with spinal cord effacement but without cord signal change (Fig. 14.6). Since the lesion was eccentric to the left and involved the ribs with significant invasion of the vertebral body, the decision was made to perform a lateral extracavitary approach from the left taking the T6–T7 ribs and over half the vertebral bodies. Preoperative angiography was not indicated due to the eccentricity of pathology. Because of her kyphosis and involvement of two levels, instrumentation was planned from T3 to T9 (three above, two below). On the day of surgery, her neurologic exam had further declined to a T6 sensory level with motor movements of 1–2 out of 5 in her bilateral lower extremities.

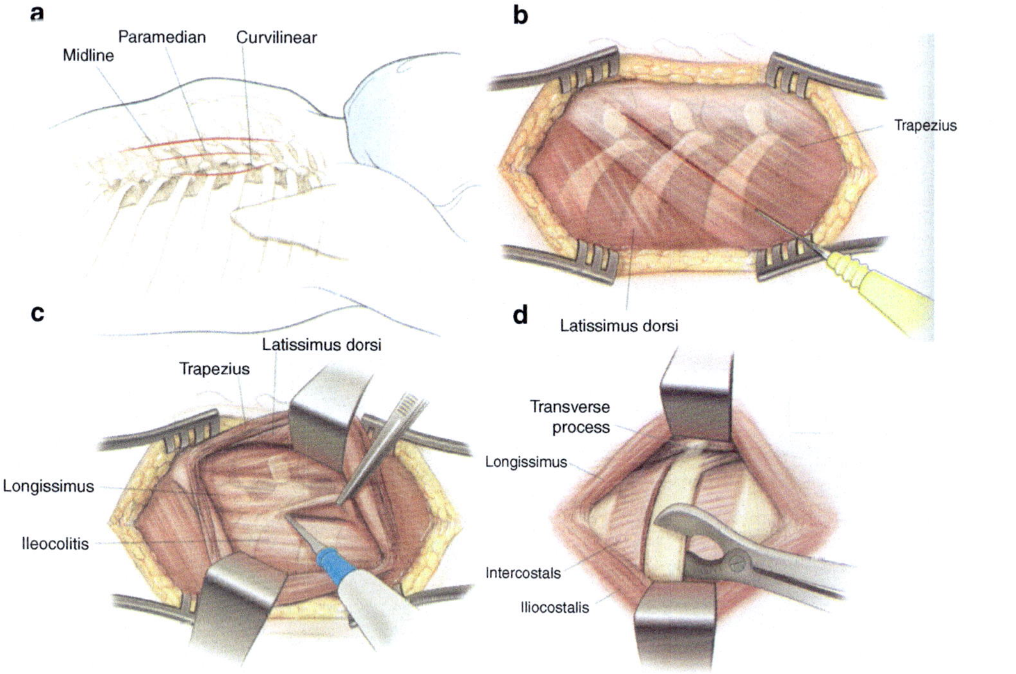

Fig. 14.2 Skin incision and rib exposure for lateral extracavitary approach to the thoracic spine (**a**–**d**). (Reprinted with permission from Miller et al. [14].)

Fig. 14.3 Lateral extracavitary approach. A. Rib disarticulation. B. Extracavitary retraction. (Reprinted with permission from Miller et al. [14].)

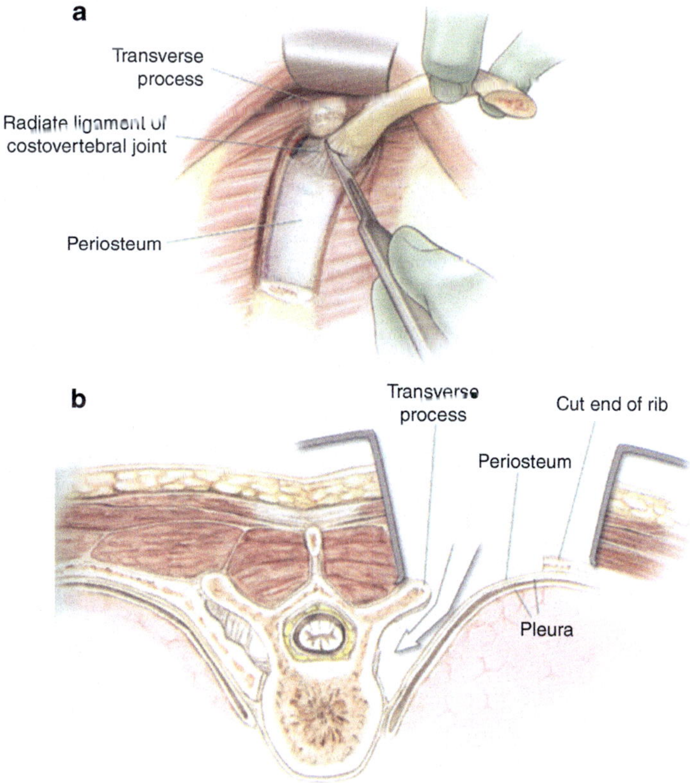

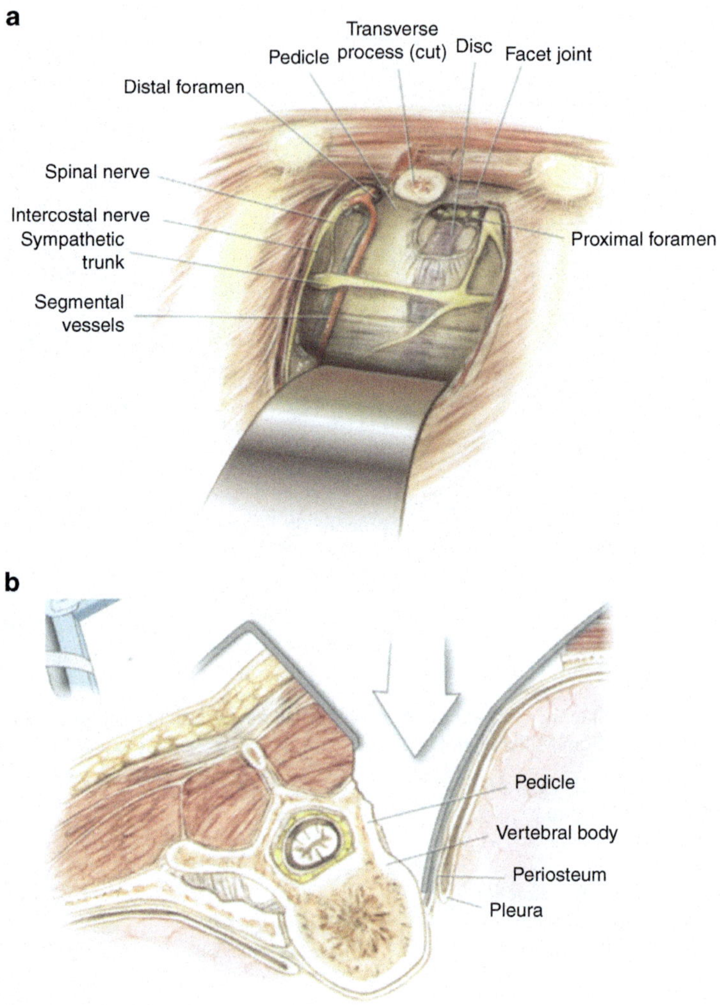

Fig. 14.4 Lateral extracavitary retraction to expose the thoracic vertebral body (**a**, **b**). (Reprinted with permission from Miller et al. [14].)

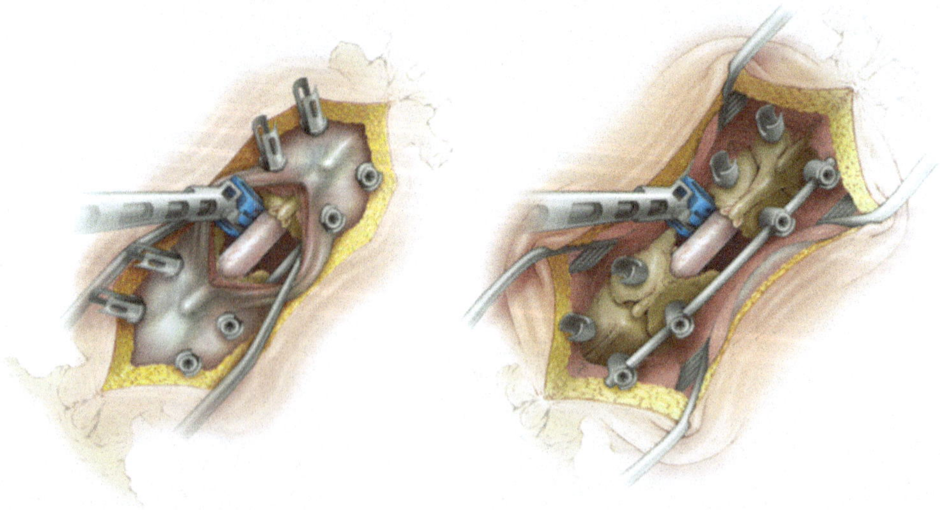

Fig. 14.5 Mini-open and open anterior column reconstruction for thoracic tumor resection. (Reprinted with permission from Lau and Chou [15])

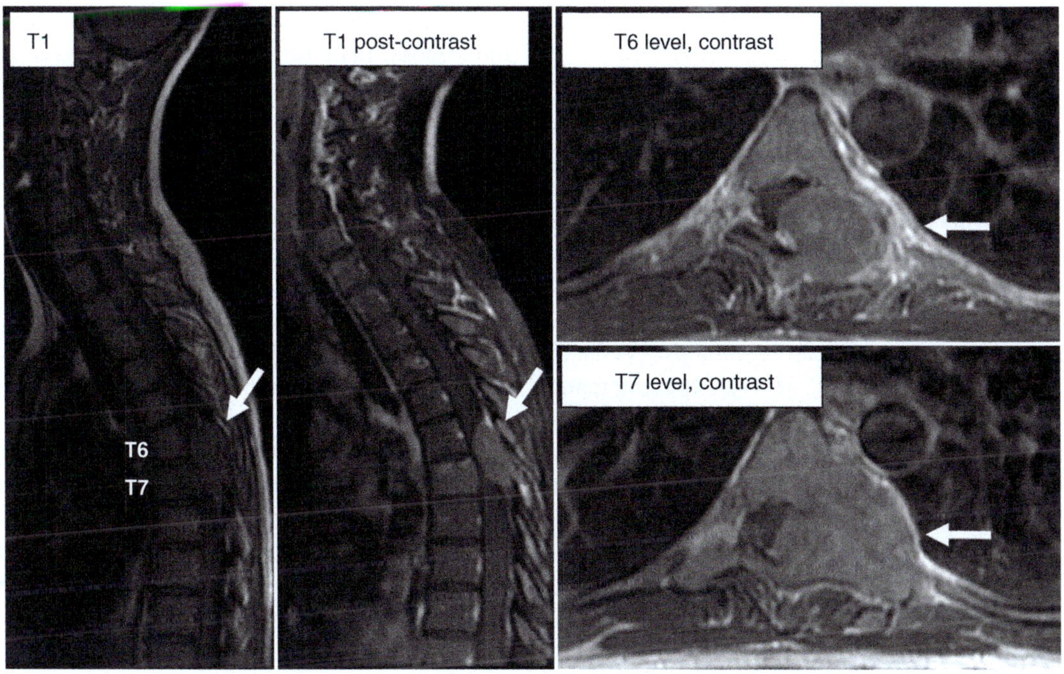

Fig. 14.6 Preoperative MRI of patient with metastatic breast cancer to T6–T7. Sagittal pre–/post-contrast images (left panels) show the lesion posterior to the canal (arrows). Axial T1 cuts at each vertebral level (T6 top, T7 bottom) show extent of tumor involvement into the vertebral body

Procedure

Outline of Steps

The following steps are carried out for the LECA procedure:

- Preoperative image review and surgical planning
- Positioning
- Neuromonitoring
- Incision
- Pedicle screws
- Transverse process dissection
- Rib dissection and resection
- Laminectomy
- Pars and facets
- Temporary rod placement
- Coring out pedicle
- Nerve root sacrifice for wider access
- Corpectomy
- Cage placement
- Complete instrumented fusion

Preoperative Image Review and Surgical Planning

The preparation of a posterior approach for anterior access of the thoracic spine requires careful review of the patient's MRI and CT scan. One needs to determine how much bone needs to be removed, the laterality of the approach to the anterior spine, and how much stabilization is required. In certain situations, a preoperative angiogram may be appropriate as well. For instance, for lesions in the T6–T9 region, the artery of Adamkiewicz should be identified, both its level and laterality to avoid injury if approached from that side. In ~20% of thoracic spinal metastasis, the lesion occurs at the level of Adamkiewicz [11]. Second, for patients where you suspect renal cell carcinoma, thyroid cancer, or other bloody metastases, preoperative embolization can greatly reduce intraoperative bleeding. We recommend admitting the patient for embolization the day before surgery so collateral circulation does not have time to develop.

Positioning

Position the patient on a rotating Jackson table with thigh and hip pads. This is a critical step because this rotation (25–40°) provides enhanced visualization necessary for cross-midline resections without the need for additional lateral dissection to achieve line of sight. Further, Jackson tables are less dense (less radio-opaque), and hence they improve intraoperative imaging and ease of location via fluoroscopy. For larger patients, a minimum of two circumferential straps are required to secure the patient from falling or slipping at higher-angle rotations. In high thoracic lesions (T1–T6), we prefer to tuck the arms. Placing the patient with arms extended forces the surgeon to cantilever their body over the arm board in an uncomfortable position.

Neuromonitoring

Neuromonitoring, both motor-evoked potential (MEP) and somatosensory-evoked potential (SSEP), is highly recommended for cases where the nerve root is to be sacrificed or deformity corrections are planned. We also include anal sphincter EMG as it is very sensitive to neurological changes. In the surgical description below, we describe their use in preparing to sacrifice the nerve root.

Localization

Localization can be extremely challenging in the thoracic spine. Preoperative assessment of upright plain films and CT should be carefully reviewed. Count the total number of ribs and lumbar vertebra to note any abnormalities. Rib numbers and morphologically unique deformities can be useful to ensure correct levels are identified. It may be necessary to incrementally count up from T12/L1 or down from T1 with several fluoroscopy shots, optionally resting a radiopaque instrument on the patient's back or inserting a spinal needle down to the spinous process for landmarks. In some cases, the index level will have a pathological fracture easily recognized on lateral fluoroscopy. In obese or muscular patients, intraoperative rib counting can be especially difficult. Consider using lateral fluoroscopy counting from the sacral prominence to be sure.

Incision

The incision is marked linearly over the midline and centered on the level of metastasis (index level). Retract the skin in a diamond shape, with the apex over the rib at the index level. This diamond shape allows for the largest corridor of approach over the index body once the rib and transverse process have been removed. The incision can be extended to enable further lateral retraction to see down the surgical corridor. In contrast to the "hockey-stick" incision [10], this midline incision does not transect the paraspinal muscles which improve postoperative pain and recovery. With the use of a rotating bed, we have found this midline incision adequate for visualization throughout the case.

Pedicle Screw Placement

Pedicle screws are placed in standard fashion before dissecting the transverse process and rib to minimize blood loss. Screws are placed a minimum of two levels above and below the index level. Thoracic pedicle screws can be placed free hand, under fluoro, or using O-arm navigation depending on comfort level. Free-hand screws are started by removing the cortex from the junction of the transverse process (TP) and the lamina 3 mm medial to the lateral margin of the pars and beneath the inferior facet of the level above. This hole places the starting point of the pedicle probe within the inferior aspect of the pedicle. This cortex can be most easily removed with a Leksell rongeur or if comfortable a high-speed drill. If the bite is placed correctly, cancellous bone will be visible with bleeding emanating most briskly from the pedicle. The starting point of your Lenke ball-tip probe should be placed in this location. An angle perpendicular to the lamina and in the sagittal plane and medialized about 15° should be used with gentle pressure to bore through the pedicle into the body; this tract should be palpated for breaches and tapped followed by screw placement. Fluoroscopy can be of great assistance in patients with small pedicles in finding the cranial to caudal starting position and orientation of trajectory for screw placement. When available, an O-arm can be helpful to avoid intraoperative breaches from the pedicle. Juxtapedicular or extrapedicular screw placement can be considered acceptable in the case where the screws breach laterally and the patient has small pedicles. This type of screw trajectory is typically used in pediatrics and scoliosis, particularly at the T4–T8 levels where the pedicles are the most narrow. In the case where there is a lateral breach, making additional passes in order to obtain a true transpedicular trajectory can further weaken the bone and result in low pull-out strength [12, 13].

Bone Removal

The approach and setup for corpectomy proceeds in the following order: resection of transverse process, rib, and lamina, coring out of the pedicles, removal of inferior facet of the index level, and removal of the superior facet of the thoracic body one level below.

Rib Dissection

The midline incision allows for a completely subperiosteal dissection and avoids transecting the erector spinae musculature as is often done with curvilinear or "hockey-stick" incisions classically described [10]. Limiting muscular dissection reduces blood loss, pain, length of stay, and recovery needs. The subperiosteal dissection begins from the spinous process carried down and over the lamina to the pars and up over the lateral aspect of the transverse process. This is repeated bilaterally at the index level as well as two above and two below, e.g., five total levels if a single-index level. Additional fixation may require a longer exposure. After removal of the muscular attachment to the lateral aspect of the TP at the index level, the tops of the TP itself can be removed with a rongeur Leksell. This allows for easier musculature dissection and retraction of and over the ribs. This maneuver with aggressive removal of the TP will also help detach the TP from the rib by cutting through the costotransverse ligament connecting the transverse costal facet of the TP and the tubercle of the rib. Use bone wax for hemostasis on any open bone surfaces. At the index level, the dissection will continue lateral and inferior to the transverse process so as to expose the connected rib. The rib should be dissected in the same subperiosteal plane pushing the erector spinae musculature lateral in one clean layer. This lateral dissection should be continued until you reach the angle of the rib (the most posterior inflection). This is typically 4–6 cm lateral to the transverse process.

Rib Resection

Once screws have been placed the rib is exposed out to the angle in the same subperiosteal plane. Circumferential dissection of the soft tissue is needed for rib removal. At the angle, dissect the periosteum off the rib edge superiorly and inferiorly using a Penfield 1. At the margins, switch to a curved curette to remove the periosteal plane over the edge and under the rib. The neurovascular bundle will be displaced from the costal groove without injury and you will not violate the pleura. It is critical that the hot electrocautery not be used over the margin of the rib edge to avoid damage to the neurovascular bundle. Once you have circumferential exposure, a Doyen rib stripper can be used to separate the remaining soft tissue from the rib proximally. If the patient has bulky musculature, it may be necessary to perform a partial rib exposure and release the musculature at adjacent level ribs. This allows additional lateral retraction without resorting to transection of the erector spinae.

At the superior rib margin, the pleura will lie just deep to the intercostal musculature, and it can be easy to create a plural defect. If a defect occurs, it is possible to repair first by removal of the rib as part of the surgery followed by primary repair using a 4.0 Vicryl suture. If necessary, a muscle patch can also be sutured similar to a dural patch. Once the pleura is mostly closed, you can place a small red rubber catheter into the thoracic cavity purse string around the catheter. A Valsalva maneuver will force the air from the pleural space. Once evacuated, pull the red rubber and synch the purse string. Serial chest X-rays should be followed postoperatively. The patient will likely have a small pneumothorax; however, as long as no violation of the visceral pleura occurs, the small pneumothorax will remain stable and should require no further intervention and resolve spontaneously.

At the inferior rib margin, the neurovascular bundle is located within the costal grove. The structures are in the order superior to inferior: vein, artery, nerve. At this margin, it can be easy to cause significant bleeding if either the vein or artery is injured. These arteries are fed via the posterior intercostal artery from the aorta and the anterior intercostal arteries via the internal thoracic/internal mammary artery.

Rib Disarticulation

After the soft tissue is dissected circumferentially, the rib can be removed. At the angle (distal cut), use a Kerrison 4 or 5 punch to cleanly cut through the rib. We find this preferable to a rib cutter that can be cumbersome and cause pleural defects. Use bone wax to seal the distal stump.

The proximal rib articulates posteriorly at two locations. First, the costotransverse ligament connects the transverse costal facet of the transverse process to the tubercle of the rib. This is easily cut during the removal of the transverse process as described above. Second, radiate ligaments connect the rib head to the superior and inferior costal facets of the vertebra (costovertebral joint). This is the final attachment of the rib to the body after the completion of the above steps. To free the rib, dissect between the rib and the body of the vertebra using a Penfield 4. Using firm but controlled pressure allows for disruption of this ligament from the vertebral bodies. Once free, the rib can be posteriorly elevated and the final periosteal layer on the underside close to the body can be further dissected using a Kittner and Penfield 1. If completed properly, the rib will freely elevate from the cavity without damage to the neurovascular bundle or tear in the pleura.

Laminectomy

In unilateral approaches, the laminectomy should be completed with no more than half of the pars removed from the contralateral side of the exposure. This will ensure increased stability of the posterior elements, with ample room for a posterior fusion bed if desired. In bilateral approaches or to accomplish a more complete corpectomy, a bilateral laminectomy can be carried lateral through both pars. The removal of lamina should also be carried out in the adjacent levels to provide further decompression and the room needed for ventral decompression.

Pars and Facets

By drilling through of the pars, the inferior facet of the index level will be detached (Gill fragment). In cases of severe compression, rotational removal of this fragment is not safe and should not be attempted. These freed fragments should be carefully removed using a Kerrison. Once the inferior facet is removed, the superior facet of the inferior body should be drilled to expose the neuroforamen at the index level. If residual transverse process remains, this can be removed with a Leksell or as part of the pedicle resection using a 3-mm drill.

Temporary Rod

Once pedicle screws are placed and before proceeding with the destabilizing facetectomy and corpectomy, it is important to place a temporary rod on the contralateral side from the ventral approach. If this is not in place prior to anterior and middle column removal, the patient's spine may collapse on the table and kink their spinal cord resulting in devastating neurologic injury. The rod does not require final tightening. The rod can be moved from one side to another side if a bilateral corpectomy approach is desired; however, a second rod must be placed prior to the first rod removal when switching sides. At all times, there must be at least one rod for support.

Transpedicular Resection

Once the neuroforamen is completely exposed, a 3-mm drill bit can be used to burr down the cancellous cavity of the pedicle. This drilling can continue into the body of the bone. Once the cancellous bone is removed, drilling can be continued circumferentially until the bone is egg shelled. The remaining cancellous bone can be outfractured away from the cord or removed with a mastoid rongeur.

Corpectomy

At this point, all dorsal elements obstructing the ventral pathology have been completely removed. The corpectomy proceeds in stages: sacrifice nerve root for greater access, radiographic identification of resection limits, completion of a periosteal dissection, removal of tumor mass, and placement of graft.

Nerve Root

In order to perform a resection of the ventral tumor and place an anterior construct, it is necessary to sacrifice a nerve root at the level of the lesion (Fig. 14.7). Each posterior intercostal artery supplies a spinal artery; this joins the nerve root and contributes to the anterior and posterior radicular artery. These segmental radicular arteries join the anterior and posterior spinal arteries feeding the spinal cord. To sacrifice a root, there are several steps. First, ensure mean arterial pressure is greater than 90 mmHg during this aspect of the case. An arterial line is essential (not cuff pressure). Prior to manipulating the vascular supply, assess baseline MEP and SSEP readings. Instead of proceeding to cut the nerve root, use silk tie to temporarily ligate the candidate nerve root. Neuromonitoring should be observed for a minimum of 5 min to ensure blood supply lost from the radicular artery within the root is not critical for spinal cord perfusion. If no changes are seen in MEPs, or SSEPs, permanent ligation should be safe. It is important to ligate the nerve proximal to the dorsal root ganglion (pre-DRG). Cutting the nerve root pre-DRG removes the nerve cell bodies, while transecting post-DRG causes permanent radiculopathy from the retained body. If significant neuromonitoring changes are seen, cut the suture to free the nerve root and switch to the contralateral side.

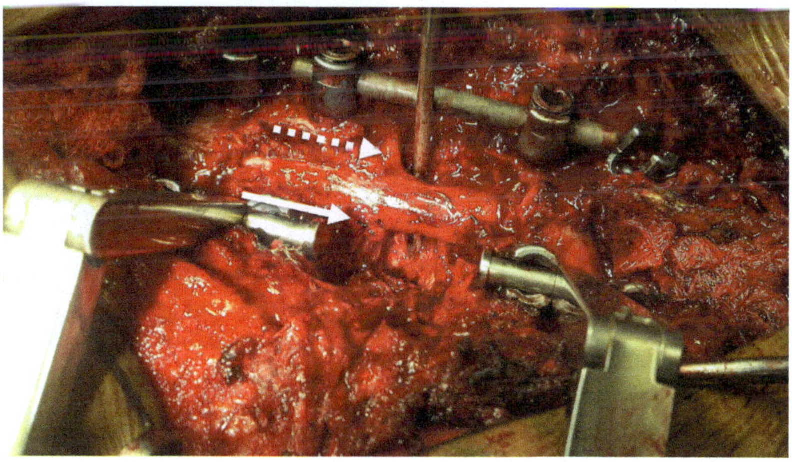

Fig. 14.7 Nerve root ligation (solid arrow), retraction from pedicle tulips, and contralateral temporary rod. For additional bone removal and better cage placement, optionally approach from the contralateral side while leaving the contralateral nerve intact (dashed arrow)

Boundary Localization

Once the nerve root is mobilized, it is critical to identify the resection boundaries. In the cranial/caudal axis, use a lateral fluoroscopic view placing Penfield 4 in the disc space above and below the index level to mark the endplates of the cranial and caudal bodies. In metastatic disease, a fractured body at the index level can cause conformational changes that greatly displace these margins. These gross deformities can lead to inadvertently entering and damaging the endplates of the adjacent body.

Boundary Dissection

Once the cranial/caudal limits are identified, dissection of the periosteal plane must be completed to ensure a safe anterior (ventral) displacement of the pleura and vascular structures during resection. In the same plane created from the removal of the rib, gently dissect along vertebral body until the ventral midline is reached using a Kittner and Penfield 1 as needed. This will displace the aorta and pleura away from the bone. Once free, a retractor system can be placed between the bone and the viscera to protect these structures from your drill.

Resection of Vertebral Body

After defining the ventral, cranial, and caudal margins, and once a rod is in place for structural support, it is then possible to begin resection of the vertebral body/tumor mass. In soft tumors, a pituitary can be used to begin debulking the mass centrally. Once the bulk of the tumor is removed, curettes can be used to fracture the mass ventral to the cord into the resection cavity. In areas where the tumor is firm or significant bone remains, a high-speed drill is employed to remove the mass. As your dissection progresses, the line of sight is maintained through rotation of the Jackson table up to 30°. Through rotating the table, a larger exposure with greater rib resection is avoided. In this process we aim to remove the bulk of the mass and vertebral body. We prefer to leave a rim of bone in the contralateral and ventral sides to protect the contralateral pleura and vascular structures. To remove the contralateral tumor from an ipsilateral costotransverse or LECA corridor, a dental mirror can be used to see under and around the spinal cord (Fig. 14.8). In addition to visualization under the cord, these circular mirrors can also be used as a probe, if turned perpendicular, to ensure the cavity is large enough for cage placement.

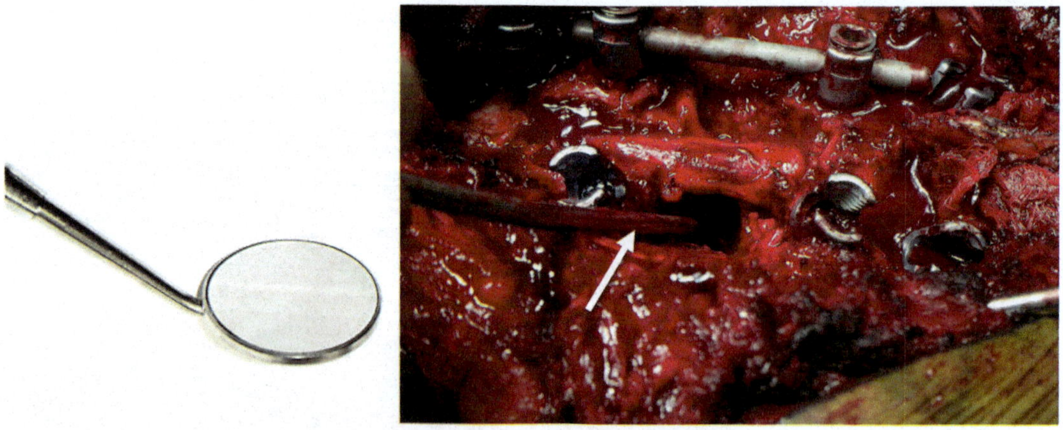

Fig. 14.8 Use a standard dental mirror (left) to visualize the cavity contralateral and posterior bone (right). White solid arrow indicates mirror placed in the space. Turned sideways, this tool doubles as a circular probe with the diameter of the mirror as your cage width. This step will allow you to verify that the corpectomy site is sufficient to fit the cage

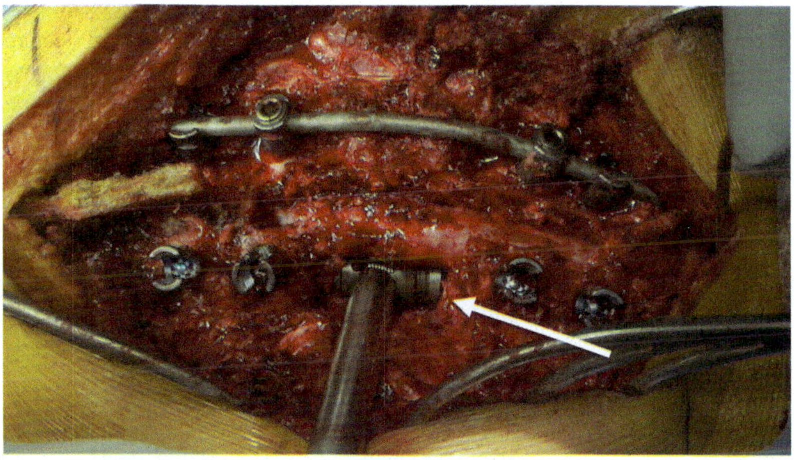

Fig. 14.9 Placement of a two-level expandable cage (arrow) with temporary rod placement shown. Cage selection is critically important to correct any kyphotic deformity from the pathological fracture

Fusion and Cage Placement

Since resection is often followed by radiation therapy, every effort must be made to prepare the fusion beds and obtain good purchase in hardware placement. Once the tumor is removed/debulked, proper endplate preparation is required. This ensures seating the cage, graft, and a fusion bed. A curette should be used to remove all disc and ligamentous material from the endplate of the bodies above and below the index level.

Cage Placement

We prefer to use a packed titanium expandable cage when possible; this allows for deformity correction typically seen in these patients. Neuromonitoring should be used while expanding the cage; if changes are noted, less distraction will be required. In cases where there is endplate damage, a metal expandable cage will often subside and the deformity will worsen over time. In our experience in these cases, a solid strut graft of humerus or tibia packed with bone is preferred for the anterior construct. In these cases, the bone will incorporate better and we have less subsidence with progressive kyphosis. To pack our cages or strut graft we prefer to have the rib graft removed during access, which is typically not involved in the tumor. Placement of the cage should be midline within the anterior column, without any of the cage seen in the posterior limit of the body in a lateral X-ray (Fig. 14.9).

Posterior Instrumentation

Once the cage is placed and expanded, the final rods should be placed one at a time. This is particularly true in patients with iatrogenic pars defects from the exposure. If a strut graft was used, the rods should be compressed to ensure it is under pressure and will not retropulse into the spinal cord. Place and finally tighten the posterior rods and locking screws. In patients with unilateral removal of rib, it is not necessary to place a cross-link.

A final Valsalva should be performed to check the nerve root stump as well as the ventral dura for leaks.

Case Follow-Up

Pathology from the patient presented at the start of the chapter was estrogen receptor-positive metastatic carcinoma. She underwent a T6–T7 LECA with instrumented fusion from T3 to T9. The procedure required only ipsilateral nerve root sacrifice. Her postoperative course was uneventful, and she was transferred on day 7 to acute rehabilitation. Adjuvant therapy included external beam radiation and continued tamoxifen.

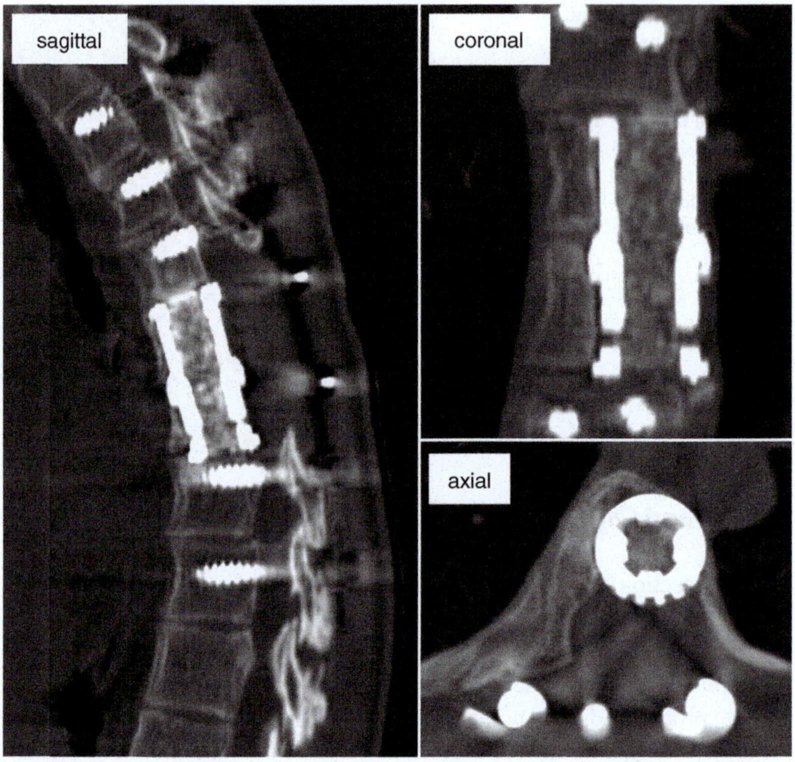

Fig. 14.10 Follow-up CT at 1 year showing good hardware placement and progression of bony formation in the interbody cage at T6–T7

At 5 months, she had significant return of strength in her lower extremities and was ambulating without assistance. A 6-month PET scan was negative in the thoracic region. At 1-year follow-up, the patient had good hardware placement and progression of bony fusion (Fig. 14.10).

Discussion and Conclusion

Mastering the lateral extracavitary approach is a technical and critical skill needed for resection of large ventral lesions. The techniques described above allow for the maximal exposure of the contralateral spine through a posterior ipsilateral approach. Near-complete vertebrectomy can be performed safely through this technique. Limitations to LECA include visualization of the contralateral vertebral body, sacrifice of the ipsilateral nerve root, and temporary destabilization of the spine. The visual limitations are dependent on the approach angle. Muscular or obese patients typically restrict your vision, even with extensive soft tissue dissection and rib resection. In morbidly obese patients, this approach may not be feasible and transthoracic exposures may prove to be more practical. Requirements of ipsilateral nerve root ligations can lead to spinal cord stroke. Due to this, neuromonitoring is critical, and preoperative angiograms are recommended for both identification of artery of Adamkiewicz and preoperative embolization from T6 to T9. Through exposure and resection using LECA, significant removal of bone in both anterior and posterior elements occurs. Operative consideration for both temporary and permanent hardware is needed, and a postsurgical goal of fusion should be a primary surgical aim. In our experience, with good endplate preparation and placement of appropriate construct/graft, these patients will have a high rate of fusion, despite receiving postoperative adjuvant chemotherapy and radiation.

Using the techniques for LECA, the extent of exposure can be scaled back for smaller lesions eccentric to a side. With reduction in total rib removal (less than 4 cm), the approach would be defined as a costotransversectomy, which enables partial exposure across midline. If the approach is restricted to removal of the transverse process, lamina, and pedicle, the approach would be defined as transpedicular, which limits resection of lesions to the lateral recess of the spinal canal. Transpedicular approaches are a typical approach used for calcified thoracic discs. These approaches should be viewed as in a continuum, and by utilizing the same incision a surgeon should be able to expand or restrict the extent of dissection to ensure adequate visualization to accomplish the goals of surgery without jeopardizing critical structures.

References

1. Herkowitz HN, Rothman RH, Simeone FA. Rothman-Simeone, the spine. 5th ed. Philadelphia: Saunders Elsevier; 2006.
2. Larson SJ, Holst RA, Hemmy DC, Sances A. Lateral extracavitary approach to traumatic lesions of the thoracic and lumbar spine. J Neurosurg. 1976;45(6):628–37.
3. Ohgiya Y, Oka M, Hiwatashi A, Liu X, Kakimoto N, Westesson PL, et al. Diffusion tensor MR imaging of the cervical spinal cord in patients with multiple sclerosis. Eur Radiol. 2007;17(10):2499–504.
4. Patchell RA, Tibbs PA, Regine WF, Payne R, Saris S, Kryscio RJ, et al. Direct decompressive surgical resection in the treatment of spinal cord compression caused by metastatic cancer: a randomised trial. Lancet (London, England). 2005;366(9486):643–8.
5. Bilsky M, Smith M. Surgical approach to epidural spinal cord compression. Hematol Oncol Clin North Am. 2006;20(6):1307–17.
6. Laufer I, Rubin DG, Lis E, Cox BW, Stubblefield MD, Yamada Y, et al. The NOMS framework: approach to the treatment of spinal metastatic tumors. Oncologist. 18. Durham, NC, USA, 2013. p. 744–51.
7. Bilsky MH, Laufer I, Fourney DR, Groff M, Schmidt MH, Varga PP, et al. Reliability analysis of the epidural spinal cord compression scale. J Neurosurg Spine. 2010;13(3):324–8.
8. Gerszten PC, Mendel E, Yamada Y. Radiotherapy and radiosurgery for metastatic spine disease: what are the options, indications, and outcomes? Spine (Phila Pa 1976). 2009;34(22 Suppl):S78–92.
9. Moussazadeh N, Laufer I, Yamada Y, Bilsky MH. Separation surgery for spinal metastases: effect of spinal radiosurgery on surgical treatment goals. Cancer Control: J Moffitt Cancer Center. 2014;21(2):168–74.
10. Lubelski D, Abdullah KG, Steinmetz MP, Masters F, Benzel EC, Mroz TE, et al. Lateral extracavitary, costotransversectomy, and transthoracic thoracotomy approaches to the thoracic spine: review of techniques and complications. J Spinal Disord Tech. 2013;26(4):222–32.
11. Champlin AM, Rael J, Benzel EC, Kesterson L, King JN, Orrison WW, et al. Preoperative spinal angiography for lateral extracavitary approach to thoracic and lumbar spine. Am J Neuroradiol. 1994;15(1):73.
12. Dvorak M, MacDonald S, Gurr KR, Bailey SI, Haddad RG. An anatomic, radiographic, and biomechanical assessment of extrapedicular screw fixation in the thoracic spine. Spine (Phila Pa 1976). 1993;18(12):1689–94.
13. Cruz LC Jr, Domingues RC, Gasparetto EL. Diffusion tensor imaging of the cervical spinal cord of patients with relapsing-remising multiple sclerosis: a study of 41 cases. Arq Neuropsiquiatr. 2009;67(2B):391–5.
14. Miller MD, Chhabra AB, Hurwitz HR, et al. Posterior extracavitary/costotransversectomy/posterolateral approach to the thoracic spine. In: Orthopaedic surgical approaches. Philadelphia: Saunders/Elsevier; 2008. p. 296–303.
15. Lau D, Chou D. Posterior thoracic corpectomy with cage reconstruction for metastatic spinal tumors: comparing the mini-open approach to the open approach. J Neurosurg Spine. 2015;23(2):217–27.

Antero/Anterolateral Thoracic Access and Stabilization from a Posterior Approach, Costotransversectomy, and Lateral Extracavitary Approach, En Bloc Resection

15

Akash A. Shah and Joseph H. Schwab

Introduction

The purpose of this chapter is to illustrate the reasons why a posterior approach to tumors located in the anterior column of the thoracic spine can be advantageous. The chapter will focus on the technical aspects of posterior approaches, and two cases will be utilized to illustrate variations on the posterior approach. It is important to understand that the most common osseous tumor of the spine encountered is metastatic from another organ system and, therefore, the majority of surgical approaches should be geared toward palliation of symptoms rather than en bloc resection for cure. The two cases discussed in this chapter outline technical aspects of en bloc resection for primary spinal tumors. While the treatment of primary tumors is generally more technically complex – and much less commonly encountered – the anatomic, physiologic, and technical aspects of these approaches are translatable to the treatment of metastatic lesions. The vast majority of surgically indicated metastatic lesions of the spine can be successfully approached posteriorly, and the approaches described here can help form the basis for these – albeit with divergent clinical goals.

A. A. Shah · J. H. Schwab (✉)
Massachusetts General Hospital, Department of Orthopaedic Surgery, Boston, MA, USA
e-mail: jhschwab@partners.org

One of the main advantages of a posterior approach to tumors of the thoracic spine is that "normal" dura uninvolved with tumor is more accessible from this approach. This is useful when the surgeon is trying to avoid contact with the tumor in the case of primary tumors or when trying to develop tissue planes to separate the dura from a bulky, vascular tumor in the case of metastatic disease. In an anterior approach to the spine, the removal of the vertebral bodies would be necessary to visualize the dura above or below the tumor. Furthermore, a posterior approach allows 360° access to the dura with anterior column reconstruction; this is not possible in a solely anterior approach (Figs. 15.1 and 15.2). Accessing the ventral surface of the dura can be accomplished indirectly by a transpedicular approach; direct visualization can occur with wide removal of the posterior rib segments in order to allow a lateral view as opposed to a posterior or posterolateral view. An added advantage of a posterior approach is that it allows reconstruction of both the anterior and posterior columns through the same approach. The primary disadvantage of a posterior approach is that the great vessels are not easily accessible, making vascular control potentially difficult should an injury occur. While not appropriate for all spinal tumors, a posterior-only approach can be used to manage the majority of metastatic tumors and select primary tumors (Fig. 15.3).

D. M. Sciubba (ed.), *Spinal Tumor Surgery*, https://doi.org/10.1007/978-3-319-98422-3_15

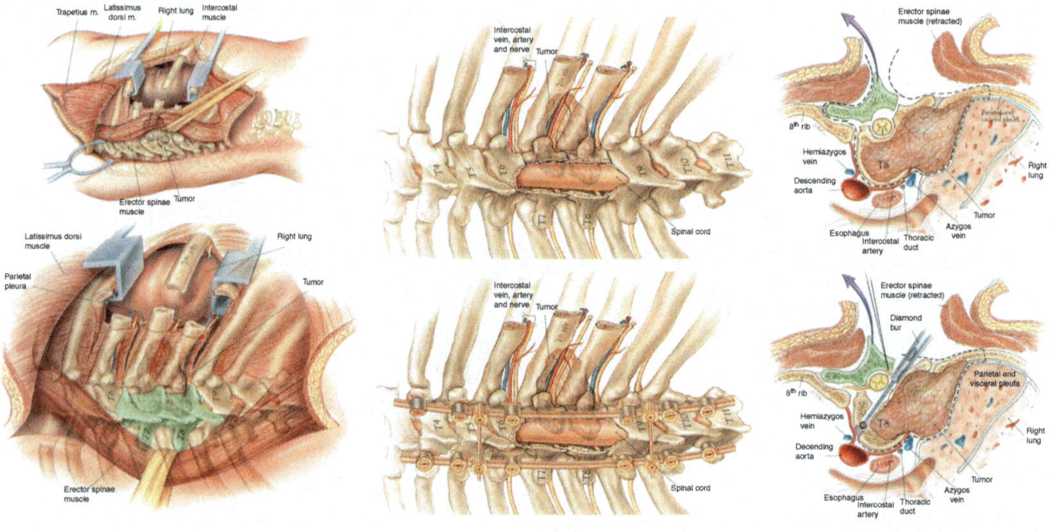

Fig. 15.1 En bloc resection of primary thoracic spinal tumor, artist illustration. (Reprinted with permission from Fourney et al. [25])

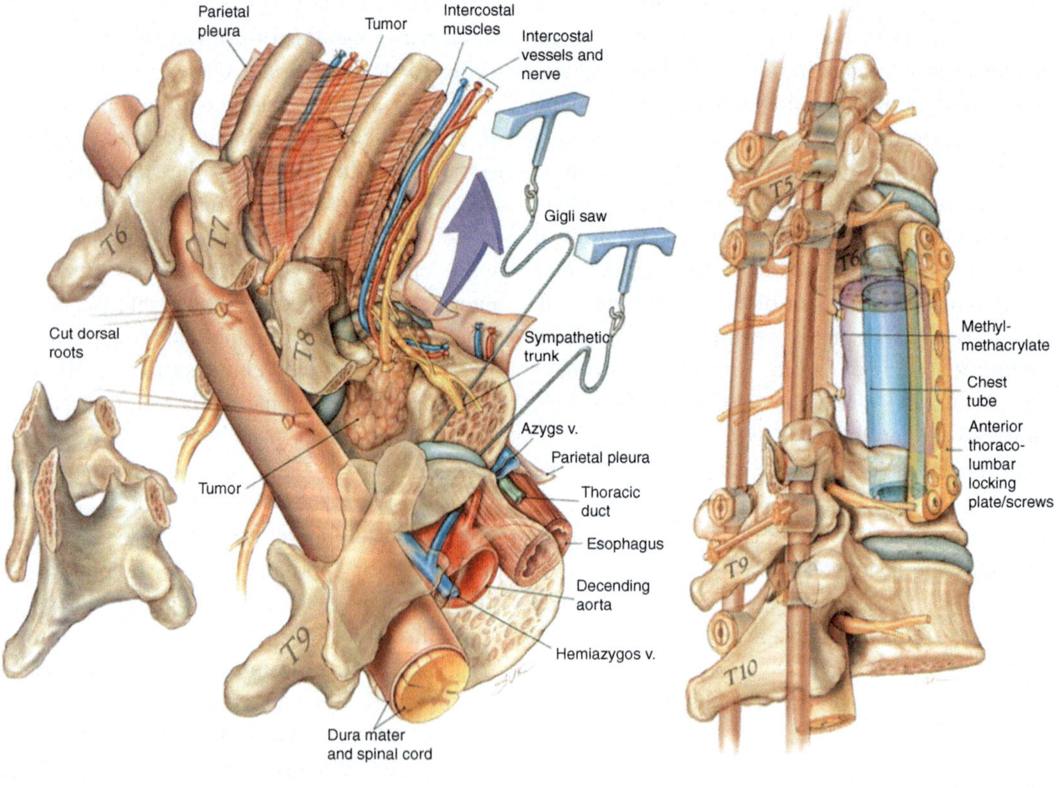

Fig. 15.2 Artist illustration and anterior column reconstruction. (Reprinted with permission from Fourney et al. [25])

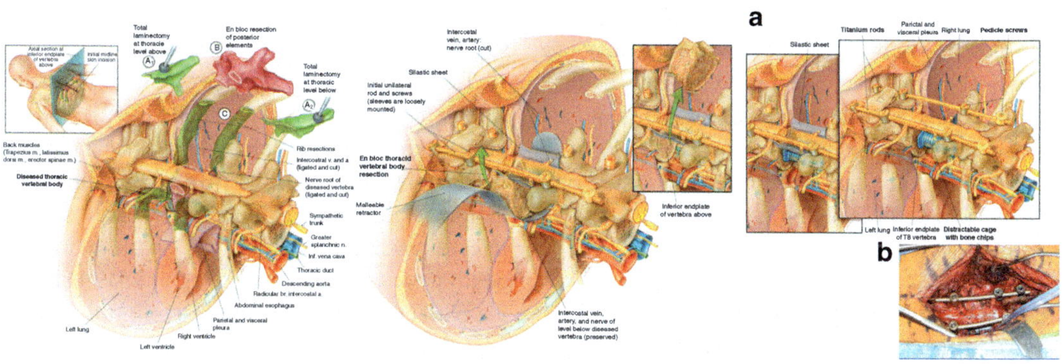

Fig. 15.3 Posterior approach for en bloc spondylectomy of primary thoracic spine tumor. (Reprinted from Hsieh et al. [30], by permission of Oxford University Press)

Anatomy

The vascular anatomy of the thoracic spine must be considered in any approach to this region. In the thoracic spine, segmental vessels originate from the aorta or the subclavian artery and continue on as intercostal arteries. The azygos vein provides the primary venous drainage of the returning intercostal veins; this structure must be respected despite its small caliber, as venous injury can be difficult to manage from a posterior approach. These segmental vessels typically divide into paired radicular arteries and veins that provide inflow and outflow for the thoracic spinal cord. The radicular arteries that supply the anterior spinal artery – and thus the anterior two-thirds of the spinal cord – are named anterior radiculomedullary vessels. Anterior radiculomedullary arteries are generally not paired at any given level. The anterior spinal artery experiences both anterograde and retrograde flow from the radiculomedullary vessels. There are fewer radiculomedullary arteries in the thoracic spine, and they are more spread out than in other parts of the spine. As a result, there is poor collateral circulation potential in this region [1]. One or two anterior radiculomedullary vessels supply the anterior spinal artery of the thoracolumbar spine. The dominant vessel is the artery of Adamkiewicz and is most commonly found on the left side between T9 and T12 [2, 3]. It gives off a dominant descending branch and a smaller ascending branch as it joins the anterior spinal artery. While the anterior spinal artery is continuous throughout the thoracic spine, its caliber considerably narrows as it approaches the artery of Adamkiewicz. Taken together, these factors contribute to the sensitivity of the anterior thoracic spinal cord to ischemic insult [1].

Posterior approaches to the thoracic spine often require wide lateral exposure including removal of posterior ribs. Removal of the ribs is necessary when a lateral extracavitary approach is utilized. The length of the rib removed depends upon the location of the tumors and desired exposure of the ventral surface of the spinal cord. As the ribs approach their attachment to the spine, they run anterior and directly adjacent to the paired transverse processes. The rib head then attaches to the costal facets on the vertebral body. The intercostal muscles attach to the ribs and must be untethered to provide access to the underlying neurovascular bundle. The corresponding segmental nerve and subcostal vessels travel inferior to the rib and are readily seen once the intercostal muscles are detached. The parietal pleura lies deep to the neurovascular bundle. The pleura can be incised with dissecting scissors, allowing access to the thoracic cavity. It is not always necessary to violate the pleura; it can be utilized as a margin in the approach to a primary tumor. In other cases, the pleura can be bluntly elevated off the lateral border of the vertebral bodies until the surgeon can palpate and visualize the anterolateral aspect of the vertebral body with the great vessels. It is in this location that one can best visualize the segmental vessels as they approach the aorta and azygos vein. One can gain an appreciation for the disposition of these vessels and whether they appear tethered or are otherwise at risk for avulsion.

Case 1: Posterior-Only En Bloc Spondylectomy for Giant-Cell Tumor of Bone

The patient is a 41-year-old male who initially presented to the emergency department with atypical ongoing chest pain. A computed tomography (CT) scan of the chest demonstrated collapse of the T6 vertebral body as well as an expansile soft tissue mass within the vertebral body that invades the central canal and narrows the neural foramina bilaterally, likely causing radicular chest pain. An MRI of the cervical, thoracic, and lumbar spine demonstrated marrow-replacing lesions involving the vertebral body and posterior elements of T6 and T7. A pathologic compression fracture of the T6 vertebral body was observed. A soft tissue mass was seen extending posteriorly into the spinal canal, with mild mass effect on the thecal sac. There was severe right and mild left neural foraminal stenosis at T6–T7 (Fig. 15.4). A CT-guided core needle biopsy of the T6 collapsed vertebral body was obtained and was consistent with giant-cell tumor of the bone.

The patient was started on monthly denosumab therapy, which he tolerated well. It is our practice to treat giant-cell tumor with neoadjuvant denosumab for 6 months [4]. A CT scan of the thoracic spine after 5 months of therapy showed interval increased ossification of the extraosseous portions of the tumor (Fig. 15.5). Although the patient had an expected response to neoadjuvant therapy, the tumor remained Enneking Stage III. It is our practice to consider en bloc resection for cases of Enneking Stage III giant-cell tumor owing to the high local recurrence rate with intralesional resection in these tumors [5].

Posterior Exposure

The patient was placed in a prone position on a Jackson table with the arms tucked at their sides. A midline thoracic incision was made from T4 through T8, and the paraspinal muscles were carefully dissected to expose the posterior osseous elements in a subperiosteal fashion. Pedicle screws were placed at T8 and T9 as well as at T4 and T5 using anatomic technique for their insertion.

In order to provide sufficient access to the ventral surface of the vertebrae, we planned on removing the sixth, seventh, and eighth paired

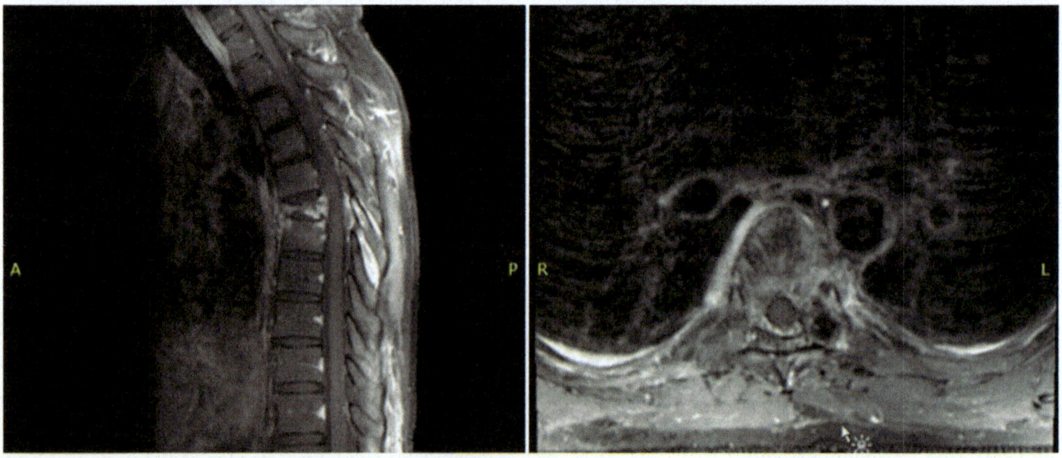

Fig. 15.4 Pre-treatment T1-weighted post-contrast MRI of thoracic spine, sagittal and axial views

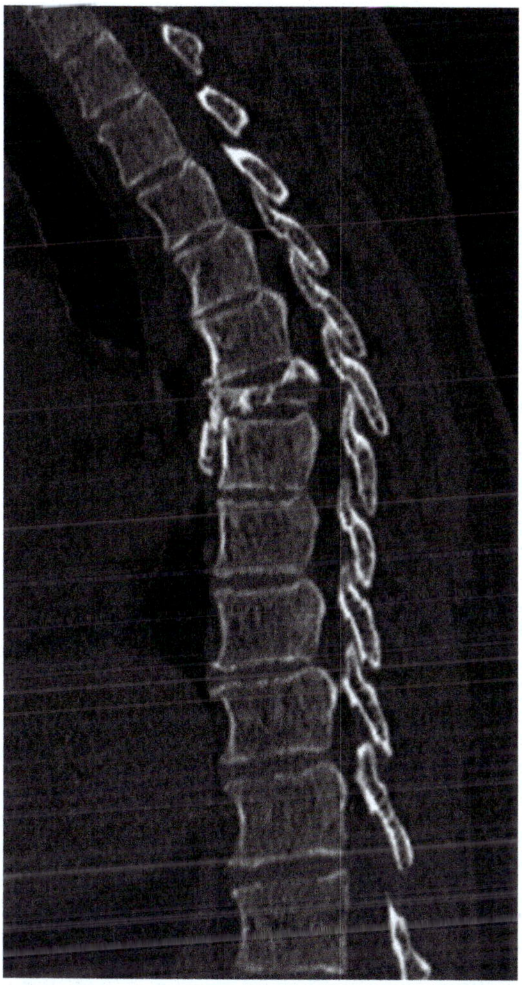

Fig. 15.5 CT thoracic spine after 5 months of denosumab therapy, sagittal view

thoracic ribs with our rib transection occurring approximately 7 cm lateral to the transverse process of the corresponding vertebrae. The transverse processes of T8 were also removed to facilitate access to the thoracic cavity. At this time, an assessment can be made regarding the accessibility ventral to the vertebrae; additional ribs (T5 and T9) can be removed if necessary. The intercostal muscles were dissected away from their insertion onto the rib, allowing a right-angle clamp or rib stripping instrument to be placed ventral to the rib but in the extra-pleural space. This plane was then developed to approximately 2 cm lateral to the planned rib transection point. The rib was then transected laterally and then again at the junction with the transverse process. The rib can be used as bone graft if it is not involved with tumor. The intervening intercostal muscles with underlying neurovascular vessels must be transected laterally at the level of the rib transection and again medially.

After these tissues are removed from the field, one can visualize the parietal pleura and develop a plane between it and the vertebrae. This dissection can be performed bluntly. As the pleura is elevated away from the vertebrae, one can gain additional appreciation of the segmental vessels as they branch from the aorta and azygos vein.

Passage of Saws

Passage of the threadwire saws requires that a plane ventral to the vertebral body and dorsal to the great vessels be developed. This is done in part with blunt finger dissection and in part with long curved vascular forceps depending upon the size of the patient's vertebrae. In this case, most of the dissection was done bluntly with our fingers. Several traversing segmental vessels at T6, T7, and T8 were identified and ligated under direct visualization using 2–0 silk ties or vascular clips. Figure 15.6 illustrates the technique using blunt finger dissection to develop the interval ventral to the vertebra bodies but dorsal to the aorta and azygos vein. One of the risks in this portion of the technique is tearing of a segmental vessel or avulsion off of its root from the aorta or azygos vein, due to undue or unrecognized tension on the vessel. For this reason, one must take time to optimize exposure and inspect the segmental vessels to ensure that they have been properly ligated and are not in harm's way. Furthermore, dissection should remain closely approximated to the vertebral body and the anterior longitudinal ligament.

The plane was slowly enlarged enough to accommodate a large vascular clamp with a half-circle clamp configuration. Once the tip of the clamp can be visualized on the contralateral side of the vertebrae, a quarter-inch Penrose drain was delivered to the clamp with forceps. In this case, the Penrose drain was positioned at the

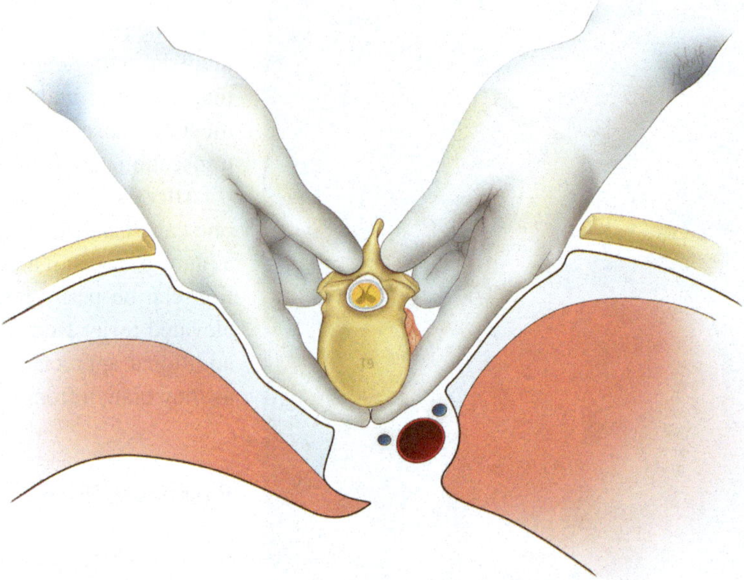

Fig. 15.6 Blunt dissection is performed to develop a plane between the vertebral body and the great vessels. (Reprinted with permission from Shah et al. [29])

level of T5/T6. Similarly, another Penrose drain was passed at the level of T7/T8. At this point, the Penrose drains had both free ends in the field, and they were looped ventral to the vertebral body but dorsal to the great vessels. It is advisable to perform this portion of the procedure with a plan in place if the great vessels become injured. The anesthesiologist must be well aware of the risk in order to be prepared in case rapid resuscitation is needed. We generally pass the Penrose drains with the assistance of our thoracic surgery colleagues in case rapid repositioning with subsequent thoracotomy is required to gain control of bleeding.

Two multifilament diamond threadwire saws as described by Tomita and colleagues were then passed through the Penrose drains (Fig. 15.7) [6, 7]. We generally utilize two saws at each level, as it is not uncommon for them to break during the vertebral osteotomy. Each of the pairs was sutured together at either end to facilitate passage through the drain. The saws were passed through the Penrose drain until they were visualized on the other end of the drain. The Penrose drains were then removed, leaving the saws in position.

The next step was to remove the posterior elements of the spine to allow passage of the saws ventral to the thecal sac and dorsal to the vertebral bodies. In order to adequately expose the thecal sac and nerve roots, decompressive laminectomies with removal of the posterior elements of T5, T6, T7, and T8 were performed using a high-speed burr and Kerrison rongeurs. The T6, T7, and T8 nerve roots were then ligated and transected near their origin to allow for removal of the T6/T7 tumor. The potential space ventral to the dura and dorsal to the vertebral bodies was carefully developed using gentle blunt dissection along with sharp incision of soft tissue attachments encountered between the posterior longitudinal ligament and the dura. There is also a rich venous plexus in this plane that must be dealt with using bipolar electrocautery. Once the potential space has been developed, a right-angle clamp was passed deep to the dura and one end of the threadwire saw was passed to the clamp. The saws were pulled through this plane to the contralateral side, effectively lassoing the vertebral body (Fig. 15.8). This was performed at the T5/T6 and T7/T8 levels. The saws were now in position to allow for the osteotomies.

Osteotomies and Reconstruction

The paired threadwire saws were separated, and both ends of one saw were clamped together.

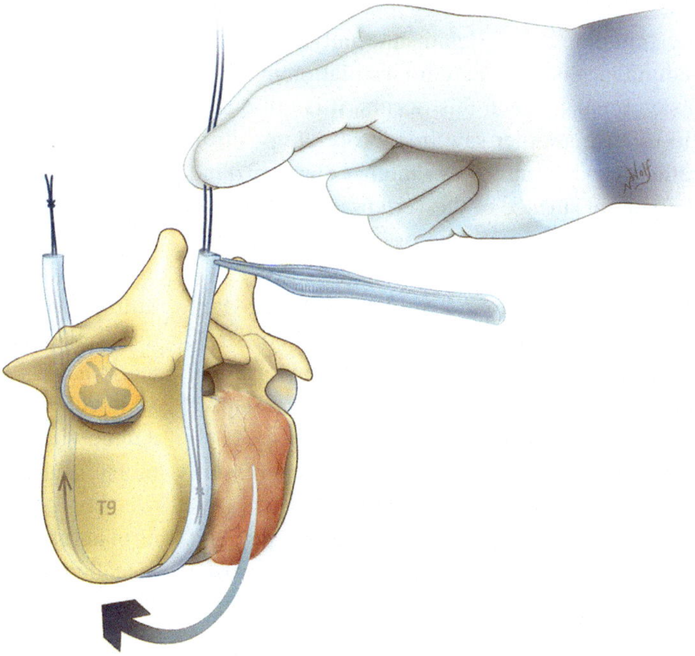

Fig. 15.7 Following dissection, a Penrose drain is passed anterior to the vertebral body but posterior to the great vessels. Then, threadwire saws are passed into the sheath and tied together. This is performed both cephalad and caudal to the tumor. (Reprinted with permission from Shah et al. [29])

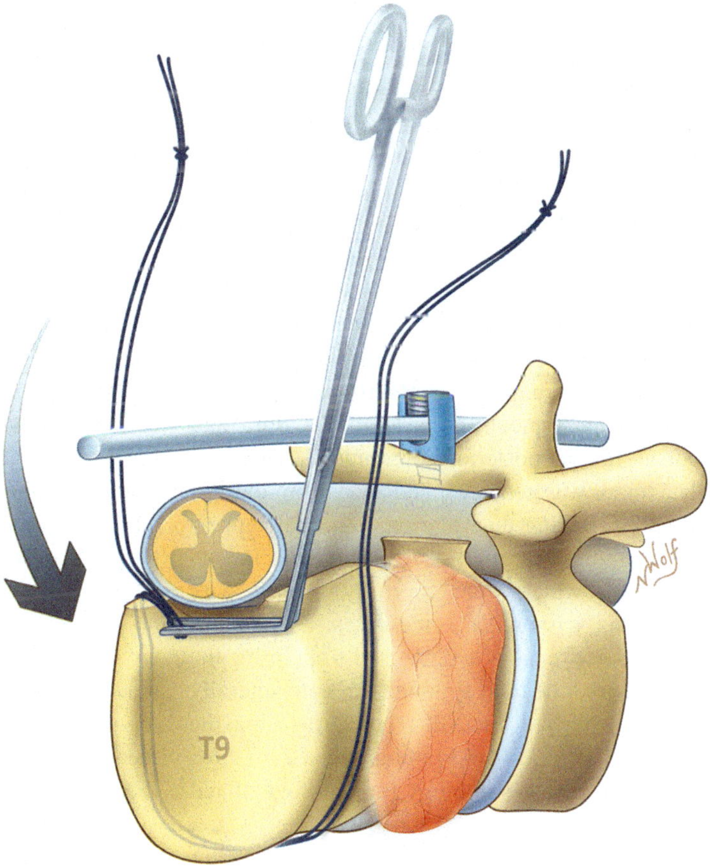

Fig. 15.8 A plane is developed anterior to the thecal sac and posterior to the vertebral body. One end of each threadwire saw is passed through this plane, and the saws are lassoed around the vertebral body. (Reprinted with permission from Shah et al. [29])

The clamp was carefully placed away from the remaining saw. Again, the purpose of this redundancy is to prepare for a situation in which a saw breaks. When this occurs, it is quite useful to have another saw in appropriate position rather than having to pass another clamp around the ventral surface of the vertebrae. The threadwire saws chosen for the osteotomy were then attached to their respective handles. Note that these saws are now posterolateral to the dura and are on the ipsilateral side of one another. It is best to cross one's hands prior to sawing. The challenge here is to protect the ventral aspect of the dura where the traversing saw exits. It is helpful to have an assistant place pressure on the saw to keep it from irritating the dura. This can be done with various instruments, and there are pulleys that can be used to assist. It should be noted that this portion of the procedure is associated with some risk and must be performed with an assistant who understands the risk in order to mitigate potential complications. In this case, we performed the osteotomy in sequential fashion starting at the T5/T6 level and then proceeding to the T7/T8 level. It is not uncommon to encounter significant bleeding from the vertebral body during the osteotomy. We usually cut the vertebrae immediately adjacent to the disc space. In this case, our cuts were through T5 just above the T5/T6 disc space in order to ensure we did not enter the tumor. Similarly, the caudal cut was through T8 just caudal to the T7/T8 disc space.

The tumor was now free of its osseous attachments, but there usually remain some soft tissue attachments typically ventral to the dura and dorsal to the posterior longitudinal ligament. The tumor was gently rotated away from the spinal cord. During this rotation, it became apparent that further soft tissue attachments indeed remained, which were carefully incised with dissecting scissors. In some cases, the remaining threadwire saws can be used to help lift the tumor out of the field although this can generally be accomplished manually. After releasing the specimen en bloc, it was radiographed with three views and sent to pathology for histological and margin analysis (Fig. 15.9). Complete anterior and posterior decompression of the spinal cord was achieved.

After the pathologist confirmed that the margins appear grossly negative, the wound was thoroughly irrigated, and we began spinal reconstruction. The resected specimen or the remaining space between T5 and T8 can be measured in order to facilitate reconstruction. We decided to utilize a humeral allograft because of our access to a robust bone bank, because of the immediate structural benefits of utilizing the said graft, and because the graft can be easily cut to fit the defect. The rib graft that we harvested earlier was morselized and packed into the allograft bone. We then gently impacted the graft from a posterolateral approach on the left side of the spine, visualizing the spinal cord and also palpating the position of the graft relative to the vertebral bodies.

Once confident that the graft is in the appropriate position, we contoured titanium rods to fit into the pedicle screws we had previously placed. A rod was first placed into the pedicle screws without a temporary rod in position. Once that rod was placed, the contralateral temporary rod was replaced with a permanent rod. After placing appropriately sized rods, we tightened the distal set-screws. The proximal set-screws were loosened sufficiently to allow for compression of the graft.

Proximally, we placed set-screws but did not tighten them at this point. We clamped the rod and compressed the rods at the cephalad portion of the construct. The purpose of this was to compress down on the allograft. After compressing on the left and right sides, we palpated the graft and confirmed that it was solidly fixed. An additional rod was added to each side of the posterior reconstruction for added stability. Close inspection of the pleura was performed to ensure no parenchymal injury has occurred and that no air leak is detected. Two 19 Blake drains were placed into the thoracic cavity on either side of the spine, and the remaining wound was closed in layers. A post-operative radiograph is provided (Fig. 15.10).

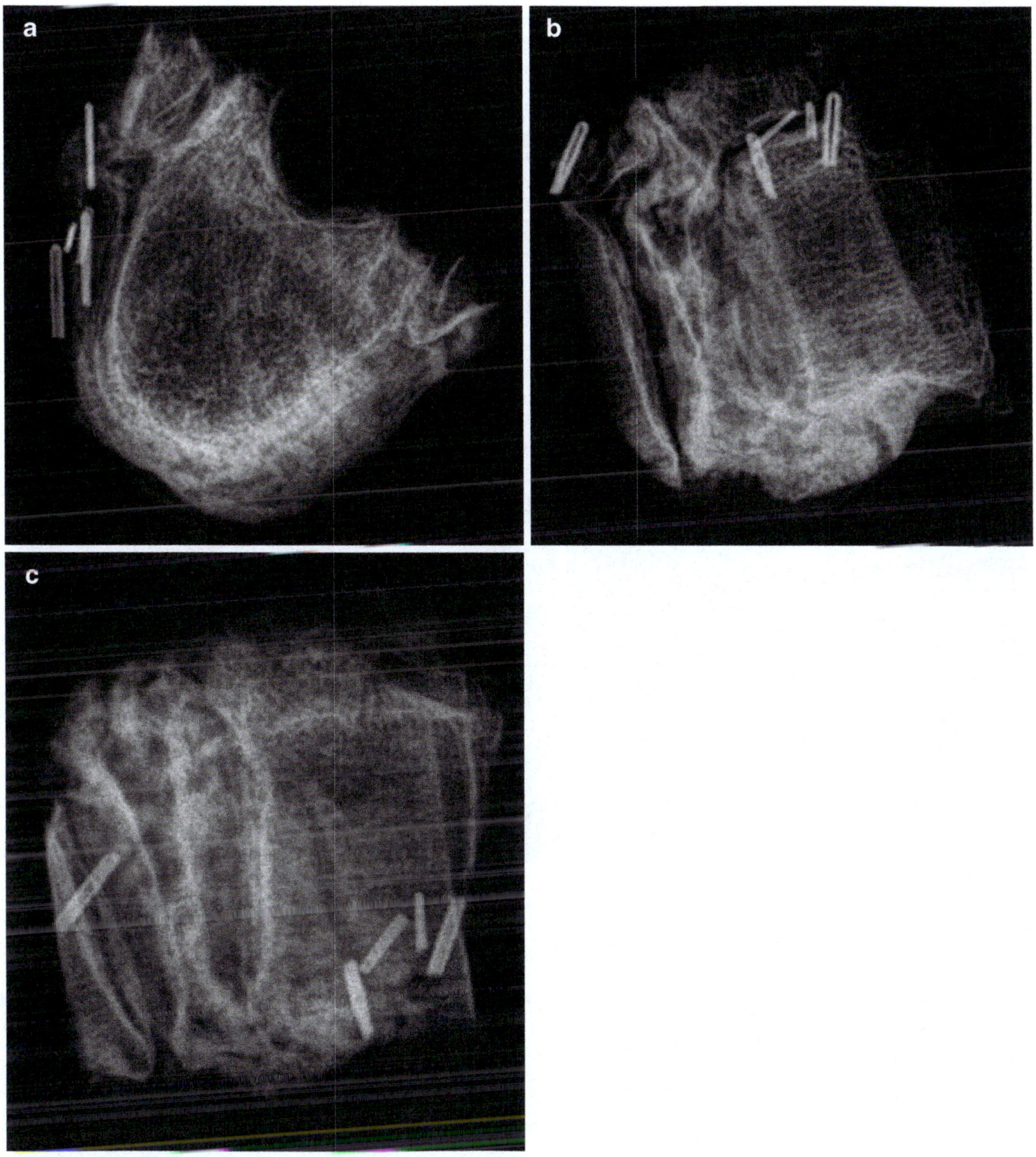

Fig. 15.9 Specimen radiograph. (**a**) Anteroposterior view. (**b**) Lateral view. (**c**) Swimmer's view

Case 2: En Bloc Spondylectomy with Chest Wall Excision for Ewing's Sarcoma

The patient is a 27-year-old male with progressively worsening right-sided flank and back pain initially thought to be related to muscle spasm. When his pain symptoms did not improve, a CT chest scan demonstrated a soft tissue mass adjacent to or arising from the area of the right 10th rib. MRI of the thoracic spine demonstrated that the mass medially abuts the T10 and T11 ribs and vertebral bodies, with epidural extension into the right T10–T11 neural foramen (Fig. 15.11). Tissue biopsy confirmed Ewing's sarcoma. He was started on a 3-month course of neoadjuvant chemotherapy with seven cycles of alternating vincristine/adriamycin/cyclophosphamide and ifosfamide/etoposide therapy.

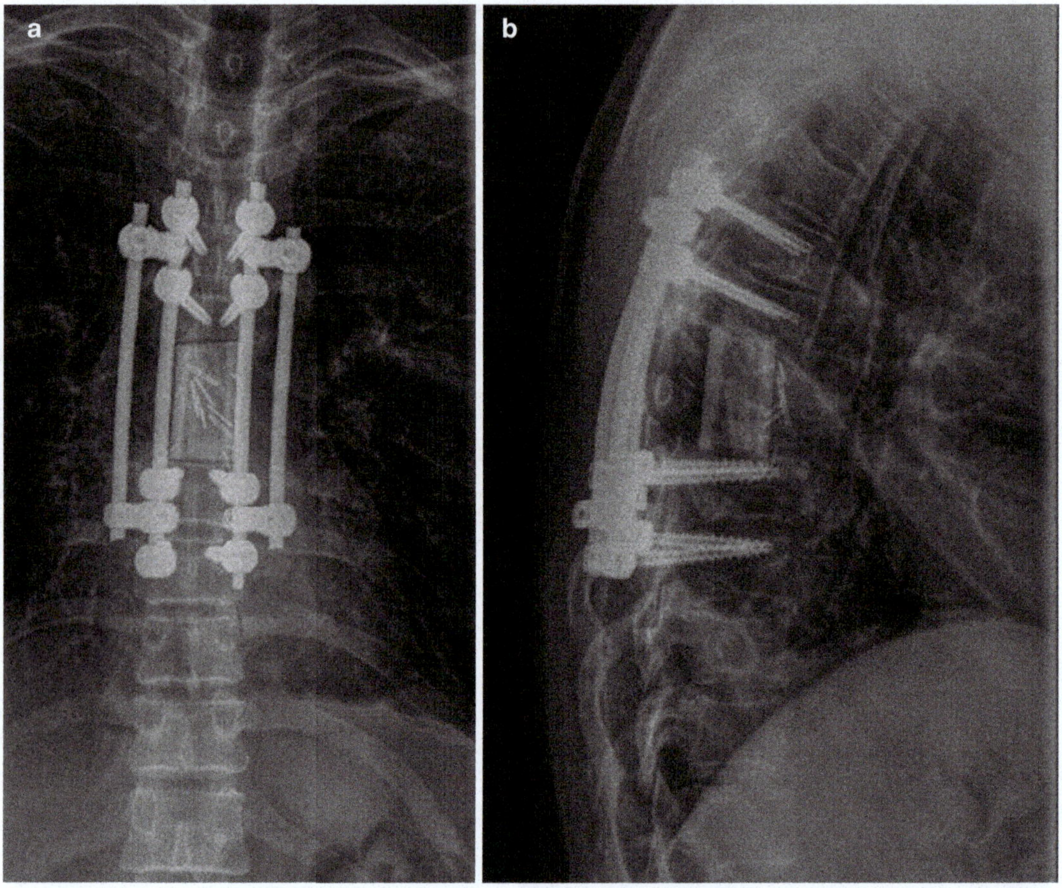

Fig. 15.10 Post-operative radiograph. (**a**) Anteroposterior view. (**b**) Lateral view

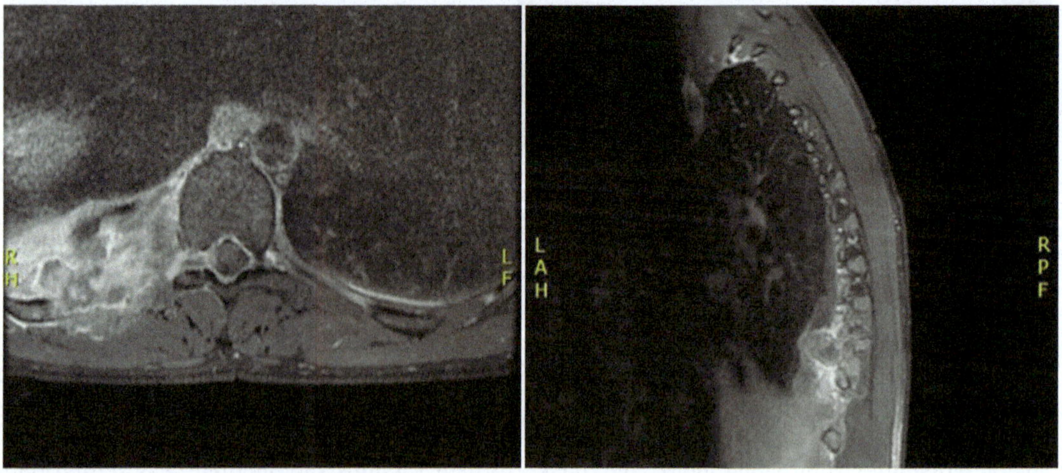

Fig. 15.11 Pre-treatment T1-weighted fat-suppressed MRI of thoracic spine, axial and sagittal views

In his case, the patient was not treated with neoadjuvant radiation. One reason to forego radiation is that negative margins can be predictably obtained with acceptable morbidity. Furthermore, it is important to avoid the risk of secondary malignancy in a young patient treated with chemotherapy and radiation. If no radiation is utilized, however, the surgeon must resect the pre-chemotherapy tumor volume rather than the post-chemotherapy volume as demonstrated in [8].

This case illustrates issues surrounding partial vertebrectomy with sagittal vertebral osteotomy and associated chest wall excision. In these cases, one must dissect far laterally on the chest wall in order to osteotomize the rib safely away from the tumor. In this case, the tumor emanated from the rib and the vertebra is secondarily involved. Some of the same issues exist for this surgery as in the last regarding the great vessels and pleura. In this case, however, the parietal pleura was resected with the specimen in order to provide an adequate margin. Furthermore, the vertebrae were not completely excised as they were not completely involved with tumor. For this reason, a sagittal osteotomy was chosen.

The exposure to this case is slightly different, and a long longitudinal incision is made from T6 to L3 in order to allow sufficient retraction of the paraspinal muscles to allow the far-lateral rib osteotomies. We removed the paraspinal musculature adjacent to the vertebrae and the paraspinal musculature adjacent to the ribs at T10 and T11 to ensure that we moved all gross total disease from the pre-neoadjuvant MRI. We dissected laterally until we identified the T12 rib and skeletonized the T12 rib but left its neurovascular bundle intact. We incised the pleural parallel to the T12 rib from just lateral to the vertebral body. We transected the T10 and T12 ribs and identified the segmental vessels and cauterized them. Once the ribs are transected, the parietal pleura is incised in line with the rib cuts. Cephalad to T10, we continued to dissect through the intercostal musculature and the pleura until we arrived at the T9 rib. Transverse dissection through the intercostal musculature was deepened through the parietal pleura until the soft tissue dissection meets the vertebral bodies.

At this point, posterior laminectomies were required to expose the thecal sac and allow transection of the ipsilateral involved nerve roots. Once the laminae and nerve roots were removed, a transverse bony cut was made through the pars interarticularis cephalad and caudal to the tumor. At this point, we utilized intra-operative navigation (Stealth, Medtronic, Minneapolis, MN) combined with intra-operative O-arm imaging (O-arm, Medtronic, Minneapolis, MN). The reason for this is that it allows us to make a sagittal cut through the body in precisely the intended area to help us achieve a negative margin while preventing us from unnecessarily removing the healthy bone. We utilized a 6-mm diamond burr (Legend, Medtronic, Minneapolis, MN) to perform our bone cuts. We used this burr tip because the diamond action helps cauterize bone bleeding, facilitating better visualization. We also used the 6-mm tip because the wider tip better facilitates visualization. Once the bone cuts are complete, the anterior longitudinal ligament was apparent through the 6-millimeter trough made by the burr. Now the specimen is attached to the ligament and the ipsilateral segmental vessels. The specimen can be gently mobilized into the chest cavity, which further widens the trough created by the burr. Now one can apply large vascular clips starting at the caudal soft tissue attachment. After a clip is applied, the soft tissues lateral to the clips (on the specimen side) were incised with dissection scissors. This allows another clip to be applied slightly more cephalad than the first clip. Each time a clip is applied, the soft tissues lateral to the clip were incised until all of the soft tissue attachments were ligated and the specimen was removed. The specimen was radiographed and sent to pathology (Fig. 15.12). In this case, the spine was stabilized with posterior instrumentation but no anterior reconstruction is required. The T12 rib, which was removed to facilitate exposure, was used for bone graft posterolaterally. The wound was closed in layers. Post-operative radiographs are provided (Fig. 15.13).

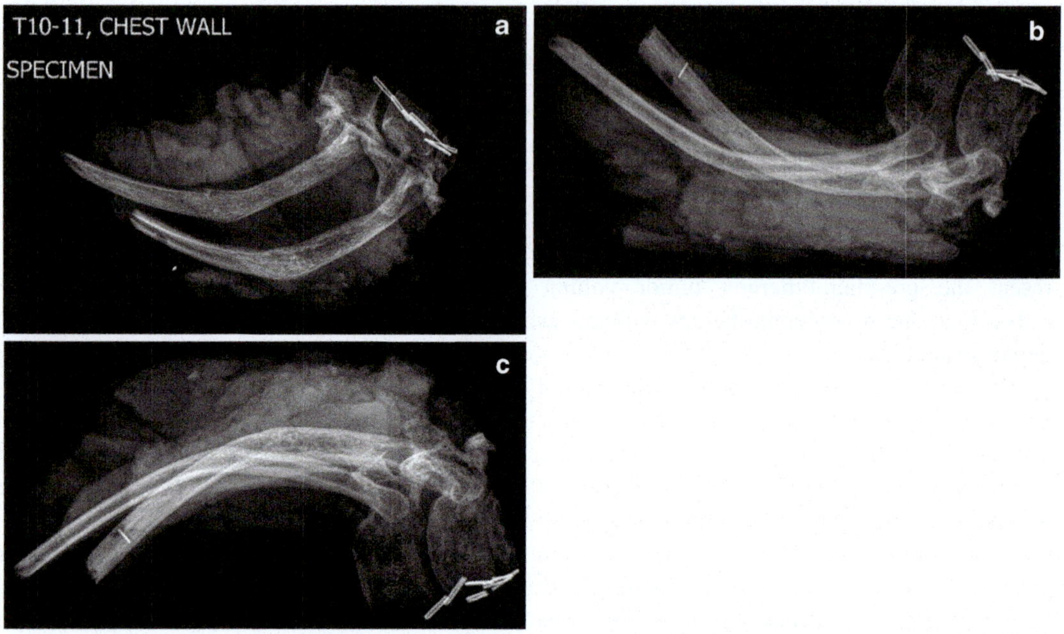

Fig. 15.12 Specimen radiograph. (**a**) Posteroanterior view. (**b**) Oblique view. (**c**) Lateral view

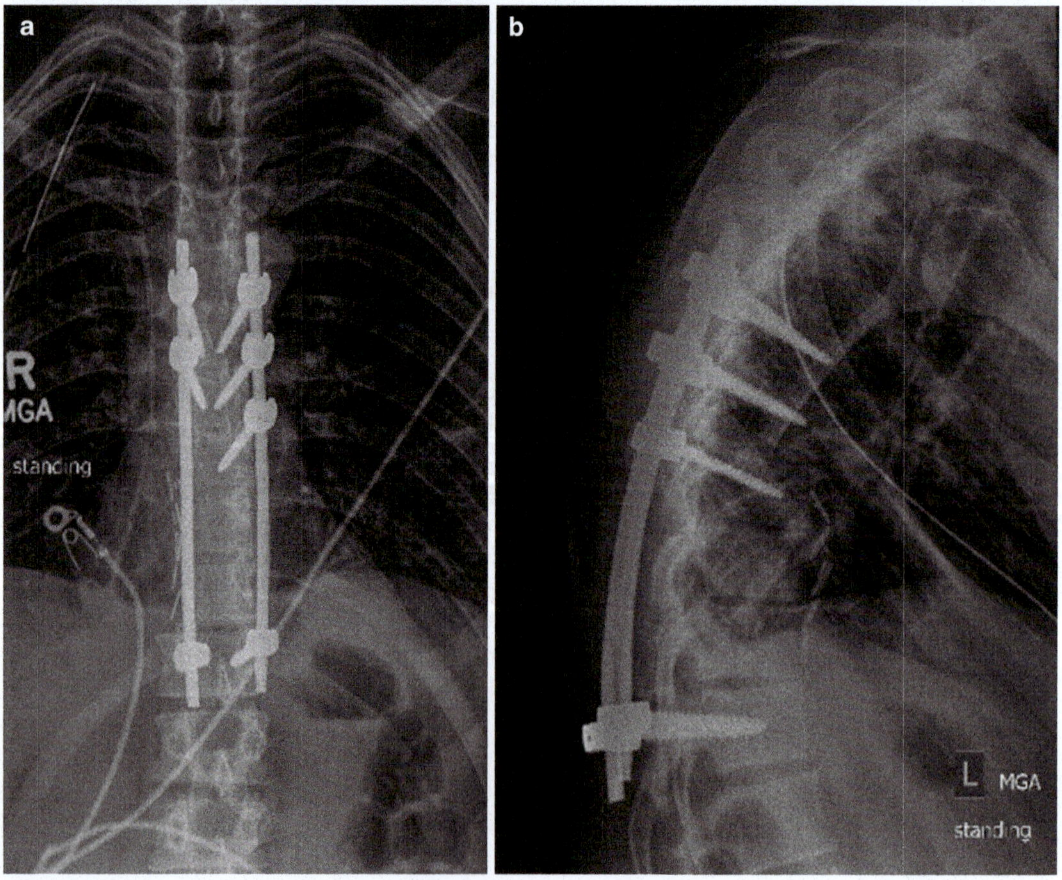

Fig. 15.13 Post-operative radiograph. (**a**) Anteroposterior view. (**b**) Lateral view

Discussion

The management of tumors of the thoracic spine is challenging, as the proximity of critical neurovascular structures makes it considerably difficult to achieve negative tumor margins in this region. Since Roy-Camille and Stener first described spondylectomy for spinal tumors in the late 1960s and early 1970s [9–11], there have been considerable advances in the surgical management of spinal tumors. Multiple studies have demonstrated that total en bloc spondylectomy (TES) – complete resection of the tumor in a single piece, fully encased in a layer of healthy tissue – improves survival and reduces local recurrence rates compared with intralesional piecemeal resection for primary tumors and solitary metastases of the spine [12–20]. Since TES was first reported in 1994 [21, 22], many TES approaches have been described varying in number of stages as well as instruments used to perform the vertebral osteotomies [23–29]. Here we describe two cases in order to demonstrate techniques utilized for posterior en bloc spondylectomy. In one case, we used threadwire saws for our osteotomy and in the other we used a 6-millimeter diamond burr. Both cases sought to achieve a negative margin in a safe manner. These surgeries mandate planning for the worst-case scenario as there is significant risk associated with these procedures. A clear understanding of the anatomy is required and appropriate pre-operative imaging is crucial for planning purposes. An MRI is most useful for planning resection levels as it helps identify the extent of the tumor. A contrast-enhanced CT is also important as it helps one understand the venous vessels about the region of the planned resection. It is useful to work with colleagues in other specialties such as vascular surgery or thoracic surgery should their services be required expeditiously. While most surgeons will not perform en bloc resections, an understanding of the issues related to them is useful to those surgeons who may manage the more common metastatic lesions even though they rarely require spondylectomy.

Conclusion

Posterior approaches to the spine offer several advantages in the operative management of malignant tumors of the spine. Ease of direct access to the "normal" dura above and below the segments involved with tumor and direct 360° visualization of the dura are two key advantages. The en bloc approaches emphasized in this chapter can help to form the basis of understanding the technical, anatomic, and physiologic aspects of these approaches.

References

1. Colman MW, Hornicek FJ, Schwab JH. Spinal cord blood supply and its surgical implications. J Am Acad Orthop Surg. 2015;23(10):581–91.
2. Koshino T, Murakami G, Morishita K, Mawatari T, Abe T. Does the Adamkiewicz artery originate from the larger segmental arteries? J Thorac Cardiovasc Surg. 1999;117(5):898–905.
3. Lazorthes G, Gouaze A, Zadeh JO, Santini JJ, Lazorthes Y, Burdin P. Arterial vascularization of the spinal cord. Recent studies of the anastomotic substitution pathways. J Neurosurg. 1971;35(3):253–62.
4. Raskin KA, Schwab JH, Mankin HJ, Springfield DS, Hornicek FJ. Giant cell tumor of bone. J Am Acad Orthop Surg. 2013;21(2):118–26.
5. Boriani S, Bandiera S, Casadei R, Boriani L, Donthineni R, Gasbarrini A, et al. Giant cell tumor of the mobile spine: a review of 49 cases. Spine (Phila Pa 1976). 2012;37(1):E37–45.
6. Tomita K, Kawahara N. The threadwire saw: a new device for cutting bone. J Bone Joint Surg Am. 1996;78(12):1915–7.
7. Tomita K, Kawahara N, Murakami H, Demura S. Total en bloc spondylectomy for spinal tumors: improvement of the technique and its associated basic background. J Orthop Sci. 2006;11(1):3–12.
8. Foulon S, Brennan B, Gaspar N, Dirksen U, Jeys L, Cassoni A, et al. Can postoperative radiotherapy be omitted in localised standard-risk Ewing sarcoma? An observation study of the Euro-E.W.I.N.G group. Eur J Cancer. 2016;61:128–36.
9. Lièvre JA, Darcy M, Pradat P, Camus JP, Bénichou C, Attali P, et al. Giant cell tumor of the lumbar spine; total spondylectomy in 2 states. Rev Rhum Mal Osteoartic. 1968;35(3):125–30.
10. Stener B. Total spondylectomy in chondrosarcoma arising from the seventh thoracic vertebra. J Bone Joint Surg Br. 1971;53(2):288–95.
11. Stener B, Johnsen OE. Complete removal of three vertebrae for giant-cell tumour. J Bone Joint Surg Br. 1971;53(2):278–87.

12. Boriani S, Chevalley F, Weinstein JN, Biagini R, Campanacci L, De Lure F, et al. Chordoma of the spine above the sacrum. Treatment and outcome in 21 cases. Spine (Phila Pa 1976). 1996;21(13):1569–77.
13. Boriani S, De lure F, Bandiera S, Campanaci L, Biagini R, Di Fiore M, et al. Chondrosarcoma of the mobile spine: repot on 22 cases. Spine (Phila Pa 1976). 2000;25(7):804–12.
14. Boriani S, Bandiera S, Biagini R, Bacchini P, Boriani L, Cappuccio M, et al. Chordoma of the mobile spine: fifty years of experience. Spine (Phila Pa 1976). 2006;31(4):493–503.
15. Melcher I, Disch AC, Khodadadyan-Klostermann C, Tohtz S, Smolny M, Stöckle U, et al. Primary malignant bone tumors and solitary metastases of the thoracolumbar spine: results by management with total en bloc spondylectomy. Eur Spine J. 2007;16(8):1193–202.
16. Schwab J, Gasbarrini A, Bandiera S, Boriani L, Amendola L, Picci P, et al. Osteosarcoma of the mobile spine. Spine (Phila Pa 1976). 2012;37(6):E381–6.
17. Schoenfeld AJ, Hornicek FJ, Pedlow FX, Kobayashi W, Raskin KA, Springfield D, et al. Chondrosarcoma of the mobile spine: a review of 21 cases treated at a single center. Spine (Phila Pa 1976). 2012;37(2):119–26.
18. Kato S, Murakami H, Demura S, Yoshioka K, Kawahara N, Tomita K, et al. More than 10-year follow-up after total en bloc spondylectomy for spinal tumors. Ann Surg Oncol. 2014;21(4):1330–6.
19. Amendola L, Cappuccio M, De lure F, Bandiera S, Gasbarrini A, Boriani S. En bloc resections for primary spinal tumors in 20 years of experience: effectiveness and safety. Spine J. 2014;14(11):2608–17.
20. Cloyd JM, Acosta FL Jr, Polley MY, Ames CP. En bloc resection for primary and metastatic tumors of the spine: a systematic review of the literature. Neurosurgery. 2010;67(2):435–44.
21. Tomita K, Toribatake Y, Kawahara N, Ohnari H, Kose H. Total en bloc spondylectomy and circumspinal decompression for solitary spinal metastasis. Paraplegia. 1994;32(1):36–46.
22. Fidler MW. Radical resection of vertebral body tumours. A surgical technique used in ten cases. J Bone Joint Surg Br. 1994;76(5):765–72.
23. Tomita K, Kawahara N, Murakami H, Demura S. Total en bloc spondylectomy for spinal tumors: improvement of the technique and its associated basic background. J Orthop Sci. 2006;11(1):3–12.
24. Sundaresan N, DiGiainto GV, Krol G, Hughes JEO. Spondylectomy for malignant tumors of the spine. J Clin Oncol. 1989;7(10):1485–91.
25. Fourney DR, Abi-Said D, Rhines LD, Walsh GL, Lang FF, McCutcheon IE, et al. Simultaneous anterior-posterior approach to the thoracic and lumbar spine for the radical resection of tumors followed by reconstruction and stabilization. J Neurosurg. 2001;94(2 Suppl):232–44.
26. Kawahara N, Tomita K, Murakami H, Demura S. Total en bloc spondylectomy for spinal tumors: surgical techniques and related basic background. Orthop Clin North Am. 2009;40(1):47–63:vi.
27. Kawahara N, Tomita K, Murakami H, Demura S, Yoshioka K, Kato S. Total en bloc spondylectomy of the lower lumbar spine: a surgical technique of combined posterior-anterior approach. Spine (Phila Pa 1976). 2011;36(1):74–82.
28. Sciubba DM, De la Garza RR, Goodwin CR, Xu R, Bydon A, Witham TF, et al. Total en bloc spondylectomy for locally aggressive and primary malignant tumors of the lumbar spine. Eur Spine J. 2016;25(12):4080–7.
29. Shah AA, Pereira NRP, Pedlow FX, Wain JC, Yoon SS, Hornicek FJ, et al. Modified en bloc spondylectomy for tumors of the thoracic and lumbar spine. Surgical technique and outcomes. J Bone Joint Surg Am. 2017;99(17):1476–84.
30. Hsieh PC, Li KW, Sciubba DM, Suk I, Wolinsky JP, Gokaslan ZL. Posterior-only approach for total en bloc spondylectomy for malignant primary spinal neoplasms: anatomic considerations and operative nuances. Oper Neurosurg. 2009;65:ons173–81.

16 Anterior/Anterolateral Thoracic Access and Stabilization from Posterior Approach, Transpedicular, Costotransversectomy, Lateral Extracavitary Approaches via Minimally Invasive Approaches, Minimal Access and Tubular Access

Rodrigo Navarro-Ramirez,
Juan Del Castillo-Calcáneo, Roger Härtl,
and Ali Baaj

Introduction

Minimally invasive spine surgery (MISS) involves accessing the spine through small corridors and achieving the same results as in open surgery, thereby minimizing damage to other tissues [1].

The main areas of opportunity for MISS include reduced blood loss during operation, decreased postoperative recovery time and pain, and less disruption to the paraspinal muscles and ligaments that contribute to the maintenance of proper spine biomechanics, all of which are important advantages since they could reduce complications in patients undergoing surgery for spinal tumors [1].

Tumors associated with the spinal cord can have devastating effects on patient function and quality of life. They have been traditionally approached with large open surgeries and fusion procedures with the objective of providing oncological control, decompression, and stabilization to ultimately improve both neurological and oncological prognosis. However, in the past years, the use of MISS has been on the rise mainly due to its ability to decrease the amount of surgical trauma, which translates into improved recovery and return to productive life. We also have to consider that oncologic patients have different perioperative complications than degenerative or deformity patients, such that posterior MISS approaches may be better tolerated for them.

In this chapter, we summarize the less disruptive approaches that are available in treating thoracic tumor pathologies (Fig. 16.1).

Preoperative Evaluation

As a general rule, all spinal tumor cases which will undergo MISS must have at least a preoperative contrasted MRI, a CT scan of the area of interest, and scoliosis films in order to evaluate and ultimately compare their sagittal alignment.

R. Navarro-Ramirez (✉) · R. Härtl · A. Baaj
New York Presbyterian, Weill Cornell Brain and Spine Center, Department of Neurological Surgery, New York, NY, USA
e-mail: ron2006@med.cornell.edu

J. Del Castillo-Calcáneo
National Autonomous University of Mexico, Department of Neurosurgery, Mexico City, Mexico

D. M. Sciubba (ed.), *Spinal Tumor Surgery*, https://doi.org/10.1007/978-3-319-98422-3_16

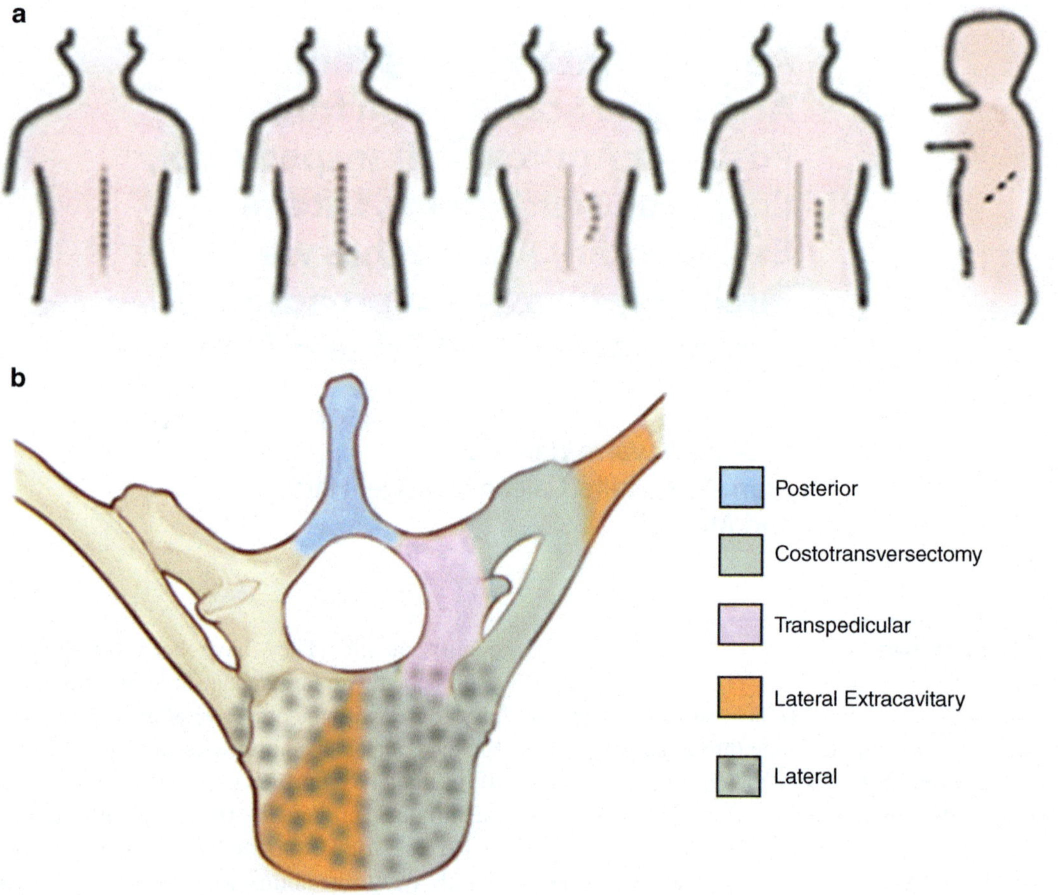

Fig. 16.1 (**a**) Types of positions and incisions (dotted lines) for thoracic approaches. (**b**) Surgical scope for the posterior thoracic surgical approaches

In patients in whom metastasis is suspected, a thorough oncological evaluation of the primary site should be performed in case there is no neurological dysfunction that requires immediate decompression of the spinal cord. The use of corticosteroids has been standard in such patients as a temporizing measure to improve or stabilize neurologic function until definitive treatment. Corticosteroids may result in a rapid improvement of neurological function, but their long-term benefits are limited, and there is no evidence that they improve survival [2].

Since surgery for spine tumors appears to be associated with a higher incidence of surgical site infections (SSIs) than non-tumor spine surgery [3], we recommend the use of intraoperative and postoperative antibiotics.

The spinal neoplastic instability score has proven to be useful in the surgical decision-making process and as a prognostic tool and is recommended [4].

Every patient should be examined and stratified using the American Spinal Injury Association (ASIA) classification before undergoing surgery. Neurophysiological monitoring is not mandatory but it is recommended; motor- and somatosensory-evoked potentials are also useful and sometimes set a baseline for the neurological activity before the actual surgical procedure.

Surgical Techniques

Mini-Open Transpedicular Approach

Indications

- Biopsy
- Dorsal, ipsilateral, and laterally located lesions

Patient Positioning

After anesthetic induction, the patient is positioned in a prone position over a Jackson table. Preoperative x-rays are obtained to localize the indexed spinous process and the corresponding pedicle for the indexed level; alternatively, intraoperative CT with navigation can be used. Percutaneous pedicle screws can be placed two levels above and below the affected vertebral body, depending on surgeons' preference. We prefer to place the percutaneous screws using a navigated guide tube and "total navigation" or sometimes using K-wires and fluoroscopy or using a free-hand technique and fluoroscopic confirmation.

Surgical Details and Special Considerations

Transpedicular corpectomy is performed through a midline approach, and a complete 360° decompression is the primary goal. The uniqueness of this approach in the thoracic spine is that the rib head is left intact [5].

The skin is incised in the midline along with the fascia over the indexed level. A tubular retractor system is then placed and docked over the articulating process of the level of interest, and confirmation is obtained using either navigation or intraoperative fluoroscopy.

A laminectomy with complete removal of the superior articulating process is performed. The ligamentum flavum can be preserved during the laminectomy and during the drilling process to prevent incidental durotomy.

We laterally preserve the rib heads; the discs above and below the corpectomy level are identified and marked. Identification of the pedicle with either navigation, fluoroscopy, or palpation is performed. Using a high-speed drill, a small window at the posterior cortex of the pedicle is opened and the high-speed drill is used until the "eggshell" is left (Figs. 16.2 and 16.3). After reaching the posterior vertebral body wall, an angled curette is used to carefully fracture the medial wall out laterally, exposing the lateral margin of the thecal sac. At this point, if necessary, a small window can be opened over the annulus of the disc right over its posterolateral surface and a partial discectomy can be done using pituitary rongeurs; this cavity can be used to tuck away structures that need to be removed

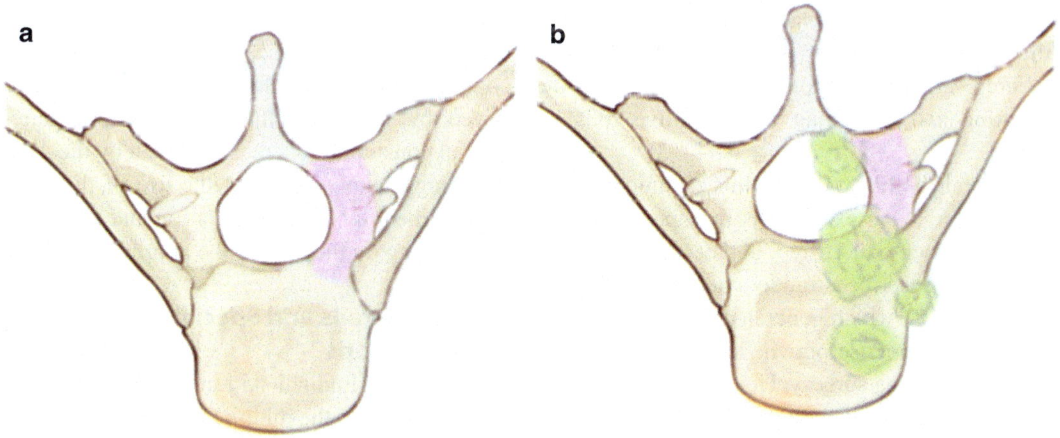

Fig. 16.2 (**a**) Surgical corridor of the transpedicular approach (pink area). (**b**) Surgical corridor of the transpedicular approach (pink area) to access tumors posterior and anterior to the spinal canal

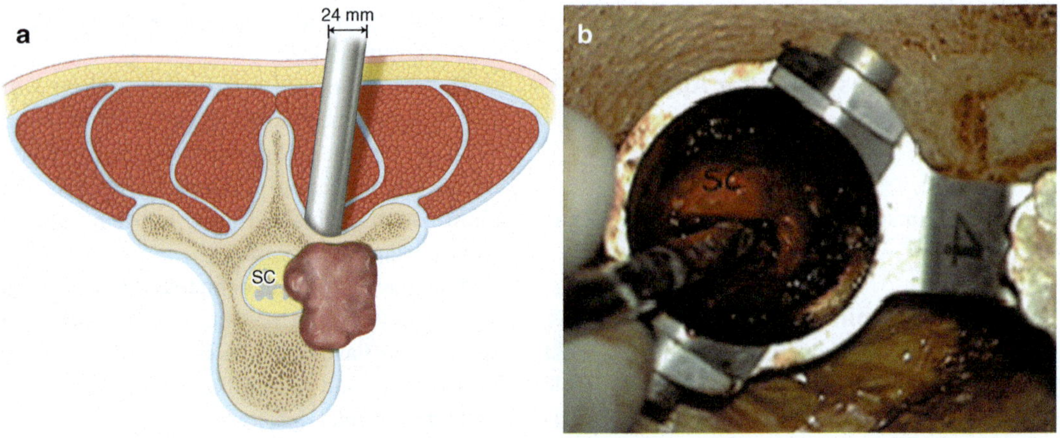

Fig. 16.3 Minimally invasive transpedicular approach. (**a**) Illustration of retractor positioning. (**b**) Intraoperative transpedicular decompression. (Reprinted with permission from Zairi et al. [7])

from the midline to avoid displacing or putting pressure on the spinal cord.

The posterior longitudinal ligament is separated from the dura very carefully; sometimes, if dural sac compression exists, adhesions may be present and incidental dural tears may complicate the procedure. Now, the discectomy is completed, the tumor is removed, and the endplate preparation is performed. The expandable cage is inserted in its collapsed configuration from lateral to medial and then moved medially and anteriorly. The cage is expanded until even contact with the superior and inferior endplate is achieved.

Once the corpectomy is completed and the cage has been put in place, a temporary rod on the contralateral side is placed and loosely secured. Finally, the construct is completed by inserting and tightening the definitive rods in place.

Several modifications to this technique have been adopted. An example is the open vs mini-open approach cohort by Chou et al. using their previously described trapdoor technique for rib osteotomy [6], which generated favorable results for the mini-open group in terms of estimated blood loss during surgery. However, these results must be interpreted with caution because there was a significant difference in age groups, where the MISS option was offered more frequently to younger patients [5].

MISS Costotransversectomy Approach

Indications

- Dorsal and laterally located lesions
- Centrally located lesions with soft consistency
- Paraspinal nerve-sheath tumors

Patient Positioning

The patient is placed in prone position on a Jackson table, and the level of interest is marked under fluoroscopic guidance or neuronavigation.

Neuromonitoring of somatosensory-evoked potentials and motor-evoked potentials is of paramount importance for this approach.

For this specific procedure, the most common complication is neurological deterioration, followed by hemo/pneumothorax. For the latter, special considerations must be taken by the anesthesiology team, including the use of divergent endotracheal tubes for ventilation and for deflating the lung on the side of the approach.

Surgical Details and Special Considerations

A 2.5-cm longitudinal skin incision is performed 3–5 cm lateral to the midline and ipsilateral to the tumor. The paramedian musculature can be retracted laterally. After the lateral transverse process is identified, a K-wire is inserted into the

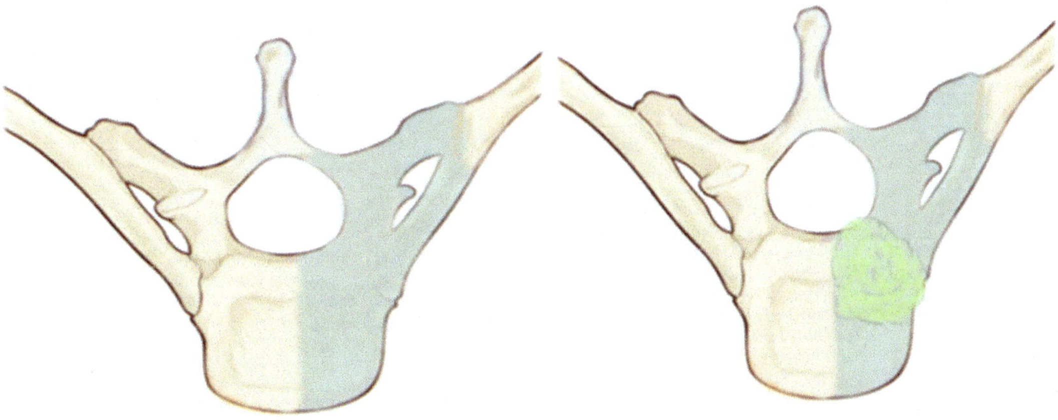

Fig. 16.4 Surgical corridor for the costotransversectomy approach

bone under fluoroscopic control to be docked at the costotransverse process junction. After this, a series of tubular retractors is guided into the area of interest which involves the interlaminar space, adjacent laminae, transverse process, and the adjacent rib (Fig. 16.4).

The transverse process and the ribs are resected using a high-speed drill and/or Kerrison rongeurs in order to achieve better visualization. From this approach, it is possible to verify the integrity of the nerve root as well as the decompression of the thecal sac. Once the goal of decompression or biopsy has been achieved, the tubular or blade retractor is removed and the fascia and skin are closed.

MISS Lateral Extracavitary Approach

Patient Positioning

After anesthetic induction, the patient is positioned prone in a Jackson table over a frame. Fluoroscopic guidance is used to identify the level of the lesion, and the skin incision is marked 4–5 cm lateral to the midline.

Surgical Details and Special Considerations

After the incision is made, blunt dissection, usually with the surgeon's finger, is performed all the way to the transverse process in an oblique lateral extracavitary trajectory in order to insert a working portal. Percutaneous pedicle screw insertion above and below the corpectomy level is performed using 3-D navigation or fluoroscopy and K-wires.

The accurate position of the screws is confirmed by AP and lateral x-rays. The patient is then rotated away from the surgeon to compensate for the obliquity of the approach. The surgical microscope is introduced to the field, the inferior transverse process and facet are freed, and the transverse process is removed using a high-speed drill. The lateral aspect of the laminae is decompressed from lateral to medial with a high-speed drill and Kerrison rongeurs. At this point, the ligamentum flavum becomes visible and is removed in order to access the spinal canal to perform the required operation. The oblique trajectory allows for an excellent bilateral decompression of the cord through a unilateral approach.

This approach allows for an excellent visibility of the vertebral body and discs. The rib heads are preserved. The pedicles at the pathological level are removed. The discs above and below the vertebral body are identified. A high-speed drill is used to begin the corpectomy on one side. After a significant amount of vertebral body has been removed, a holding rod is placed and locked. If a rib head is maintained as trapdoor, no pleural dissection will be necessary.

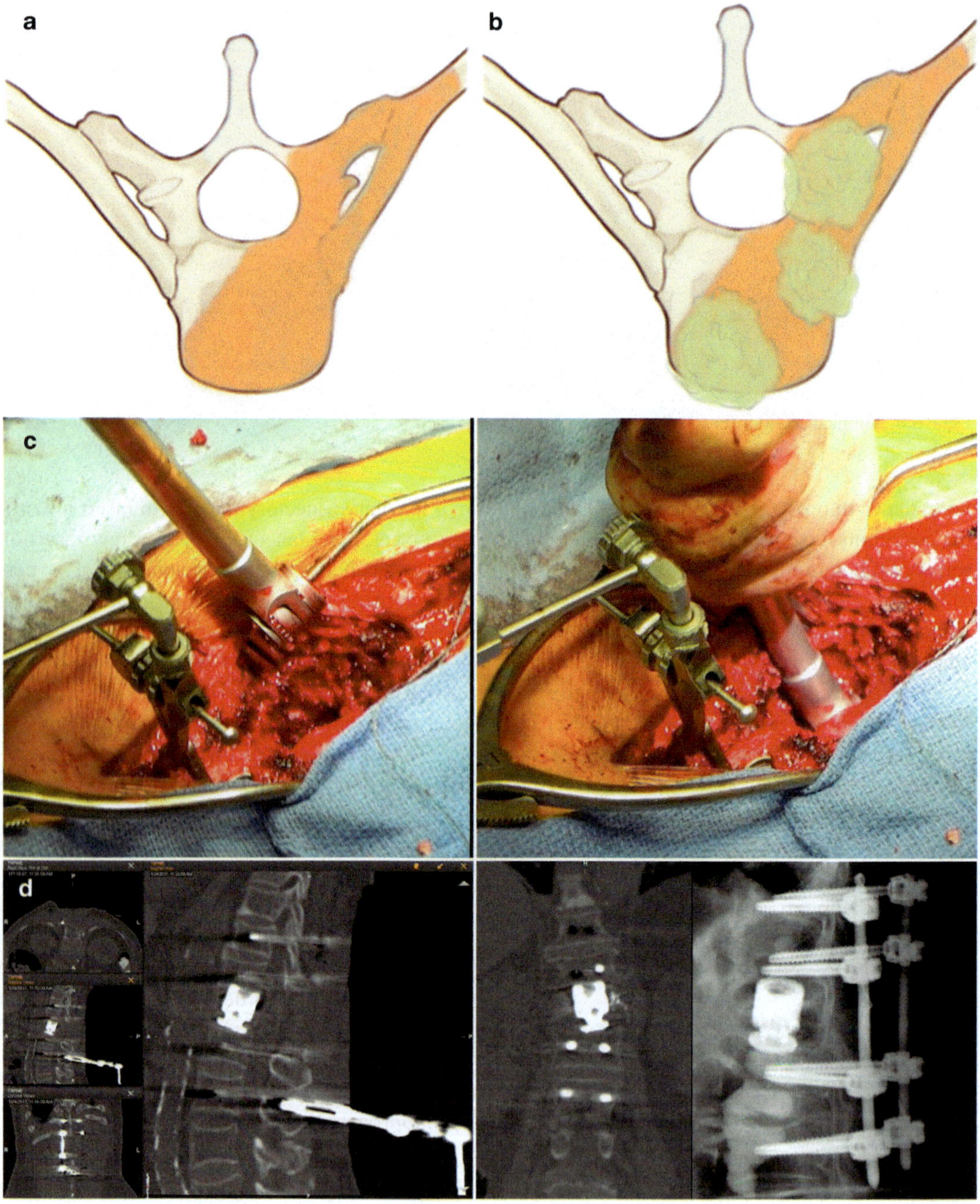

Fig. 16.5 (**a**, **b**) Surgical corridor for the thoracic lateral extracavitary approach. (**c**) Intraoperative images of the insertion of the collapsed expandable cage through the lateral corridor. (**d**) Intraoperative navigation images of the cage placement and final location on fluoroscopic images

Depending on the type of operation, an expandable cage can be introduced and expanded to fit once positioned (Fig. 16.5).

The contralateral rod is then put in place and fixed, and additional crosslinks are placed for circumferential arthrodesis.

Lateral Approach

Patient Positioning

The patient is intubated using a dual-lumen tube to allow for selective bronchi ventilation and in case it is necessary to collapse the lung on the operative side (see Fig. 16.5). The patient is placed in the lateral position with the side of the targeted pathology facing up. If the pathology is located near the midline, the right side is preferred in order to reduce the risk of vascular injury.

Surgical Details and Special Considerations

Under fluoroscopic guidance, the skin is marked on the level of interest; the incision is marked parallel to the contour of the rib cage. The incision is then made and subperiosteal blunt dissection is done with preservation of the neurovascular bundle located under each rib. The parietal pleura is opened, and the first dilator is swept along the rib to approach the level of the pathology. If necessary, 3–4 cm of the rib can be resected to achieve maximal exposure. Sometimes this part of the procedure is performed by cardio-thoracic surgeons.

The dilators are then progressively placed until the necessary exposure is achieved, and the microscope is placed over the operating field.

With this approach, the placement of cages or corpectomy implants can be easily performed.

After resection of pathology and stabilization are achieved, a chest tube is placed and closure of the fascia and skin is performed.

Postoperative Care

- Obtain immediate postoperative chest x-rays to rule out pneumothorax or hemothorax.
- Strict pain control to prevent shallow ventilation postoperative is mandatory.
- Frequent and scheduled neurological checks for 24-h postoperative window. Patients should be evaluated in the immediate postoperative period in all aspects of the ASIA classification to establish if any additional damage occurred during the surgery despite the neurophysiological monitoring.
- Urgent MRI should be considered if new neurological symptoms are present.
- Routine postoperative imaging is not required.
- Corticosteroid dose should be tapered down in the weeks following surgical management of the spinal tumor to avoid complications related to its use [2].

Conclusion

MISS posterolateral approaches to the thoracic spine for tumor surgery are feasible and safe if certain rules are followed. For instance, if subtotal resections are the goal, the posterior, transpedicular, extracavitary, and lateral approaches are good options. However, for pathologies extending anteriorly and closer to the midline, only the lateral extracavitary or lateral approaches are recommended.

References

1. Härtl R, Korge A. Minimally invasive spine surgery. Stuttgart: Thieme; 2012.
2. National Institute for Health and Clinical Excellence. Metastatic spinal cord compression: diagnosis and management of patients at risk of or with metastatic spinal cord compression. London: NICE; 2008.
3. Omeis IA, Dhir M, Sciubba DM, Gottfried ON, McGirt MJ, Attenello FJ, et al. Postoperative surgical site infections in patients undergoing spinal tumor surgery: incidence and risk factors. Spine. 2011;36(17):1410–9.
4. Fisher CG, DiPaola CP, Ryken TC, Bilsky MH, Shaffrey CI, Berven SH, et al. A novel classification system for spinal instability in neoplastic disease: an evidence-based approach and expert consensus from the Spine Oncology Study Group. Spine. 2010;35(22):E1221–9.
5. Chou D, Lu DC. Mini-open transpedicular corpectomies with expandable cage reconstruction. J Neurosurg Spine. 2011;14(1):71–7.
6. Chou D, Wang VY. Trap-door rib-head osteotomies for posterior placement of expandable cages after transpedicular corpectomy: an alternative to lateral extracavitary and costotransversectomy approaches. Technical note. J Neurosurg Spine. 2009;10:40–5.
7. Zairi F, et al. Minimally invasive decompression and stabilization for the management of thoracolumbar spine metastasis. J Neurosurg Spine. 2012;17(1):19–23.

Posterolateral Approach to Thoraco-Lumbar Metastases - Separation Surgery

17

Ori Barzilai, Ilya Laufer, and Mark H. Bilsky

Introduction

Twenty to 40% of all cancer patients develop spinal metastases with microscopic evidence of spinal disease found in up to 90% [2, 3], and with modern cancer therapies and improved survival times, these numbers are likely to grow. Metastases most commonly affect the thoracic spine (70%) and are typically found in the vertebral body with or without extension into the posterior elements [4]. Further, up to 20% of patients diagnosed with spinal metastases can progress to symptomatic cord compression [5, 6]. The most frequent histologic types of cancer that give rise to bone metastases are breast, prostate, and lung cancer [7].

Treatment goals for patients with spine metastases are palliative and include preservation or restoration of neurological function, maintenance of spinal stability, palliation of pain, and durable local tumor control. Treatment options include surgery, radiation therapy (RT), and systemic treatment including chemotherapy and biologics or combinations of these modalities. Selecting the most favorable treatment strategy is challenging in light of recent advances, particularly the development of SSRS.

Case Presentation

A 90-year-old female presented with recently diagnosed stage IV non-small-cell lung cancer (NSCLC). Her past medical history was significant for prior smoking, well-controlled hypertension, and a heart murmur treated with baby aspirin. She underwent a systemic workup for her newly diagnosed lung cancer and was found to have spine metastases with epidural extension. Retrospectively, she recalled experiencing thoracic back pain radiating around the chest bilaterally for several weeks. She did not endorse extremity weakness, numbness, paresthesias, gait disturbances, or bowel and bladder issues.

Diagnostic Workup

Recent technological and scientific advancements have introduced a plethora of new, promising, systemic agents and spine technologies that are fundamentally changing cancer care. Specifically for treatment of spinal metastases, the integration of SSRS has revolutionized the approach to treatment. As these new therapies and modalities become available, tailoring the appropriate treat-

O. Barzilai
Memorial Sloan Kettering Cancer Center, Department of Neurosurgery, New York, NY, USA

I. Laufer · M. H. Bilsky (✉)
Memorial Sloan Kettering Cancer Center, Department of Neurosurgery, New York, NY, USA

Department of Neurological Surgery, Weill Cornell Medical College, New York, NY, USA
e-mail: bilskym@mskcc.org

D. M. Sciubba (ed.), *Spinal Tumor Surgery*, https://doi.org/10.1007/978-3-319-98422-3_17

ment to the individual patient is becoming increasingly challenging. To this end, the NOMS framework was created [8]. NOMS serves as a template for the analysis of important clinical and radiological data and is not wedded to any particular treatment or technology. As treatments and technologies progress, so too will the treatment modalities utilized within NOMS. The framework is comprised of four major domains from which clinical information is assessed: neurologic, oncologic, mechanical, and systemic.

The neurologic assessment determines clinically the presence of myelopathy and functional epidural spinal cord compression (ESCC) as has been previously described [9] (Fig. 17.1, *ESCC*). The oncologic assessment consists of determining the expected histology-specific tumor response to treatments including radiation therapy, chemotherapy, biologics, or checkpoint inhibitors. Mechanical instability serves as an independent factor prompting surgical intervention even for radiosensitive tumors since radiotherapy and systemic therapy do not restore mechanical stability of the spine. The mechanical assessment is facilitated by the Spinal Instability Neoplastic Scoring (SINS) system [10]. SINS considers multiple factors important for biomechanical spinal integrity: location, pain, lesion character, radiographic spinal alignment, degree of vertebral body collapse, and the degree of posterolateral spinal element involvement. The last consideration is the systemic assessment which incorporates the patient's overall burden of disease and medical co-morbidities. The ultimate task is to determine the patient's capacity to tolerate a surgical intervention and sufficiently recover in order to become a candidate for continued systemic therapy. This involves knowledge of the complex interplay of tumor biology, molecular markers, and targeted therapies. As knowledge increases, so does complexity in decision-making and hence warrants a multidisciplinary team approach comprised of spine surgeons, medical and radiation oncologists, interventional radiologists, pain specialists, and rehabilitation experts.

During the patients' workup, a chest CT was performed which demonstrated a right lower lobe (RLL) lung mass, moderate left pleural effusion and pericardial effusion, and a mass invading the T5 vertebra. To further investigate this thoracic spine tumor, a total spine MRI was performed. *It is important to obtain a total spine MRI* at presentation with spine metastases as multiple lesions are present, which may influence the treatment plan. In this case, the MRI (Fig. 17.2) demonstrated multilevel, multifocal osseous metastases and epidural disease, worst at T3–T6 with high-grade circumferential epidural spinal cord compression (ESCC

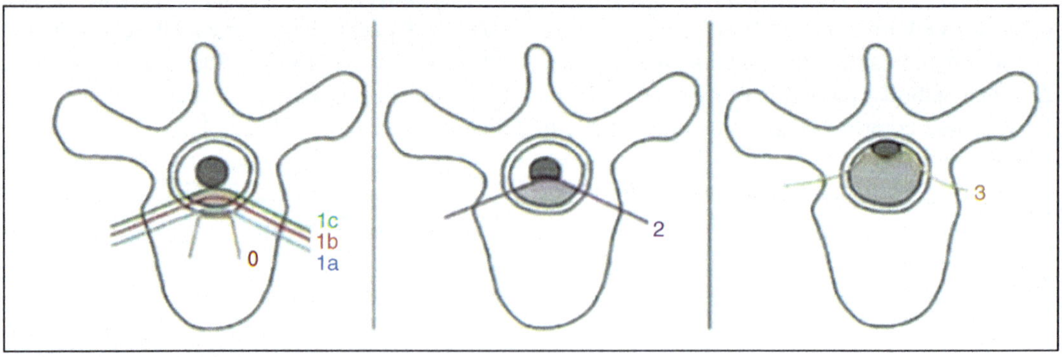

Schematic representation of the 6-point ESCC grading scale.

Grade 0	Bone-only disease
Grade 1a	Epidural impingement, without deformation of thecal sac
Grade 1b	Deformation of thecal sac, without spinal cord abutment
Grade 1c	Deformation of thecal sac, with spinal cord abutment, without cord compression
Grade 2	Spinal cord compression, with cerebral spinal fluid (CSF) visible around the cord
Grade 3	Spinal cord compression, no CSF visible around the cord

Fig. 17.1 Epidural spinal cord compression score [9]. (Reproduced with permission from Bilsky et al. [9])

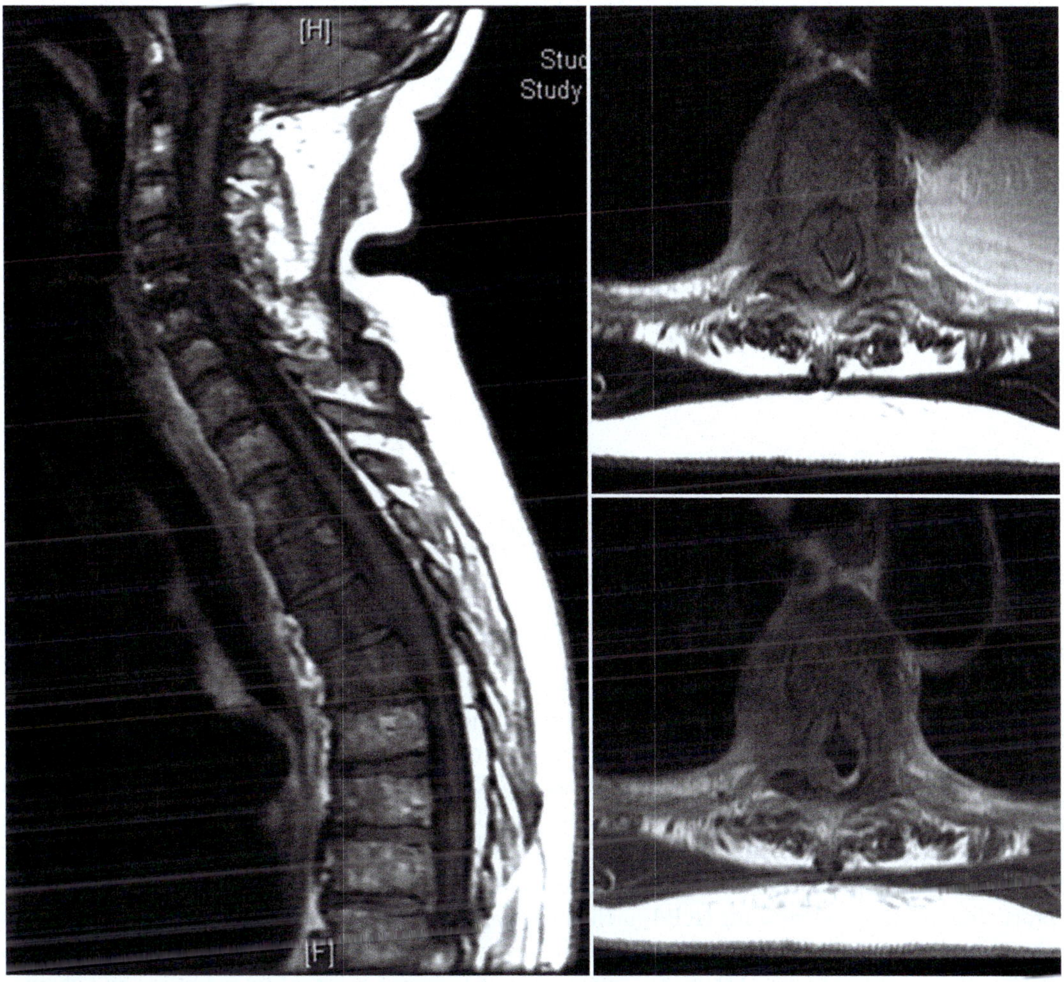

Fig. 17.2 Pre-operative MRI. Left: Sagittal T1 non-contrast enhancing demonstrates multilevel hypointense tumor infiltration. Top right: axial T2. Bottom right: axial T1 with contrast enhancement demonstrating high-grade metastatic epidural spinal cord compression (ESCC 3)

3) and at T5–T6 paraspinal extension and bilateral foraminal involvement. Additionally noted were T12 vertebral body involvement with minor epidural extension (ESCC 1b) and C3 vertebral body infiltration with no epidural extension (ESCC 0).

This patient was evaluated by a multidisciplinary team. Neurologically and oncologically, she was intact with high-grade ESCC from a radioresistant tumor. The high-grade ESCC precluded the delivery of SSRS as definitive therapy. Mechanically, her calculated SINS score was 10 (i.e., indeterminate/pending instability). Systemically, despite advanced age, there were no major co-morbidities, and she was in good clinical condition. Considering all NOMS criteria, surgery for decompression of the thoracic lesion was deemed the best initial management step. In patients with metastatic cancer, the goals of surgery must include short operative times and minimal blood loss in order to reduce the risks of perioperative complications. Prior to surgery, the vascularity of the tumor must be taken into consideration. For example, renal cell carcinoma (RCC) represents a highly vascular tumor, and pre-operative embolization is imperative in order to avoid massive intraoperative blood loss [11].

She underwent *separation surgery*, which included a circumferential decompression of T5–T6 with T3–T8 fusion through a posterolateral approach (Fig. 17.3).

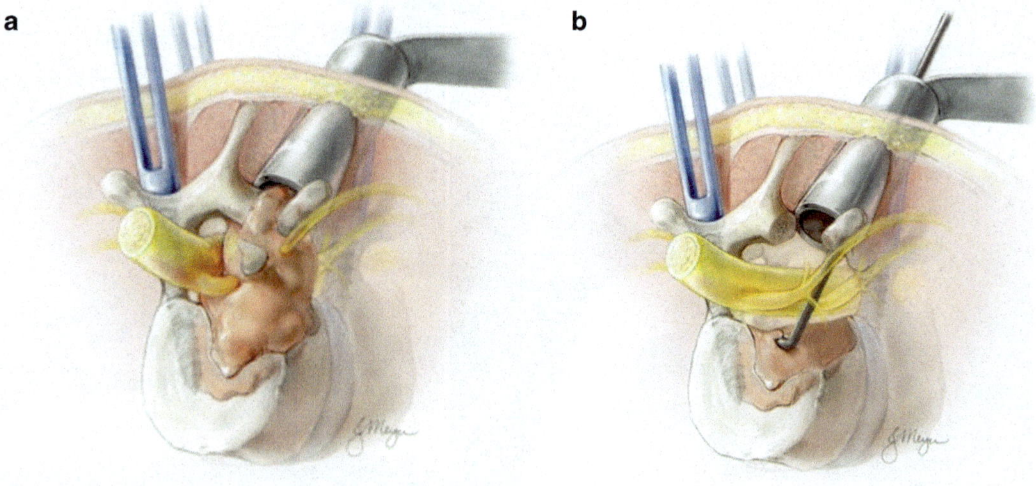

Fig. 17.3 Artist illustration of minimally invasive separation surgery. (**a**) Percutaneous stabilization is performed and the tube is guided for decompression. (**b**) Tumor is resected from the thecal sac and pushed anteriorly to create space between the soft tissue lesion and the anterior thecal sac. (Reprinted from Nasser et al. [37], Copyright (2018), with permission from Elsevier)

Surgery

The patient was put under general anesthesia with placement of an arterial line and Foley catheter. Intraoperative electrophysiological electrodes were placed, and the patient was positioned prone. Intraoperative monitoring (IOM) included electromyography (EMG) to the lower extremities and lower sacral root distributions, somatosensory evoked potentials (SSEPs), and motor evoked potentials (MEPs). IOM provides neurophysiologic feedback which can be used to adjust intraoperative strategies to reduce or reverse neurological deficits. The target levels are localized and the incision planned using fluoroscopy. The surgical site was prepped and draped in typical sterile fashion.

Following a midline linear skin incision, the posterior spinal elements were exposed using monopolar cautery. Prior to canal decompression, pedicle screw and rod constructs were placed. Spinal navigation systems [12] are currently widely utilized, yet, to date, standard "free-hand" instrumentation is definitely acceptable as well. All patients who undergo separation surgery will require instrumentation as not only are the osseous structures typically compromised by tumor invasion, but decompression requires removal of the laminae and pedicle/joint complex and is thus destabilizing. Instrumenting prior to decompression is safer than placing hardware over an unprotected spinal canal. The potential for arthrodesis is severely compromised in oncologic patients due to poor bone quality, radiation, and chemotherapy [13]. Long-segment fixation, normally two levels above and two levels below the index tumor level, has been previously described with low complication rates [14]. This patient was instrumented two levels above and two levels below the decompression site (Fig. 17.4).

Next, the posterior elements were resected with a high-speed 3-mm matchstick bur. Adequate circumferential separation of the tumor from the thecal sac is critical in order to facilitate post-operative SSRS. The pedicles and facet joints are drilled bilaterally, creating a corridor to the ventral epidural space. The tumor dissection off the dura was the preformed. This was initiated from normal dural planes toward the site of maximal compres-

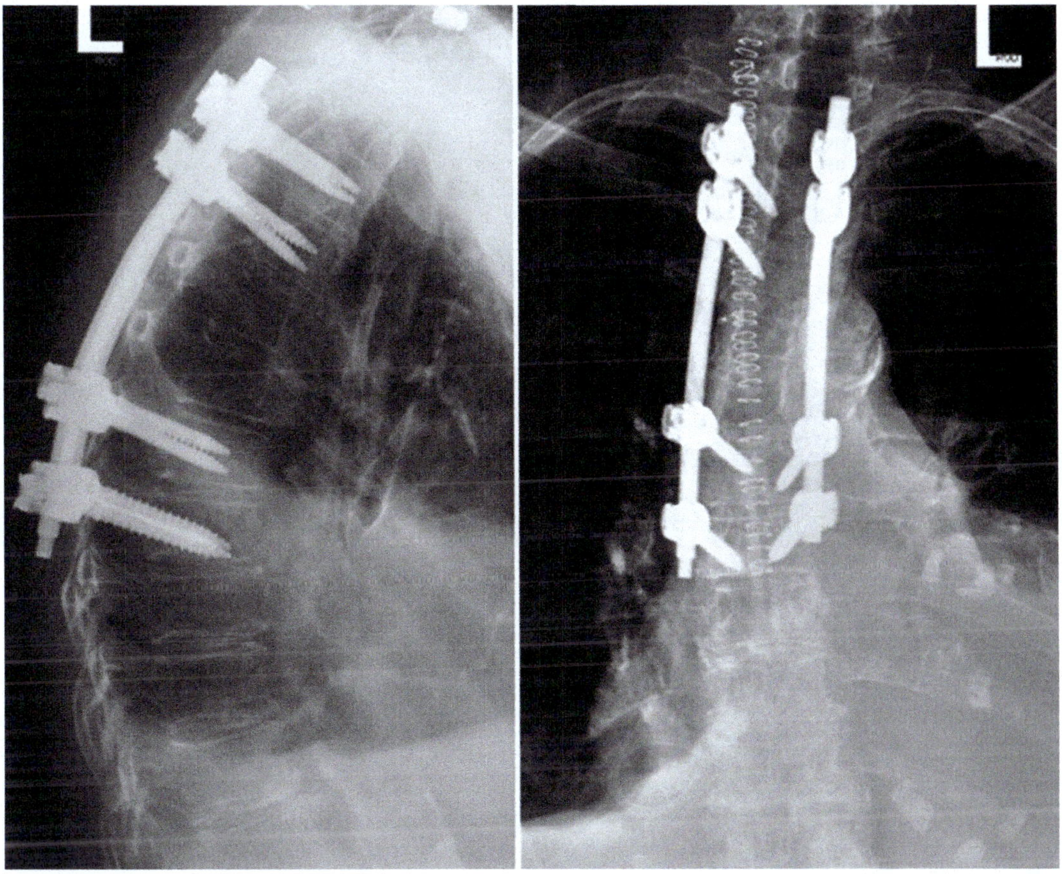

Fig. 17.4 Sagittal (left) and anterior posterior (right) post-operative standing x-rays demonstrating the stabilizing construct

sion. Following resection of the posterior longitudinal ligament, the ventral component of the tumor including the ligament of Hoffman was dissected ventrally (i.e., away from the spinal cord). In this case, a small ventral cavity was created within the vertebral body and a "Woodson" dissector used to depress the epidural component ventrally. If a large portion of the vertebral body is removed, anterior support can be achieved by inserting poly-methyl-methacrylate (i.e., PMMA bone cement) into the cavity (deemed unnecessary in the current case). Hemostasis was achieved and the wound was irrigated copiously. To optimize arthrodesis, the facet joints and transverse processes were decorticated, and autologous bone graft was placed posteriorly to initiate bony fusion. Variable fusion rates in this population are reported (36–100%), and various options for bone graft are used according to surgeon's preference [15]. A drain was placed in the epidural space, the surgical site sutured in layers, and a sterile dressing applied. The patient was flipped back to the supine position, INM electrodes were removed, and the patient was extubated. It is important to acknowledge that *no attempt for gross total tumor removal was attempted since post-operative SSRS will effectively provide local tumor control.*

Post-operatively, while still admitted, a CT myelogram was preformed demonstrating reconstitution of the thecal sac (Fig. 17.5). This was done in the post-operative setting to facilitate rapid radiosurgery treatment planning.

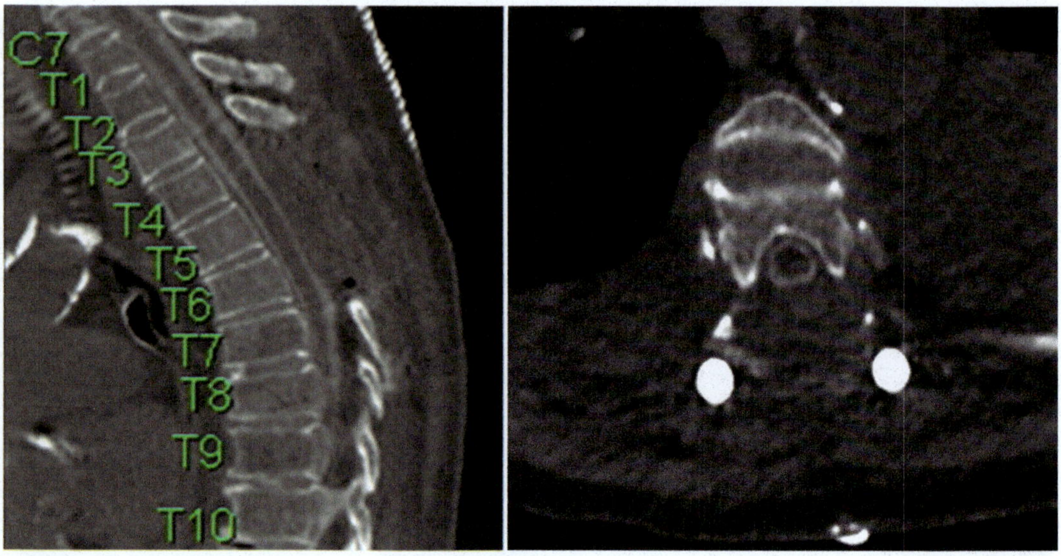

Fig. 17.5 Post-operative CT myelogram demonstrating complete re-constitution of the thecal sac. Left: sagittal. Right: axial at T6 level

Discussion

Separation surgery was first described in 2000 as a single-stage posterolateral trans-pedicle approach for spondylectomy, epidural decompression, and circumferential fusion for treatment of spinal metastases [16]. The goal of decompression is neurologic preservation or recovery but also to provide an ablative target for SSRS within spinal cord constraints. Data evaluating the safety, efficacy, and adverse effects of this surgery have since been established and discussed extensively [14, 17, 18]. Our detailed technique for separation surgery has been previously described elsewhere. The implementation of spinal sterotactic radiosrgery (SSRS) for treatment of spinal metastases is a result of technological advancements in non-invasive patient immobilization, intensity-modulated image-guided radiation therapy (IGRT) delivery systems, and sophisticated planning software [19, 20]. These technical advancements facilitated the integration of SSRS into treatment paradigms and have been a true paradigm changer for the treatment of spinal metastases.

SSRS treatment failures occur when less than 15 Gy is delivered to a portion of the clinical treatment volume (CTV) [21], and this dose cannot be delivered to the entire tumor margin without risking spinal cord injury unless a safe distance between the tumor and the spinal cord is created [22]. To safely deliver an appropriate radiation dose, patients with high-grade ESCC caused by radioresistant tumors undergo separation surgery [8, 23]. Historically, treatment responses for osseous tumors to systemic therapies were limited, and, thus, conventional external beam radiation therapy (cEBRT), often defined as 30 Gy in 10 fractions, was the mainstay of treatment for spinal tumors [24–26]. Based on the treatment response to cEBRT, tumors are classified as either radioresistant or radiosensitive. Moderately to highly radiosensitive tumors to cEBRT include most hematologic malignancies (i.e., lymphoma, multiple myeloma, and plasmacytoma), as well as selected solid tumors (i.e., breast, prostate, ovarian, and neuroendocrine carcinomas and seminoma) [13, 27]. However, most solid tumors are radioresistant to cEBRT including renal cell carcinoma (RCC); colon, non-small-cell lung (NSCLC), thyroid, and hepatocellular carcinoma; melanoma; and sarcoma [13, 25–27].

Recent data demonstrate that SSRS yields a clinical benefit regardless of tumor histology and volume, providing high local-control rates and durable symptomatic responses [28–30]. Evidence shows excellent outcomes with SSRS for traditionally radioresistant histologies such as renal cell carcinoma [31–33], sarcoma [34], and melanoma [35]. Hence, high-dose SSRS for radioresistant tumors overcomes the radioresistance seen in cEBRT. Still, the setting of high-grade spinal cord compression from a radioresistant tumor, as presented in the case described herein, requires separation surgery to allow delivery of a cytotoxic radiosurgery dose. This method of hybrid therapy (i.e., separation surgery-radiosurgery) has been previously shown to be safe and effective [18, 36]. Recently, this has also been shown to improve patients' health-related quality of life as analyzed using patient-reported outcome tools [1].

Conclusion

Patients with high-grade spinal cord or cauda equina compression, from a radioresistant tumor, require surgical decompression creating space for concomitant SSRS. SSRS overcomes traditional radioresistance when high enough doses are delivered and provides durable symptomatic relief and tumor control. Separation surgery is a posterolateral approach that provides circumferential spinal cord decompression and stabilization. Ventral separation through bilateral pedicle and joint removal is crucial. Patient and treatment selection are a multidisciplinary task and are facilitated by the NOMS framework.

References

1. Barzilai O, Amato MK, McLaughlin L, Reiner AS, Ogilvie SQ, Lis E, Yamada Y, Bilsky MH, Laufer I. Hybrid surgery-radiosurgery therapy for metastatic epidural spinal cord compression: a prospective evaluation using patientreported outcomes. Neurooncol Pract. 2018;5(2):104–13. https://doi.org/10.1093/nop/npx017. Epub 2017 Jul 22.
2. Cobb CA 3rd, Leavens ME, Eckles N. Indications for nonoperative treatment of spinal cord compression due to breast cancer. J Neurosurg. 1977;47(5):653–8.
3. Wong DA, Fornasier VL, MacNab I. Spinal metastases: the obvious, the occult, and the impostors. Spine (Phila Pa 1976). 1990;15(1):1–4.
4. Sciubba DM, Petteys RJ, Dekutoski MB, Fisher CG, Fehlings MG, Ondra SL, et al. Diagnosis and management of metastatic spine disease. A review. J Neurosurg Spine. 2010;13(1):94–108.
5. Klimo P Jr, Schmidt MH. Surgical management of spinal metastases. Oncologist. 2004;9(2):188–96.
6. North RB, LaRocca VR, Schwartz J, North CA, Zahurak M, Davis RF, et al. Surgical management of spinal metastases: analysis of prognostic factors during a 10-year experience. J Neurosurg Spine. 2005;2(5):564–73.
7. Greenlee RT, Murray T, Bolden S, Wingo PA. Cancer statistics, 2000. CA Cancer J Clin. 2000;50(1):7–33.
8. Laufer I, Rubin DG, Lis E, Cox BW, Stubblefield MD, Yamada Y, et al. The NOMS framework: approach to the treatment of spinal metastatic tumors. Oncologist. 2013;18(6):744–51.
9. Bilsky MH, Laufer I, Fourney DR, Groff M, Schmidt MH, Varga PP, et al. Reliability analysis of the epidural spinal cord compression scale. J Neurosurg Spine. 2010;13(3):324–8.
10. Fisher CG, DiPaola CP, Ryken TC, Bilsky MH, Shaffrey CI, Berven SH, et al. A novel classification system for spinal instability in neoplastic disease: an evidence-based approach and expert consensus from the Spine Oncology Study Group. Spine (Phila Pa 1976). 2010;35(22):E1221–9.
11. Nair S, Gobin YP, Leng LZ, Marcus JD, Bilsky M, Laufer I, et al. Preoperative embolization of hypervascular thoracic, lumbar, and sacral spinal column tumors: technique and outcomes from a single center. Interv Neuroradiol. 2013 Sep;19(3):377–85.
12. Costa F, Dorelli G, Ortolina A, Cardia A, Attuati L, Tomei M, et al. Computed tomography-based image-guided system in spinal surgery: state of the art through 10 years of experience. Neurosurgery. 2015;11(Suppl 2):59–67; discussion –8.
13. Rades D, Fehlauer F, Schulte R, Veninga T, Stalpers LJ, Basic H, et al. Prognostic factors for local control and survival after radiotherapy of metastatic spinal cord compression. J Clin Oncol. 2006;24(21):3388–93.
14. Amankulor NM, Xu R, Iorgulescu JB, Chapman T, Reiner AS, Riedel E, et al. The incidence and patterns of hardware failure after separation surgery in patients with spinal metastatic tumors. Spine J. 2014;14(9):1850–9.
15. Elder BD, Ishida W, Goodwin CR, Bydon A, Gokaslan ZL, Sciubba DM, et al. Bone graft options for spinal fusion following resection of spinal column tumors: systematic review and meta-analysis. Neurosurg Focus. 2017;42(1):E16.
16. Bilsky MH, Boland P, Lis E, Raizer JJ, Healey JH. Single-stage posterolateral transpedicle approach for spondylectomy, epidural decompression, and circumferential fusion of spinal metastases. Spine (Phila Pa 1976). 2000;25(17):2240–9; discussion 250.
17. Bilsky M, Smith M. Surgical approach to epidural spinal cord compression. Hematol Oncol Clin North Am. 2006;20(6):1307–17.

18. Laufer I, Iorgulescu JB, Chapman T, Lis E, Shi W, Zhang Z, et al. Local disease control for spinal metastases following "separation surgery" and adjuvant hypofractionated or high-dose single-fraction stereotactic radiosurgery: outcome analysis in 186 patients. J Neurosurg Spine. 2013;18(3):207–14.
19. Alongi F, Arcangeli S, Filippi AR, Ricardi U, Scorsetti M. Review and uses of stereotactic body radiation therapy for oligometastases. Oncologist. 2012;17(8):1100–7.
20. Chang BK, Timmerman RD. Stereotactic body radiation therapy: a comprehensive review. Am J Clin Oncol. 2007;30(6):637–44.
21. Lovelock DM, Zhang Z, Jackson A, Keam J, Bekelman J, Bilsky M, et al. Correlation of local failure with measures of dose insufficiency in the high-dose single-fraction treatment of bony metastases. Int J Radiat Oncol Biol Phys. 2010;77(4):1282–7.
22. Yamada Y, Bilsky MH, Lovelock DM, Venkatraman ES, Toner S, Johnson J, et al. High-dose, single-fraction image-guided intensity-modulated radiotherapy for metastatic spinal lesions. Int J Radiat Oncol Biol Phys. 2008;71(2):484–90.
23. Joaquim AF, Powers A, Laufer I, Bilsky MH. An update in the management of spinal metastases. Arq Neuropsiquiatr. 2015;73(9):795–802.
24. Gerszten PC, Mendel E, Yamada Y. Radiotherapy and radiosurgery for metastatic spine disease: what are the options, indications, and outcomes? Spine (Phila Pa 1976). 2009;34(22 Suppl):S78–92.
25. Mizumoto M, Harada H, Asakura H, Hashimoto T, Furutani K, Hashii H, et al. Radiotherapy for patients with metastases to the spinal column: a review of 603 patients at Shizuoka Cancer Center Hospital. Int J Radiat Oncol Biol Phys. 2011;79(1):208–13.
26. Maranzano E, Latini P. Effectiveness of radiation-therapy without surgery in metastatic spinal-cord compression – final results from a prospective trial. Int J Radiat Oncol. 1995;32(4):959–67.
27. Rades D, Fehlauer F, Stalpers LJ, Wildfang I, Zschenker O, Schild SE, et al. A prospective evaluation of two radiotherapy schedules with 10 versus 20 fractions for the treatment of metastatic spinal cord compression: final results of a multicenter study. Cancer. 2004;101(11):2687–92.
28. Yamada Y, Katsoulakis E, Laufer I, Lovelock M, Barzilai O, McLaughlin LA, et al. The impact of histology and delivered dose on local control of spinal metastases treated with stereotactic radiosurgery. Neurosurg Focus. 2017;42(1):E6.
29. Yamada Y, Lovelock DM, Yenice KM, Bilsky MH, Hunt MA, Zatcky J, et al. Multifractionated image-guided and stereotactic intensity-modulated radiotherapy of paraspinal tumors: a preliminary report. Int J Radiat Oncol Biol Phys. 2005;62(1):53–61.
30. Gerszten PC, Burton SA, Ozhasoglu C, Welch WC. Radiosurgery for spinal metastases: clinical experience in 500 cases from a single institution. Spine (Phila Pa 1976). 2007;32(2):193–9.
31. Ghia AJ, Chang EL, Bishop AJ, Pan HY, Boehling NS, Amini B, et al. Single-fraction versus multi-fraction spinal stereotactic radiosurgery for spinal metastases from renal cell carcinoma: secondary analysis of phase I/II trials. J Neurosurg Spine. 2016;24(5):829–36.
32. Gerszten PC, Burton SA, Ozhasoglu C, Vogel WJ, Welch WC, Baar J, et al. Stereotactic radiosurgery for spinal metastases from renal cell carcinoma. J Neurosurg Spine. 2005;3(4):288–95.
33. Zelefsky MJ, Greco C, Motzer R, Magsanoc JM, Pei X, Lovelock M, et al. Tumor control outcomes after hypofractionated and single-dose stereotactic image-guided intensity-modulated radiotherapy for extracranial metastases from renal cell carcinoma. Int J Radiat Oncol Biol Phys. 2012;82(5):1744–8.
34. Chang UK, Cho WI, Lee DH, Kim MS, Cho CK, Lee SY, et al. Stereotactic radiosurgery for primary and metastatic sarcomas involving the spine. J Neuro-Oncol. 2012;107(3):551–7.
35. Gerszten PC, Burton SA, Quinn AE, Agarwala SS, Kirkwood JM. Radiosurgery for the treatment of spinal melanoma metastases. Stereotact Funct Neurosurg. 2005;83(5–6):213–21.
36. Moulding HD, Elder JB, Lis E, Lovelock DM, Zhang Z, Yamada Y, et al. Local disease control after decompressive surgery and adjuvant high-dose single-fraction radiosurgery for spine metastases. J Neurosurg Spine. 2010;13(1):87–93.
37. Nasser R, Nakhla J, Echt M, et al. Minimally invasive separation surgery with intraoperative stereotactic guidance: a feasibility study. World Neurosurg. 2018;109:68–76.

Minimally Invasive Stabilization Alone (Thoracic and Lumbar): Cement Augmentation

18

Zoe Zhang, Ahmed Mohyeldin, Ulas Yener, Eric Bourekas, and Ehud Mendel

Introduction

Seventy percent of patients with cancer develop metastatic disease, and spinal involvement occurs in up to 40% of these patients. The majority of metastases occur in the thoracic and lumbar spine [1–3]. The indications of minimally invasive surgery include mechanical instability, refractory pain, and neurologic deficits.

In this chapter, we discuss minimally invasive surgical techniques for lumbar and thoracic spinal stabilization. After describing the general methods, each application will be illustrated by a representative case. Compared with traditional open surgery, in selective cases, minimally invasive techniques have a smaller blood loss, shorter hospital stay, faster functional recovery, and fewer complications. Especially for the fragile patients with spine metastasis, the reduction in operative time and surgical trauma is critical.

In recent years, tremendous improvements have been made for the minimally invasive surgeries that include the following: (a) better percutaneous surgical tools for approach and exposure and improved visualization through better microscopes and endoscopes; (b) improved implant devices, instrumentation, and augmentative materials; and (c) improved intraoperative image guidance and robot-assisted modalities. With these advancements and the cumulative experience, minimally invasive surgical technologies are valuable tools for treating patients with spinal tumors.

Patient Selection

Preoperative laboratory and imaging tests need to be studied to assess the tumor spread by Tomita scoring system [4]. Also recommended is consideration of the Tokuhashi or neoplastic (spinal instability neoplastic score [SINS]) scores, depending on the tumor type, degree of spinal instability, and metastatic and functional status [5, 6]. By these scoring systems, the overall condition of a patient, tumor growth rate, and location of the tumor may help the surgeon make treatment decisions and anticipate the prognosis of the patient. Cement augmentation is the least invasive procedure, suitable for treating patients with painful pathologic fractures secondary to

Z. Zhang · A. Mohyeldin · U. Yener
Ohio State University Medical Center, Department of Neurosurgery, Columbus, OH, USA

E. Bourekas
Ohio State University Wexner Medical Center, Department of Radiology, Columbus, OH, USA

E. Mendel (✉)
The Ohio State Neurological Society, Columbus, OH, USA

OSU Spine Research Institute, Columbus, OH, USA

Wexner Medical Center at The Ohio State University/ The Arthur James Cancer Hospital, Columbus, OH, USA
e-mail: ehud.mendel@osumc.edu

D. M. Sciubba (ed.), *Spinal Tumor Surgery*, https://doi.org/10.1007/978-3-319-98422-3_18

spinal metastases, especially those who cannot tolerate open surgery or who may have poor bone quality for traditional instrumentation. However, it may not be appropriate for use in tumors that mainly involve the pedicle and posterior elements. Percutaneous pedicle screw fixation alone or its combination with vertebral augmentation yields more versatile treatments in patients with significant destabilization who will not tolerate extensive open surgical approaches [7].

Minimally Invasive Methods and Case Studies

Cement Augmentation

Cement augmentation is a key technique in the minimally invasive treatment of painful spinal metastatic fractures (Figs. 18.1 and 18.2). It creates internal stabilization in the affected vertebra [8]. Bone cement injection into spine tumors is an effective way to relieve severe pain by mechanical stabilization, destruction of the sensitive nerves, and induction of necrosis of tumor cells [9]. Typically cement augmentation such as kyphoplasty or vertebroplasty is suitable for patients with painful pathologic fractures without cord compression and primary diseases of the bone such as multiple myeloma [10].

The most common material used is polymethylmethacrylate (PMMA); brand names include Kyphon (Medronic), SpinePlex (Stryker), AVAmax (Care Fusion), and Osseoperm (Aegis Spine). PMMA is freshly prepared in liquid form for injection through a needle in the target. After solidification, the cement supports the bone structurally and prevents mechanical pain by stabilizing the fracture fragments. The approach is generally transpedicular (unilateral or bilateral) but may be extrapedicular as well. Cement extrusion into the spinal canal with neurologic compromise is the most feared and immediate risk; however, with slow injection under continuous careful imaging (fluoroscopy), this risk can be minimized. Other risks include infection, pulmonary embolism, bleeding, rib fractures, or adjacent vertebral fractures.

PMMA cement augmentation is one of the least invasive procedures capable of quickly supporting and stabilizing a defect. However, it has been found that over time, with bone reconstruction, osteoclasts appear at the cement-bone interface, resulting in bone loss. Therefore, PMMA cement augmentation may not be a long-term solution. Improvement in the bone cement material is critical in improving its efficacy and duration [11].

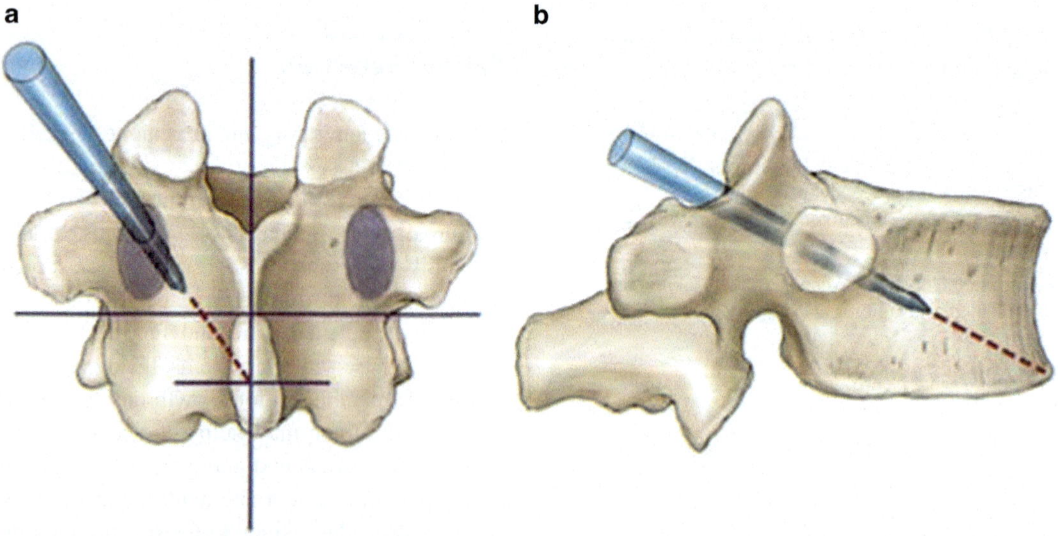

Fig. 18.1 (**a**, **b**) Artist illustration of needle trajectory for vertebroplasty and kyphoplasty. (Reprinted with permission from Fourney et al. [19])

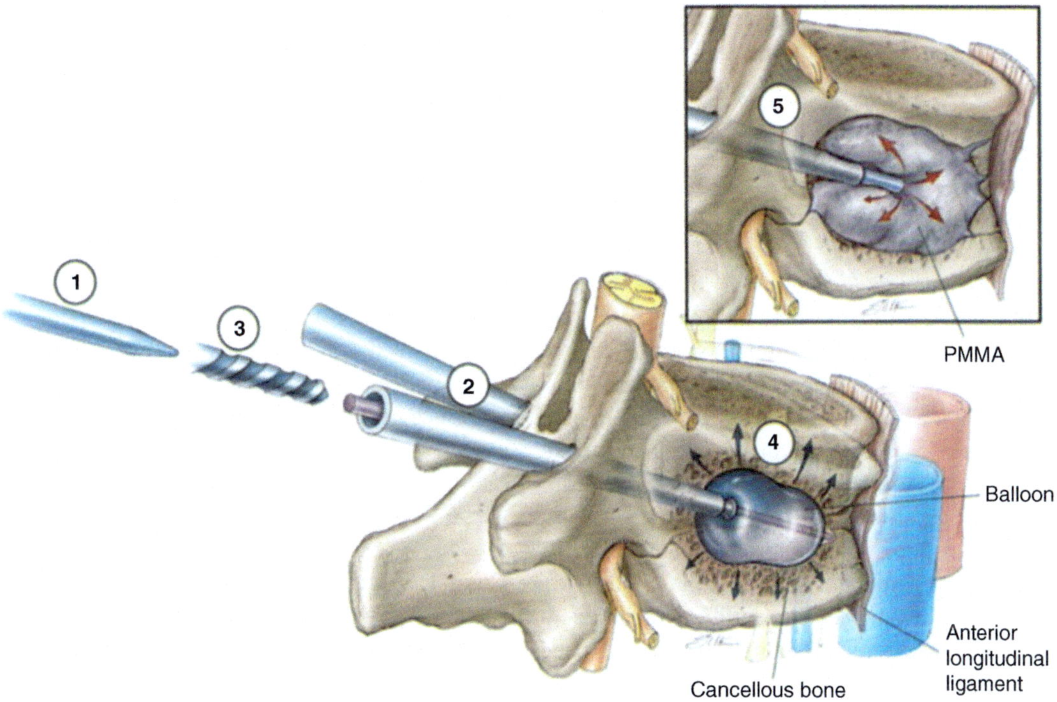

Fig. 18.2 Artist illustration of kyphoplasty technique. (Reprinted with permission from Fourney et al. [19])

Percutaneous Screws and Fixation Systems

In patients with metastatic disease involving the posterior elements, the use of cement augmentation alone may not be adequate. Extensive open surgery may similarly not be suitable in light of limited life expectancy. The dilemma of spinal stabilization in this situation can be solved by using pedicle screw fixation in a minimally invasive fashion followed by cement augmentation. The application of rigid instrumentation at healthy vertebrae above and below to bridge the diseased segment has proven to be more lasting than cement augmentation alone. Instrumentation can also be used to realign the spine in addition to stabilizing it. There are many brand names in the market such as Viper® Synthes, ES2 Spinal System, Vertelink's KOBRA, MIS posterior fixation systems, and many more; the principle fixation mechanism of all of them is the same.

Using muscle dilation rather than electrocautery dissection, trauma and blood loss are reduced. Because the incisions are small, bony landmarks are not exposed and the angulation and placement of the screw are dependent on fluoroscopic guidance. Once the pedicle screws are placed, rods are passed through small stab incisions and secured with cap screws via towers. These towers also allow reduction and correction of deformity. However, because there is no exposure, arthrodesis cannot be performed and the rates of fusion are decreased.

Lumbar spine fusions have long been used for the treatment of degenerative disorders. A posterolateral instrumentation is supplemented by further anterior support in the form of transforaminal lumbar interbody fusion (TLIF), posterior lumbar interbody fusion (PLIF), lateral lumbar interbody fusion (LLIF), anterior lumbar interbody fusion (ALIF), and axial lumbar interbody fusion (AxiaLIF). With advances in technology, almost all of these can be performed in minimally invasive ways. PLIF and TLIF are the common techniques performed in the thoracic and lumbar regions [12]. TLIFs may be more advantageous than PLIFs due to unilateral approach and decreased nerve root and dural retraction. ALIFs can be performed from a laparoscopic transperitoneal approach, mini-open retroperitoneal approach, or endoscopic lateral retroperitoneal approach.

Combination Techniques

Use of cement augmentation in conjunction with percutaneous instrumentation can be accomplished in a number of different ways. A cement augmentation of a vertebral body can be done at the level of a pathologic fracture. If needed, pedicle screws can be placed in a percutaneous fashion, adding posterior stabilization to the anterior stabilization afforded by the cement.

Due to poor bone quality in many patients with spine tumors, complications of fixation include screw loosening, pullout, or adjacent fractures. Cement augmentation can be used concurrently with pedicle screw fixation to decrease these risks by reducing induced bone stress [13, 14].

The combination of percutaneous pedicle screw fixation and cement augmentation is perhaps the optimal option in patients with significant neoplastic destabilization who will not tolerate more extensive and open surgical approaches [15, 16].

Associated Procedures

Treatment of patients with spine tumors is rarely a matter of stabilization alone. Tumor resection can identify the source of malignancy and molecular markers of the tumor to support ongoing radiation therapy, chemotherapy, or laser ablation [17]. Spinal cord decompression is another goal of surgery to reverse, halt, or prevent neurological deficits [18]. Prior to procedures of spine stabilization by cement augmentation and instrumented fusion, the need for tumor resection and spinal cord decompression must be determined. The use of minimally invasive transpedicular vertebrectomies or laminectomies can be approached with unique retractors and dilating systems such as METRx (Medtronic), Pipeline/Spotlight (DePuy), Luxor (Stryker), Atavi (Zimmer), MaXcess (NuVasive), or MIRA (Synthes). There are slight differences in shape and size; some come with illumination or other additional attachments, but the main function of exposure is the same: after the retractor is inserted through the fascial incision toward the affected target, it is expanded sequentially until there is appropriate exposure for dissection, decompression, and other types of tissue manipulation. Though the use of minimally invasive procedures to remove the tumor is not the theme of this chapter, it is a useful tool in spine stabilization.

Case Presentations

Case 1: Vertebroplasty for Compression Fractures in the Setting of Multiple Myeloma

This is a 68-year-old male with a history of multiple myeloma with good disease control who presents with a T11 compression fracture and severe back pain. MRI revealed no cord compression, and the CT scan demonstrated poor bone density (thoracic CT scan with compression fracture at T11, Fig. 18.3a). The patient complained of mechanical back pain, worse with standing and not relieved by oral pain medication. The patient was initially managed with a vertebroplasty with good pain control (thoracic x-ray after vertebroplasty at T11, Fig. 18.3b). Within months, the patient developed two new fractures at L1 and L2 (thoracic CT scan with compression fractures at L1 and L2, Fig. 18.3c), and MRI revealed no thecal sac compression. The nature of the pain was similar in character and localized to the upper lumbar region. The patient was managed with a two-level vertebroplasty with excellent pain control (thoracic x-ray after vertebroplasty at L1 and L2, Fig. 18.3d). It is critical during intraoperative planning that adequate anteroposterior (AP) and lateral images of the spine and level of interest are obtained (intraoperative x-ray of vertebral body visualization, Fig. 18.4a). The vertebral body is localized, and under fluoroscopic guidance, an 11-gauge

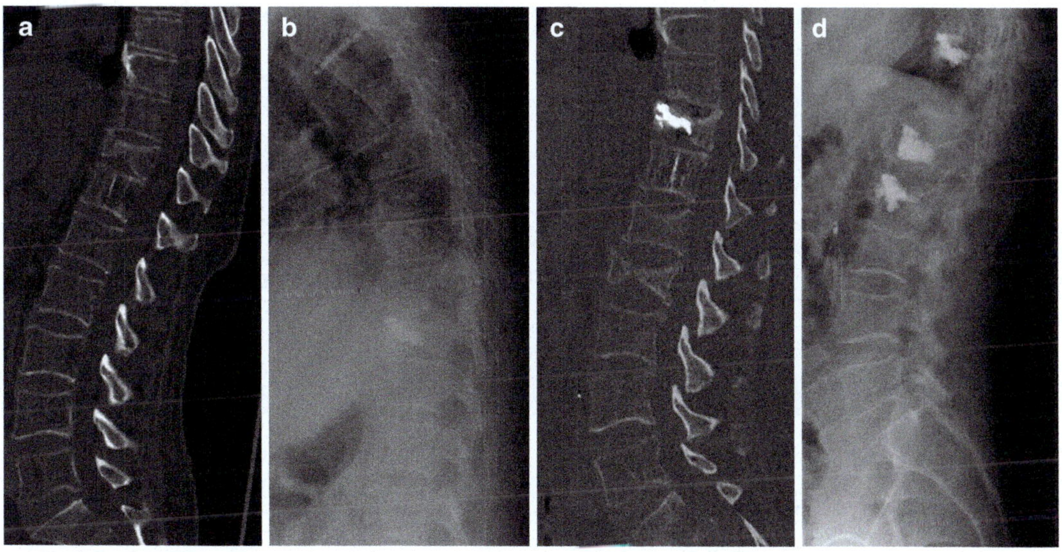

Fig. 18.3 A 68-year-old male with a history of multiple myeloma and a T11 compression fracture and severe back pain. Displayed are thoracic CT scans (**a** and **c**) and thoracic x-rays (**b** and **d**). Refer to Case 1

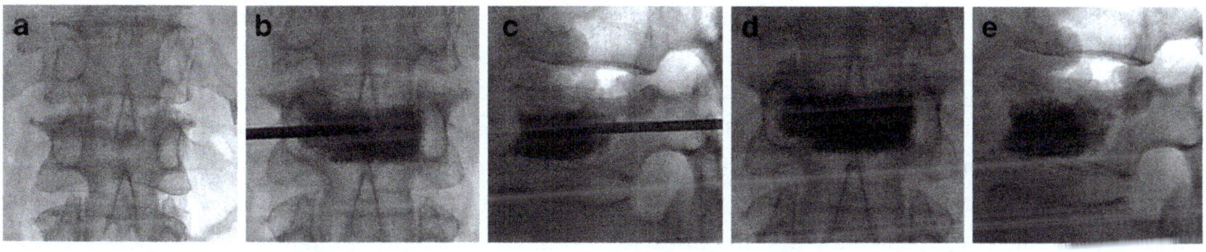

Fig. 18.4 (**a–e**) Intraoperative x-rays of vertebral body visualization in a 68-year-old male with a history of multiple myeloma and a T11 compression fracture undergoing vertebroplasty. Refer to Case 1

12 cm needle is introduced and advanced through the pedicle into the anterior aspect of the vertebral body with the needle tip crossing the midline to the right (intraoperative x-ray of vertebral body visualization and cement filling Fig. 18.4b–e). This allows for safe and symmetric filling of the vertebral body with a unipedicular approach.

Case 2: Fenestrated Screw Placement with Cement Augmentation for Osteopenic Bone in the Setting of Spine Metastasis

This is a 61-year-old male who presented with severe back pain and radicular pain shooting across his chest. The MRI revealed a suspected carcinoma which was biopsied and consistent with a squamous cell carcinoma of lung origin. The MRI showed severe compression of the spinal cord, both of the canal and of the nerve roots. The CT scan demonstrated severe osteopenia (MRI thoracic spine with contrast Fig. 18.5a, b). The patient was managed surgically, and a complete pediculectomy and partial vertebrectomy at T9 with 30% removal of the T9 vertebral body were performed with adequate decompression of the spinal cord. To perform the posterior pedicle screw fixation in the setting of osteopenic bone from T6 to T11, we relied on utilizing cannulated fenestrated and non-cannulated screws for our construct (preoperative thoracic CT scan and postoperative thoracic CT, Fig. 18.5c–e). Fenestrated screw technology has provided a controlled mechanism to deliver cement to the vertebral body to provide column support and

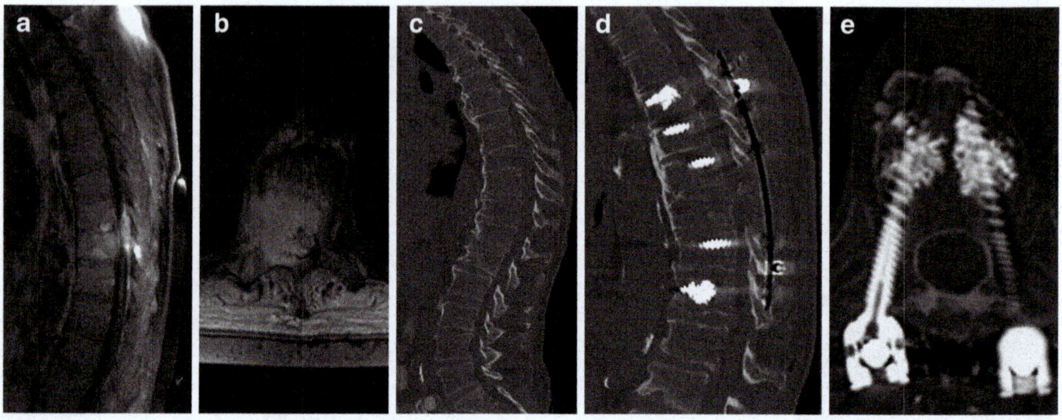

Fig. 18.5 A 61-year-old male who presented with severe back pain and radicular pain shooting across his chest (**a**, **b**, **c**). MRI of the thoracic spine with contrast and preoperative CT scan of the thoracic spine demonstrating severe osteopenia (**d**, **e**). Postoperative CT scans demonstrating cement augmentation of the construct. Refer to Case 2

increase pullout strength of screws with weak bone purchase. Intraoperative vertebroplasty with cement injected through the cannulated screws at T6 and T11 for purpose of augmenting the proximal and distal end of the construct was performed. It is important, during cement delivery, that this be performed under live fluoroscopy to avoid any retrograde injection of cement toward the canal and/or into the nerve root foramina (intraoperative surgical setup and injection of cement using cannulated screws, Fig. 18.6a, and live fluoroscopy images of sequential cement injection, Fig. 18.6b–d).

Case 3: Cement Augmentation with Pedicle Screws to Correct Kyphotic Deformity in the Setting of Spine Cancer

This is a 73-year-old female who was diagnosed with lung cancer with metastatic disease of the posterior elements of the C7 vertebrae. She underwent previous laminectomy with cervicothoracic fixation from C4 to T3 (cervical x-ray, Fig. 18.7a). She had done well for a while but then developed acute onset of upper back pain. X-ray films (cervical thoracic x-ray, Fig. 18.7b) and a CT scan (cervical thoracic CT, Fig. 18.8a) revealed hardware failure at the distal portion of the construct with a pathologic fracture of the T3 vertebra and severe kyphotic deformity. To revise this, a posterior pedicle screw fixation was performed from T4 to T9 utilizing fenestrated screws, and the instrumentation system was connected to the previous rod for a total fixation construct from C4 to T9. Intraoperative vertebroplasty was performed through cannulated fenestrated screws placed at the T9 vertebral body for the purpose of cement augmenting the screws under live fluoroscopic guidance (intraoperative thoracic x-ray with cement augmentation at the distal construct, Fig. 18.8b). This allowed for open reduction and internal fixation and correction of severe spinal deformity centered at the T3 vertebral body (cervical thoracic CT, Fig. 18.8c). Angulation of the kyphotic deformity was dramatically improved with preservation of neurological function.

Case 4: Vertebrectomy and Reconstruction of the Vertebral Column with Cement Augmentation

This is a 40-year-old female with a history of breast carcinoma who presented with several weeks' history of severe mid-thoracic back pain with a radicular component across her chest. A CT scan (thoracic CT, Fig. 18.9a) and MRI (thoracic MRI, Fig. 18.9b) ultimately revealed severe pathologic fracture with kyphosis and

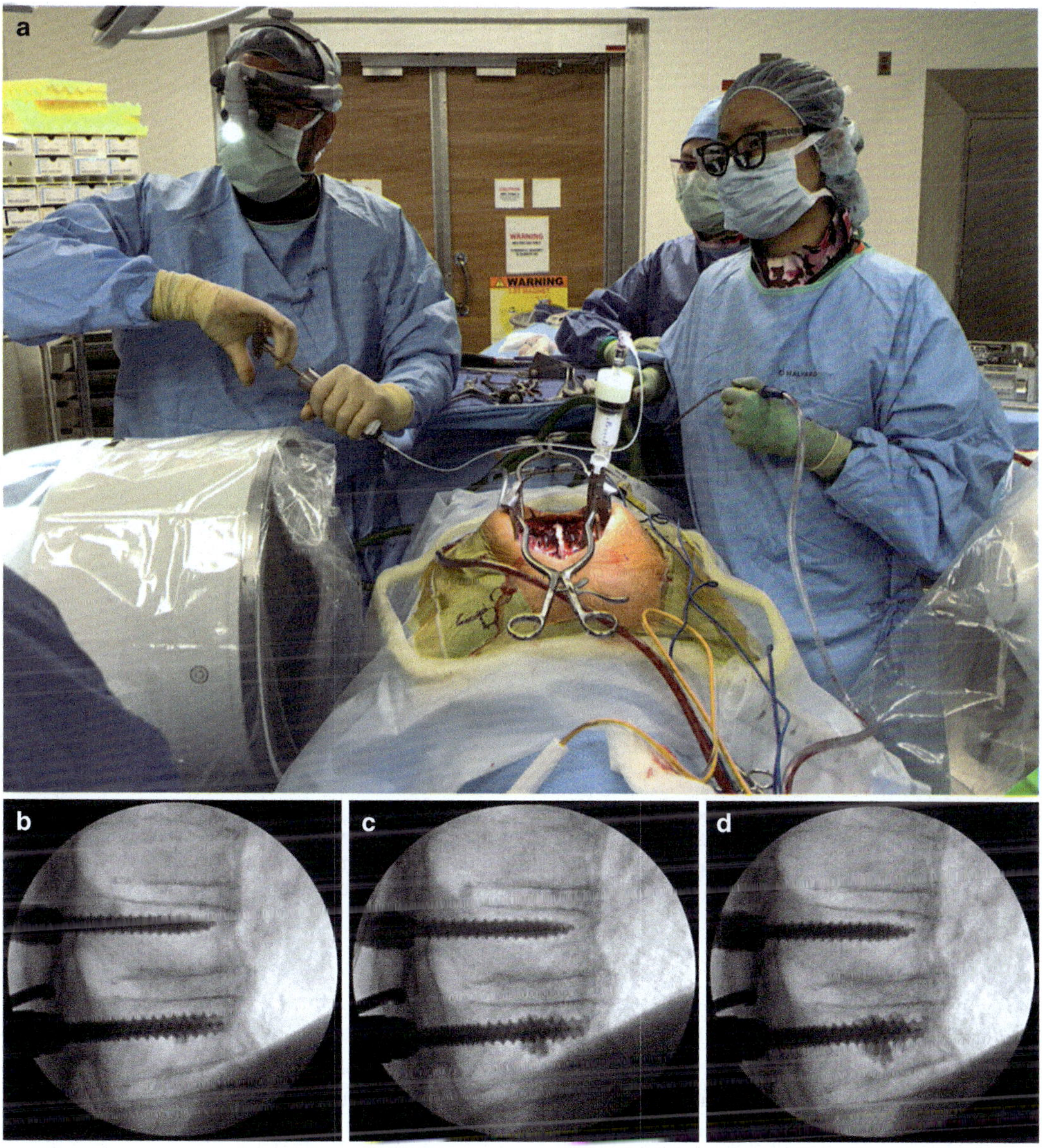

Fig. 18.6 (**a**) Intraoperative surgical setup and injection of cement using cannulated screws. (**b–d**) Live fluoroscopy images of sequential cement injection. Refer to Case 2

severe cord compression at T9 from suspected metastatic disease. The imaging revealed severe retropulsion anteriorly and posteriorly with extensive epidural involvement along the ventral and dorsal aspect of the thecal sac, significantly narrowing the canal and causing cord compression with abnormal signal change within the spinal cord. The patient underwent a transpedicular T9 vertebrectomy with removal of approximately 80% of the T9 vertebral body and decompression of the spinal cord and posterior pedicle screw fixation from T6 to T12 (thoracic CT, Fig. 18.9c, and thoracic XR, Fig. 18.9d). Reconstruction of the anterior column at T9 was done utilizing polymethylmethacrylate cement placed at T9 between the T8 and the T10 vertebral bodies for the purpose of anterior column support.

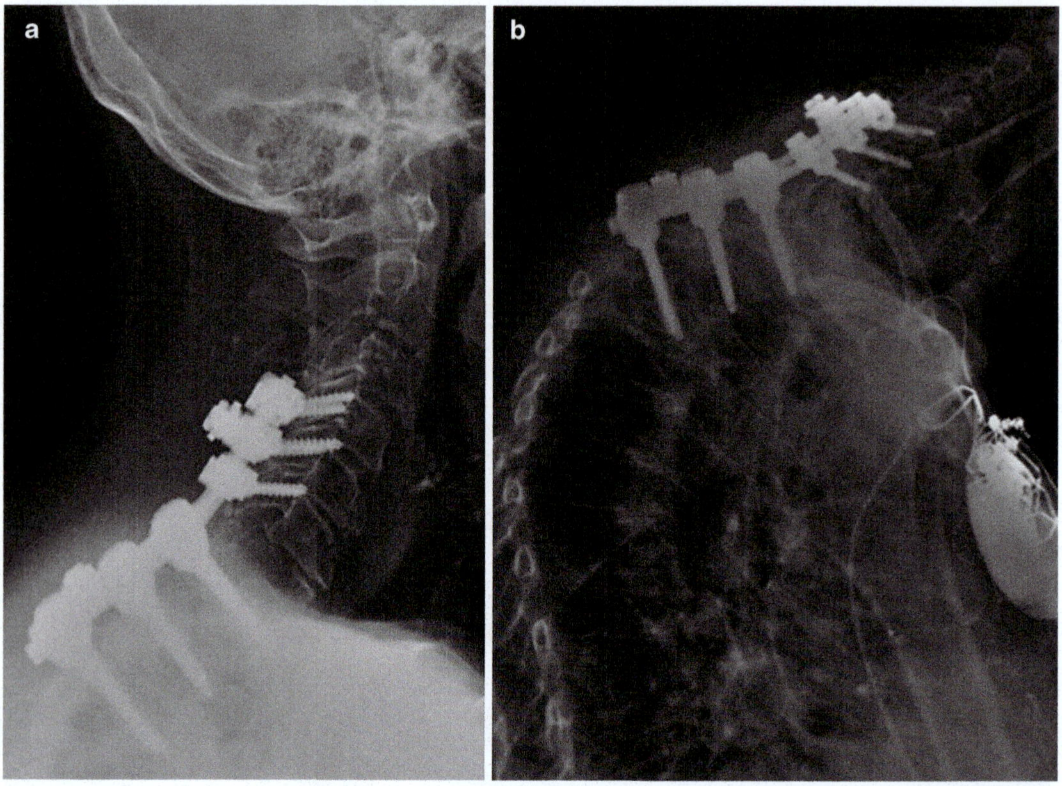

Fig. 18.7 (**a**, **b**) A 73-year-old female who was diagnosed with lung cancer with metastatic disease of the posterior elements of the C7 vertebrae. She underwent previous laminectomy with cervicothoracic fixation from C4 to T3. Displayed are x-ray images demonstrating revealed hardware failure at the distal portion of the construct with a pathologic fracture of the T3 vertebra and severe kyphotic deformity. Refer to Case 3

Discussion and Conclusion

In patients with primary or metastatic spine cancer, the tumor cells infiltrate into the vertebral body, causing displacement and biological pain. It can also cause pathologic fractures leading to instability and/or refractory pain. The primary surgical goal for this group of patients is improvement of their pain as well as preservation of neurologic function for the best quality of life. Non-surgical methods include opioids, steroids, local nerve blocks, and bracing.

In the past decade, minimally invasive techniques have become increasingly popular in treating metastatic spine disease in patients who either are poor candidates for open surgery or have a limited life expectancy. These minor surgical procedures coupled with low morbidity become an optimal treatment option that may benefit a patient's quality of life while maintaining cost-effectiveness in surgery and postoperative cares. The selection of specific procedure depends on the condition of the patient, life expectancy, bone quality, instability or deformity, degree of neural compression, instrumentation availability, and surgeon preference.

A cement augmentation procedure such as a vertebroplasty or kyphoplasty (in the absence of neural compression) could be considered to provide relief from intractable pain even in the most advanced conditions. Cement alone is not usually an effective treatment for unstable spinal metastases especially with extension into the posterior elements. The use of concurrent minimally

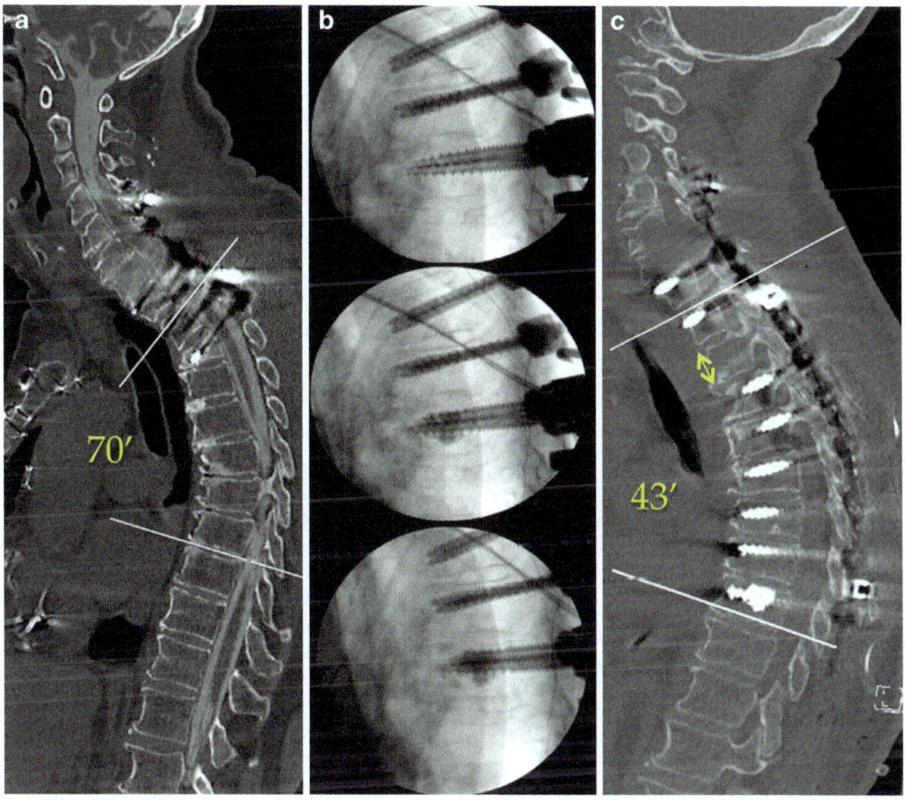

Fig. 18.8 A 73-year-old female who was diagnosed with lung cancer with metastatic disease of the posterior elements of the C7 vertebrae. She underwent previous laminectomy with cervicothoracic fixation from C4 to T3 with a subsequent pathologic fracture of the T3 vertebra and a severe kyphotic deformity. Displayed are (**a**) preoperative CT scans; (**b**) intraoperative x-ray images during cement augmentation; and (**c**) postoperative scans. Refer to Case 3

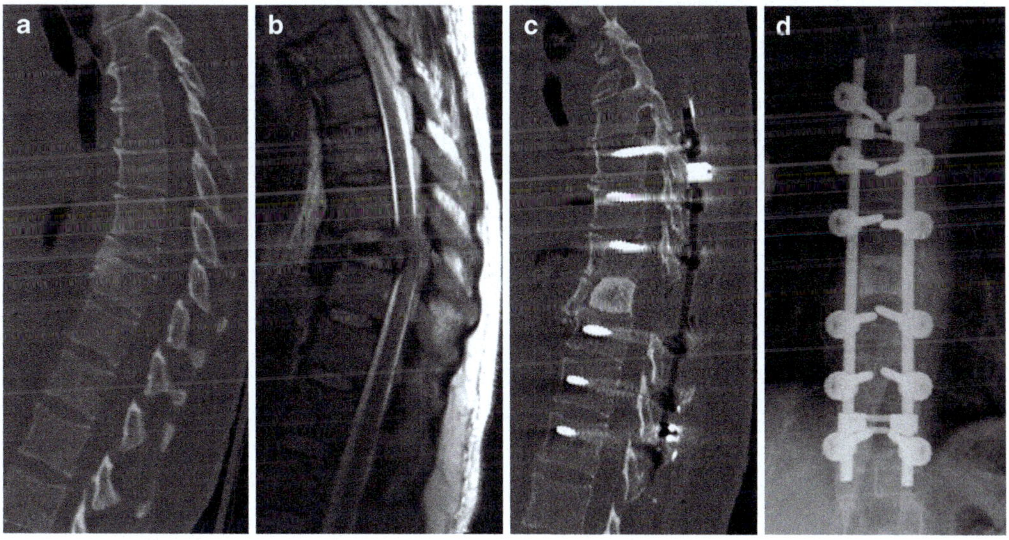

Fig. 18.9 A 40-year-old female with a history of breast carcinoma who presented with several weeks' history of severe mid-thoracic back pain with a radicular component across her chest. Displayed is preoperative MRI (**a**) and CT (**b**) of thoracic spine demonstrating severe pathologic fracture with kyphosis and severe cord compression at T9. Also displayed are postoperative CT scans and x-rays (**c**, **d**) of the thoracic spine. Refer to Case 4

invasive instrumentation techniques may be considered. Cement-augmented screws also provide increased pullout strength in osteoporotic bone with tumor burden.

With new developments in material and accuracy of computer navigation along with stringent surgical training, minimally invasive surgical techniques have proved effective in the field of spine tumor management. Though open surgeries are still dominating the field, minimally invasive techniques offer a viable alternative for this patient population.

Conflict of Interest We declare no conflict of interest.

References

1. Binning MJ, Gottfried ON, Klimo P Jr, Schmidt MH. Minimally invasive treatments for metastatic tumors of the spine. Neurosurg Clin N Am. 2004;15:459–65.
2. Gerszten PC, Welch WC. Current surgical management of metastatic spinal disease. Oncology (Williston Park). 2000;14:1013–24.
3. Sciubba DM, Petteys RJ, Dekutoski MB, Fisher CG, Fehlings MG, Ondra SL, et al. Diagnosis and management of metastatic spine disease. A review. J Neurosurg Spine. 2010;13:94–108.
4. Murakami H, Kawahara N, Demura S, Kato S, Yoshioka K, Tomita K. Total en bloc spondylectomy for lung cancer metastasis to the spine. J Neurosurg Spine. 2010;13:414–7.
5. Tokuhashi Y, Matsuzaki H, Oda H, Oshima M, Ryu J. A revised scoring system for preoperative evaluation of metastatic spine tumor prognosis. Spine (Phila Pa 1976). 2005;30:2186–91.
6. Fourney DR, Frangou EM, Ryken TC, Dipaola CP, Shaffrey CI, Berven SH, et al. Spinal instability neoplastic score: an analysis of reliability and validity from the spine oncology study group. J Clin Oncol. 2011;29:3072–7.
7. Kim CH, Chung CK, Sohn S, Lee S, Park SB. Less invasive palliative surgery for spinal metastases. J Surg Oncol. 2013;108:499–503.
8. Bartolozzi B, Nozzoli C, Pandolfo C, Antonioli E, Guizzardi G, Morichi R, et al. Percutaneous vertebroplasty and kyphoplasty in patients with multiple myeloma. Eur J Haematol. 2006;76:180–1.
9. Ha KY, Min CK, Seo JY, Kim YH, Ahn JH, Hyun NM, et al. Bone cement augmentation procedures for spinal pathologic fractures by multiple myeloma. J Korean Med Sci. 2015;30:88–94.
10. Tosi P. Diagnosis and treatment of bone disease in multiple myeloma: spotlight on spinal involvement. Scientifica (Cairo). 2013;2013:104546.
11. Quan R, Ni Y, Zhang L, Xu J, Zheng X, Yang D. Short- and long-term effects of vertebroplastic bone cement on cancellous bone. J Mech Behav Biomed Mater. 2014;35:102–10.
12. Tatsui CE, Belsuzarri TA, Oro M, Rhines LD, Li J, Ghia AJ, et al. Percutaneous surgery for treatment of epidural spinal cord compression and spinal instability: technical note. Neurosurg Focus. 2016;41:E2.
13. Fan HT, Zhang RJ, Shen CL, Dong FL, Li Y, Song PW, et al. The biomechanical properties of pedicle screw fixation combined with trajectory bone cement augmentation in osteoporotic vertebrae. Clin Spine Surg. 2016;29(2):78–85. https://doi.org/10.1097/BSD.0b013e3182a14870.
14. Moussazadeh N, Rubin DG, McLaughlin L, Lis E, Bilsky MH, Laufer I. Short-segment percutaneous pedicle screw fixation with cement augmentation for tumor-induced spinal instability. Spine J. 2015;15:1609–17.
15. Kim P, Kim SW. Bone cement-augmented percutaneous screw fixation for malignant spinal metastases: is it feasible? J Korean Neurosurg Soc. 2017;60:189–94.
16. Hariri O, Takayanagi A, Miulli DE, Siddiqi J, Vrionis F. Minimally invasive surgical techniques for management of painful metastatic and primary spinal tumors. Cureus. 2017;9:e1114.
17. Abi LG, Abi JS. Role of surgery in the management of vertebral metastases. General revue. Cancer Radiother. 2016;20:484–92.
18. Hamad A, Vachtsevanos L, Cattell A, Ockendon M, Balain B. Minimally invasive spinal surgery for the management of symptomatic spinal metastasis. Br J Neurosurg. 2017:1–5.
19. Fourney DR, et al. Percutaneous vertebroplasty and kyphoplasty for painful vertebral body fractures in cancer patients. J Neurosurg. 2003;98(1 suppl):21–30.

19 Percutaneous Stabilization

Ori Barzilai, Mark H. Bilsky, and Ilya Laufer

Introduction

Treatment goals for metastatic spine disease include restoration or preservation of neurologic function and spinal column stability, pain relief, and local tumor control. Therapies are directed toward improvement of patients' quality of life and are, in general, of palliative nature. With the aging overall population, improved diagnostics, and improved survivals of cancer patients due to modern cancer treatments, the number of people requiring treatment for spinal metastatic tumors continues to increase. In-depth knowledge of surgical, radiotherapy, and systemic therapy options aids in tailoring the optimal treatment strategy. Experience with minimally invasive spine techniques in the degenerative and deformity settings has facilitated the implementation of these techniques into cancer care. The current chapter focuses on percutaneous stabilization of pathological fractures from diagnosis, surgical decision-making, and workup to technical nuances.

O. Barzilai
Memorial Sloan Kettering Cancer Center, Department of Neurosurgery, New York, NY, USA

M. H. Bilsky · I. Laufer (✉)
Memorial Sloan Kettering Cancer Center, Department of Neurosurgery, New York, NY, USA

Department of Neurological Surgery, Weill Cornell Medical College, New York, NY, USA
e-mail: lauferi@mskcc.org

Case Presentation

A 34-year-old female patient presented with worsening back and right hip pain. She was recently diagnosed with metastatic intraductal breast carcinoma (ER+, HER2+). This was diagnosed with breast FNA and subsequent right pelvic biopsy. She had known radiological evidence of lesions in her spine, right hip, and lymph nodes. At presentation she was treated with THP (THP: Docetaxel, Trastuzumab and Pertuzumab) and was planned for radiation treatment to T9 and to the right hip.

She presented with progressive, intractable back pain along with abdominal pain, nausea, and vomiting. Back pain had been present for several months but had progressively worsened with increased pain medication requirement. Further, the pain had worsened 2 days prior to presentation since she had been nauseated and unable to swallow oral pain medications. She also endorsed abdominal pain; however, this had been present for months, even before her diagnosis of cancer. Her back pain increased with movement and posture changes. She had extreme difficulty lying flat in bed. She denied noticing weakness of her arms or legs, gait disturbances, numbness or tingling in her legs, and bowel or bladder dysfunction.

D. M. Sciubba (ed.), *Spinal Tumor Surgery*, https://doi.org/10.1007/978-3-319-98422-3_19

Diagnostic Workup

Neurological exam at presentation was remarkable for mild bilateral lower-limb hyperreflexia but otherwise neurologically intact. Laboratory findings were within normal limits.

Diagnostic imaging exams play key roles in the workup evaluation of oncological patients. Since metastases may affect any organ, imaging techniques most commonly involve bone scintigraphy (frequently ordered by medical oncologists and is useful as a reference but has significant diagnostic limitations), computed tomography (CT), and magnetic resonance imaging (MRI). CT imaging of the chest, abdomen, and pelvis or whole-body PET imaging is often used to evaluate the systemic tumor burden. MRI provides the greatest sensitivity for detection of osseous metastases of the spine, with equivalent specificity when compared to multi-detector CT. CT provides valuable information about the bony structure and may be useful in evaluation of fractures. Upon diagnosis of a spinal lesion, it is important to obtain radiologic images of the *whole spine*, preferably an MRI scan with contrast enhancement. Many patients will present with multiple spinal lesions. Early diagnosis facilitates timely treatment or close monitoring of these often asymptomatic lesions.

A total spine MRI with contrast enhancement was performed and demonstrated diffuse metastatic infiltration of T9 with increased collapse deformity (Fig. 19.1). Ventral and right lateral epidural disease causes cord compression (epidural spinal cord compression [1] (ESCC) grade 2). Additionally noted on this scan was increased metastatic infiltration of T12 and L4 with minor ventral epidural disease at both levels.

Treatment Approach

The goals of treatment for patients with spinal metastases are palliative and include neurological functional preservation, maintenance of spinal stability, palliation of pain, and durable local tumor control. There are several treatment options including surgery, radiation therapy (RT), systemic therapy, or combinations of these modalities. Recent advancements in cancer care such as the evolution of radiosurgery and the emergence of a myriad biologic agents complicate treatment paradigms. Optimally, the approach to spine cancer patients is multidisciplinary comprising of surgeons, radiation oncologists, medical oncologists, interventional radiologists, and pain specialists.

NOMS is a decision-making framework designed to facilitate and guide therapeutic decisions for patients with spinal metastases [2]. It provides a guide for integration of important clinical data and as such is not bound to any particular treatment or technology. NOMS consists of four main considerations: Neurologic, Oncologic, Mechanical, and Systemic. The Neurologic and Oncologic considerations are often combined in order to determine whether or not the patient requires surgical intervention for spinal cord or nerve root decompression. This decision is made based on the neurological examination and degree of spinal cord compression as well as on the predicted tumor sensitivity to the current available treatments [3, 4]. Historically, the best available treatment modality for local control of spinal metastases was external beam radiation therapy, yet with the improvement in radiosurgical techniques the concept of radiosensitivity is being challenged [5]. The mechanical consideration serves as an independent indication for intervention, since spinal instability represents a mechanical problem requiring mechanical repair, such as cement augmentation or instrumented stabilization. In order to ease the assessment of mechanical stability and to unify reporting, the SOSG developed a scoring system: the Spinal Instability Neoplastic Score (SINS) [6]. SINS accounts for six parameters: location, pain, alignment, lesion character (i.e., lytic vs. blastic), vertebral body collapse, and posterior element involvement (Table 19.1). The systemic consideration accounts for the patient's estimated survival, extent of overall metastatic tumor burden, and medical comorbidities in order to determine whether they can tolerate the proposed treatment plan.

In summary, the current patient presented with (*N*) mild hyperreflexia, ESCC grade 2 compression; (*O*) metastatic breast cancer, a radiosensitive solid malignancy [7], with local failure

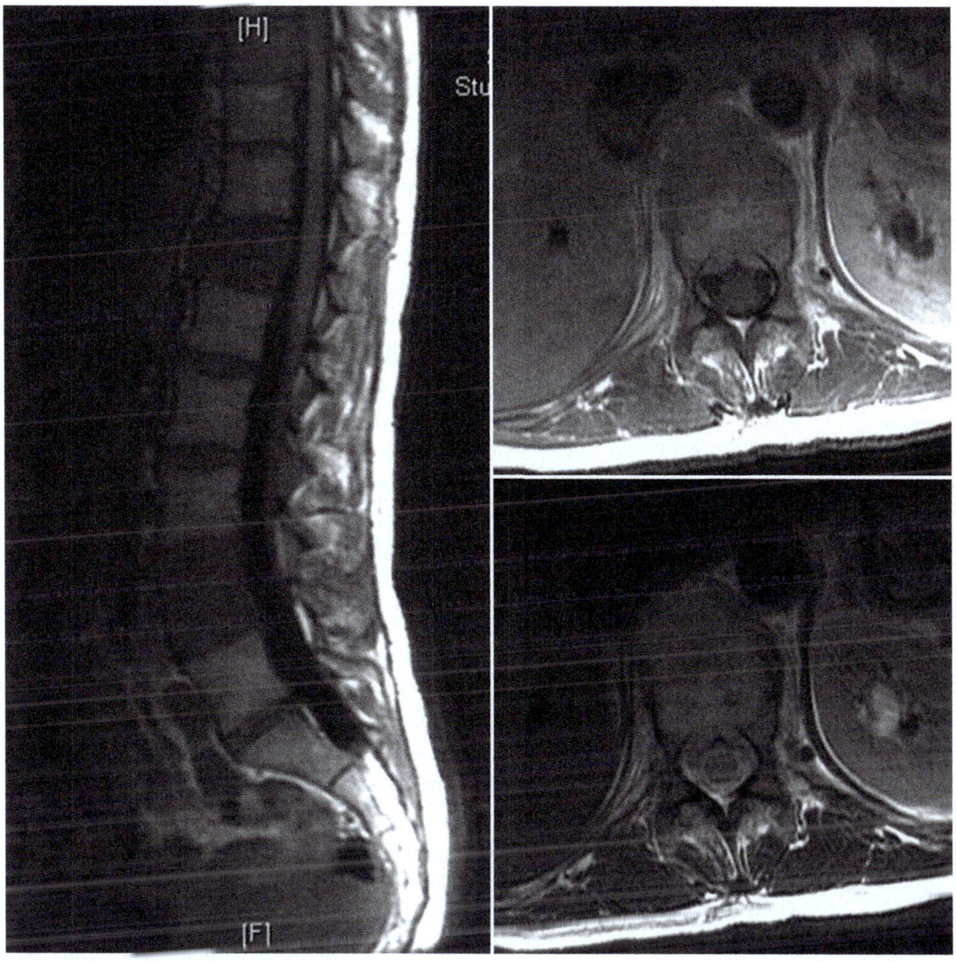

Fig. 19.1 Preoperative MRI of the thoracolumbar spine. Left: Sagittal T1, non-contrast enhanced, demonstrating multiple hypointense vertebral tumor infiltration. A compression fracture <25% of vertebral body height with a minimal kyphotic deformity is noted at T9 (top of the image) and T12. Top right: Axial T1 with contrast enhancement at T9 level demonstrating an ESCC grade 1c compression. Bottom right: Axial T2 at T9 level demonstrating an ESCC grade 1c compression

despite adequate systemic therapy, (*M*) significant mechanical back pain with SINS score of 14; and (*S*) 34-year-old with no major comorbidities. As this patient presents with no neurological deficits, with a radiosensitive tumor, there is no need to decompress the spinal cord. Tumor control is likely to be effectively controlled with radiation. However, she presents with frank spinal instability that is disabling and uncontrolled with analgesia. As mentioned, spinal instability serves as an independent surgical indication, and thus this patient is likely to benefit from surgical stabilization with pedicle screws and rods. Further, the multilevel lytic involvement complicates achievement of pain relief, and in this particular case, the authors decided to complement the stabilizing construct with multilevel kyphoplasty.

Surgery

All patients are placed under general anesthesia, typically with an arterial line and Foley catheter. Percutaneous instrumentation is considered a relatively bloodless surgery, and the use of blood products is typically unnecessary. Intraoperative nerve monitoring (IOM) is often helpful as the generated feedback can be used to modify intraoperative maneuvers to reduce or reverse iatro-

Table 19.1 The Spinal Instability Neoplastic Score (SINS) [6]

SINS component		Score
Location	Junctional (occiput–C2, C7–T2, T11–L1, L5–S1)	3
	Mobile spine (C3–C6, L2–L4)	2
	Semi-rigid (T3–T10)	1
	Rigid (S2–S5)	0
Pain	Yes	3
	Occasional pain but not mechanical	1
	Pain-free lesion	0
Bone lesion	Lytic	2
	Mixed (lytic/blastic)	1
	Blastic	0
Radiographic spinal alignment	Subluxation/translation present	4
	De novo deformity (kyphosis/scoliosis)	2
	Normal alignment	0
Vertebral body collapse	>50% collapse	3
	<50% collapse	2
	No collapse with >50% body involved	1
	None of the above	0
Posterolateral involvement of spinal elements	Bilateral	3
	Unilateral	1
	None of the above	0
Total	Stable	0–6
	Indeterminate	7–12
	Unstable	13–18

genic neurological deficits. IOM electrodes are placed, and monitoring includes EMG to the lower extremities and lower sacral root distributions, somatosensory-evoked potentials (SSEPs), and motor-evoked potentials (MEPs). The patient is then positioned prone and prepped in the typical fashion.

Traditionally, percutaneous surgery is performed using fluoroscopy, but in recent years, with the widespread use of intraoperative CT or fluoroscopy-based navigation systems, there appears to be a trend toward utilization of navigation systems. These provide real-time image guidance while limiting radiation exposure to operating room staff. The principle goal using intraoperative navigation systems is to track surgical instruments and anatomy in the operative field relative to a registered reference point. The most commonly used method is by optical tracking using cameras that project and detect reflected infrared light from reflecting spheres or light-emitting diodes [8]. A reference frame is tightly attached to a bony surface, typically either a spinous process below the lowest planned instrumented level or, when operating in the lower lumbar area, this can be docked on the iliac crest. The registration process following patient positioning is crucial, as inaccurate registration with the use of image guidance and computer-assisted navigation potentially has multiple sources of error. This necessitates frequent validation and accuracy assessment on a continuous basis [9]. This can be accomplished by placing the navigation probe on a known anatomical location (i.e., expected midline, spinous process, skin, etc.). Once accurate image guidance is confirmed, local entry points for screw placement are determined. Local anesthesia is injected, and a 0.5–1 inch incision is made. The underlying fascia is next incised using either a 10″ blade or monopolar cautery. A navigated Jamshidi needle is inserted into the wound, and an optimal entry point and trajectory are found while looking at the navigation screen. The Jamshidi needle is lightly tapped and carefully advanced to cannulate the pedicle into the vertebral body. Once the target depth is reached, a guide wire is inserted and placed in the vertebral body and the Jamshidi needle is carefully removed. *It is important to ensure throughout the procedure that the guide wire maintains accurate position and is not unintentionally pulled out with removal of other instruments.* Serial dilators are next inserted in standard minimally invasive muscle-sparing techniques, and a large-diameter working channel is placed on the bony surface of the cannulated entry point. A tap is inserted over the guide wire and the pedicle is tapped appropriately. Once the pedicles have been tapped, the screws are next inserted over the guide wire until secured and tightened. The guide wire should be removed prior to tightening of the pedicle screw or it may be difficult to pull out. Fluoroscopy is used to confirm the correct location of the screws. When used, fenestrated screws allow injection of poly-methylmethacrylate (PMMA) or "bone cement" through the pedicle screws to augment the stabilizing construct. The cement is injected under fluoroscopic guidance with care taken to avoid retropulsion of cement to the spinal canal or extravasation into blood vessels.

Once all pedicle screws have been placed and secured, the rod length is measured (the technique will vary based on the system used, but typically a caliper is inserted into the towers overlaying the screws and the rod length is measured). The rod is then advanced through one of the incisions, under the fascia, and advanced until it is placed on both screws. Once the rod is placed, caps are tightened and the rod is secured. When all screws and rods have been tightened and secured, the towers and rod holders are disconnected and removed.

The surgical sites are irrigated copiously, meticulously sutured layer by layer, and a sterile dressing is applied. The patient is then rolled back to the supine position, IOM electrodes are removed, and the patient is extubated.

There are several procedure-specific complications that must be considered. When dealing with navigation systems, accuracy must constantly be evaluated. This can be done by repeatedly identifying and placing the navigation probe on known anatomical landmarks including midline and the skin. Screw malpositioning with navigation is rare, but performing this surgery without intraoperative radiological confirmation of proper pedicle cannulation and screw placement is not recommended. Cord or nerve root injuries are rare, and intraoperative neural monitoring is a useful aid in early recognition and reversal of potential neural compromise. It is important to evaluate and familiarize with all parts of the percutaneous system used, as each system has advantages and pitfalls and, once placed below the skin, troubleshooting the hardware (loose caps, misplaced rods, etc.) can be a complicated task.

In the current case, the patient underwent T8–T10 percutaneous screw fixation with cement augmentation and T9, T12 kyphoplasty (Figs. 19.2, 19.3, and 19.4).

Discussion

Surgical indications for the treatment of spinal metastases include restoration of mechanical stability and decompression the spinal cord or nerve roots [4]. The growing use of minimal access sur-

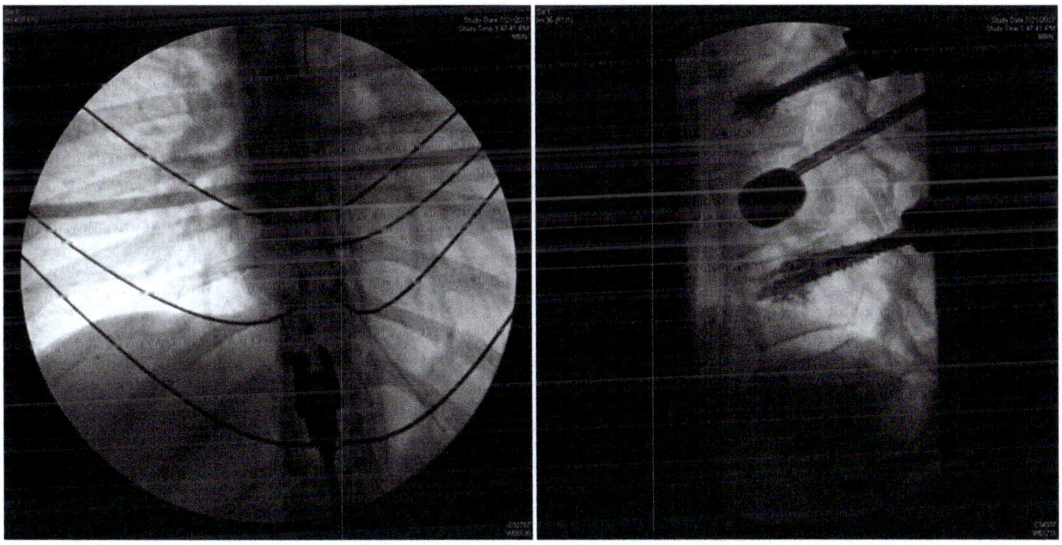

Fig. 19.2 Intraoperative fluoroscopy for confirmation of appropriate pedicle cannulation. Left: AP view showing k-wires inserted into target pedicles. Bilateral cannulation was performed at T8 (top) and T10 for insertion of pedicle screws, as well as unilateral cannulation at T9 and bilateral at T12 for kyphoplasty. Note the slightly exaggerated lateral to medial trajectory used in T9 to enable adequate filling at the midline. Also notable is the navigation reference frame clamped on the spinous process of T10. Right: Lateral view demonstrating the pedicle screws at T8 and T10 with cement injected through fenestrated screws. At T9 note the kyphoplasty balloon with contrast dye

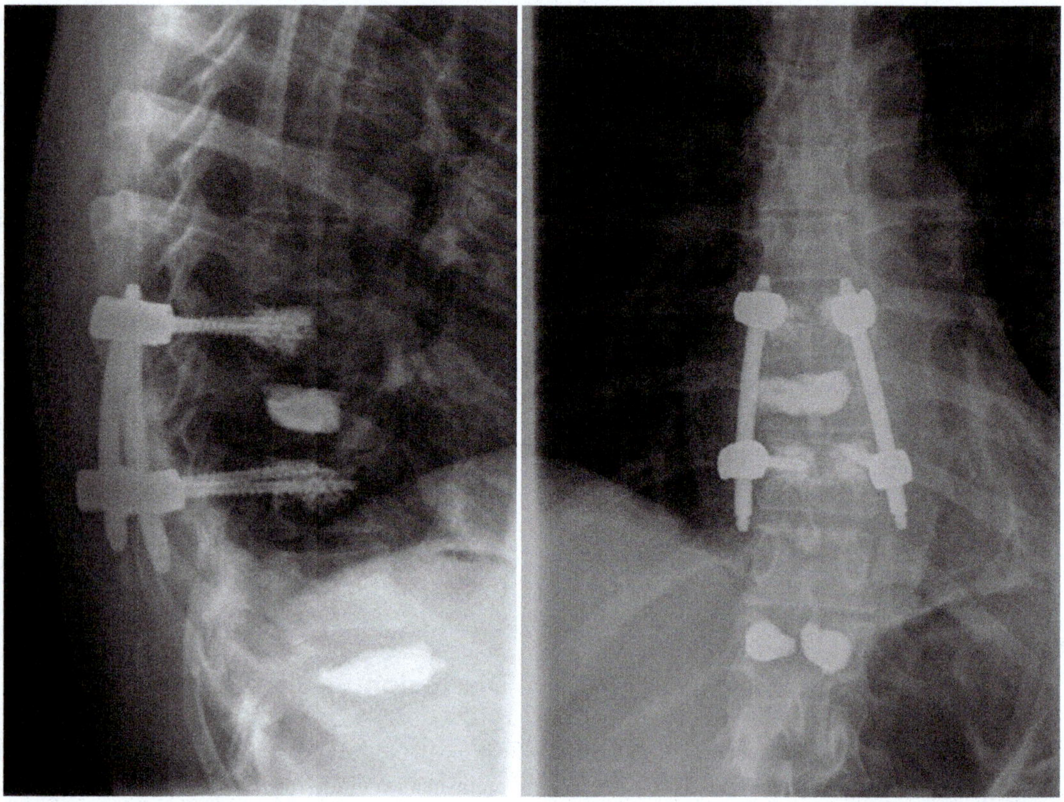

Fig. 19.3 Postoperative standing thoracic spine x-rays. Lateral view (left) and AP view (right) demonstrating the stabilizing construct. Notice the cement augmentation of the pedicle screws as well as the kyphoplasty at T9 and T12 providing anterior column support

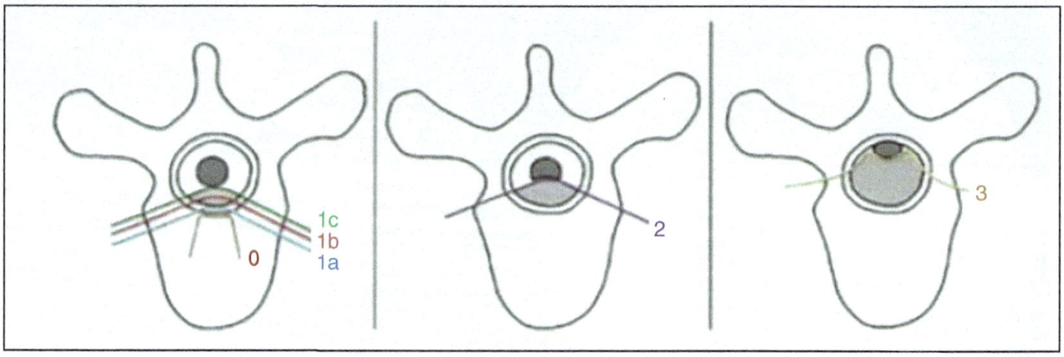

Schematic representation of the 6-point ESCC grading scale.

Grade 0	Bone-only disease
Grade 1a	Epidural impingement, without deformation of thecal sac
Grade 1b	Deformation of thecal sac, without spinal cord abutment
Grade 1c	Deformation of thecal sac, with spinal cord abutment, without cord compression
Grade 2	Spinal cord compression, with cerebral spinal fluid (CSF) visible around the cord
Grade 3	Spinal cord compression, no CSF visible around the cord

Fig. 19.4 Epidural spinal cord compression score. (Reproduced with permission from Bilsky et al. [1])

gery (MAS) in the treatment of degenerative and traumatic spinal disorders has led to the exploration of the role of MAS in the treatment of spinal tumors. Percutaneous pedicle screw placement techniques provide spinal stabilization with preservation of muscle attachments (Fig. 19.5). Several studies have shown decreased blood loss, transfusion rates, and hospitalization length with MAS stabilization techniques [10–13]. The technique described herein provides a minimally invasive alternative to traditional open surgeries in restoring the posterior tension band and main-

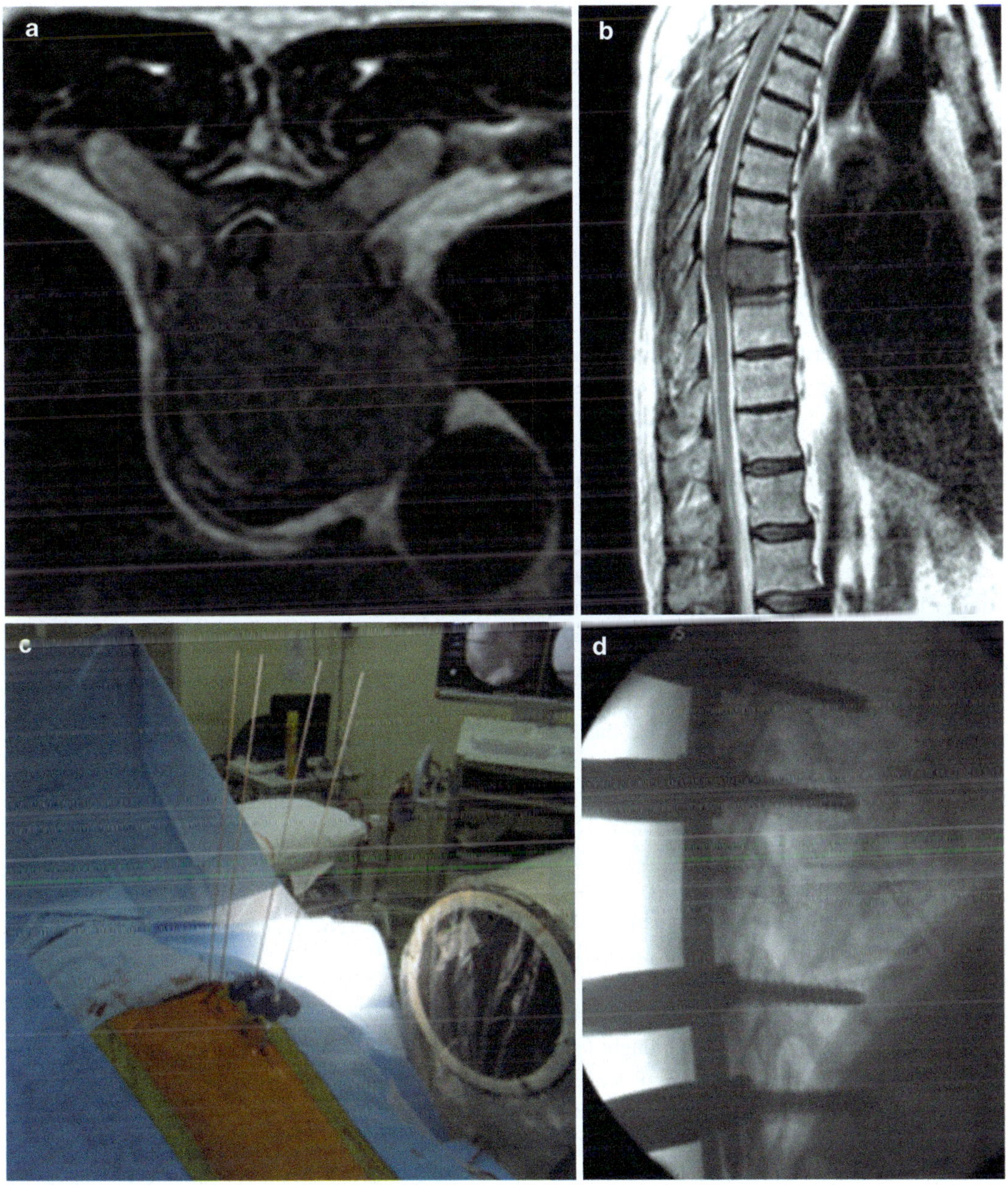

Fig. 19.5 Representative case of minimally invasive thoracic stabilization for metastatic spine disease. (**a**) Axial MRI. (**b**) Sagittal MRI. (**c**) Insertion of percutaneous K-wires under fluoroscopic guidance. (**d**) Lateral radiograph of instrumentation. (Reproduced with permission from Zairi et al. [26])

taining spinal stability. Patients with spinal tumors generally require a combination of surgical, radiation, and systemic therapies, making prompt postoperative healing and return to treatment essential. This is one of the greater benefits of MAS such as percutaneous stabilization. With this technique, radiation can occasionally be started within a week after surgery, unlike open surgeries where the risk of wound complications frequently delays radiation therapy [14, 15].

Since the majority of cancer patients have poor bone quality, we routinely employ pedicle screw cement augmentation, as screw pullout or pedicle fracture in a short construct can be potentially catastrophic [16]. Preliminary reports demonstrate safety and efficacy of radiation using both PEEK [17] and PMMA [18] materials. For some pathologic compression fractures, evidence strongly supports kyphoplasty for symptomatic relief and to provide structural support [19–21]. As seen in the case presented herein, fractures with evidence of posterior element disease often require augmentation of the posterior tension band through the use of pedicle screws and connecting rods. Combining vertebral cement augmentation and percutaneous instrumentation provides stabilization of both the anterior and posterior columns of the spine. At our practice these are often performed in concert. It is important to understand that in patients presenting with high-grade spinal cord or cauda equina compression, these constructs are placed without addition of kyphoplasty at the index level in order to avoid iatrogenic tumor retropulsion into the spinal canal.

Traditionally, percutaneous stabilization was performed using intraoperative fluoroscopic guidance. Using standard insertion techniques, the rate of misplaced pedicle screws ranges from 14% to 55%, with as many as 7% of these misplaced screws resulting in neurological injuries [22, 23]. Recent technological advancements have brought forth the utilization of three-dimensional (3D) image guidance systems. The routine use of these systems has been shown to improve the accuracy and safety of pedicle screw placement, especially in more complex spinal deformities [22–25], and pitfalls and shortcomings have been established [9]. With the current prolonged survival in cancer patients owed to modern cancer therapies, along with recent advancements in engineering, new spine construct materials, and the introduction of robotic surgery, it is likely that the role of minimally invasive percutaneous spinal tumor surgery will grow.

Conclusion

Patients with spinal instability require surgical stabilization as systemic therapies and radiation do not restore stability. MAS techniques are increasingly utilized in spine tumor treatment and, with proper indications, offer multiple advantages over open surgery. The greatest advantage of MAS for spine metastases is the ability to rapidly return to systemic and radiation therapy. Percutaneous stabilization of pathologic fractures improves patients' pain control and overall quality of life. It is likely that the role of minimally invasive percutaneous spinal tumor surgery will grow owing to prolonged survivals and improved surgical technology. Surgeons must be familiar with the technical aspects of minimally invasive surgery including complication avoidance, staff radiation safety, and technical troubleshooting.

References

1. Bilsky MH, Laufer I, Fourney DR, Groff M, Schmidt MH, Varga PP, et al. Reliability analysis of the epidural spinal cord compression scale. J Neurosurg Spine. 2010;13(3):324–8.
2. Laufer I, Rubin DG, Lis E, Cox BW, Stubblefield MD, Yamada Y, et al. The NOMS framework: approach to the treatment of spinal metastatic tumors. Oncologist. 2013;18(6):744–51.
3. Barzilai O, Laufer I, Yamada Y, Higginson DS, Schmitt AM, Lis E, et al. Integrating evidence-based medicine for treatment of spinal metastases into a decision framework: neurologic, oncologic, mechanicals stability, and systemic disease. J Clin Oncol. 2017;35(21):2419–27. https://doi.org/10.1200/JCO.2017.72.7362.
4. Bilsky MH, Laufer I, Burch S. Shifting paradigms in the treatment of metastatic spine disease. Spine (Phila Pa 1976). 2009;34(22 Suppl):S101–7.
5. Yamada Y, Katsoulakis E, Laufer I, Lovelock M, Barzilai O, McLaughlin LA, et al. The impact of his-

tology and delivered dose on local control of spinal metastases treated with stereotactic radiosurgery. Neurosurg Focus. 2017;42(1):E6.

6. Fisher CG, DiPaola CP, Ryken TC, Bilsky MH, Shaffrey CI, Berven SH, et al. A novel classification system for spinal instability in neoplastic disease: an evidence-based approach and expert consensus from the spine oncology study group. Spine (Phila Pa 1976). 2010;35(22):E1221–9.
7. Rades D, Fehlauer F, Schulte R, Veninga T, Stalpers LJ, Basic H, et al. Prognostic factors for local control and survival after radiotherapy of metastatic spinal cord compression. J Clin Oncol. 2006;24(21):3388–93.
8. Holly LT, Foley KT. Intraoperative spinal navigation. Spine (Phila Pa 1976). 2003;28(15 Suppl):S54–61.
9. Rahmathulla G, Nottmeier EW, Pirris SM, Deen HG, Pichelmann MA. Intraoperative image-guided spinal navigation: technical pitfalls and their avoidance. Neurosurg Focus. 2014;36(3):E3.
10. Hansen-Algenstaedt N, Kwan MK, Algenstaedt P, Chiu CK, Viezens L, Chan TS, et al. Comparison between minimally invasive surgery and conventional open surgery for patients with spinal metastasis: a prospective propensity score-matched study. Spine (Phila Pa 1976). 2017;42(10):789–97.
11. Hikata T, Isogai N, Shiono Y, Funao H, Okada E, Fujita N, et al. A retrospective cohort study comparing the safety and efficacy of minimally invasive versus open surgical techniques in the treatment of spinal metastases. Clin Spine Surg. 2017;30(8):E1082–E1087.
12. Rao PJ, Thayaparan GK, Fairhall JM, Mobbs RJ. Minimally invasive percutaneous fixation techniques for metastatic spinal disease. Orthop Surg. 2014;6(3):187–95.
13. Kumar N, Malhotra R, Maharajan K, Zaw AS, Wu PH, Makandura MC, et al. Metastatic spine tumor surgery: a comparative study of minimally invasive approach using percutaneous pedicle screws fixation versus open approach. Clin Spine Surg. 2017;30(8):E1015–E1021.
14. Disa JJ, Smith AW, Bilsky MH. Management of radiated reoperative wounds of the cervicothoracic spine: the role of the trapezius turnover flap. Ann Plast Surg. 2001;47(4):394–7.
15. Yang Z, Yang Y, Zhang Y, Zhang Z, Chen Y, Shen Y, et al. Minimal access versus open spinal surgery in treating painful spine metastasis: a systematic review. World J Surg Oncol. 2015;13:68.
16. Burval DJ, McLain RF, Milks R, Inceoglu S. Primary pedicle screw augmentation in osteoporotic lumbar vertebrae: biomechanical analysis of pedicle fixation strength. Spine (Phila Pa 1976). 2007;32(10):1077–83.
17. Jackson JB 3rd, Crimaldi AJ, Peindl R, Norton HJ, Anderson WE, Patt JC. Effect of polyether ether ketone on therapeutic radiation to the spine: a pilot study. Spine (Phila Pa 1976). 2017;42(1):E1–7.
18. Barzilai O, DiStefano N, Lis E, Yamada Y, Lovelock DM, Fontanella AN, et al. Safety and utility of kyphoplasty prior to spine stereotactic radiosurgery for metastatic tumors: a clinical and dosimetric analysis. J Neurosurg Spine. 2017:1–7.
19. Mendel E, Bourekas E, Gerszten P, Golan JD. Percutaneous techniques in the treatment of spine tumors: what are the diagnostic and therapeutic indications and outcomes? Spine (Phila Pa 1976). 2009;34(22 Suppl):S93–100.
20. Papanastassiou ID, Filis AK, Gerochristou MA, Vrionis FD. Controversial issues in kyphoplasty and vertebroplasty in malignant vertebral fractures. Cancer Control. 2014;21(2):151–7.
21. Berenson J, Pflugmacher R, Jarzem P, Zonder J, Schechtman K, Tillman JB, et al. Balloon kyphoplasty versus non-surgical fracture management for treatment of painful vertebral body compression fractures in patients with cancer: a multicentre, randomised controlled trial. Lancet Oncol. 2011;12(3):225–35.
22. Vaccaro AR, Rizzolo SJ, Balderston RA, Allardyce TJ, Garfin SR, Dolinskas C, et al. Placement of pedicle screws in the thoracic spine. Part II: an anatomical and radiographic assessment. J Bone Joint Surg Am. 1995;77(8):1200–6.
23. Laine T, Lund T, Ylikoski M, Lohikoski J, Schlenzka D. Accuracy of pedicle screw insertion with and without computer assistance: a randomised controlled clinical study in 100 consecutive patients. Eur Spine J. 2000;9(3):235–40.
24. Tian NF, Huang QS, Zhou P, Zhou Y, Wu RK, Lou Y, et al. Pedicle screw insertion accuracy with different assisted methods: a systematic review and meta-analysis of comparative studies. Eur Spine J. 2011;20(6):846–59.
25. Laudato PA, Pierzchala K, Schizas C. Pedicle screw insertion accuracy using O-Arm, robotic guidance or freehand technique: a comparative study. World J Surg Oncol. 2015;13:68.
26. Zairi F, Arikat A, Allaoui M, et al. Minimally invasive decompression and stabilization for the management of thoracolumbar spine metastasis. J Neurosurg Spine. 2012;17(1):19–23.

20 Posterior Lumbar and Sacral Approach and Stabilization: Intralesional Lumbar Resection

John H. Shin and Ganesh M. Shankar

Introduction

Many types of tumors can affect the spinal column and the structural integrity of the spine, leading to severe pain and disability [1, 2]. The main types of tumors that involve the spinal column are metastatic cancers and primary tumors of the spine (chordoma, chondrosarcoma, osteosarcoma, etc.). Though primary tumors of the spine are rare, the resection and oncologic strategies are completely different from that of metastatic tumors [3, 4]. In these tumors, en bloc or excisional-type resections with wide margins are often planned and attempted for durable long-term local control as part of multi-modal treatment planning, often with a combination of radiation and/or chemotherapy [5].

However, most tumors affecting the spinal column are metastases from other primary sites such as the lung, breast, kidney, and prostate [6]. In these cases, patients may present with pain related to pathologic fracture of the vertebrae from metastatic involvement of the bone marrow, which may ultimately extend into the epidural space and lead to nerve root and spinal cord compression [7]. Any part of the spinal column can be affected by tumor and cause compression, including the facets and posterolateral elements. However, since the bone marrow within the vertebral body is usually the site of metastases, compression is usually ventral to the dura. The technical challenge is to separate the tumor and retropulsed bone from the ventral dura without disrupting the dura or excessively retracting the nerve roots.

The lumbar spine is second only to the thoracic spine for the occurrence of metastatic disease [8]. Metastases to the affected vertebral bodies may affect the structural integrity of the vertebral body and lead to severe pain, limiting weight bearing, standing, or walking as the spine is loaded. Though these fractures can be mitigated and treated to a degree with rest, medication, and medical therapy, often, these fractures may result in severe pain. An assessment of the type of pain the patient is having needs to be performed from careful history taking and corroborating that information with the radiographic appearance of the lesion to assess the stability of the spine [9]. Patients may also have symptoms from tumor progression within and extending from the vertebral body after radiation therapy. In these situations, intralesional debulking may be required in cases of cauda equina-type symptoms or severe nerve root compression.

Goals of Surgery: Strategy and Approach Considerations

These patients may require stabilization and reconstruction which is usually performed through a posterior approach. When this occurs,

J. H. Shin (✉) · G. M. Shankar
Massachusetts General Hospital,
Department of Neurosurgery, Harvard Medical School,
Boston, MA, USA
e-mail: shin.john@mgh.harvard.edu

D. M. Sciubba (ed.), *Spinal Tumor Surgery*, https://doi.org/10.1007/978-3-319-98422-3_20

the goals of surgery are to decompress the nerve roots, separate tumor from the dura, and stabilize the spine. In the metastatic patient, this is done through an intended intralesional technique with decancellation of the vertebral body and piecemeal resection of the vertebral body and tumor [10, 11].

Because the goal of surgery is not curative resection, an intralesional strategy is safe and effective [9]. This also avoids the anterior and lateral approaches which introduce a wider spectrum of potential complications involving other soft-tissue organs and vascular structures [12–14]. As mentioned earlier, in cases of primary tumor resections where an en bloc resection is planned, staging the resection and incorporating either anterior or lateral access may be advantageous. Staging these types of operations allows for careful planning of osteotomies and intended cuts through bone and soft tissue to maximize margins of resections and the surgical visibility. In these situations, the morbidity of such approaches may be justified considering the challenges of local tumor control with transgression through the tumor. In these cases, an intralesional approach is avoided [15, 16].

For patients with cancer and metastatic disease, however, the anterior approach may not be ideal as patients may already be suffering from other side effects of chemotherapy or treatment, affecting their other organ systems. For instance, patients with liver metastases may have recurring ascites, abdominal distension, and venous hypertension, requiring frequent peritoneal drainage among other issues. Patients with diffuse adenopathy may also have venous congestion affecting venous return and circulation. For patients with previous bowel surgery or retroperitoneal surgery, the scar tissue associated with those approaches also makes the anterior approach less inviting and potentially more dangerous as dissection of the large vascular structures may prohibit safe exposure.

Similarly, the lateral approach is an excellent way to access the lumbar spine but in the metastatic patient, careful consideration of the regional anatomy is needed. The lateral approach is an excellent way to reconstruct and instrument the lumbar spine for many degenerative and traumatic spinal conditions [17]. With the development of minimal access techniques, there is certainly a role for lateral approaches to the lumbar spine in tumor cases, but this is usually more difficult at the lumbosacral junction due to the anatomical relationship of this region with the iliac crest and the iliac vessels [18–20]. Tumors that involve the lumbar vertebrae also involve the surrounding psoas muscles as well, and that is a major consideration, especially for vascular tumors, such as renal cell carcinoma. It is typically difficult to control bleeding in tumors that diffusely involve the psoas muscles. Practically, it is also technically difficult to work at L5 and S1 from this lateral position due to the position of the spine and the distance from the surgeon. It is also difficult to instrument the sacrum from this approach given the orientation and anatomy of the sacrum. The iliac crest is often in the way, limiting access to the sacrum from a lateral approach.

An Integrated Approach with Radiation Planning

With advances in radiation therapy, such as stereotactic radiosurgery, local tumor control can now be achieved through less invasive, extensive, and morbid surgery. By incorporating and planning for advanced radiation delivery like stereotactic radiosurgery post-operatively, the extent of surgery upfront can be minimized [21]. With enough decompression and separation of tumors away from the dura, surgery sets the stage for radiation by providing sufficient clearance around the critical neural structures to allow for maximal radiation dose distribution, typically 18–24 Gy in a single fraction [18]. In the cervical and thoracic spines, the dose-limiting structure is usually the spinal cord. The permitted spinal cord dose allowance varies from center to center but in the lumbar spine, it is generally agreed upon that the cauda nerve roots may tolerate more dose than the spinal cord. Nonetheless, the need for separation from the thecal sac is important not only for decompression purposes but also for radiation dose planning.

Despite these advances in radiation technology, surgeons still need to be comfortable with and able to circumferentially decompress around the thecal sac and nerve roots to maximize the efficacy of post-operative radiation. Inadequate decompression or separation of tumor and bone away from the neural elements will limit the applicable dose to the residual areas of metastatic disease in the surgical field [22, 23]. In this chapter, we take a step beyond laminectomy to describe and illustrate the nuances of intralesional tumor resection in the palliative setting.

Clinical Presentation: Spine Tumor Pain

Low back pain is the most common presenting symptom for most lumbar and lumbosacral tumors. There are several basic types of pain in patients with metastatic disease affecting the lumbar spine. These include local axial biologic pain, radicular pain, and mechanical pain. Local axial back pain is described as constant and generally does not worsen with movement or improve with recumbency. This type of pain has been attributed to several factors including the stretching of the vertebral body periosteum by the growing vertebral body mass or local cancer-related inflammation within the bone. This local axial biologic pain often improves with steroids and tends to have a diurnal variation with regard to the cycling and severity of pain. This is thought related in part to the cyclical variation in endogenous steroid production throughout the day.

Since cancer patients are to a degree immunocompromised, this explains the response of this type of pain to medical steroid treatment. Radicular pain is related to nerve root compression by the tumor in the epidural space. The source of this pain may be an extraosseous extension of the tumor, but may also include compression from venous engorgement and compression as well as bony compression from ipsilateral pedicle expansion from tumor or from retropulsed bone hitting the nerve root as it exits the foramen. This type of pain, regardless of the offending compressor, characteristically radiates in the dermatomal distribution of the compressed nerve root and is usually associated with dysesthesia.

Finally, mechanical pain is characterized by pain that is worse with changing positions, particularly sitting and standing as the spine is loaded. Radiculopathy that is prominent with standing is referred to as mechanical radiculopathy and suggests dynamic compression of the nerve roots with weight bearing given the compromise of the spinal column [24].

Radiological Evaluation

Careful analysis of imaging studies is critical in surgical planning in anticipation of intralesional resection and stabilization through a posterior approach in the lumbosacral region. Magnetic resonance imaging (MRI) is readily available and shows the extent of cauda or nerve root compression. The extent of bony metastases and marrow replacement is often readily seen as T1 hypointense changes within the marrow itself. T2 hyperintense changes within the bone marrow may reflect osseous edema within the bone marrow. The sagittal and axial T2-weighted sequences are often most helpful to study the areas of worst nerve compression and visualization of the foramen and lateral recesses. The administration of gadolinium is useful for visualizing the vascularity of these tumors, particularly the epidural component. The venous congestion in the epidural space often exaggerates the extent of actual epidural tumor extension and compression. Often, it is not possible to separate these visually by MRI.

The MRI is also useful to study the extent of tumor lateral to the vertebral bodies and extending into the psoas muscles. It is important to study these before planning surgery as bulky, and diffuse tumor within the psoas muscle may explain non-dermatomal pain and proximal weakness in a patient. This also affects surgical planning as decompression of the lumbar nerve root proximally may not result in adequate relief of pain if there is bulky tumor within the psoas and in the retroperitoneum sitting on or involving the lumbosacral plexus. Consideration of the extent of vertebral body involvement is also critical for planning the number of levels to instrument. Again, consideration of the number of vertebral bodies involved may sway one to instrument over multiple levels given anticipated challenges to fixation with pedicle screws through the weak bone. Radiation effect on the bone can also be seen on the MRI.

The vascularity of suspected tumors is often associated with the primary tumor type, as in renal cell carcinoma. Identifying flow voids or increased vascularity on MRI imaging, especially the T2 sequences needs to be analyzed before surgery as these patients may benefit from pre-operative spinal angiography and embolization. From a posterior approach in this region, access to the major iliac blood vessels and segmental vessels is not easily achieved due to the depth of field and the lumbosacral anatomy. Especially with an intralesional resection where the vertebral body is being resected piecemeal, there is no easy way to control rapid bleeding from the bone.

Analysis of computed tomography (CT) imaging is also helpful to see in greater detail the quality of the bone. Anticipating whether the bone is lytic, blastic, or sclerotic may affect surgical planning. Axial sequences can also help plan for pedicle screw width and length to maximize fixation in this challenging environment. The surgeon needs to consider that in addition to general osteopenia, the bone may be affected by radiation, marrow replacement, and lytic change, all affecting the purchase and pullout strength of the screws. Many times, these patients will have had CT of the chest, abdomen, and pelvis performed as recent staging. This can be helpful for surgical planning as the orientation and location of the iliac vessels can be seen well on axial imaging and have implications for pedicle screw fixation toward the lumbosacral junction. Assessing for any regional vascular variations may save trouble later. Also, much information can be gleaned from these staging scans as the extent of ascites or other metastases such as liver may likely influence hemostasis and intraoperative coagulation.

Finally, if patients can tolerate it, standing lumbar radiographs can be very helpful in assessing the overall alignment of the spine. This may be very difficult, however, and CT often suffices for evaluating the bony anatomy.

Case Illustration: Lumbar

This 71-year-old male was diagnosed with melanoma from a chest lesion that was resected. He was started on pembrolizumab and 1 year later was found to have multiple liver and spine lesions. He presented to oncology clinic with severe left leg pain. MRI was performed demonstrating lytic metastases at L1 and L2, with epidural disease at L2 consistent with his radicular symptoms (Fig. 20.1). He underwent laminectomy and resection of epidural tumor. This was followed by fractionated conventional external beam radiation (30 Gy in 10 fractions). The patient's left leg pain improved enough that he could reduce his pain medications over the subsequent 6 weeks.

Approximately 3 months after surgery, however, the pain returned and was significantly worse with sitting, standing, and walking. The back pain was worse with standing. The left leg pain was much worse with standing and limited ambulation to several steps. The patient had several episodes of falling due to the leg giving out. The patient was admitted for pain crisis and an increasing oral narcotic requirement and inability to manage daily tasks at home. On examination, he was unable to sit upright or stand due to severe pain.

MRI of the lumbar spine demonstrated lytic metastases involving L1 and L2 with pathologic fracture (Fig. 20.2). At both levels, there was evidence of extraosseous extension and epidural disease. At the L2 level, there was severe compression of the cauda equina with a large epidural soft-tissue component. Tumor also destroyed the left lateral wall of the vertebra and extended into the adjacent psoas muscle.

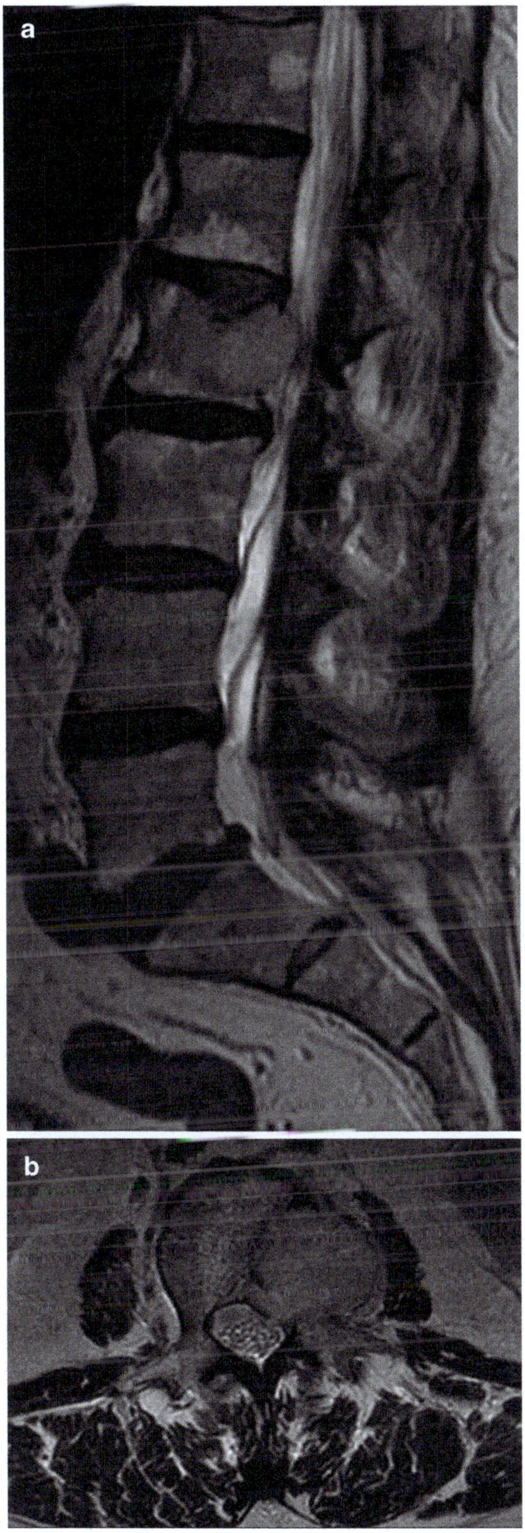

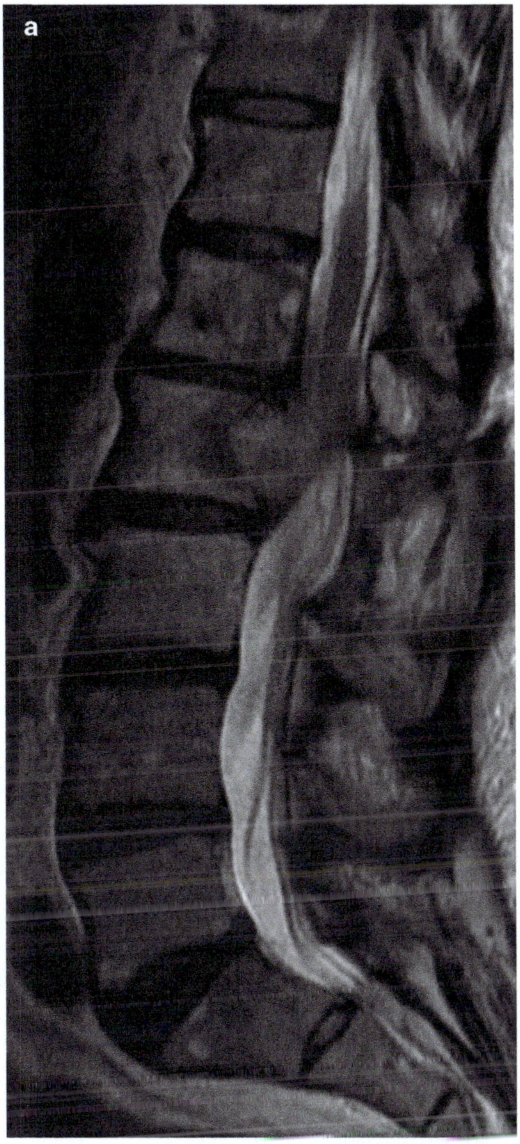

Fig. 20.2 (**a**) MRI, sagittal T2 sequence, after the initial decompression surgery and radiation therapy shows progression of disease and worse epidural compression. (**b**) Axial T2 sequence shows severe cauda equina compression and effacement of cerebrospinal fluid. There is clear progression compared to the previous MRI

Fig. 20.1 (**a**) Pre-operative MRI, sagittal T2 sequence, shows L1 and L2 vertebral body metastases with pathologic fracture and retropulsion of tumor at L2. (**b**) Pre-operative MRI, axial T2 sequence, at the level of the L2 pedicle showing the involvement of the left L2 vertebral body, pedicle, and facet with epidural extension. There is also the lateral vertebral body wall extension to the psoas muscle. The L2 and L3 nerve roots are compressed by tumor

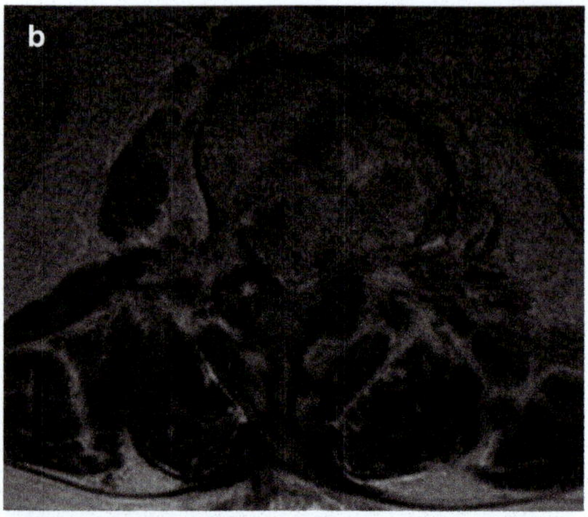

Fig. 20.2 (continued)

The patient underwent surgery with the specific goals of stabilization to address his mechanical back pain due to pathologic vertebral fractures and separation/debulking of gross epidural and bony disease given progression and now debilitating pain and function-limiting weakness. Stereotactic radiosurgery was planned after intralesional debulking for an attempt at local tumor control given his local progression. In a patient with widely metastatic disease with progression on pembrolizumab, the focus was on palliating the severe oncologic mechanical pain and decompressing the nerves in the least morbid way.

Surgical Technique: Pearls and Planning

The general familiarity and relative technical ease of posterior approaches to the lumbar spine make them appealing to most spine surgeons [25–27]. With the posterior approach, multiple levels of the spine can be accessed, making multi-level decompression and stabilization with instrumentation feasible through a single approach. With the more liberal handling characteristics of the cauda equina, satisfactory intralesional decompression of metastatic tumors can be achieved regardless of whether the posterior elements or structures ventral to the thecal sac are involved. Ventral decompression and access to that space is easily achieved by removal of the facets and pedicles as needed. Transpedicular drilling allows access to the vertebral body and the ventral epidural space.

In this case, the patient was brought to the operating room with the plan for multi-level decompression and stabilization. With prone positioning, it is important that the abdomen lies free with all pressure points sufficiently padded to minimize increasing the abdominal venous pressure which then affects the epidural bleeding. A prone Jackson table is extremely useful for this purpose. For cases not involving the cervical or thoracic spinal cord, intraoperative neurophysiologic recording (motor-evoked potentials, somatosensory-evoked potentials) is not routinely used, though it is an option based on surgeon preference. Adequate intravenous access and arterial lines are secured with the arms toward anesthesia.

A midline incision is made and Bovie electrocautery used to perform the dissection. In patients with spinal metastases, the soft tissue including muscle is often edematous and may weep fluid. Similarly, the muscle may tend to bleed based on the patient's underlying coagulopathy, immunosuppression, and poor hematologic reserve. Dissection is performed lateral to the facet joints to expose the lateral tips of the transverse processes. In this case, the exposure was performed from T11 to L4. The areas of concern were at L1 and L2, and multiple points of fixation were planned given the poor bone quality.

The tumor at L2 was known to affect the transverse process, pedicle, and facets. Pedicle screw instrumentation was placed at each level using anatomic landmarks and free-hand technique. Instrumentation is performed prior to decompression. This allows for stabilization if the surgery must be aborted for medical or other reasons. Another advantage to placing the instrumentation first is that the anatomy is not distorted and obscured by further bone and soft-tissue bleeding which tends to accumulate as the case goes on.

In this case, fenestrated screws were used from T11 to L4 to allow for cement-augmented screw placement (Fig. 20.3). The fenestrated

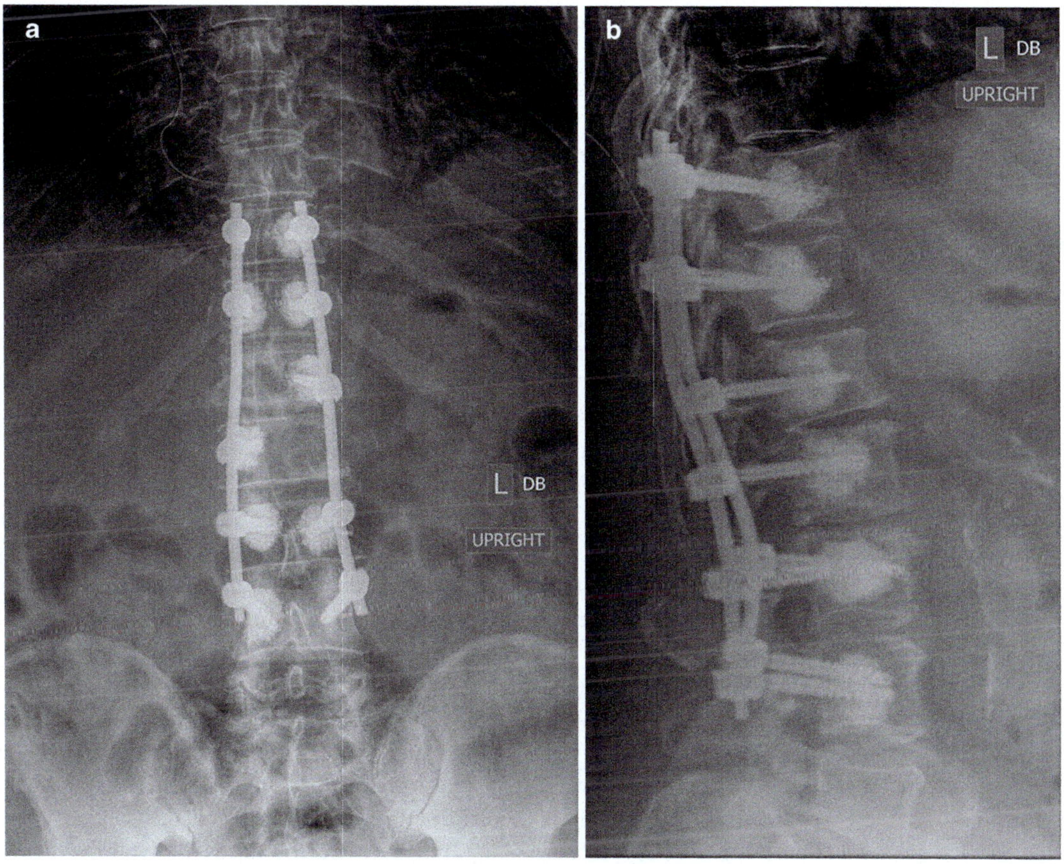

Fig. 20.3 (**a**) AP standing lumbar x-ray showing the construct from T11 to L4. The right L1 and left L2 pedicles were not instrumented due to gross pedicle destruction. (**b**) Lateral standing lumbar x-ray. The endplate-to-endplate fill of cement of each vertebral body is shown

screws allow for controlled delivery of cement through the actual pedicle screw at any time after screw placement. In this workflow, the screws are placed using free-hand technique, and the placement of the screws is verified using anteroposterior (AP) and lateral x-ray. The O-arm or any other type of intraoperative imaging modality can be used to verify the position of the screws. It is important to confirm the accuracy of screw placement so that when the cement is injected, it goes into the vertebral body and not into the epidural space. To maximize workflow efficiency, the scrub tech can start mixing and preparing the cement while the verification x-rays are being performed. This allows enough time for the cement to be ready and time to set up the screws for cement injection. Once the position of the screws is confirmed, the cement is injected into each pedicle using intraoperative fluoroscopy.

After the screws were placed, laminectomy was performed removing all the dorsal elements of L1 and L2. Laminectomy was performed wide to the medial wall of the pedicles of L1, L2, and L3. This is achieved using the cutting burr and Kerrison rongeurs. The instability of the spine was obvious, and the facet of L1–L2 was grossly incompetent. Knowing that the L2 pedicle and the L1–L2 facet on the left side were involved, Leksell rongeurs were used to bite and resect as much of the L1–L2 facet until the cancellous stump of the L2 pedicle on the left side was visualized and identified. The tumor had destroyed the pedicle, facet, and transverse process. The L2 and L3 nerve roots were not visualized yet as they were buried under epidural tumor which displaced the nerve roots. A dental instrument was used to follow the dura from the midline and out to where the foramen for L2 and L3 should be. Once that plane was dissected, the tumor was then resected using pituitary and Kerrison rongeurs. To facilitate complete L2 and L3 nerve root decompression and epidural tumor resection, the pars interarticularis of L2 was also resected by using the cutting burr to drill across the pars immediately caudal to the L2 pedicle. It is helpful to take a dental instrument and palpate and visualize the medial wall of the pedicle. With an assistant holding the dental along the inferior border of the pedicle and directly underneath the pars, the cutting burr can be used to drill directly over the pars medial to lateral, drilling all the bone away until the dental. This allows for resection of the pars as well as the inferior articulating process of L2, which then helps visualize the L3 nerve root.

With resection of the pars, the L2 nerve root is completely visualized and all tumors can be resected out to the intertransverse fascia. The transverse process of L2 is then drilled away, which isolates the L2 pedicle. The L2 pedicle is then drilled down into the vertebral body which is already partially destroyed by the tumor. It is unnecessary to dissect along the lateral aspect of the vertebral body wall at the level of pedicle resection as the tumor had essentially destroyed this lateral wall and this area tends to be extremely vascular. Since this is an intralesional resection, the goal is to stay within the vertebral body cavity that is entered through the pedicle on that side. Once the vertebral body tumor cavity is encountered, this is usually quickly and easily vacuated using a combination of tumor forceps, curettage, and suction. If the dissection stays within the vertebral body in an intralesional technique, there should be no danger to the great vessels coursing ventral to the vertebral body. Similarly, the retroperitoneal structures should not be a factor through this surgical corridor. As seen on the MRI, the tumor had destroyed a significant portion of the vertebral body.

Aggressive decancellation and evacuation of tumor and marrow contents can be performed through this approach. The last critical step of this technique is resection of the posterior vertebral body wall and removal of tumor immediately ventral to the thecal sac, including the posterior longitudinal ligament. This can be done by gently mobilizing the dura here with a dental or Penfield #4 instrument while the operating surgeon uses a down-angled curette to push down the remaining vertebral body wall down into the vertebrectomy defect. This can be done unilaterally or from both sides. Especially if stereotactic radiosurgery is planned post-operatively, it is critical to establish a clear ventral epidural space with separation and clearance of tumor and bone away from the dura. Great care must be taken to identify the plane between the posterior longitudinal ligament and the ventral dura. In tumor cases, the posterior longitudinal ligament is often able to be dissected away from the dura as tumor does not usually disrupt this structure, unlike in trauma. This plane may be harder to identify in cases like this one where the patient previously underwent radiation. Ventral durotomies can be challenging to fix, and it is at this point of the operation that surgery slows down somewhat to ensure safe dissection of this plane. The posterior longitudinal ligament needs to be resected to fully reconstitute the ventral thecal sac and ensure circumferential decompression.

During the intralesional resection, bleeding may be an issue. In cases of hypervascular tumors such as renal cell carcinoma, pre-operative embolization can be very helpful, though such embolization does not mean that the tumor or vertebral body will not bleed during surgery. In this case of metastatic melanoma, the tumor did not bleed significantly during this piecemeal resection, but generous epidural bleeding was encountered as anticipated. Such bleeding can be controlled by using thrombotic agents, gelfoam, and hydrogen peroxide.

Following intralesional resection, reconstruction of the anterior column is an option but not mandatory. In this case, anterior column reconstruction was not performed as the entire vertebral body was not resected (Fig. 20.4). In cases where there is a significant vertebral body defect, anterior column reconstruction with cement secured with either Steinman pins or the chest

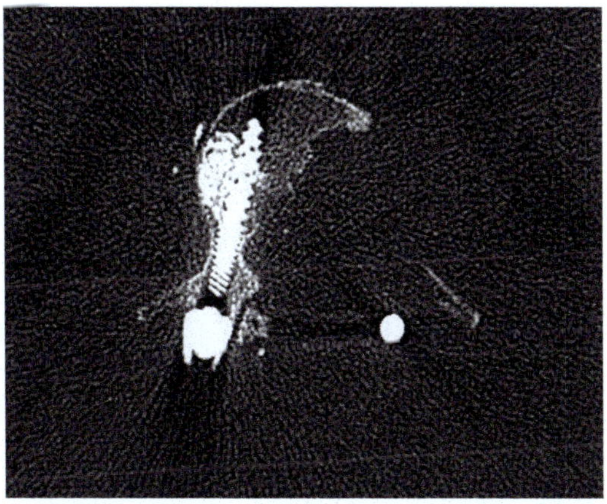

Fig. 20.4 Post-operative CT, axial image, at the level of the L2 vertebral body, shows the cement-augmented pedicle screw on the right side. There is no screw on the left side as the left facet, pedicle, and lateral portion of the vertebral body have been resected using an intralesional technique

tube technique can be performed. It is difficult to use devices such as structural allograft and/or expandable cages due to the limitations of the space and the ability to safely insert and manipulate such devices within the ventral lumbar epidural space. Unlike the thoracic spine, where nerve root sacrifice greatly facilitates being able to navigate such implants into the ventral epidural space, lumbar nerve root sacrifice is not an acceptable morbidity in an intralesional, palliative strategy.

Case Illustration: Lumbosacral

This intralesional technique is particularly useful for metastases at the lumbosacral junction as the morbidity of the posterior approach is relatively low compared to the anterior transperitoneal approach. The major potential complication to consider is wound healing in the lumbosacral region. Patients who have pain localized to this region are often immobile and spend most of their time lying on their back and buttocks. This is an area that is high risk for infection as well as wound dehiscence, particularly if the patient had previous radiation or is undergoing active cancer therapy [28]. Though a cage or graft can be maneuvered into this space, the fixation for such anterior support is challenging as is demonstrated in this case. In these cases, fixation to the pelvis is critical to provide additional support across the lumbosacral junction.

A 67-year-old male with metastatic rectal carcinoma was admitted to the oncology service with severe back pain limiting any movement. He was known to have metastases to the sacrum. He developed urinary retention, saddle anesthesia, and so much pain that he laid flat in bed for weeks. He was treated with conventional external beam radiation to the sacrum approximately 8 weeks prior to admission. The radiation did not help his pain, and his narcotic requirement steadily increased. He underwent several cryoablation therapy treatments by interventional radiology to alleviate the pain which localized to the buttocks, particularly on the right side.

MRI showed severe sacral nerve root compression, epidural tumor, and diffuse sacral destruction at S1 due to tumor (Fig. 20.5). CT also showed the extent of the bony metastases and destruction within the sacrum. The bony involvement extended to the sacro-iliac joints bilaterally (Fig. 20.6).

Surgery was performed with the intent of stabilizing across the sacrum from L3 to the pelvis. The patient had a degenerative spondylolisthesis at L4–L5, so the instrumentation was extended to L3 to maximize the points of fixation. Given the concern for stability across the sacro-iliac joint, two iliac screws were placed on each side into the pelvis. An extensive sacral laminectomy was performed, decompressing the sacral nerve roots. The bone quality was poor, and a large cavity within the sacrum was eventually created by intralesional resection. On the right side of the sacrum, between the right L5, S1, and S2 nerve roots, a large gap was created by taking apart the sacral ala and drilling down the right S1 pedicle (Fig. 20.7). The bone did not bleed and the tumor itself was not vascular. It did not take much to curette the cancellous bone of the sacrum away from the ventral thecal sac and the S1, S2, S3, and S4 nerve roots. As seen on the pre-operative imaging, most of the compression was on the right side and this is where the bone was the

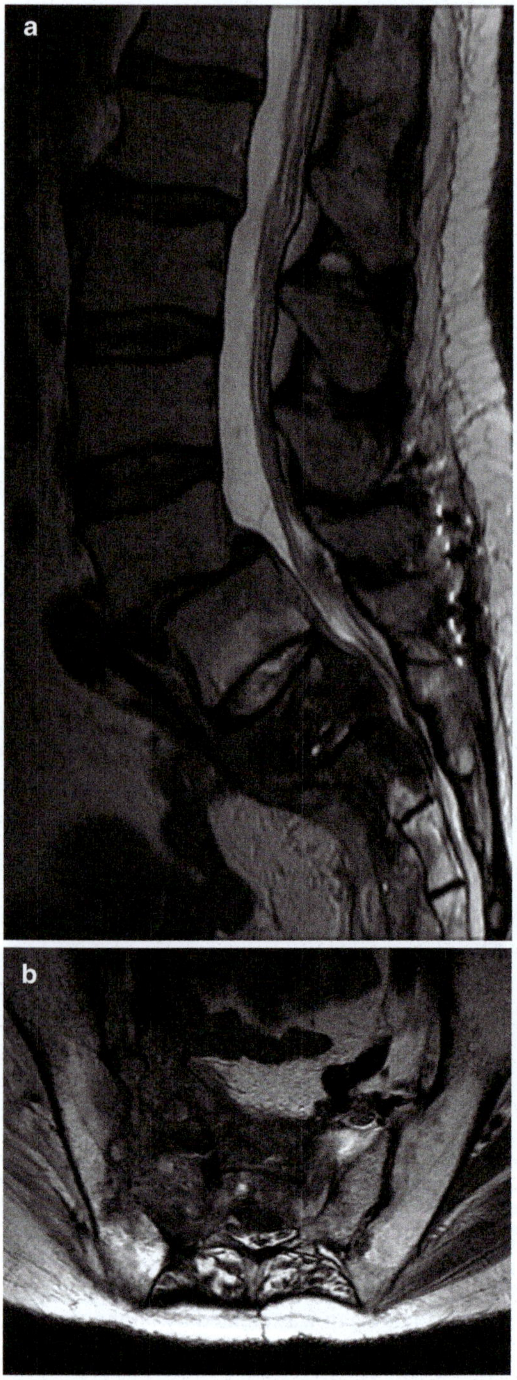

Fig. 20.5 (**a**) Pre-operative MRI, sagittal T2 sequence, shows metastases involving L5 and the sacrum with severe destruction of S1. There is a degenerative spondylolisthesis and stenosis at L4–L5. (**b**) Pre-operative MRI, axial T2 sequence, shows extensive sacral involvement and sacral nerve root compression from epidural extension

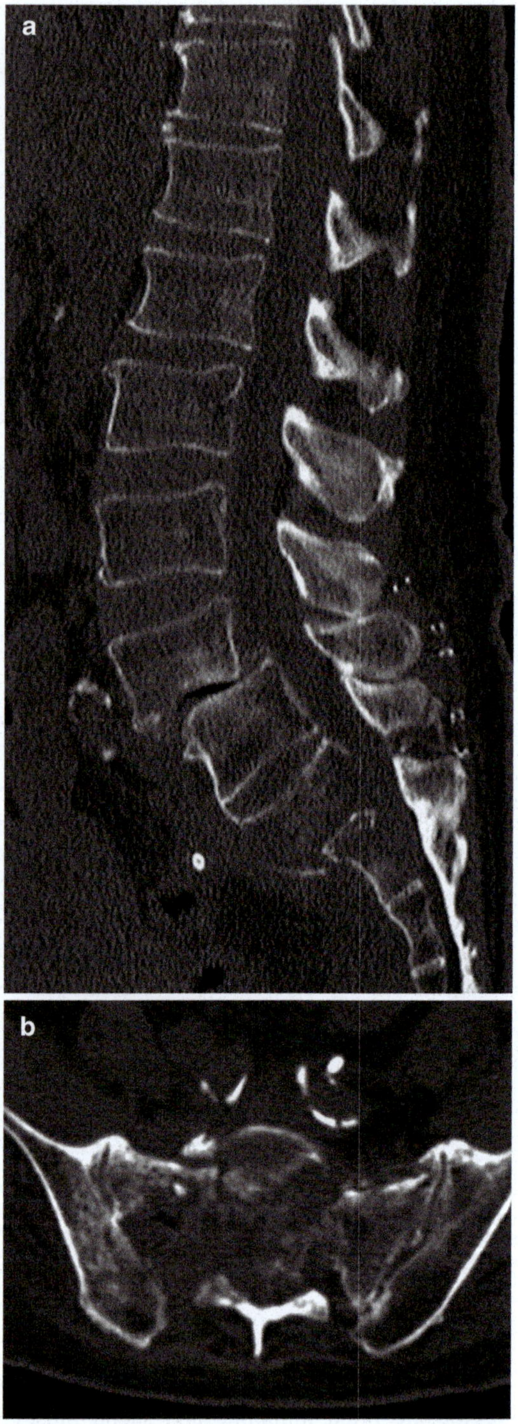

Fig. 20.6 (**a**) Pre-operative CT, sagittal, shows the extent of bone destruction in the sacrum and (**b**) pre-operative CT, axial, shows the extent of sacral tumor involvement to the sacro-iliac joints

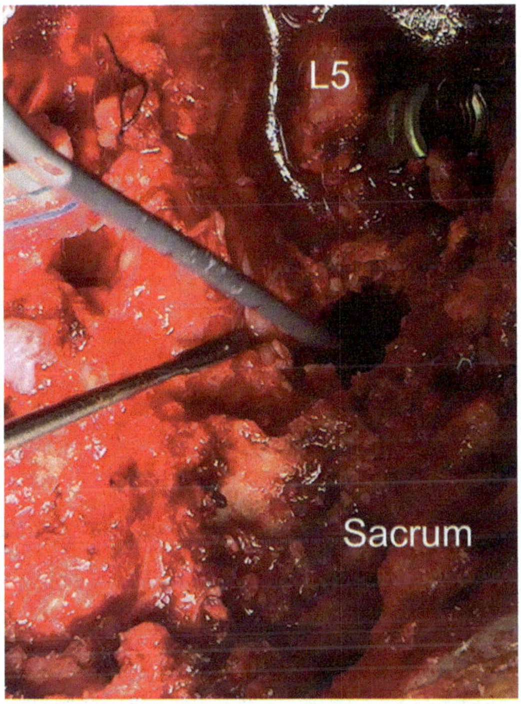

Fig. 20.7 Intraoperative photo, surgeon's view. The Penfield #4 instrument is retracting the right S1 nerve root. The right pedicle of S1 has been drilled down into the body of S1. The suction catheter is shown deep in this cavity

weakest. The right S1 pedicle was drilled down into the body of the sacrum. Various curettes were used to remove tumor and bone piecemeal away from the sacral nerve roots.

After the debulking was complete, the space ventral to the dura was reconstructed with a mesh titanium cage. This is typically not possible but with the lytic nature of bone, a cage was navigated between the nerve roots and into this space. An attempt was made to fill the gap between the inferior endplate of L5 and the stump of the remaining sacrum to provide some ventral support given the extensive destruction. Because so much of the lateral wing of the sacrum and iliac crest were destroyed by bone, a cage could be passed between the S1 and S2 nerve roots after being carefully sized. The cage was inserted perpendicular to the dura and then rotated 90 degrees once in the space between L5 and S2. The cage was wedged in as tightly as possible, but the purchase and fit on the inferior end was poor. This was due to the small shelf of bone at the S2 level and the size of the cage (Fig. 20.8).

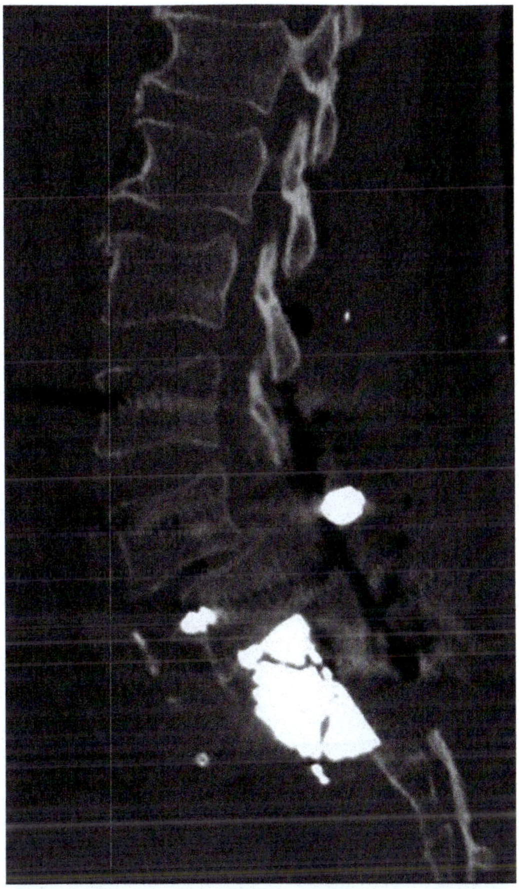

Fig. 20.8 Post-operative CT, sagittal, shows the construct and the cage sitting on the stump of S2. The sacrum, S1, was resected with an intralesional technique. Cement fills the cage

Cement was used to fill the cage and the area around the cage to provide additional stability. Cement was used instead of bone to fill the cage as arthrodesis was highly unlikely here given the previous radiation and the extent of cancer. Rods were contoured and locked in standard fashion (Fig. 20.9). An epidural pain catheter was inserted intraoperatively, and the patient had significant pain relief in subsequent days. The patient discharged to rehab where he could sit, stand, and take steps with a walker. This improvement was maintained for approximately 3 months at which time he passed due to cancer progression.

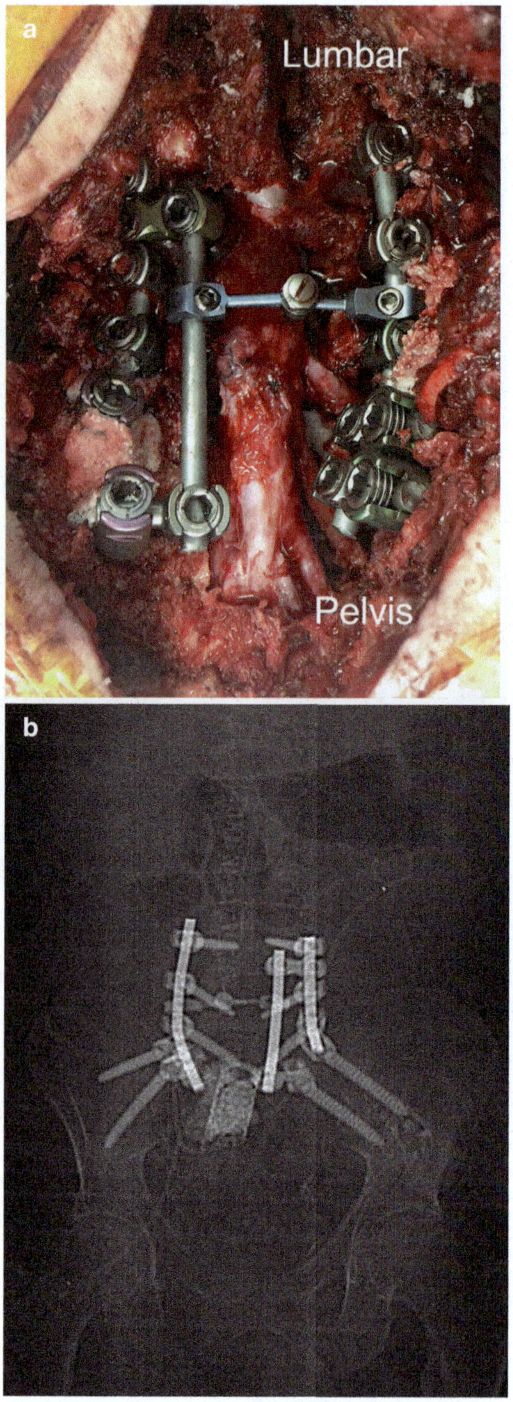

Fig. 20.9 (**a**) Intraoperative photo of the final surgical construct. The right S1, S2, 3, and S4 nerve roots are seen. The left-side sacral nerve roots are obscured by the rod. For orientation, this is a surgeon's view. The right side of the patient is on the right. The cement around the cage is seen between the S1 and S2 nerve roots on the right side. (**b**) Post-operative AP lumbar scout film from CT shows the multiple points of fixation. (**c**) Post-operative lateral lumbar scout film from CT

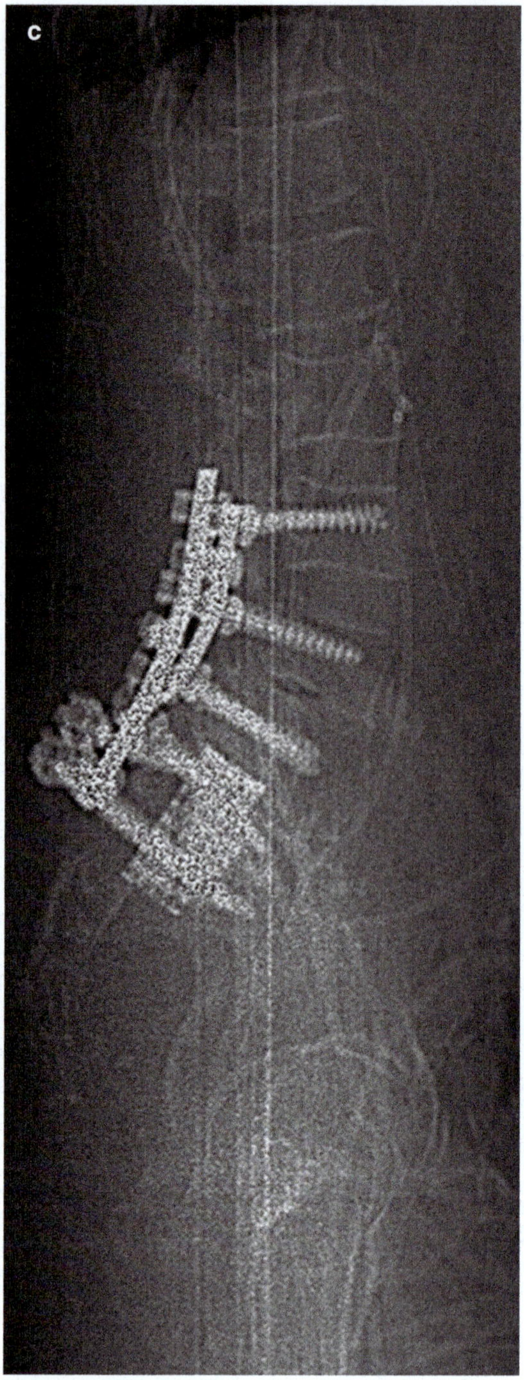

Fig. 20.9 (continued)

Conclusion

Intralesional tumor resection in the lumbar spine is the workhorse approach in the surgical treatment of spinal metastases where the goals of surgery are decompression and stabilization. Careful consideration to approach-related morbidity, particularly in the context of patients enduring cancer treatments, is critical to minimizing surgical complications and maximizing the benefit of spine surgery in this region.

References

1. Dea N, Charest-Morin R, Sciubba DM, Bird JE, Disch AC, Mesfin A, et al. Optimizing the adverse event and HRQOL profiles in the management of primary spine tumors. Spine (Phila Pa 1976). 2016;41(Suppl 20):S212–S7.
2. Laufer I, Zuckerman SL, Bird JE, Bilsky MH, Lazary A, Quraishi NA, et al. Predicting neurologic recovery after surgery in patients with deficits secondary to MESCC: systematic review. Spine (Phila Pa 1976). 2016;41(Suppl 20):S224–S30.
3. Glennie RA, Rampersaud YR, Boriani S, Reynolds JJ, Williams R, Gokaslan ZL, et al. A systematic review with consensus expert opinion of best reconstructive techniques after osseous en bloc spinal column tumor resection. Spine (Phila Pa 1976). 2016;41(Suppl 20):S205–S11.
4. Altaf F, Weber M, Dea N, Boriani S, Ames C, Williams R, et al. Evidence-based review and survey of expert opinion of reconstruction of metastatic spine tumors. Spine (Phila Pa 1976). 2016;41(Suppl 20):S254–S61.
5. Pennicooke B, Laufer I, Sahgal A, Varga PP, Gokaslan ZL, Bilsky MH, et al. Safety and local control of radiation therapy for chordoma of the spine and sacrum: a systematic review. Spine (Phila Pa 1976). 2016;41(Suppl 20):S186–S92.
6. Fehlings MG, Nater A, Tetreault L, Kopjar B, Arnold P, Dekutoski M, et al. Survival and clinical outcomes in surgically treated patients with metastatic epidural spinal cord compression: results of the prospective multicenter AOSpine study. J Clin Oncol. 2016;34(3):268–76.
7. Choi D, Fox Z, Albert T, Arts M, Balabaud L, Bunger C, et al. Rapid improvements in pain and quality of life are sustained after surgery for spinal metastases in a large prospective cohort. Br J Neurosurg. 2016;30(3):337–44.
8. Klimo P Jr, Schmidt MH. Surgical management of spinal metastases. Oncologist. 2004;9(2):188–96.
9. Laufer I, Rubin DG, Lis E, Cox BW, Stubblefield MD, Yamada Y, et al. The NOMS framework: approach to the treatment of spinal metastatic tumors. Oncologist. 2013;18(6):744–51.
10. Tomita K, Kawahara N, Kobayashi T, Yoshida A, Murakami H, Akamaru T. Surgical strategy for spinal metastases. Spine (Phila Pa 1976). 2001;26(3):298–306.
11. Chaichana KL, Pendleton C, Wolinsky JP, Gokaslan ZL, Sciubba DM. Vertebral compression fractures in patients presenting with metastatic epidural spinal cord compression. Neurosurgery. 2009;65(2):267–74. discussion 74-5.
12. Hu Y, Xia Q, Ji J, Miao J. One-stage combined posterior and anterior approaches for excising thoracolumbar and lumbar tumors: surgical and oncological outcomes. Spine (Phila Pa 1976). 2010;35(5):590–5.
13. Villavicencio AT, Oskouian RJ, Roberson C, Stokes J, Park J, Shaffrey CI, et al. Thoracolumbar vertebral reconstruction after surgery for metastatic spinal tumors: long-term outcomes. Neurosurg Focus. 2005;19(3):E8.
14. Walsh GL, Gokaslan ZL, McCutcheon IE, Mineo MT, Yasko AW, Swisher SG, et al. Anterior approaches to the thoracic spine in patients with cancer: indications and results. Ann Thorac Surg. 1997;64(6):1611–8.
15. Shankar GM, Clarke MJ, Ailon T, Rhines LD, Patel SR, Sahgal A, et al. The role of revision surgery and adjuvant therapy following subtotal resection of osteosarcoma of the spine: a systematic review with meta-analysis. J Neurosurg Spine. 2017;27(1):97–104.
16. Ailon T, Torabi R, Fisher CG, Rhines LD, Clarke MJ, Bettegowda C, et al. Management of locally recurrent chordoma of the mobile spine and sacrum: a systematic review. Spine (Phila Pa 1976). 2016;41(Suppl 20):S193–S8.
17. Salzmann SN, Shue J, Hughes AP. Lateral lumbar interbody fusion-outcomes and complications. Curr Rev Musculoskelet Med. 2017;10(4):539–46.
18. Zuckerman SL, Laufer I, Sahgal A, Yamada YJ, Schmidt MH, Chou D, et al. When less is more: the indications for MIS techniques and separation surgery in metastatic spine disease. Spine (Phila Pa 1976). 2016;41(Suppl 20):S246–S53.
19. Massicotte E, Foote M, Reddy R, Sahgal A. Minimal access spine surgery (MASS) for decompression and stabilization performed as an out-patient procedure for metastatic spinal tumours followed by spine stereotactic body radiotherapy (SBRT): first report of technique and preliminary outcomes. Technol Cancer Res Treat. 2012;11(1):15–25.
20. Muhlbauer M, Pfisterer W, Eyb R, Knosp E. Minimally invasive retroperitoneal approach for lumbar corpectomy and anterior reconstruction. Technical note. J Neurosurg. 2000;93(1 Suppl):161–7.
21. Ho JC, Tang C, Deegan BJ, Allen PK, Jonasch E, Amini B, et al. The use of spine stereotactic radiosurgery for oligometastatic disease. J Neurosurg Spine. 2016;25(2):239–47.
22. Moulding HD, Elder JB, Lis E, Lovelock DM, Zhang Z, Yamada Y, et al. Local disease control after decompressive surgery and adjuvant high-dose

single-fraction radiosurgery for spine metastases. J Neurosurg Spine. 2010;13(1):87–93.
23. Laufer I, Iorgulescu JB, Chapman T, Lis E, Shi W, Zhang Z, et al. Local disease control for spinal metastases following "separation surgery" and adjuvant hypofractionated or high-dose single-fraction stereotactic radiosurgery: outcome analysis in 186 patients. J Neurosurg Spine. 2013;18(3):207–14.
24. Hussain I, Barzilai O, Reiner AS, DiStefano N, McLaughlin L, Ogilvie S, et al. Patient-reported outcomes after surgical stabilization of spinal tumors: symptom-based validation of the spinal instability neoplastic score (SINS) and surgery. Spine J. 2017;18(2):261–7.
25. Street J, Fisher C, Sparkes J, Boyd M, Kwon B, Paquette S, et al. Single-stage posterolateral vertebrectomy for the management of metastatic disease of the thoracic and lumbar spine: a prospective study of an evolving surgical technique. J Spinal Disord Tech. 2007;20(7):509–20.
26. Sundaresan N, Galicich JH, Lane JM, Bains MS, McCormack P. Treatment of neoplastic epidural cord compression by vertebral body resection and stabilization. J Neurosurg. 1985;63(5):676–84.
27. Eleraky M, Setzer M, Vrionis FD. Posterior transpedicular corpectomy for malignant cervical spine tumors. Eur Spine J. 2010;19(2):257–62.
28. Mesfin A, Sciubba DM, Dea N, Nater A, Bird JE, Quraishi NA, et al. Changing the adverse event profile in metastatic spine surgery: an evidence-based approach to target wound complications and instrumentation failure. Spine (Phila Pa 1976). 2016;41(Suppl 20):S262–S70.

Lumbar En Bloc Resection

21

A. Karim Ahmed, Daniel M. Sciubba,
and Stefano Boriani

Introduction

The Enneking staging system [1] is a valid and reproducible tool for understanding and staging the biological behavior of bone and soft tissue tumors and for deciding the appropriate surgical procedure from an oncological point of view. This system is based on histological diagnosis and on clinical, laboratory, and imaging studies. One of the most relevant issues is also proposing a common terminology to the multidisciplinary team who take care of these diseases. Throughout this chapter, we make reference to Enneking's oncological terminology.

En bloc resection can be defined as a surgical procedure aiming to remove a tumoral mass in its entirety, fully covered by a continuous shell of healthy tissue. This shell is called "margin" and qualifies the procedure from an oncological point of view, affecting the local and systemic prognosis [2, 3]. This procedure became the golden standard in the treatment of bone tumors of the limbs in the 1970s, after the introduction of the protocols of neo-adjuvant chemotherapy. The effects of these new drugs on the tumoral mass (volume reduction, harder consistency) allowed development of techniques of surgical resection of the tumor without sacrificing the limb (so-called "limb salvage procedures") [4].

The problems to be faced in planning to perform in the spine a procedure fulfilling the same oncological criteria are included in the definition. Spinal cord, cauda equina, nerve roots, aorta, cava, vertebral artery, and so on can run inside the tumor margin or be involved by the tumor. These anatomical constraints can prevent a tumor-free margin en bloc resection, unless relevant sacrifices are accepted and important structures representing the margins are resected in the same specimen (Fig. 21.1).

Further, it should be considered that the epidural space is continuous from the foramen magnum to the sacrum, thus preventing not only a "radical" resection according to Enneking's terminology [4] (defined as en bloc removal of the tumor together with the whole compartment of origin) but even a difficult evaluation of the margins if the tumor encroaches the canal (Fig. 21.2).

Electronic Supplementary Material The online version of this chapter (https://doi.org/10.1007/978-3-319-98422-3_21) contains supplementary material, which is available to authorized users.

A. Karim Ahmed · D. M. Sciubba
Department of Neurosurgery, The Johns Hopkins Hospital, Baltimore, MD, USA

S. Boriani (✉)
IRCCS Galeazzi Orthopedic Institute, Spine Surgery Unit, Milan, Italy
e-mail: sb@stefanoboriani.eu

D. M. Sciubba (ed.), *Spinal Tumor Surgery*, https://doi.org/10.1007/978-3-319-98422-3_21

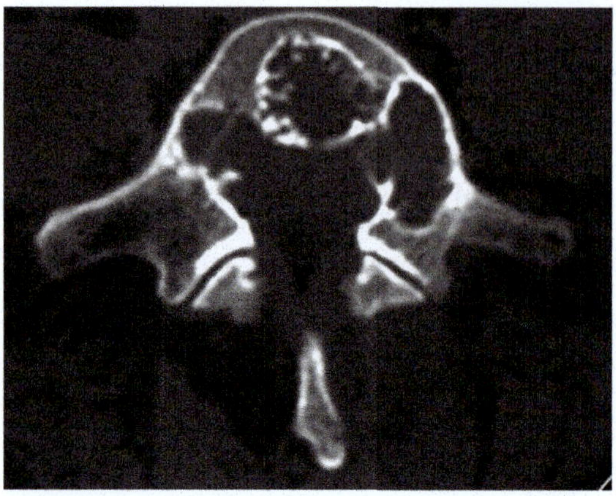

Fig. 21.1 CT scan of a chordoma of L5. The posterior wall is no longer visible; the margin at the canal is presumably very thin, if present at all

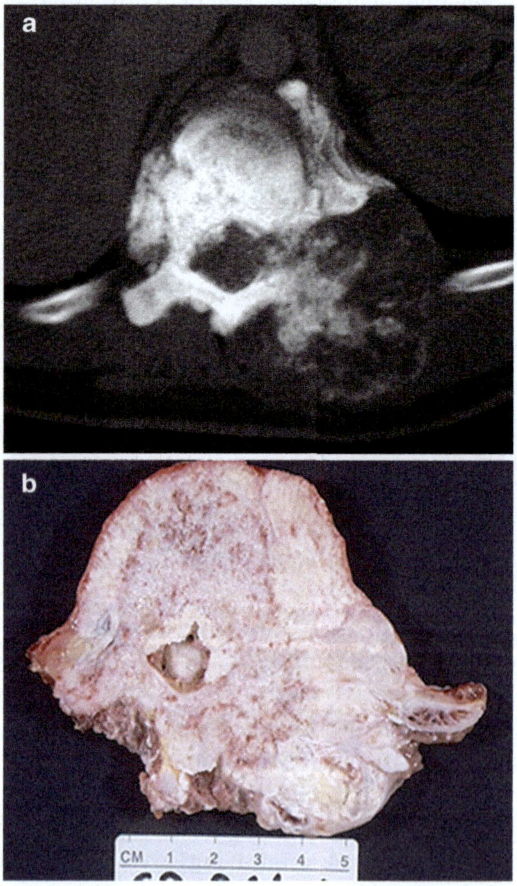

Fig. 21.2 (**a**) CT scan of T12 of an osteosarcoma T11–L1. Notwithstanding chemotherapy, the tumor involves the whole vertebra. (**b**) Specimen of the same case. To achieve a tumor-free margin, the vertebrae were resected together with the soft-tissue neoplastic content in the canal

Indications and Margins

En bloc resection is recommended in cases of benign aggressive (Enneking stage 3) tumors (i.e., osteoblastomas and giant-cell tumors) and low-grade malignant tumors (Enneking stage IA and B) like chordomas and chondrosarcomas. In high-grade malignancies (Enneking stage II) like osteosarcoma and Ewing sarcoma, chemotherapy and radiotherapy (RT) have a very relevant and essential role.

Once the resection is performed, the pathologist must carefully evaluate the tumor margins [2, 5], defined as "wide" (a relevant barrier like a fascia or at least healthy bone 1-cm thick), "marginal" (a thin barrier like periosteum), or "intralesional".

"Intralesional" resection is defined as when the surgeon incidentally or intentionally violates the tumor. Violation of the margins significantly worsens the prognosis [6]. Intentional intralesional resection may be an option when obtaining a surgical margin requires resection of functionally relevant tissue that is closely contiguous to the tumor or has been infiltrated by the tumor [7].

In cases where the tumor is growing in the epidural space, one may consider resecting the dura together with the tumor to achieve a tumor-free margin resection [8]. Dura covering the scar is only expected when the epidural space is occupied by scar, a frequent finding in cases of tumor recurrence. A cost-benefit assessment is required in situations where diagnosis and staging indicate the need for a wide margin that includes a structure such as a nerve root, whose sacrifice will result in functional or neurological compromise. The patient must be fully informed regarding the expected functional loss as well as the risk of recurrence with intentional intralesional resection. Specific techniques of en bloc resection have been published with the sacrifice of these structures: dura [8], cervical nerve roots [9, 10], cauda equina [11], spinal cord [12], major vascular structures, and visceral organs [13].

In addition, the decision-making process should also consider that the rates of complications and tumor recurrence are significantly higher for revision surgery [14, 15]. If the patient opts for preservation of the critical structure, adjuvant therapy is indicated. In patients with spinal metastases, surgery may be indicated in cases where tumors are resistant to radiation-based treatment and/or chemotherapy or there is current or impending risk of spinal instability or cord compression [16, 17]. En bloc resection with the primary goal of achieving complete local control should only be performed in selected cases of spinal metastases [18, 19]. The primary goal in these patients is to preserve or improve function and quality of life without unnecessary morbidity; thus, in principle, no functionally significant nerve root, for example, should be sacrificed when resecting a metastasis. In the authors' experience, the indication to en bloc resection is appropriate in single localizations, with full tumor control at the primary site and no involvement of visceral organs, best after long-term, disease-free evolution [20]. The key point in this decision is the lack of sensitivity to medical oncology or radiation oncology treatments; alternatively, less aggressive surgery could be combined with these treatments, reducing the surgical morbidity without reducing the possibility to local cure.

Surgical Planning

Surgical planning of en bloc resection in the spine, as in any other skeletal location, should be decided on a case-by case basis, related to the tumor extension and to the need of margin appropriate to the tumor aggressiveness. Bertil Stener was the first to apply to the spine the oncologic principles generally accepted for gastrointestinal tumors [21, 22]. His detailed reports of the surgical planning of en bloc resections are still an extremely useful and exhaustive guide to this procedure.

Conversely, Roy-Camille [23] and Tomita [24] popularized the techniques of en bloc resection by posterior approach without a specific concern on tumor extension and margin fulfilling. The Weinstein-Boriani-Biagini (WBB) surgical system for staging extensions of primary bone tumors of the spine (Fig. 21.3) was proposed in 1997 [25], adopted in several spine oncology centers and subjected to clinical evaluations [26]. More recently, the WBB system has been submitted to a study of reliability and validity by an international multidisciplinary group of spine tumor experts [27], resulting in a moderate interobserver reliability and substantial intraobserver reliability. The WBB staging system [25] focuses on the extent and location of the tumor. In the transverse plane, the vertebra is divided into 12 radiating zones (numbered 1 to 12 in an anti-clockwise order) and into five layers from the prevertebral to the dural involvement (A to E). The longitudinal extent of the tumor is recorded by identifying the specific vertebrae involved. This system allows for a more rational approach to the surgical planning, provided that all efforts are made to perform surgery along the required margins.

The WBB staging system [25] can be helpful in standardizing the surgical planning of en bloc resection according to the region of the spine and the tumor extent and location. The great variability of these two parameters dictates that the same surgical procedure as proposed by Roy-Camille [23] and Tomita [24] cannot be performed in all

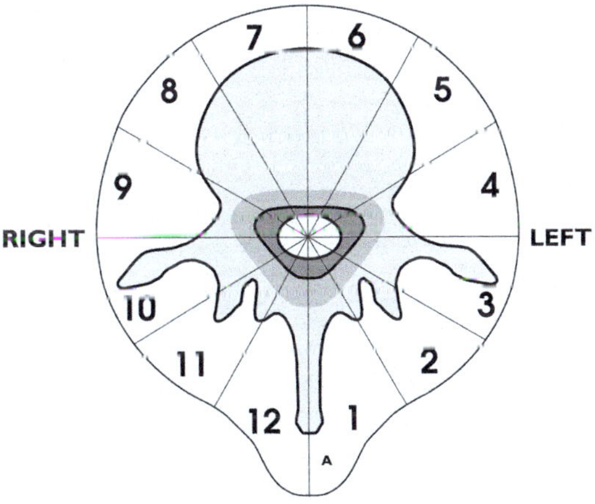

Fig. 21.3 WBB surgical staging system. In the transverse (axial) plane, the vertebra is divided into 12 radiating zones (numbered 1 to 12 in a counterclockwise order) and 5 layers ((**a**) extracompartmental peripheral tumor; (**b**) outer intracompartmental tumor; (**c**) inner intracompartmental tumor; (**d**) tumor inside the epidural space; (**e**) intradural tumor)

cases and that surgical planning is usually different for each case [28].

The WBB-guided planning of en bloc resection for spine tumors identifies 7 types of procedures, with several subgroups, ending in a total of 10 different surgical strategies. The types are defined by the approach or the combination of approaches: single anterior approach (type 1); single posterior approach (type 2) including three subtypes (a, b, c); anterior and then posterior approach (type 3) with three subtypes (a, b, c); first posterior approach, followed by both side anterior approaches (type 4); first posterior approach and then simultaneous anterior and re-opening of posterior approach (type 5); anterior, posterior, and then simultaneous anterior (contralateral) and re-opening of posterior approach (type 6, mostly performed for L5); and posterior approach as the first step and anterior approach as the second step (type 7, Fig. 21.4).

Type 1

The single anterior approach (Fig. 21.5) allows one to perform en bloc resection only of small tumors of the thoracic and lumbar vertebral bodies. These must be enclosed inside sectors 8–5, arising from layer A and B but not extending to layer C. In this case, in fact, a posterior approach is required to provide an appropriate margin under direct visual control by entering the canal and releasing the dura. This approach involves three steps. First, provide the appropriate margin over the anterior tumor growth by releasing the anterior structures from the tumor pseudocapsule or leaving the selected anatomical structures as margin (I). These are also the cases of direct bone invasion by contiguous tumor. Second, perform an osteotomy between the tumor and the posterior wall (II). Third, finalize the en bloc resection (III).

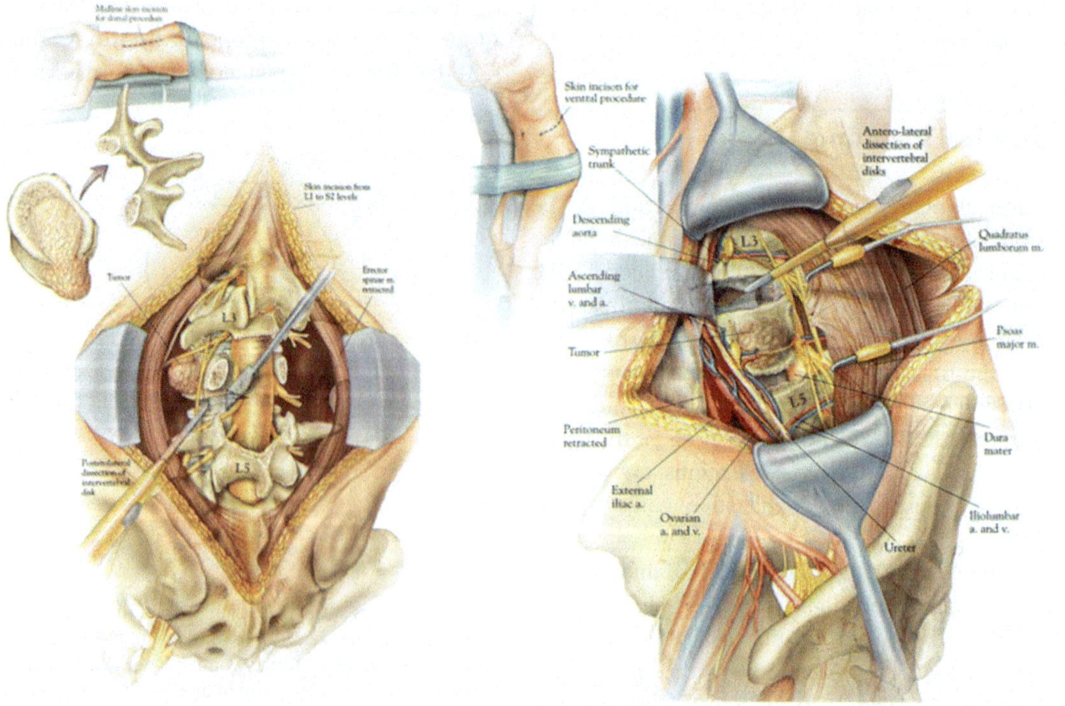

Fig. 21.4 En bloc lumbar spondylectomy with posterior decompression and anterior tumor resection. (Reprinted with permission from Marmor et al. [41])

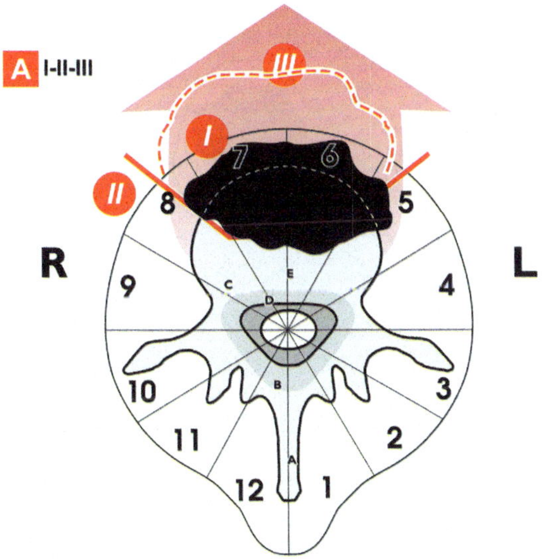

Fig. 21.5 Type 1 WBB-based en bloc resection. A single anterior approach allows one to perform en bloc resection of small tumors of the thoracic and lumbar vertebral bodies. These must be enclosed inside sectors 5–8, arising from layers A and B, without extension into layer C. In this case, a posterior approach is required to provide an appropriate margin, under direct visual control by entering the canal and releasing the dura. There are three steps: first, provide the appropriate margin over the growing anterior tumor by releasing the anterior structures from the tumor pseudocapsule (I); these are also the cases of direct bone invasion by contiguous tumor. Second, perform an osteotomy between the tumor and the posterior wall (II). Third, finalize the en bloc resection with removal of the tumor (III)

Type 2

The single posterior approach allows one to perform many different en bloc resections on tumors occurring in the posterior elements, either in the vertebral body or eccentrically located.

Type 2a

The single posterior approach is the obvious strategy to remove by en bloc resection a tumor arising in the posterior arch (Fig. 21.6a) in the cervical, thoracic, and lumbar spine. Criteria to achieve appropriate margins include sector 9 and 4 free from tumor. If the tumor grows in layer D, the margin will become intralesional during the release from the dura. This approach involves three steps: first, provide the appropriate margin over the tumor posteriorly growing by resecting inside the posterior muscles covering the tumor mass if it is expanding in layer A (I). The second step includes piecemeal excision of sectors 9 and 4 or osteotomy by wire saw or chisel or high-speed burr or ultrasound osteotome (II). This is obviously particularly delicate in the cervical spine, with higher risk of incidental violation of the margins. Once a transverse laminotomy is performed above and below, the tumor is released from the dura and the specimen is resected en bloc (III).

Type 2b

The single posterior approach with different surgical sequences allows removal by en bloc resection of a tumor arising in the vertebral body of a thoracic vertebra (Fig. 21.6b). Criteria to achieve an appropriate margin include sector 9 or 4 free from tumor. If the tumor grows in layer D, the margin will become intralesional during the release from the dura. If the tumor grows in layer A, the margin will become intralesional during the release from the anterior structures. This is the most popular technique of en bloc resection of a spine tumor, described by Roy-Camille [23] and later by Tomita [24]. This technique involves two steps: first, piecemeal excision of the posterior arch not involved by the tumor. At least four sectors are required, starting from sector 4 or from sector 9 (I). Release from the dura and section the nerve root(s) involved by the tumor. Second, blunt dissection of the anterior part of the vertebral body from the mediastinum, osteotomy, or discectomy above and below the tumor, full release from the dura, and finalizing the resection (II). The same technique described in Fig. 21.6b is difficult to apply to lumbar vertebrae. Digital blunt dissection of the anterior circumference is demanding or impossible due to the psoas muscle, the dimension of the vertebral body, and the major vessels kept closely connected to the spine by the transverse segmental vessels running between vertebral body and

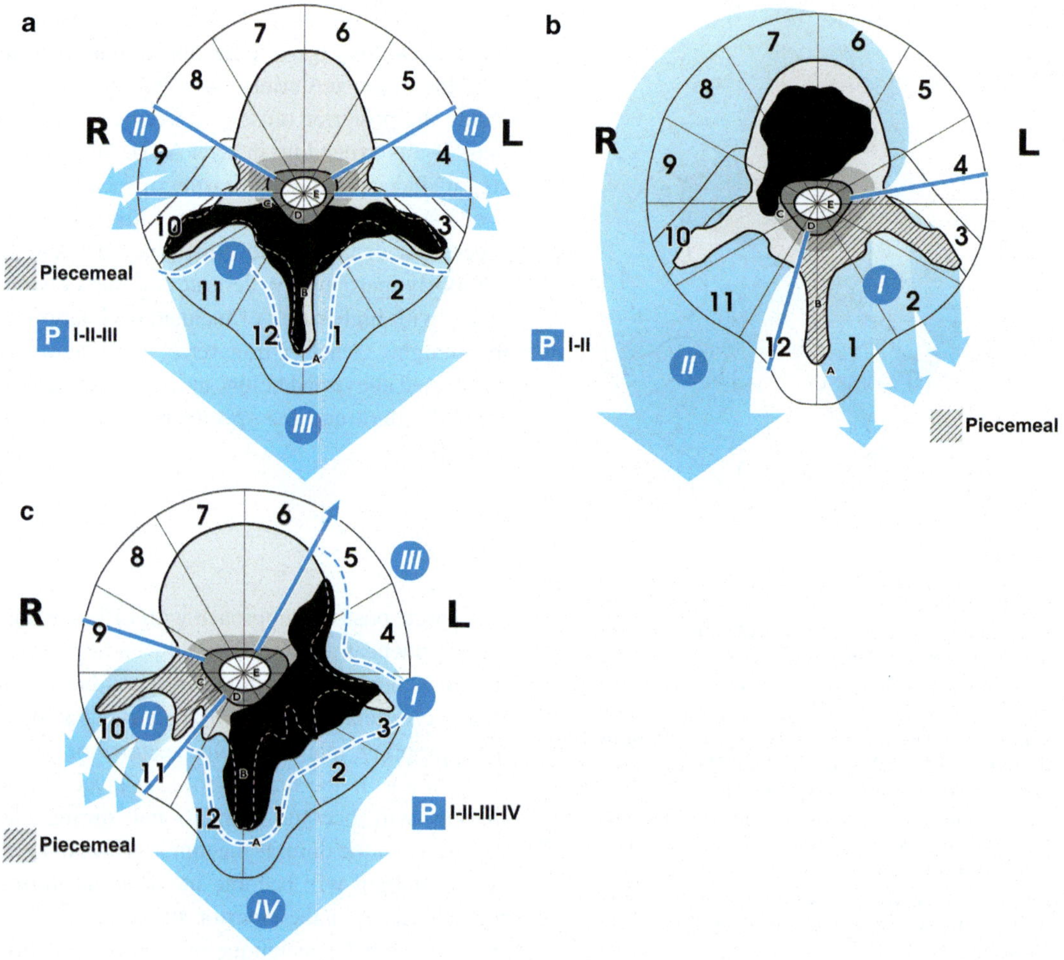

Fig. 21.6 (**a**) Type 2a WBB-based en bloc resection. Single posterior approach is the best strategy to facilitate en bloc resection of a tumor arising from the posterior arch. Criteria to achieve an appropriate margin include sector 9 and 4 free from tumor. If the tumor grows in layer D, the margin will become intralesional during the release from the dura. There are three steps: first, provide the appropriate margin over the tumor growing posteriorly by resecting inside the posterior muscles covering the tumor mass if it is expanding in layer A (I); second, piecemeal excision of sectors 9 and 4 or osteotomy by wire saw, chisel, high-speed burr, or ultrasound osteotome (II). After performing a transverse laminotomy above and below, the tumor is released from the dura and the specimen is resected en bloc (III). (**b**) Type 2b WBB-based en bloc resection, single posterior approach. It allows removal by en bloc resection of a tumor arising in the vertebral body of a thoracic vertebra. Criteria to achieve appropriate margins include sector 9 or 4 free from tumor. If the tumor grows in layer D, the margin will become intralesional during the release from the dura. If the tumor grows in layer A, the margin will become intralesional during the release from the anterior structures. There are two steps. The first includes piecemeal excision of the posterior arch not involved by the tumor. At least four sectors are required, starting from sector 4 or from sector 9(I). Release from the dura and section of the nerve root(s) involved by the tumor. Second, blunt dissection of the anterior part of the vertebral body from the mediastinum, osteotomy, or discectomy above and below the tumor, full release from the dura, and finalizing the resection (II). (**c**) Type 2c WBB-based en bloc resection. Single posterior approach with sagittal osteotomy. A tumor eccentrically growing in thoracic or lumbar spine (Fig. 21.9) can be removed en bloc by single posterior approach, provided the body is not involved over sector 5 at left and over sector 8 at right. At least three sectors posteriorly must not be involved by the tumor (from 4 to 1–2 or from 12–11 to 9). There are four steps: first, provide appropriate margin over the tumor posteriorly growing by resecting inside the posterior muscles covering the tumor mass if it is expanding in layer A (I). The release will proceed laterally until the lateral side of the vertebral body. In the thoracic spine (Fig. 21.7), the pleura can be left on the tumor; in the lumbar spine (Fig. 21.9), the posterior part of the psoas must be dissected but the segmental vessels must be found and ligated. The second step is piecemeal excision of the posterior arch not involved by the tumor. Approach the canal, release the dura from the tumor (if the tumor grows in layer D, the margin will become intralesional), and section the nerve root(s) involved by the tumor. The third step includes carefully displacing the dura and performing an osteotomy from posterior to anterior in sector 8 or 5. The specimen is finally removed (IV)

psoas. In these cases, the approaches defined as types 3b and c (Fig. 21.7b, c) and 5 (Fig. 21.9) or 7 (see Fig. 21.11) seem more appropriate and safe.

Type 2c

The single posterior approach with sagittal osteotomy is illustrated above (Fig. 21.6c). A tumor eccentrically growing in thoracic and lumbar spine can be removed en bloc by the single posterior approach (type 2c), provided the body is not involved over sector 5 at left and over sector 8 at right. At least three sectors posteriorly must be not involved by the tumor (from 4 to 1–2 or from 12 11 to 9). This approach involves four steps. First provide appropriate margin over the tumor posteriorly growing by resecting inside the posterior muscles covering the tumor mass if it is expanding in layer A (I). The release will proceed laterally until one reaches the lateral side of the vertebral body. In the thoracic spine, the pleura can be left on the tumor; in the lumbar spine, the posterior part of the psoas must be dissected, and the segmental vessels must be found and ligated. The second step is piecemeal excision of the posterior arch not involved by the tumor. It involves approach to the canal, release of the dura from the tumor (if the tumor grows in layer D, the margin will be intralesional), and section of the nerve root(s) involved by the tumor. The third step includes displacing the dura carefully and performing osteotomy from posterior to anterior in sector 8 or 5. The specimen is finally removed (IV).

Type 3a

Besides anterior approach first, posterior second should also be considered in cervical spine tumors partially occupying the vertebral body (not involving sector 6 and 7—otherwise type 4 is suggested) and the posterior arch (at least three sectors not involved) (Fig. 21.7a). The anterior approach is first performed to leave healthy tissue over the tumor growing in the lateral masses (I) and to perform a sagittal groove till the epidural space in the vertebral body (II).

Discectomies or transverse grooves in vertebral bodies are performed to define the upper and lower margins, including ligation of the vertebral artery. The second stage is a posterior approach. The third step provides appropriate margin over the tumor posteriorly growing by resecting inside the posterior muscles covering the tumor mass if it is expanding in layer A. The fourth step is a piecemeal excision of the posterior arch not involved by the tumor. At least three sectors are required, starting from sector 4 or from sector 9. This allows release of the dura from the tumor and section of the nerve root(s) involved by the tumor. Finally, the specimen is removed—once the upper and lower discectomies or osteotomies have been finalized—by rotating around the dural sac (V).

Type 3b

A sequential combination of two approaches (anterior first, posterior second) in the thoracic and in the lumbar spine is proposed (Fig. 21.7b) when the vertebral body tumor grows anteriorly in layer A; in this case, an anterior approach must be performed as the first step to provide a wide/marginal margin under visual control. In case of tumors mostly occupying the vertebral body, the anterior approach can be the first step to release from mediastinum in the thoracic spine or retroperitoneal in the lumbar spine, eventually leaving involved structures as margin (I). A sheet of silastic or similar can be left as protection. Second stage, posterior approach: piecemeal excision of the posterior arch not involved by the tumor (II). At least three to four sectors are required, starting from sector 4 or from sector 9. Release the dura from the tumor, section the nerve root(s) involved by the tumor, and then provide appropriate margin over the tumor posteriorly growing by resecting inside the posterior muscles covering the tumor mass if it is expanding in layer A (III). Finally, the specimen is removed by rotating around the dural sac (IV). This technique requires

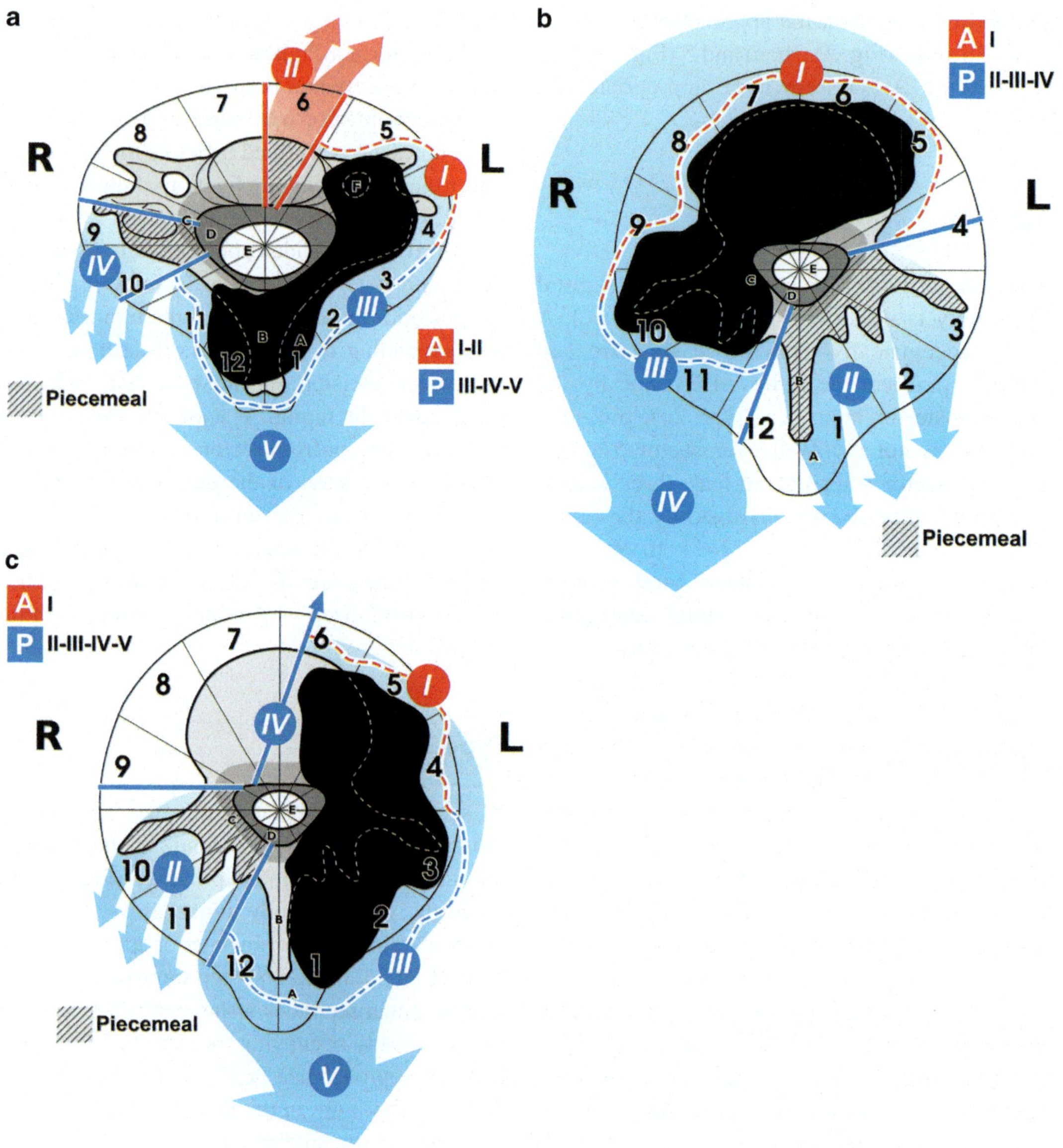

Fig. 21.7 (**a**) Type 3a WBB-based en bloc resection. When the tumor is growing anteriorly (layer A), an anterior approach must be performed as a first step to provide a wide/marginal margin under visual control. In tumors mostly occupying the vertebral body, the anterior approach can be the first step to release from mediastinum or retroperitoneal, eventually leaving involved structures as margin (I). A sheet of silastic or similar material can be left as protection. The second stage, posterior approach, involves piecemeal excision of the posterior arch not involved by the tumor (II). At least three to four sectors are required, starting from sector 4 or from sector 9. Release the dura from the tumor, section the nerve root(s) involved by the tumor, then provide the appropriate margin over the posteriorly growing tumor by resecting inside the posterior muscles covering the tumor mass if it is expanding in layer A (III). Finally, the specimen is removed by rotating around the dural sac (IV). (**b**) Type 3b WBB-based en bloc resection. In the cervical spine, three approaches can be required: posterior, anterior contralateral to the tumor side, and anterior on the tumor side. The combined simultaneous second and third approaches are required if the tumor is particularly huge, extending over the midline
The first step is in the prone position and involves piecemeal excision of the posterior arch not involved by the tumor. At least three sectors are required, starting from sector 4 or from sector 9(I). In case of tumor growing posteriorly and invading layer A, an appropriate margin must be provided by resecting inside the posterior muscles covering the tumor mass (II). Then release the dura from the tumor (if the tumor grows in layer D, the margin will become intralesional) and section the nerve root(s)

sectioning at least a nerve root in order to rotate the specimen around the thecal sac when removing from the posterior approach. If the nerve roots are not involved by the tumor and are functionally relevant, it is better to plan a type 5 resection (Fig. 21.8).

Type 3c

The same sequence of approaches is followed: anterior first and posterior second in case of tumor eccentrically growing in the thoracic and lumbar spine (Fig. 21.7c) when sagittal osteotomy is considered safe for appropriate margin, without the need to remove the whole vertebral body. In the first step the anterior approach provides a wide/marginal margin under visual control, releasing from mediastinum in the thoracic spine or from peritoneal in the lumbar spine, eventually leaving involved structures as margin (I). Discectomies or transverse grooves in vertebral bodies are performed to define the upper and lower margins. A sheet of silastic or any other tissue can be left as protection, to be removed during the final tumor removal. Second stage, posterior approach: piecemeal excision of the posterior arch not involved by the tumor. At least three sectors are required, starting from sector 4 or from sector 9 (II). Then provide the appropriate margin over the tumor posteriorly growing by resecting inside the posterior muscles covering the tumor mass if it expands in layer A (III). Release of the dura from the tumor, section of the nerve roots crossing the tumor, and osteotomy posterior to anterior at some distance from the tumor in order to leave uninvolved bone as margin comprise step IV. The resected specimen can be finally removed (V) once the upper and lower discectomies or osteotomies are finalized.

Type 4

In some huge tumors of the cervical spine, extending over the midline, three approaches are required for a safe and oncologically appropriate surgery: first posterior; second anterior contralateral to the tumor side; and third anterior on the tumor side (Fig. 21.8). First step in the prone position: piecemeal excision of the posterior arch not involved by the tumor. At least three sectors are required, starting from sector 4 or from sector 9 (I). In case of tumor posteriorly growing, and invading layer A, an appropriate margin must be provided by resecting inside the posterior muscles covering the tumor mass (II). Then release the dura from the tumor (if the tumor grows in layer D, the margin will be intralesional) and section the nerve root(s) crossing the tumor. Second and third steps are in supine position, second stage. A sagittal grove is performed in the vertebral body not occupied by the tumor (III) till the vertebral artery, which must be saved, as the other is involved by the tumor and must be sacrificed. The anterior margin is provided by leaving healthy soft tissue over the tumor mass (IV). Discectomies or transverse grooves in vertebral bodies are performed to define the upper and lower margins [29, 30]. The tumor is finally removed by the third approach (V), once the upper and lower discectomies or osteotomies are finalized, including ligation of the vertebral artery.

Type 5

Two stages—posterior approach and contemporary anterior and posterior approaches (patient positioned on the side) —can be the most appropriate for lumbar tumors expanding anteriorly. This technique was described by Roy-Camille for lumbar tumors [31] and is associated with the

crossing the tumor. The second and third steps are in supine position. In the second stage, a sagittal groove is performed in the vertebral body not occupied by the tumor (III), until the vertebral artery, which must be saved, as the other is involved by the tumor and must be sacrificed. The anterior margin is provided by leaving healthy soft tissue over the tumor mass (IV). Discectomies or transversal grooves in vertebral bodies are performed to define the upper and lower margins. The tumor is finally removed by the third approach (V) on finalizing the upper and lower discectomies or osteotomies, including ligation of the vertebral artery.

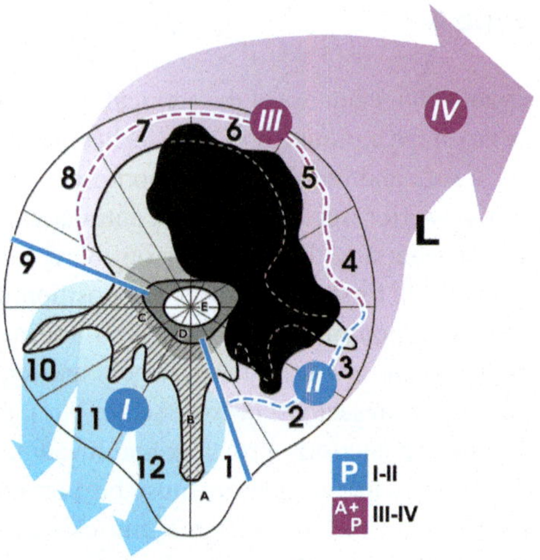

Fig. 21.8 Type 4 WBB-based en bloc resection. This is completed in two stages, first posteriorly, followed by an anterior resection. In the posterior approach, the laminae and posterior elements are removed in a piecemeal fashion to remain clear of the tumor capsule. An appropriate margin is subsequently created by resection of the surrounding soft-tissue structures. In the anterior approach the contralateral anterior column structures are resected, and an appropriate margin is made circumferentially releasing the tumor from all surrounding soft-tissue structures and underlying dura. The tumor may then be delivered, en bloc, through the anterior exposure

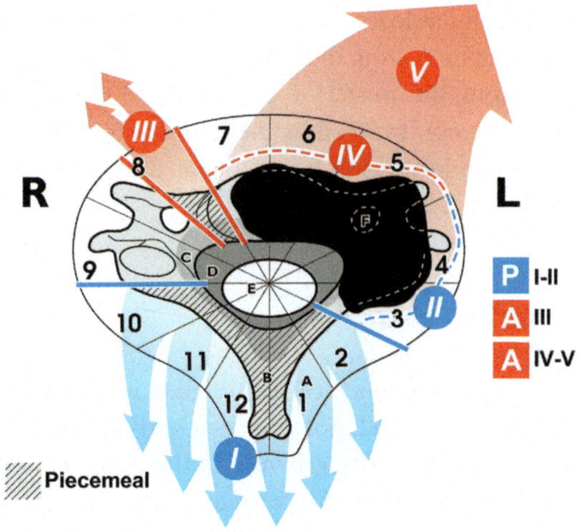

Fig. 21.9 Type 5 WBB-based en bloc resection. First steps in prone position: piecemeal excision of the posterior arch not involved by the tumor. At least three sectors are required, starting from sector 4 or from sector 9 (I). In a tumor posteriorly growing and invading layer A, an appropriate margin must be provided by resecting inside the posterior muscles covering the tumor mass (II). Then release the dura from the tumor (if the tumor grows in layer D, the margin will be intralesional) and section the nerve root(s) crossing the tumor. Discectomies or transversal grooves in vertebral bodies are performed to define the upper and lower margins. The Second stage is in lateral position. It includes antero-lateral approach (thoracotomy, thoraco-abdominal, retroperitoneal) and re-opening of the posterior approach. In order to provide appropriate margin over the tumor, it must remain covered by pleura or by psoas (III). Spiral wires are used to embolize the segmental arteries to ease the release of the aorta on the contralateral side. On finalizing the upper and lower discectomies or osteotomies, the specimen is removed by combined maneuvers (IV)

highest rate of morbidity and complications [15]. As an advantage compared to Type 3a (Fig. 21.7b), no nerve roots are sacrificed if not involved by the tumor.

First steps in prone position: piecemeal excision of the posterior arch not involved by the tumor. At least three sectors are required, starting from sector 4 or from sector 9 (I) (Fig. 21.9). In case of tumor posteriorly growing, and invading layer A, an appropriate margin must be provided by resecting inside the posterior muscles covering the tumor mass (II). Then release the dura from the tumor (if the tumor grows in layer D, the margin will be intralesional) and section the nerve root(s) crossing the tumor. Discectomies or transversal grooves in vertebral bodies are performed to define the upper and lower margins. Second stage in lateral position includes antero-lateral approach (thoracotomy, thoraco-abdominal, retroperitoneal) and re-opening of the posterior approach. In order to provide appropriate margin over the tumor, it must remain covered by pleura or by psoas (III). Spiral wires are used to embolize the segmental arteries to make easier the release of the aorta on the contralateral side. On finalizing the upper and lower discectomies or osteotomies, the specimen is removed by combined maneuvers (IV).

Type 6

Three approaches should be planned to resect a tumor of L5: first anterior on the contralateral side of the tumor; second posterior; and third contemporary anterior and posterior approaches

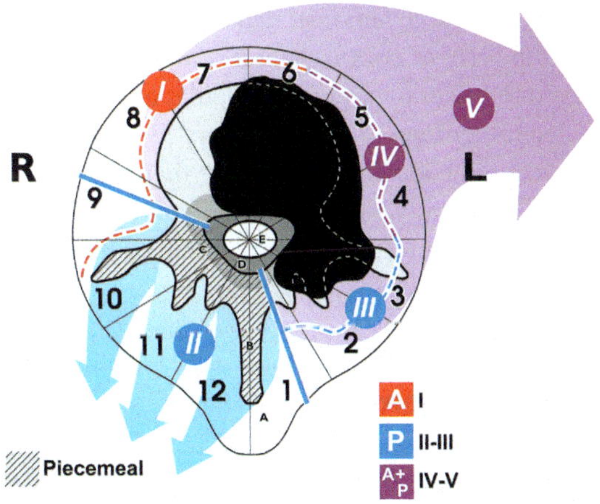

Fig. 21.10 Type 6 WBB-based en bloc resection. To perform en bloc resection of a tumor of L5, a double anterior approach is mostly required to fully release the aorta/cava bifurcation. Our technique includes (1) anterior approach on the contralateral side of the tumor, (2) posterior approach, and (3) contemporary anterior and posterior approaches. The first step in supine position involves release of the aorta/cava bifurcation and partial discectomies or osteotomies to define upper and lower margins (I). The second stage in prone position involves piecemeal excision of the posterior arch not involved by the tumor. At least three sectors are required, starting from sector 4 or from sector 9 (II). In case of tumor growing posteriorly and invading layer A, an appropriate margin must be provided by resecting inside the posterior muscles covering the tumor mass (III). Then release the dura from the tumor (if the tumor grows in layer D, the margin will be intralesional) and section the nerve root(s) crossing the tumor. Discectomies or transverse grooves in vertebral bodies are performed. The third stage in lateral position involves a retroperitoneal approach and re-opening of the posterior approach. In step 4, provide appropriate margin over the tumor by leaving it covered by psoas. Then finalize the discectomies or transverse grooves in vertebral bodies to remove the specimen by the anterior approach (V)

(Fig. 21.10). The double anterior approach is required to safely release the aorta/cava bifurcation.

First step in supine position: release the aorta/cava bifurcation and partial discectomies or osteotomies to define upper and lower margins (I). Second stage in prone position: piecemeal excision of the posterior arch not involved by the tumor. At least three sectors are required, starting from sector 4 or from sector 9 (II). In case of tumor posteriorly growing, and invading layer A, an appropriate margin must be provided by resecting inside the posterior muscles covering the tumor mass (III). Then release the dura from the tumor (if the tumor grows in layer D, the margin will be intralesional) and section the nerve root(s) crossing the tumor. Discectomies or transversal grooves in vertebral bodies are performed. Third stage in lateral position: retroperitoneal approach and re-opening of the posterior approach. The fourth stage includes providing appropriate margin over the tumor by leaving it covered by psoas. Then, finalize the discectomies or transversal grooves in vertebral bodies to remove the specimen by the anterior approach (V).

Type 7

This strategy came last in the author's 25 years' experience. It is indicated in thoracic and lumbar tumors growing anteriorly—even huge masses—in layer A without involvement of the canal (layer D) and without involvement of sectors 4 and 9 (Fig. 21.11). This strategy allows to remove huge tumors without torsion around the spinal cord but requires both pedicles free from tumor for appropriate margins. It is mandatory to achieve posteriorly a full release of posterior anatomical elements and spine–dural connection, as in supine position no access will be possible. First steps in prone position: piecemeal excision of the posterior arch and both pedicles and very careful full dura release. Discectomies or transverse grooves in vertebral bodies are performed to define the upper and lower margins. Second stage is in supine position. Step III is release of the anatomical structures from the tumor mass or even their sacrifice to provide appropriate margin under visual control. Arterial bypass can be performed in case of aorta involvement. On finalizing the upper and lower discectomies or osteotomies, the specimen is removed by combined maneuvers (IV).

In planning the surgical procedure, the cord vascularity must be considered. During these procedures, particularly when the thoraco-lumbar resection is multilevel or the tumor particularly huge, the functional integrity of the spinal cord is at risk mostly due to the manipulation of the cord during maneuvers to deliver the tumor.

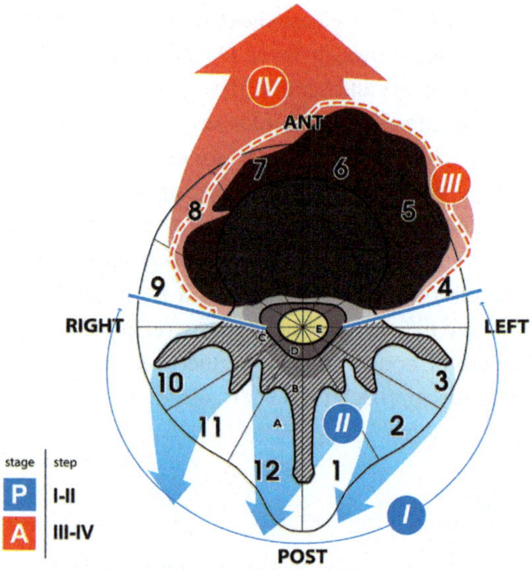

Fig. 21.11 Type 7 WBB-based en bloc resection. It is indicated in thoracic and lumbar tumors that are growing anteriorly—even huge masses—in layer A without involvement of the canal (layer D) and without involvement of sectors 4 and 9. This strategy allows removal of huge tumors without torsion around the spinal cord but requires both pedicles to be free from tumors for appropriate margins. It is mandatory to achieve by posterior approach a full release of posterior anatomical elements and spine–dural connection, as in the supine position no access will be possible. First steps in prone position are piecemeal excision of the posterior arch and both pedicles and very careful full dura release. Discectomies or transverse grooves in vertebral bodies are performed to define the upper and lower margins. The second stage is in supine position. Step 3 is release of the anatomical structures from the tumor mass or even their sacrifice to provide appropriate margin under visual control. Arterial bypass can be performed in case of aorta involvement. On finalizing the upper and lower discectomies or osteotomies, the specimen is removed by combined maneuvers (IV)

The role of the artery of Adamkiewicz as a single, exclusive feeding of the anterior spinal artery is controversial [32]. It seems reasonable that cord vascularity is not dependent on one artery. Previously we performed (unpublished data) angiographic studies before surgery to identify the radiculo-medullary artery feeding the artery of Adamkiewicz. In four cases the nerve root was sacrificed without any damage to cord vascularity. Since then, the role of such a study was felt to be less critical and did not affect the planning. Tomita and his group had the same experience and demonstrated on an animal model that the risk of cord ischemia is mostly related to the number of contiguous radicular arteries sacrificed rather than to a single artery [33–35]. It can be recommended to cut no more than three nerve roots bilaterally in the thoracic spine and avoid acute shortening or distraction during the resection [36].

Complications

The morbidity associated with en bloc resections is high, as the risks and complications of anterior spine surgery are combined with those of major posterior surgery. Tumor surgery also has specific morbidity related to the need for dissecting through muscle and not through anatomical planes; further, en bloc resection requires sacrificing not only the affected bone but also almost all connecting elements, creating full instability. Previous surgery and previous radiation therapy increase the risk of complications related to dissection. Infection is particularly threatening, due to the compromised immune status of many of these patients. Late aortic dissection is reported mostly in multi-operated cases including aorta release and submitted to monoportal high-dose conventional RT. Non-union is a common late complication due to the environment hostile to solid bony fusion. Mortality is not negligible, with a rate of 2.2% [15].

Case-Based Planning of Lumbar En Bloc Resection

A 62-year-old male presents with complaints of back pain lasting 1 year. Previous standard radiograms were reported as negative. The standard radiogram performed at admittance (Fig. 21.12a) shows both L3 endplates as partially collapsed. The cancellous bone architecture of the body is altered with a pattern similar to columnar changes. Magnetic resonance imaging (MRI) (T2 weighted) shows multiple hyperlucent images in T12, L1, L3, L4, and L5. There is pathologic fracture of L3 with protrusion in the canal

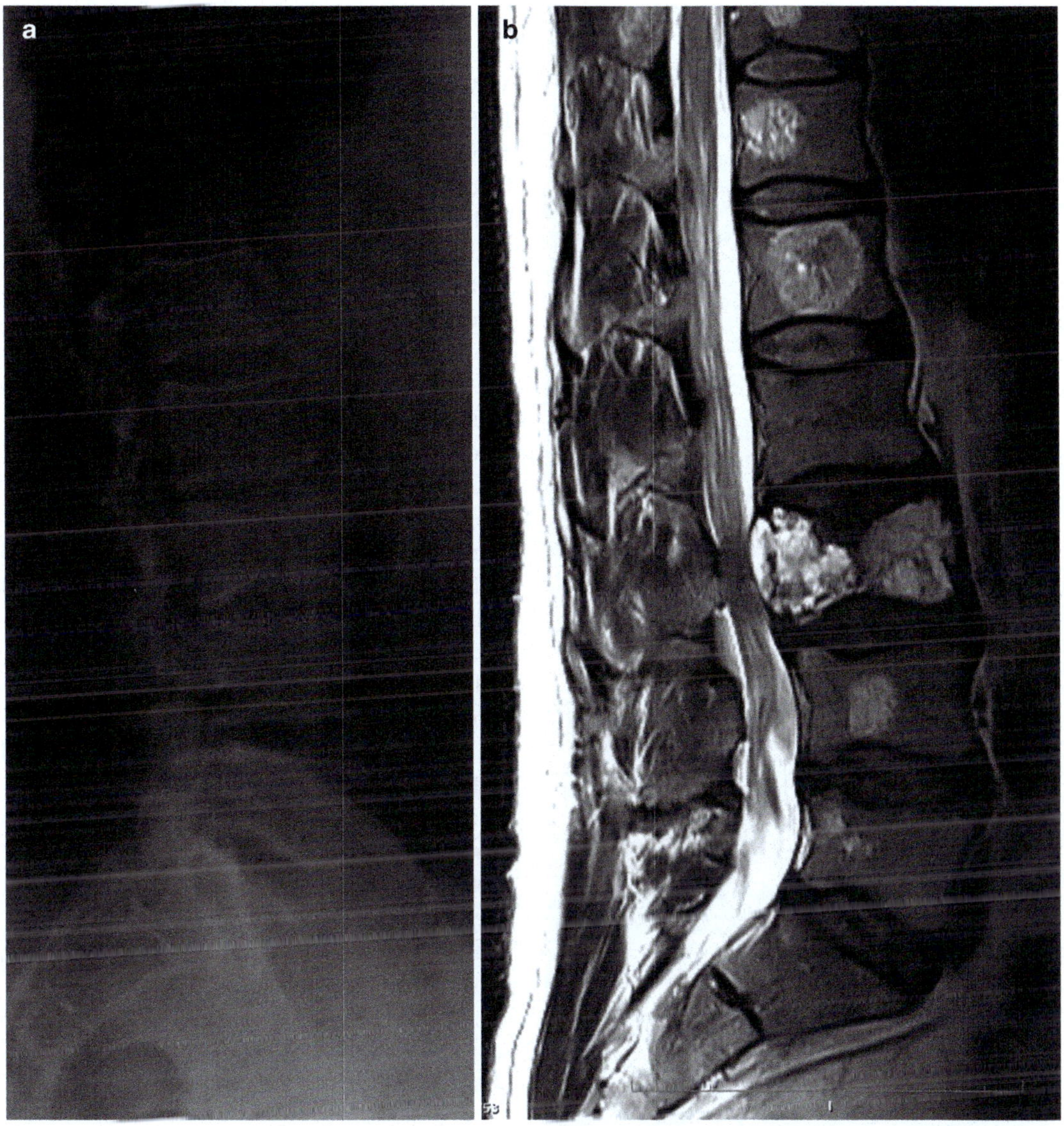

Fig. 21.12 Man, 62 years old. (**a**) Standard radiogram; (**b**) MRI T2-weighted imaging; (**c**) MRI T1-weighted imaging; (**d**) MRI T2-weighted imaging. Transverse section

(Fig. 21.12b). The T1-weighted images show that only L3 changes from hyper- to hypolucent (Fig. 21.12c), consistent with the hypothesis of hemangiomas in T12, L1, L4, and L5. The transverse section of L3 shows that the tumor erodes the periphery of the vertebral body and expands into the psoas muscle (extracompartmental in layer A) and encroaches the canal (extracompartmental or tumor bulging in layer D). Computed tomography (CT) scan confirms the lytic lesion of L3 with erosion of the cortex (Fig. 21.13a). In L1 (Fig. 21.13b) and L4 (Fig. 21.13c), the images are consistent with hemangioma. The sagittal reconstruction (Fig. 21.13d) confirms the erosion of L3 with pathologic fracture and collapse of the cranial endplate. The pattern of the images in L1 and in L4 is more consistent with hemangioma. A CT-guided biopsy (Fig. 21.14) allows the histological diagnosis of chordoma. The Enneking staging is therefore IB (low-grade malignant,

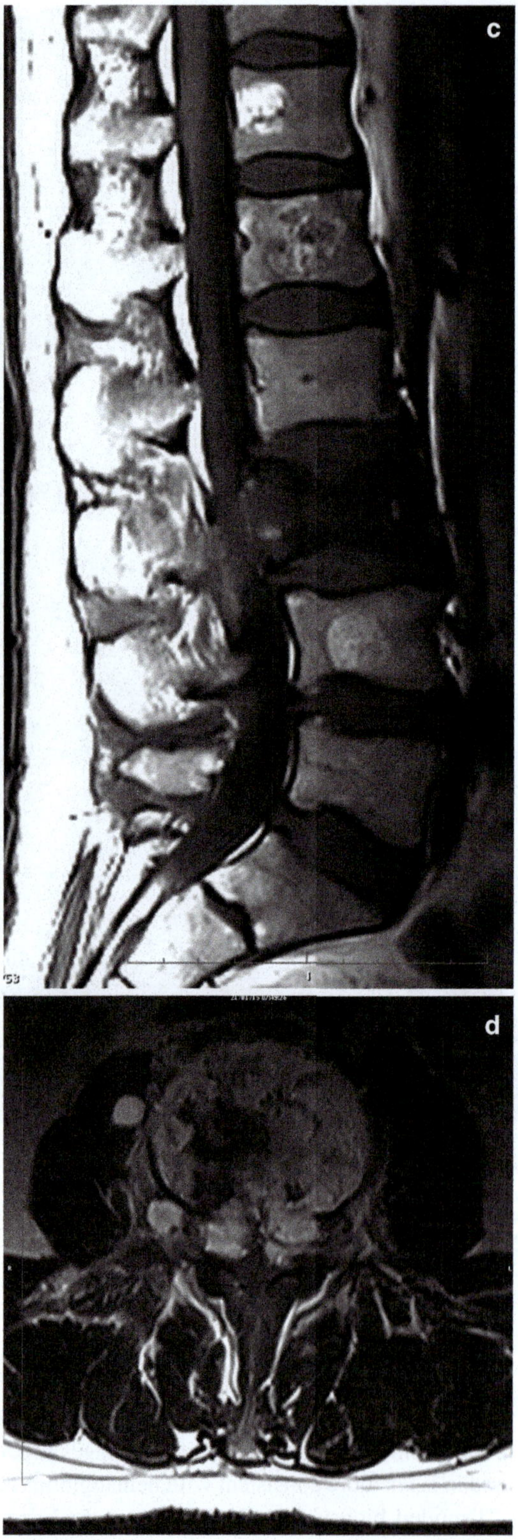

Fig. 21.12 (continued)

extracompartmental). The transverse image of the largest tumor extension is transferred on the WBB staging system. Sectors 4 to 9 to layers A to D (Fig. 21.15a). Oncological indication is en bloc tumor-free margin. To this purpose, a type 3b en bloc resection must be planned (Fig. 21.15b), including first an anterior approach in supine position to leave the appropriate margin by resection of the psoas under visual control (step I). After releasing the aorta and ligating cava, sacrifice the segmental lumbar vessels. Discectomies are performed after section of the anterior longitudinal ligaments at L2–L3 and at L3–L4. The second stage, posterior approach, involves intralesional piecemeal excision of sectors 3 to 10 (step II and III), release of the thecal sac by section of ligaments, and nerve root sacrifice, and sectioning the posterior longitudinal ligament and finalize the discectomies at L2–L3 and L3–L4. Step IV is the removal of the entire bloc.

In Video 21.1, a series of animations detail the steps of the resection—anterior approach by midline transperitoneal approach in supine position and posterior approach by midline incision in prone position. Anterior reconstruction is achieved by a stackable carbon fiber cage (Fig. 21.16) connected to a couple of posterior rods fixed by pedicular screws. The full operative time was 10 h and 17 min. The coronal and sagittal alignment is correct on the standing full-spine radiogram (Fig. 21.17a, b).

Discussion and Conclusion

En bloc resection in the spine is a very demanding surgical procedure. This operation can be safely performed and achieve oncological effectiveness if some mandatory steps are followed:

1. Diagnosis and staging must suggest that en bloc resection is the procedure of choice.

Since 30 years, the Enneking staging system has been adopted in many tumor centers, and many reports and reviews confirm its validity [37]. En bloc resection is proposed for benign aggressive (stage 3) [38] and for low-grade malignant tumors (stage I) [14]. For high-grade

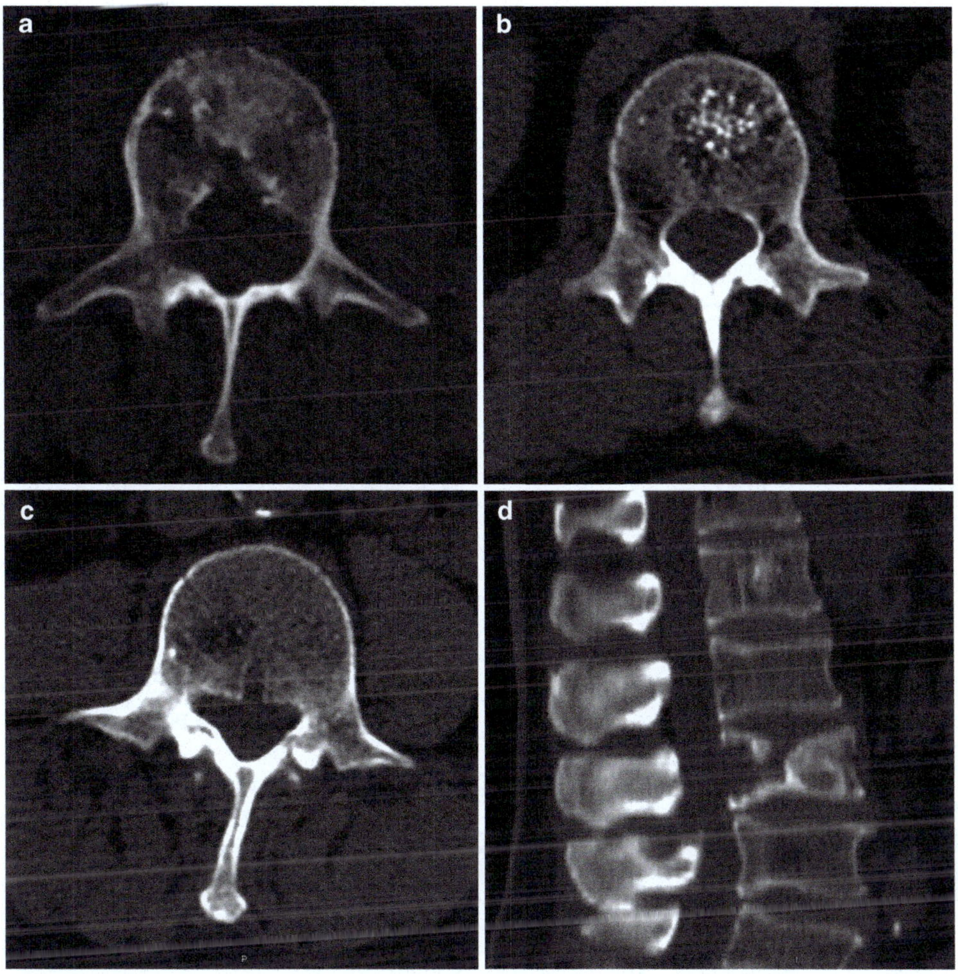

Fig. 21.13 Man, 62 years old. (**a**) L3 CT scan transverse imaging; (**b**) L1 CT scan transverse imaging; (**c**) L4 CT scan transverse imaging; and (**d**) CT scan sagittal imaging of the lumbar spine

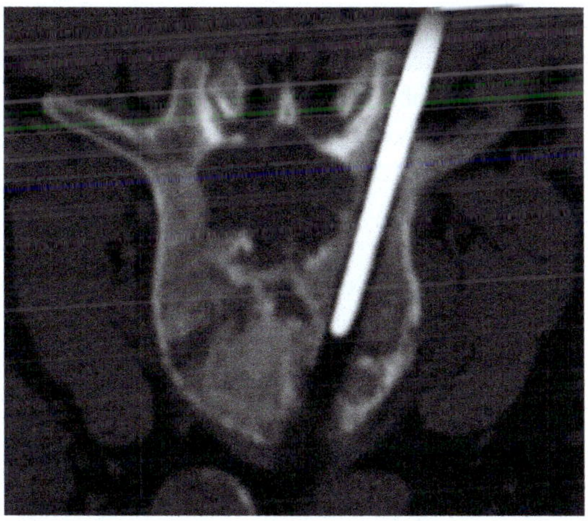

Fig. 21.14 Man, 62 years old. CT-guided trocar biopsy. The trocar is introduced through the pedicle to minimize tumor contamination in the surrounding soft tissues

malignant tumors, en bloc resection is a valid option but must always be associated with chemotherapy or radiotherapy, according to the sensitivity of the specific tumor [39, 40]. Isolated spine metastases in patients in good general status, if not sensitive to radio and chemotherapy, can be considered for en bloc resection [19].

2. Tumor extension and surgical anatomy must fulfill the criteria to perform a tumor-free margin en bloc resection safely and with acceptable functional loss.

The WBB staging system was proposed in 1997 [25] to stage primary spine tumors according to their extension, in order to easily share information on a computer-based terminology.

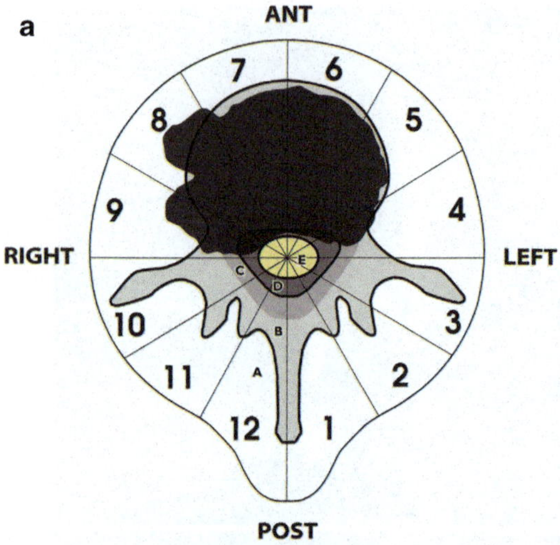

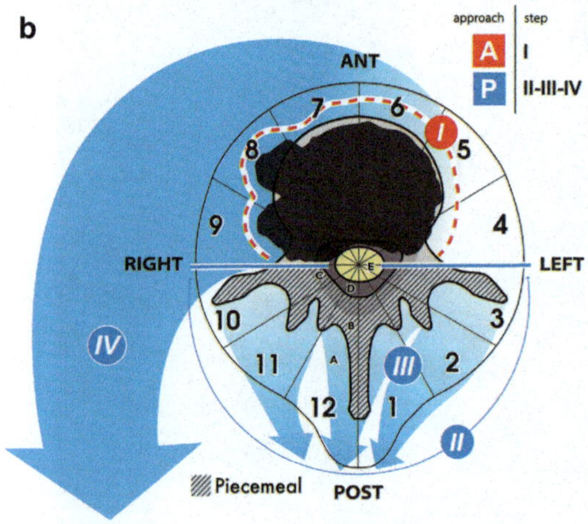

Fig. 21.15 L3 chordoma. (**a**) WBB staging of the lesion: sectors 9–4. Layers A to D and (**b**) WBB-based en bloc resection planning. The anterior growth requires visual control of the margins after releasing of the major vessels. Type 3a strategy: anterior approach first in supine position. Releasing of aorta and cava after sections of the segmental arteries and veins. Section of the psoas muscle above and below the tumor level, leaving a margin over the tumor anterior expansion. Section of the anterior longitudinal ligament and discectomies. Posterior approach as second stage in prone position, including removal of the healthy elements from sector 3–10, release of the thecal sac, section of the nerve roots involved in the tumor mass, and finalization of the discectomies and en bloc tumor removal

This system was recently validated as reliable and reproducible by a multidisciplinary group of experts in spine oncology [27]. Seven groups of strategies to plan en bloc resection have been proposed to define the criteria of feasibility of this procedure according to tumor extension.

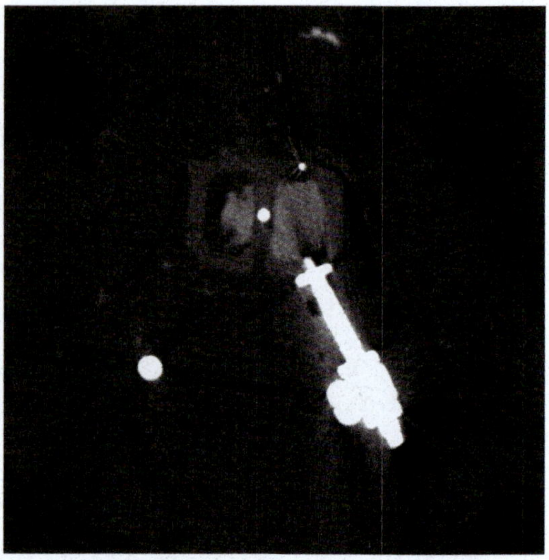

Fig. 21.16 Type 3a en bloc resection of L3 chordoma. Post-operative CT scan showing the connection between the cage and a posterior rod

3. Planning of the surgical procedure must consider the two previous points.

The surgical approach or combination and timing of approaches must be decided combining the required oncological margins and the criteria of feasibility by tumor extension and by spine region. If the margin is represented by relevant anatomical structures (dura, nerve roots, aorta, cava), a careful decision-making process will consider the improvement of prognosis versus the functional loss. In this process the patient willing will be obviously relevant. If the tumor is expanding anteriorly, the anterior approach is mandatory to leave a layer of healthy tissue over the tumor under visual control. A similar procedure must be adopted if a non-expandable anatomic structure is close to the anterior surface of the tumor. In the cervical spine and the lower lumbar spine, it is frequently necessary to combine multiple approaches due to the complexity of the anatomy.

4. Morbidity

A high morbidity rate can be expected. Intraoperative bleeding affects the risk of cardiovascular failures, post-operative hematoma, delayed wound healing, and infection. Preoperative emboli-

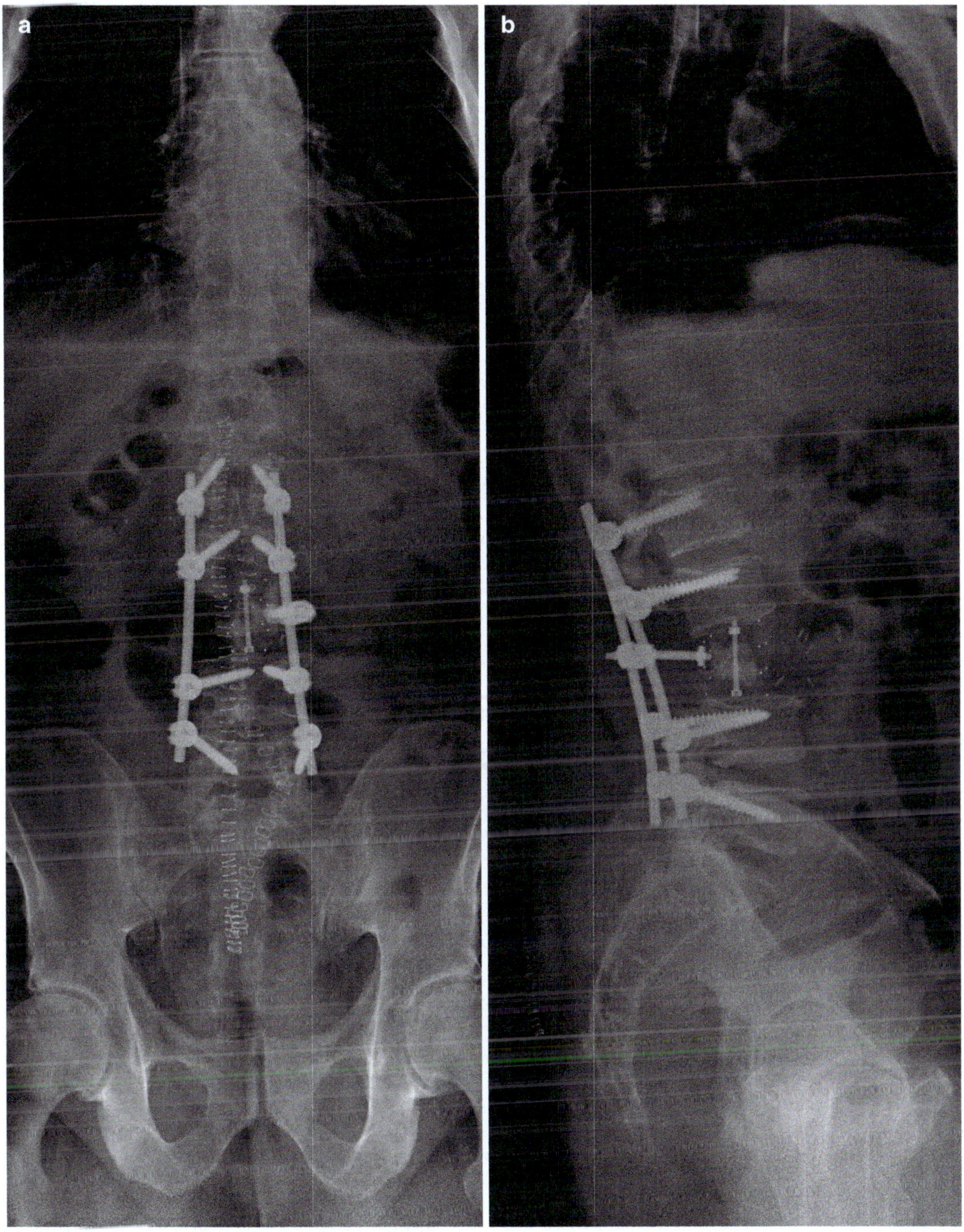

Fig. 21.17 Type 3a en bloc resection of L3 chordoma: reconstruction with carbon fiber (CF)-reinforced polyetheretherketone (PEEK) cage filled with autogenous graft and hydroxylapatite, connected with posterior implant. (**a**) Coronal orthostatic standing radiogram and (**b**) sagittal orthostatic standing radiogram confirming satisfactory 3D well-balanced reconstruction

zation is not helpful if extratumoral surgery is performed; tumor ischemia could conversely increase the vascularity on the periphery of the tumor. Patient and careful hemostasis, both of the epidural veins and of any vascular structure, is mandatory.

No more than three pairs of nerve roots should be sacrificed at the thoraco-lumbar junction in order to keep an appropriate cord vascularity. Manipulation of the dural sac, particularly at the end of these long procedures, can put the cord vascularity at risk for traction, torsion, and shortening.

Conclusion

En bloc resection in the lumbar spine is a demanding procedure, from both an oncologic and a surgical point of view. The essential surgical criteria for planning approaches and techniques are as follows.

- Visual control is essential to achieve the required margin.
- The most important anatomical structures must be released or resected for achieving an appropriate margin under visual control.
- Combined simultaneous approaches are associated with higher morbidity and should be performed only when mandatory.
- Cord vascularity must be considered in multi-segmental resections.
- Epidural bleeding can become a serious problem if underestimated.
- Removal of the specimen must be planned by the best approach to avoid tractions, torsions, and shortening of the cord.
- When intralesional surgery is planned or the risk of penetrating the tumor during resection is significant, selective arterial embolization is mandatory; however, when the surgeon anticipates a good probability of successful en bloc resection with oncological margins, tumor ischemia following embolization may induce peritumoral hyper-vascularization with increased risk of bleeding.
- Hemostasis is essential; poorly controlled epidural bleeding increases the risk of cardiovascular failure at the last steps of such a long procedure.

Acknowledgment It would not have been possible to conceive and finalize this chapter without the collaboration of Carlo Piovani. His work as an archivist and his original drawings are absolutely invaluable.

References

1. Enneking WF. Muscoloskeletal tumor surgery. New York: Churchill Livingstone; 1983. p. 69–122.
2. Simon MA. Surgical Margins. In: Simon MA, Springfield D, editors. Surgery for bone and soft tissue Tumors. Philadelphia: Lippincott-Raven; 1998. p. 77–92.
3. Talac R, Yaszemski MJ, Currier BL, Fuchs B, Dekutoski MB, Kim CW, et al. Relationship between surgical margins and local recurrence in sarcomas of the spine. Clin Orthop Relat Res. 2002;397:127–32.
4. Rosen G. Pre-operative (neo-adjuvant) chemotherapy for osteogenic sarcoma: a ten years experience. Orthopedics. 1985;8:659–70.
5. Lador R, Gasbarrini A, Gambarotti M, Bandiera S, Ghermandi R, Boriani S. Surgeon's perception of margins in spinal en bloc resection surgeries: how reliable is it? Eur Spine J. 2017 Feb 6; https://doi.org/10.1007/s00586-017-4967-0. [Epub ahead of print].
6. Boriani S, Weinstein JN. The role of "tumor-free margins" in the resection of spinal Tumors: who should be treating spine tumors? Semin Spine Surg. 2009;21:76–85.
7. Fisher CG, Saravanja DD, Dvorak MF, Rampersaud YR, Clarkson PW, Hurlbert J, et al. Surgical management of primary bone tumors of the spine: validation of an approach to enhance cure and reduce local recurrence. Spine. 2011;36(10):830–6.
8. Biagini R, Casadei R, Boriani S, Erba F, Sturale C, Mascari C, et al. En bloc vertebrectomy and dural resection for chordoma: a case report. Spine. 2003;28(18):E368–72.
9. Rhines LD, Fourney DR, Siadati A, Suk I, Gokaslan ZL. En bloc resection of multilevel cervical chordoma with C-2 involvement: case report and description of operative technique. J Neurosurg Spine. 2005;2(2):199–205.
10. Bailey CS, Fisher CG, Boyd MC, Dvorak MF. En bloc marginal excision of a multilevel cervical chordoma: case report. J Neurosurg Spine. 2006;4(5):409–14.
11. Keynan O, Fisher CG, Boyd MC, O'Connell JX, Dvorak MF. Ligation and partial excision of the cauda equina as part of a wide resection of vertebral osteosarcoma: a case report and description of surgical technique. Spine. 2005;30(4):E97–E102.
12. Murakami H, Tomita K, Kawahara N, Oda M, Yahata T, Yamaguchi T. Complete segmental resection of the spine, including the spinal cord, for telangiectatic osteosarcoma: a report of 2 cases. Spine. 2006;31(4):E117–22.
13. Druschel C, Disch AC, Melcher I, Engelhardt T, Luzzati A, Haas NP, et al. Surgical management of recurrent thoracolumbar spinal sarcoma with 4-level

total en bloc spondylectomy: description of technique and report of two cases. Eur Spine J. 2012;21(1):1–9.
14. Boriani S, Saravanja D, Yamada Y, Varga PP, Biagini R, Fisher CG. Challenges of local recurrence and cure in low grade malignant tumors of the spine. Spine. 2009;34(22 Suppl):S48–57.
15. Boriani S, Bandiera S, Donthineni R, Amendola L, Cappuccio M, De Iure F, et al. Morbidity of en bloc resections in the spine. Eur Spine J. 2010;19(2):231–41.
16. Falicov A, Fisher CG, Sparkes J, Boyd MC, Wing PC, Dvorak MF. Impact of surgical intervention on quality of life in patients with spinal metastases. Spine. 2006;31(24):2849–56.
17. Patchell RA, Tibbs PA, Regine WF, Payne R, Saris S, Kryscio RJ, et al. Direct decompressive surgical resection in the treatment of spinal cord compression caused by metastatic cancer: a randomised trial. Lancet. 2005;366(9486):643–8.
18. Yao KC, Boriani S, Gokaslan ZL, Sundaresan N. En bloc spondylectomy for spinal metastases: a review of techniques. Neurosurg Focus. 2003;15(5):E6.
19. Tomita K, Kawahara N, Kobayashi T, Yoshida A, Murakami H, Akamaru T. Surgical strategy for spinal metastases. Spine. 2001;26(3):298–306.
20. Li H, Gasbarrini A, Cappuccio M, Terzi S, Paderni S, Mirabile L, et al. Outcome of excisional surgeries for the patients with spinal metastases. Eur Spine J. 2009;18(10):1423–30.
21. Stener B, Johnsen OE. Complete removal of three vertebrae for giant-cell tumour. J Bone Joint Surg Br. 1971;53(2):278–87.
22. Stener B. Complete removal of vertebrae for extirpation of tumors. Clin Orthop Relat Res. 1989;245:72–82.
23. Roy-Camille R, Saillant G, Bisserie´ M, et al. Resection vertebrale totale dans la chirurgie tumorale au niveau du rachis dorsal par voie posterieure pure. Rev Chir Orthop. 1981;67:421–30.
24. Tomita K, Kawahara N, Baba H, Tsuchiya H, Fujita T, Toribatake Y. Total en bloc spondylectomy. A new surgical technique for primary malignant vertebral tumors. Spine. 1997,22(3):324–33.
25. Boriani S, Weinstein JN, Biagini R. Primary bone tumors of the spine. Terminology and surgical staging. Spine. 1997;22(9):1036–44.
26. Hart RA, Boriani S, Biagini R, Currier B, Weinstein JN. A system for surgical staging and management of spine tumors. A clinical outcome study of giant cell tumors of the spine. Spine. 1997;22:1773–83.
27. Chan P, Boriani S, Fourney DR, Biagini R, Dekutoski MB, Fehlings MG, et al. An assessment of the reliability of the Enneking and Weinstein-Boriani-Biagini classifications for staging of primary spinal tumors by the spine oncology study group. Spine. 2009;34(4):384–91.
28. Boriani S. Subtotal and total vertebrectomy for tumours. In: Surgical techniques in orthopedics and traumatology. 55-070-A. Paris: Editions Scientifiques et Medicales Elsevier; 2000.
29. Kawahara N, Tomita K, Baba H, Toribatake Y, Fujita T, Mizuno K, et al. Cadaveric vascular anatomy for total en bloc spondylectomy in malignant vertebral tumors. Spine. 1996;21(12):1401–7.
30. Gasbarrini A, Simoes CE, Bandiera S, Amendola L, Barbanti Brodano G, Cappuccio M, et al. Influence of a thread wire saw guide and spinal cord protector device in “en bloc” vertebrectomies. J Spinal Disord Tech. 2012;25(2):E7–12.
31. Roy-Camille R, Mazel CH, Saillant G, Lapresle PH. Treatment of malignant tumors of the spine with posterior instrumentation. In: Sundaresan N, Schmidek HH, Schiller AL, Rosenthal DI, editors. Tumors of the spine. Diagnosis and clinical management. Philadelphia: W.B.Saunders; 1990. p. 473–92.
32. Murakami H, Kawahara N, Tomita K, Demura S, Kato S, Yoshioka K. Does interruption of the artery of Adamkiewicz during total en bloc spondylectomy affect neurologic function? Spine. 2010;35(22):E1187–92.
33. Fujimaki Y, Kawahara N, Tomita K, Murakami H, Ueda Y. How many ligations of bilateral segmental arteries cause ischemic spinal cord dysfunction? An experimental study using a dog model. Spine. 2006;31(21):E781–9.
34. Kato S, Kawahara N, Tomita K, Murakami H, Demura S, Fujimaki Y. Effects on spinal cord blood flow and neurologic function secondary to interruption of bilateral segmental arteries which supply the artery of Adamkiewicz: an experimental study using a dog model. Spine. 2008;33(14):1533–41.
35. Ueda Y, Kawahara N, Tomita K, Kobayashi T, Murakami H, Nambu K. Influence on spinal cord blood flow and function by interruption of bilateral segmental arteries at up to three levels: experimental study in dogs. Spine. 2005;30(20):2239–43.
36. Kawahara N, Tomita K, Kobayashi T, Abdel-Wanis ME, Murakami H, Akamaru T. Influence of acute shortening on the spinal cord: an experimental study. Spine. 2005;30(6):613–20.
37. Fisher CG, Andersson GB, Weinstein JN. Spine focus issue. Summary of management recommendations in spine oncology. Spine. 2009;34(22 Suppl):S2–6.
38. Harrop JS, Schmidt MH, Boriani S, Shaffrey CI. Aggressive “benign” primary spine neoplasms: osteoblastoma, aneurysmal bone cyst, and giant cell tumor. Spine. 2009;34(22 Suppl):S39–47.
39. Schwab J, Gasbarrini A, Bandiera S, Boriani L, Amendola L, Picci P, et al. Osteosarcoma of the mobile spine. Spine. 2012;37(6):E381–6.
40. Sciubba DM, Okuno SH, Dekutoski MB, Gokaslan ZL. Ewing and osteogenic sarcoma: evidence for multidisciplinary management. Spine. 2009;34(22 Suppl):S58–68.
41. Marmor E, Rhines LD, Weinberg JS, Gokaslan ZL. Total en bloc lumbar spondylectomy: Case report. J Neurosurg Spine. 2001;95:264–9.

Intralesional Sacrectomy

22

A. Karim Ahmed, Zach Pennington, Ian Suk, C. Rory Goodwin, Ziya L. Gokaslan, and Daniel M. Sciubba

Anatomic Considerations

Tumors of the sacrum represent only 1–7% of spine tumors, with metastatic lesions more common than primary neoplasms [1, 2]. The sacrum plays an essential role in the biomechanical stability of the spine and houses critical neural elements. As an anchor point sustaining the load from cephalad spinal segments, the sacrum connects the spinal column to the pelvis and houses sacral nerves of the cauda equina.

Five fused vertebrae form the bony sacrum, effaced by the pelvic viscera ventrally. The paired sacral alae articulate with the ilium, forming the sacroiliac joints, and nerve roots exit laterally via sacral foramina. The ligamentous structures play opposing roles to impart structural stability on the sacrum, particularly during ambulation. Downward torque from the cephalad segment is directly opposed by tension from the sacrotuberous and sacrospinous ligaments—separating the greater and lesser sciatic foramen. This is balanced by the interosseous and dorsal sacroilial ligaments, which prevent ventral rotation of the sacrum. Inferiorly, the coccygeus and levator ani muscles contribute to the pelvic floor, with points of attachment to the sacrum.

An appreciation of vascular structures and pelvic viscera traversing the pelvic inlet is essential due to their proximity to the sacrum. The presacral fascia lines the ventral border of the sacrum, followed by retrorectal space and fascia propria of the mesorectum. The median and lateral sacral arteries provide much of the vascular supply to the sacrum, anastomosing with one another. The bifurcation of the abdominal aorta forms the common iliac arteries at ~L4 and provides the median sacral artery posteriorly. The posterior division of the internal iliac artery gives rise to the lateral sacral artery, which enters the sacral foramina. Sacral and internal iliac lymph nodes drain the pelvic viscera and sacrum.

The sacral roots contribute to the sacral plexus (L4–S4) and coccygeal plexus (S4–Co), with sensory and motor innervation. The sciatic nerve (L4–S3) is a key component of the sacral plexus, branching distally to form the tibial and common peroneal nerve. Additional contributories to the sacral plexus include the pudendal plexus (S2–S4), superior gluteal nerve (S4–S1), inferior gluteal nerve (L5–S2), nerve to obturator internus (L5–S2), nerve to superior gemellus (L5–S2), nerve to inferior gemellus (L4 – S1), nerve to quadratus femoris (L4–S1), posterior cutaneous

A. Karim Ahmed · Z. Pennington · I. Suk
D. M. Sciubba (✉)
Department of Neurosurgery, The Johns Hopkins Hospital, Baltimore, MD, USA
e-mail: dsciubb1@jhmi.edu

C. Rory Goodwin
Duke University Medical Center, Department of Neurosurgery, Durham, NC, USA

Z. L. Gokaslan
Department of Neurosurgery, Rhode Island Hospital, Warren Alpert School of Medicine at Brown University, Providence, RI, USA

D. M. Sciubba (ed.), *Spinal Tumor Surgery*, https://doi.org/10.1007/978-3-319-98422-3_22

nerve of the thigh (S1–S3), nerve to piriformis (S1, S2), perforating cutaneous nerve (S2, S3), and nerves to levator ani, coccygeus, and external anal sphincter (S4). Preganglionic parasympathetic nerves, the pelvic splanchnics (S2–S4), join the inferior hypogastric plexus for autonomic control of the pelvic viscera, bowel/bladder function, and genital arousal [3–8].

Patient Evaluation

Patients with neoplastic involvement of the sacrum may present with mechanical sacral pain, buttock pain, hip pain, leg pain, perineal numbness, neurogenic bowel/bladder dysfunction, or motor weakness [1, 2, 8–10]. Due to the large sacral canal, with the cauda equina freely floating in the thecal sac, lesions of the sacrum may grow to a large mass before becoming symptomatic or causing neurologic deficit. Motor dysfunction often occurs later in the disease course, resulting from soft-tissue extension compressing the neural elements. More commonly, patients experience pain resulting from mass effect or pathological compression fracture. Sacral metastasis occurs primarily through hematogenous spread but may also result from drop metastasis or direct extension (i.e., recurrent colorectal cancers) [10–17].

Clinical examination, imaging, biopsy, and staging are the mainstays of evaluating patients with sacral lesions. Plain x-rays are the initial form of imaging, and may demonstrate pathologic fracture, but have limited sensitivity [18–20]. Magnetic resonance imaging (MRI) is ideal for soft tissue, and neural elements, allowing for accurate localization of nerve root compression and soft-tissue neoplastic extension. The intensity, based on T1- and T2-weighted sequences, can provide insight into the diagnosis, but a pathologic diagnosis should be confirmed whenever possible. Computed tomography (CT) is unparalleled for imaging of osseous structures and can provide further insight into a lytic, blastic, or mixed process. A CT-guided needle, or core, biopsy is recommended to obtain a histopathologic diagnosis, instrumental in dictating the most appropriate treatment. Metastatic lymphoma, seminoma, and myeloma to the spine are considered as highly radiosensitive tumors and respond well to radiation without the need for surgical intervention. Radiosensitive lesions, including hematogenous (i.e., plasmacytoma, lymphoma), breast, prostate, ovarian, and neuroendocrine tumors, may be treated with radiation, in the absence of spinal instability. This is in contrast to more radioresistant lesions, including colorectal, non-small-cell lung, hepatocellular, thyroid, renal cell, and sarcoma. Nuclear imaging (i.e., positron emission tomography [PET]), or scintigraphy, is utilized for staging to identify systemic burden and other sites of osseous/visceral metastases [18–31].

Irrespective of radiosensitivity, neoplastic lesions resulting in spinal instability are only addressed with surgical stabilization [1, 2, 19, 32–36]. The Spinal Instability Neoplastic Score (SINS) [32], developed by the Spinal Oncology Study Group (SOSG), proposes a scoring framework to assess for the presence of spinal instability necessitating surgical stabilization. This scoring system accounts for factors such as location, pain, lesion type, alignment, vertebral collapse, and neural element involvement. Junctional level involvement (i.e., L5–S1) increases the risk for spinal instability, compared to lesions in rigid locations (i.e., S2–S5).

Operative Techniques

Positioning and Monitoring

General anesthesia is administered with an endotracheal tube. For a posterior approach, the patient is placed prone on a Jackson table, with the head secured in a three-point Mayfield clamp. Intraoperative monitoring consists of free-run electromyography (EMG), including the bilateral quadriceps, anterior tibialis, abductor hallucis muscles, and anal sphincter to assess for neurotonic motor discharge. Excessive neuromuscular blockade (NMB) may have reduced the sensitivity of detection of nerve root irritation, and should be appropriate, especially during critical portions of the procedure. Repetitive nerve stimulation to tibialis anterior (L5) and abductor hallicus (S1, S2), at 2.1 Hz, confirms the correct level of NMB [37, 38].

Surgical Exposure

An intraoperative x-ray is taken for localization, and a midline lumbosacral incision is made. Soft-tissue dissection is deepened to the erector spinae muscle tendon, attached to the medial crest of the sacrum, which is divided and reflected laterally to expose the sacral ala and posterior inferior iliac spine (PSIS). Subperiosteal dissection continues with removal of the supraspinous and intraspinous ligaments, using a Leksell rongeur [39–45].

Intralesional Sacrectomy for Sacral Metastasis

The extent of sacral resection is a key determinant for spinopelvic fixation. Progressive removal of caudal sacral elements increases the risk of pelvic ring failure [44, 46]. When the superior aspect of sacrectomy is between S1 and S2, or at the midpoint of the S1 vertebral body, the resulting sacropelvic structural integrity is weakened by 30% and 50%, respectively [39, 46–48]. Therefore, instrumentation should be performed early in the case, prior to tumor resection.

Iliac bolts are placed bilaterally, followed by bilateral transpedicular screws at L4, L5, and S1. For tumors located laterally with involvement of the pedicle, screw placement at the involved level may be skipped. For laterally placed tumors, one connecting rod is secured on the uninvolved side to allow for adequate decompression and ensure stability.

A high-speed burr, or ultrasonic blade, is utilized to perform laminectomies at the affected levels. The thecal sac is carefully dissected free from the ventral tumor. Attention should be paid to identify the nerve roots at each level and reflect these away with vessel loops. Tumor is subsequently debulked from the canal and foramen.

Posterior Nerve-Sparing Sacrectomy

A posterior, single-stage, sacrectomy may be performed for benign primary tumors, not requiring wide-margin en bloc resection. This technique has been described by Bydon et al. [42] for the removal of a giant-cell tumor involving the S1 and S2 vertebral bodies, in an en bloc fashion with contaminated margins.

Exposure, instrumentation, laminectomy, and separation of tumor from the ventral thecal sac proceed as described earlier for sacral metastases. The pedicles superior and inferior to the tumor are drilled bilaterally, to allow for greater tumor exposure. A high-speed burr or ultrasonic blade is utilized to make interrupted cuts between the sacral foramina, lateral to the tumor, with attention to preserve the nerve roots in between. A circumferential cut is made superior and inferior the tumor, and all interrupted cuts are connected to facilitate release of the tumor. The sacroiliac joints are drilled, bilaterally, and electrocautery is used to divide the ventral periosteum surrounding the released tumor (Fig. 22.1). A #3 Penfield dissector may be used to perform ventral organ dissection, encountering the mesorectum, which is reflected inferiorly from the tumor. At this point, the tumor is completely released and may be mobilized through a window created from the retracted nerve roots (Figs. 22.2 and 22.3) [42].

Closure

Closure is performed in the typical watertight layered fashion, with 0 Vicryl in the fascia above a subfascial Jackson-Pratt (JP) suctioning drain. The drain is tunneled with a Touhy needle and sutured to the skin. An additional suprafascial JP drain is placed for obese patients to reduce the risk of post-operative dead-space infection. The dermis is reapproximated and closed with 3–0 Vicryl, with staples on the skin surface. Due to the risk of wound infection and dehiscence in this area [49], it is advised to consult with plastic and reconstructive surgery for assistance with complex wound closure [50].

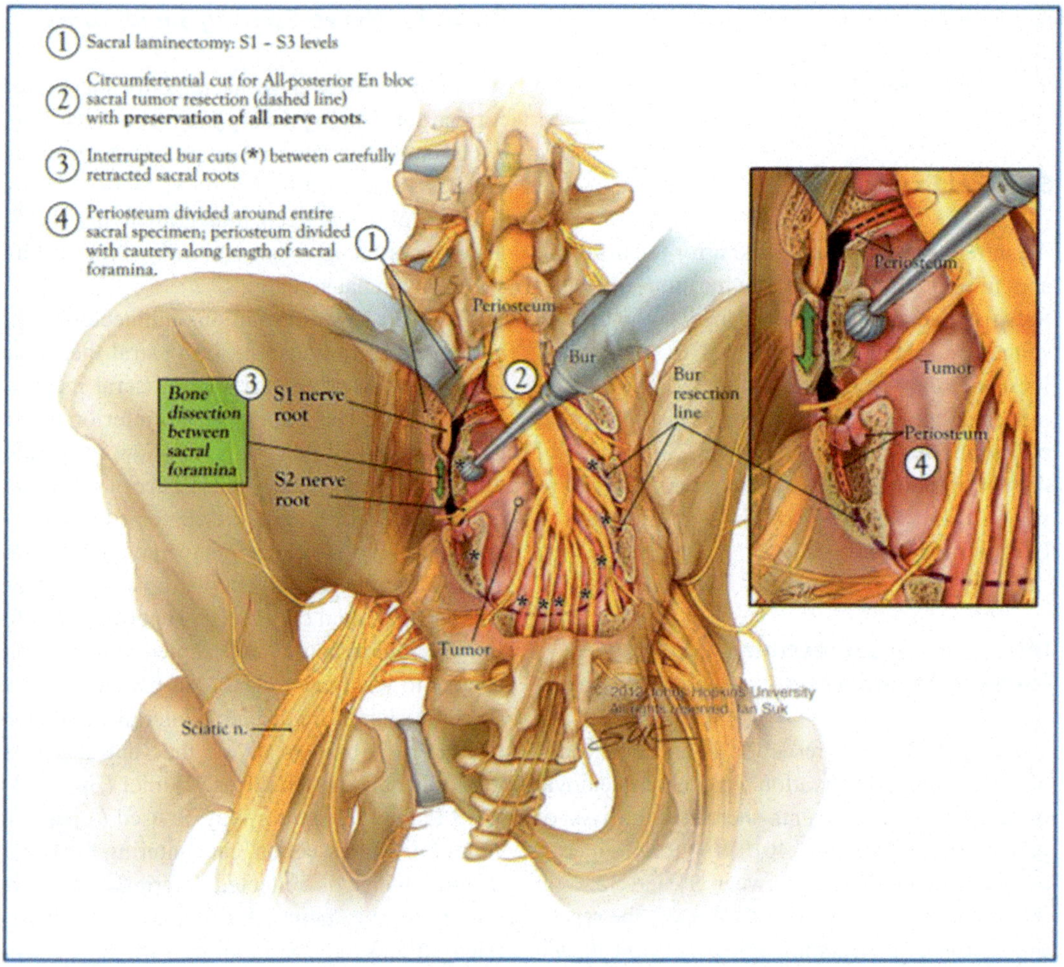

Fig. 22.1 After a wide sacral laminectomy around the tumor site (Step 1), the sacral nerve roots are exposed and mobilized. Bone dissection circumscribing the anteriorly situated tumor is done by connecting the interrupted cuts (*) between the sacral foramina (Step 2 and 3). The periosteum is divided along the length of the sacral foramina (Step 4) to release the entire tumor specimen. Dissection of the periosteum lining the foramina also helps the surgeon establish the cleavage plane between nerve roots and bone. n, nerve. (Printed with permission. Copyright 2018, The Johns Hopkins University. All Rights Reserved. Ian Suk)

Case Presentation 1

This 58-year-old female presented to the neurosurgical spine service, with a previous medical history of metastatic renal cell carcinoma, for evaluation of a large symptomatic sacral lesion. The compression fracture and soft-tissue extension resulted in mechanical pain and radiculopathy, respectively. Imaging demonstrated a compression fracture of S1, with left-sided extension into the foramina (Fig. 22.4), and CT-guided biopsy confirmed a diagnosis of renal cell carcinoma. Due to the vascular nature of this tumor, pre-operative embolization was performed by interventional neuroradiology. Tumor blush was identified arising from radicular branches of the left iliolumbar, internal iliac, and median sacral arteries. Glue embolization (n-butyl cyanoacrylate [nBCA]) resulted in 90% reduction in tumor blush (Figs. 22.5 and 22.6).

Intralesional sacrectomy was performed the following day. The patient was placed prone on a Jackson table, and an x-ray was taken for

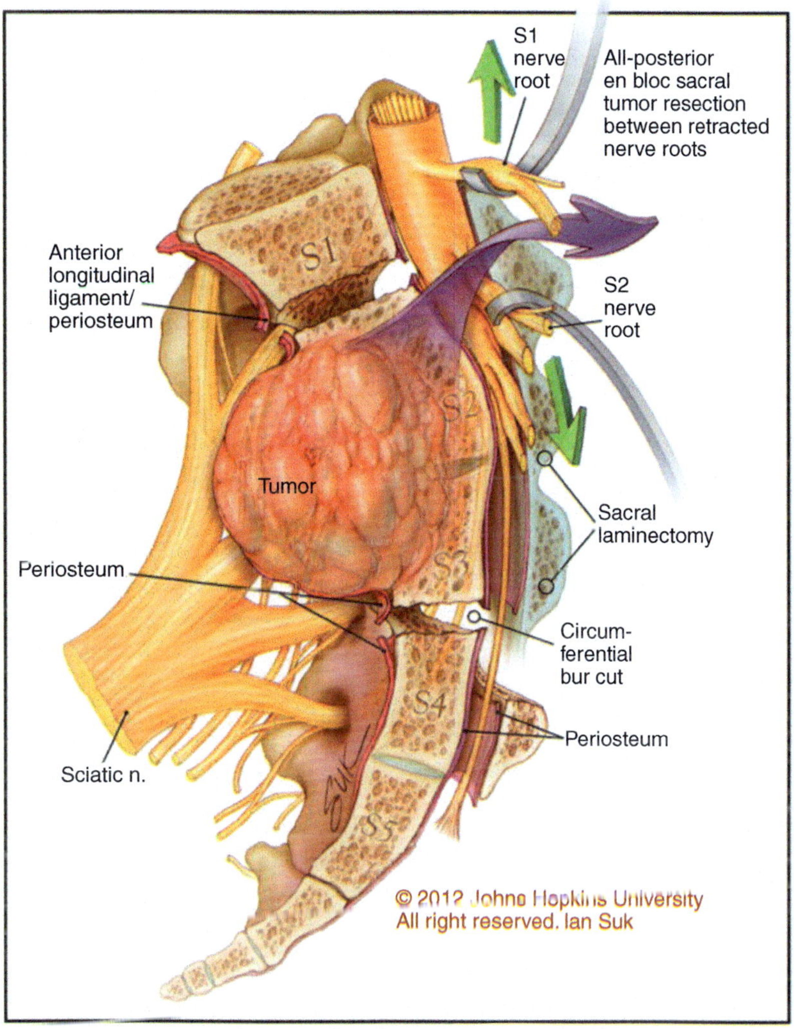

Fig. 22.2 The en bloc tumor specimen is gently mobilized by twisting it between retracted sacral nerve roots. n., nerve. (Printed with permission. Copyright 2018, The Johns Hopkins University. All Rights Reserved. Ian Suk)

localization. A midline skin incision and subperiosteal dissection were performed from L4 to S1 and the pelvis. The tumor was readily visualized bridging through the posterior aspect of S1 and sacral ala, on the left side. Using external landmarks, the pedicles of L4 and L5 were cannulated bilaterally, in addition to S1 on the right. Iliac bolts were placed, and an intraoperative CT scan (O-arm, Medtronic, Minneapolis, MN) was taken to confirm correct screw placement. Cement was administered through the fenestrated bilateral L4 and L5 screws to optimize lumbar fixation. A connecting rod was placed on the right side from L4 to S1 and the pelvis, followed by laminectomies of L5–S4. Tumor was debulked in a piecemeal fashion with attention to preserve all nerve roots. Following sufficient decompression of the neural elements, a pre-bent rod was placed on the left side, connecting L4 to the pelvis. Decortication with the placement of allografted bone chips and watertight layered closure were performed. A subfascial and suprafascial drain were placed to minimize post-operative wound infection. Intraoperative monitoring was stable throughout the case. The patient showed significant improvement in her pain and radiculopathy, post-operatively (Fig. 22.7).

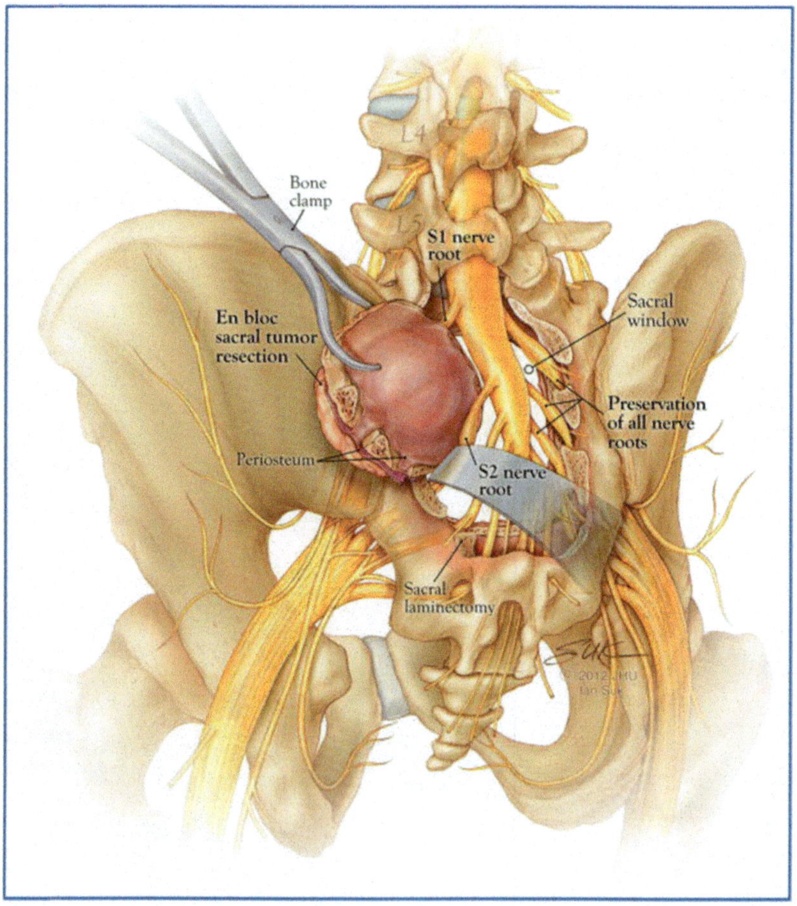

Fig. 22.3 The tumor is delivered through a sacral window, without need for nerve root sacrifice. n, nerve. Printed with permission. Printed with permission. (Copyright 2018, The Johns Hopkins University. All Rights Reserved. Ian Suk)

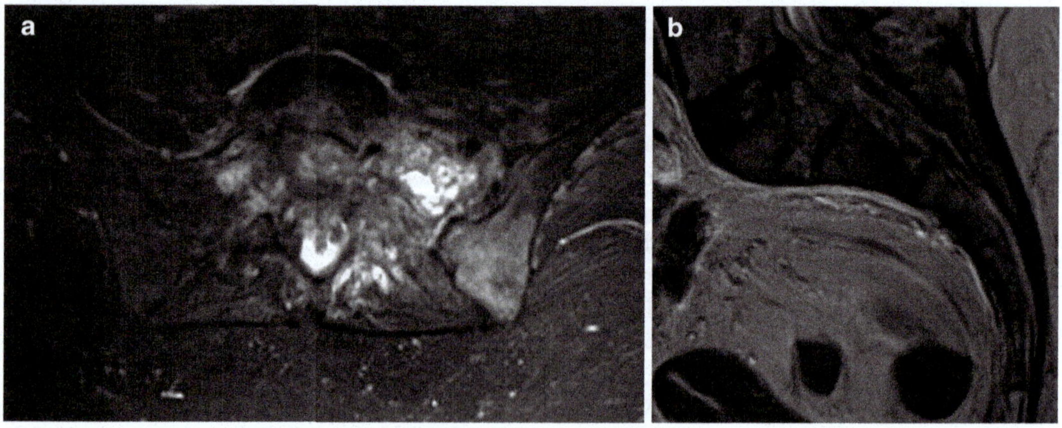

Fig. 22.4 Case presentation 1 pre-operative imaging. (**a**) Axial T2-weighted MRI. (**b**) Sagittal T2-weighted MRI

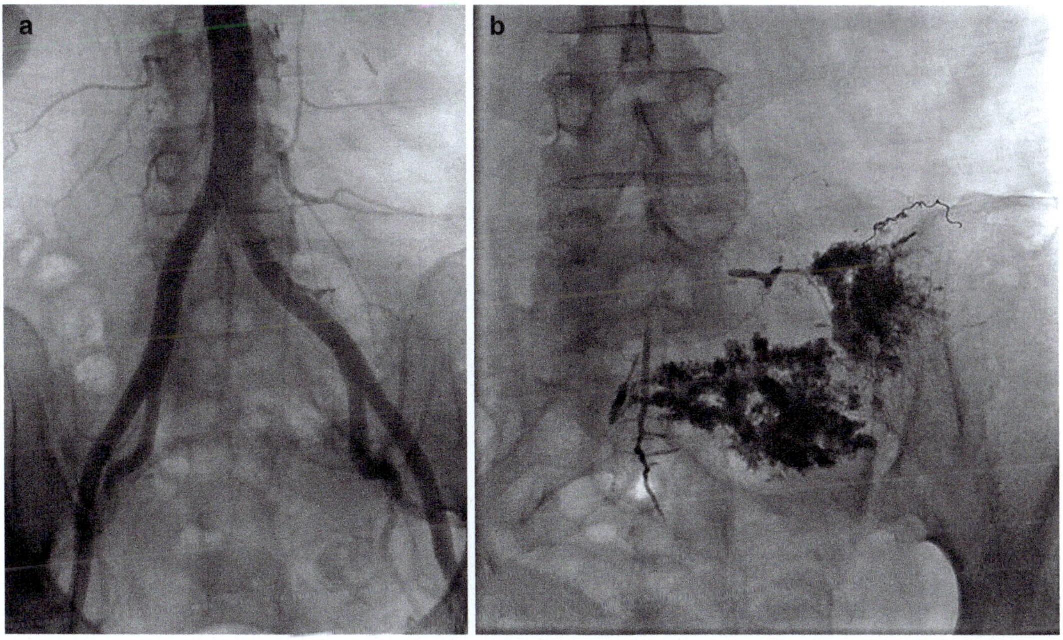

Fig. 22.5 Case presentation 1 pre-operative angiogram and embolization for metastatic renal cell carcinoma. (**a**) Angiogram. (**b**) Glue embolization with nBCA and 90% reduction in tumor blush

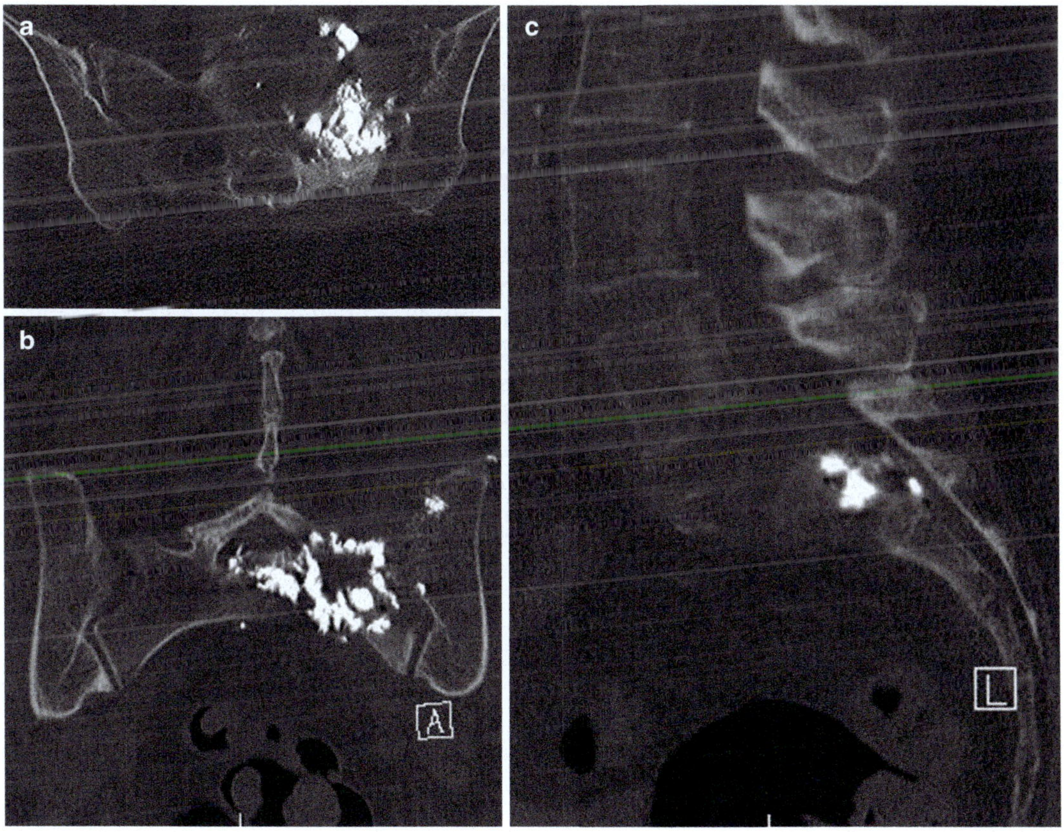

Fig. 22.6 Case presentation 1 pre-operative, post-embolization CT. (**a**) Axial CT. (**b**) Coronal CT. (**c**) Sagittal CT

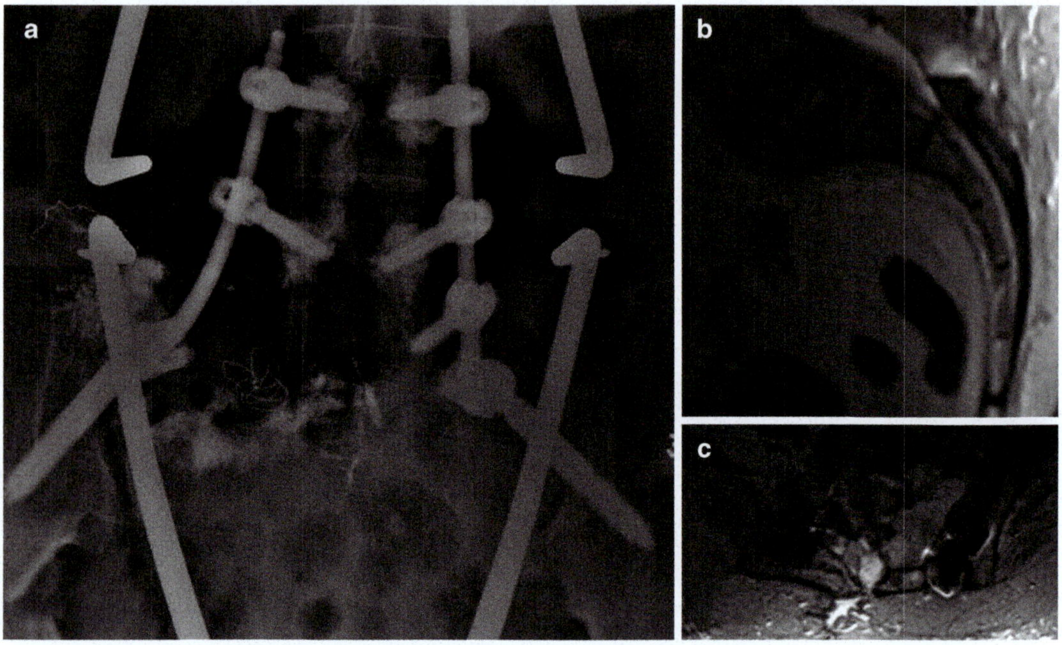

Fig. 22.7 Case presentation 1 post-operative imaging. (**a**) Intraoperative radiograph following instrumentation and tumor resection. (**b**) Post-operative T2-weighted MRI. (**c**) Coronal T2-weighted MRI

Case Presentation 2

This 33-year-old male presented with intractable back pain, with a previous medical history of multiple myeloma. Imaging demonstrated a large sacral tumor with fractures of the bilateral ala, with infiltration into the sacral foramina (Fig. 22.8). Surgical decompression was determined to be the best option due to the instability and symptomatology of the lesion.

The patient was placed prone; a midline incision and subperiosteal dissection were performed from L3 to the coccyx and the pelvis. Using external landmarks, pedicles were cannulated from L3 to L5. An x-ray was taken to confirm the correct levels. At this point, screws were placed into the pedicles, with bilateral iliac bolts. Sacral laminectomies were performed at S1–S4 to expose the tumor. The nerve roots and thecal sac were skeletonized, and the sacral tumor was completely removed with preservation of all the roots. An additional iliac bolt and rod were placed bilaterally to ensure structural stability. Complex wound closure was completed with assistance from plastic and reconstructive surgery. The patient is doing well 2 years post-operatively with resolution of his pain (Fig. 22.9).

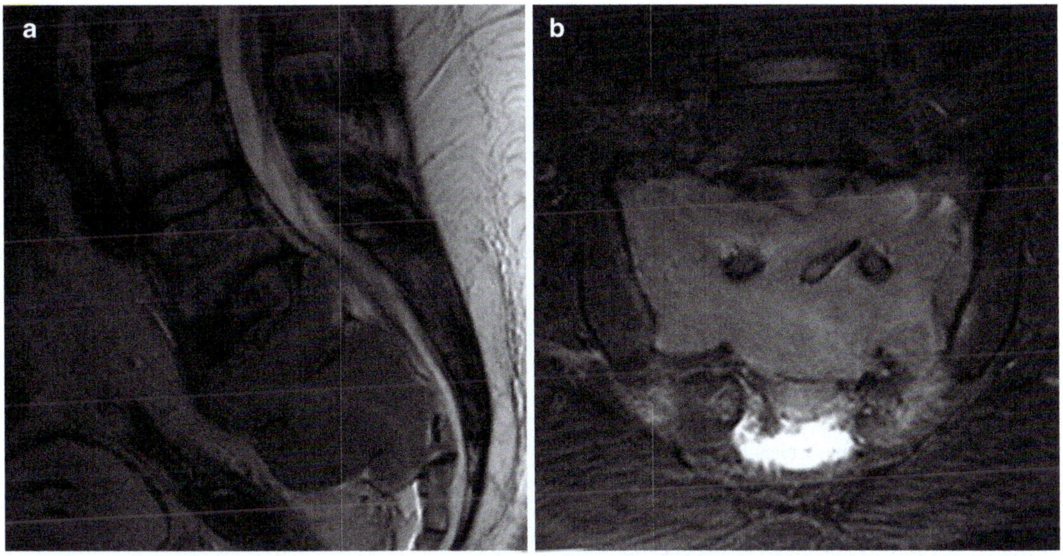

Fig. 22.8 Case presentation 2 pre-operative imaging. (**a**) T2-weighted sagittal MRI. (**b**) T2-weighted coronal MRI. (Reprinted with permission from Ahmed et al. [51])

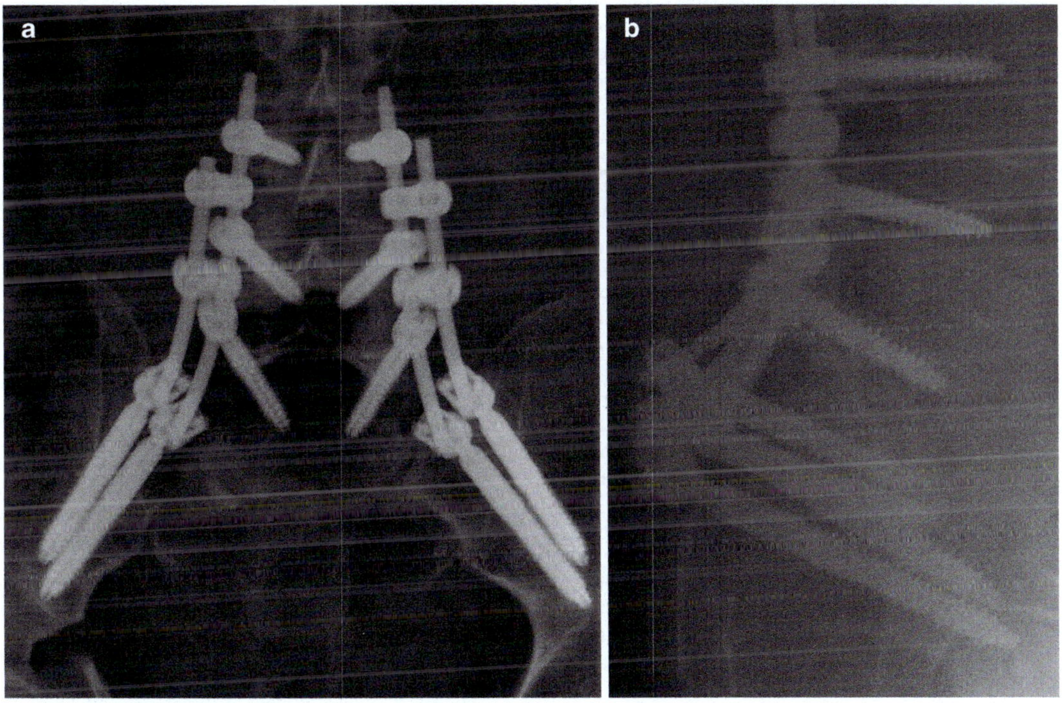

Fig. 22.9 Case presentation 2 post-operative imaging. (**a**) Anteroposterior (AP) x-ray. (**b**) Lateral x-ray. (Reprinted with permission from Ahmed et al. [51])

References

1. Quraishi NA, Giannoulis KE, Edwards KL, Boszczyk BM. Management of metastatic sacral tumours. Eur Spine J. 2012;21(10):1984–93.
2. Feiz-Erfan I, Fox BD, Nader R, Suki D, Chakrabarti I, Mendel E, et al. Surgical treatment of sacral metastases: indications and results. J Neurosurg Spine. 2012;17:285–91.
3. Bogduk N. Clinical anatomy of the lumbar spine and sacrum. 4th ed. Philadelphia: Elsevier; 2005. p. 59–76.
4. Wang T, Fielding LC, Parikh A, Kothari M, Alamin T. Sacral spinous processes; a morphologic classification and biomechanical characterization of strength. Spine J. 2015;15(12):2544–51.
5. Sae-Jung S, Khamanarong K, Woraputtaporn W, Amarttayakong P. Awareness of the median sacral artery during lumbosacral spinal surgery: an anatomic cadaveric study of its relationship to the lumbosacral spine. Eur Spine J. 2015;24(11):2520–4.
6. Zoccali C, Skoch J, Patel A, Walter CM, Maykowski P, Baaj AA. The surgical neurovascular anatomy relating to partial and complete sacral and sacroiliac resections: a cadaveric, anatomic study. Eur Spine J. 2015;24(5):1109–13.
7. Woon JT, Stringer MD. The anatomy of the sacrococcygeal corneal region and its clinical relevance. Anat Sci Int. 2014;89(4):207–14.
8. Gray H. Gray's anatomy: descriptive and applied. London: Longmans; 1967. p. 286–547.
9. Feldenzer JA, McGauley JL, McGillicuddy JE. Sacral and presacral tumors: problems in diagnosis and management. Neurosurgery. 1989;25:884–91.
10. Rhee J, Kosztowski TA, Bydon M, Gokaslan ZL. Sacral tumors: regional challenges. In: Steinmets MP, Benzel EC, editors. Spine surgery: techniques, complications, avoidance, and management. 4th ed. Philadelphia: Elsevier; 2016. p. 1061–7.
11. Fourney DR, Gokaslan ZL. Surgical approaches for the resection of sacral tumors. In: Dickman CA, Fehlings MG, Gokaslan ZL, editors. Spinal cord and spinal column tumors: principles and practice. New York: Thieme; 2006. p. 632–6.
12. Payer M. Neurological manifestation of sacral tumors. Neurosurg Focus. 2003;1(2):1–6.
13. Shah LM, Salsman KL. Imaging of spinal metastatic disease. Int J Surg Oncol. 2011;2011:1–12.
14. Fukushima T, Kasai Y, Kato K, Fujisawa K, Uchida A. Intradural squamous cell carcinoma of the sacrum. World J Surg Oncol. 2009;7:16.
15. Pain GJ. Extremities and spine-evaluation and differential diagnosis. In: Omer G, Spinner M, editors. Management of peripheral nerve problems. Philadelphia: WB Saunders; 1980. p. 169.
16. Norstrom CW, Kernohan JW, Love JG. One hundred primary caudad tumors. JAMA. 1961;178:1071–7.
17. Wilson SAK. Neurology, vol. Vol 2. London: Edward Arnold & Co; 1940. p. 1285–321.
18. Amorosa JK, Weintraub S, Amorosa LF, Safer JN, Rafii M. Sacral destruction: foraminal lines revisited. AJR. 1985;145(4):773–5.
19. Fourney DR, Gokaslan ZL. Sacral tumors: primary and metastatic. In: Dickman CA, Fehlings MG, Gokaslan ZL, editors. Spinal cord and spinal column tumors: principles and practice. New York: Thieme; 2006. p. 404–19.
20. Gerber S, Ollivier L, Leclere J, Vanel D, Missenard G, Brisse H, de Pinieux G, Neuenschwander S. Imaging of sacral tumours. Skelet Radiol. 2008;37(4):277–89.
21. Algra PR, Bloem JL, Tissing H, FAlke TH, Arndt JW, Verteboom LJ. Detection of vertebral metastases: comparison between MR imaging and bone scintigraphy. Radiographics. 1991;11(2):219–32.
22. Horger M, Bares R. The role of sing-photon emission computed tomography/computed tomography in benign and malignant bone disease. Semin Nucl Med. 2006;36(4):286–94.
23. Savelli G, Chiti A, Grasselli G, Maccauro M, Rodai M, Bombardieri E. The role of bone SPECT study in diagnosis of single vertebral metastases. Anticancer Res. 2000;20:1115–20.
24. Galasko CS. Mechanisms of lytic and blastic metastatic disease of bone. Clin Orthop Relat Res. 1982;169:20–7.
25. Laufer I, Sciubba DM, Madera M, Bydon A, Witham TJ, Gokaslan ZL, et al. Surgical management of metastatic spinal tumors. Cancer Control. 2012;19(2):122–8.
26. Babu NV, Titus VT, Chittaranjan S, Abraham G, Prem H, Korula RJ. Computed tomographically guided biopsy of the spine. Spine. 1994;19:439–44.
27. Kattapuram SV, Khurana JS, Rosenthal DI. Percutaneous needle biopsy of the spine. Spine. 1992;17:561–4.
28. Lis E, Bilsky MH, Pisinski L, Boland P, Healey JH, O'Malley B, et al. Percutaneous CT-guided biopsy of osseous lesion of the spine in patients with known or suspected malignancy. AJNR Am J Neuroradiol. 2004;25:1583–8.
29. Talamo G, Dimaio C, Abbi KKS, Pandey MK, Malysz J, Creer MH, et al. Current role of radiation therapy for multiple myeloma. Front Oncol. 2015;5(40):1–6.
30. Gerszten PC, Mendel E, Yamada Y. Radiotherapy and radiosurgery for metastatic spine disease: what are the options, indications, and outcomes? Spine. 2009;34:S78–92.
31. Laufer I, Rubin DG, Lis E, Cox BW, Stubblefield MD, Yamada Y, Bilsky MH. The NOMS framework: approach to the treatment of spinal metastatic tumors. Oncologist. 2013;18(6):744–51.
32. Fisher CG, DiPaola CP, Ryken TC, Bilsky MH, Shaffrey CI, Berven SH, et al. A novel classification system for spinal instability in neoplastic disease: an evidence-based approach and expert consensus from the spinal oncology study group. Spine. 2010;35(2):E1221–9.

33. Fourney DR, Gokaslan ZL. Spinal instability and deformity due to neoplastic conditions. Neurosurg Focus. 2003;14:E8.
34. Fourney DR, Frangou EM, Ryken TC, Dipaola CP, Shaffrey CI, Berven SH, et al. Spinal instability neoplastic score: an analysis of reliability and validity from the spine oncology study group. J Clin Oncol. 2011;29(22):3072–7.
35. Biagini R, Ruggieri P, Mercuri M, Capanna R, Briccoli A, Perin S, et al. Neurologic deficit after resection of the sacrum. Chir Organi Mov. 1997;82(4):357–72.
36. Ghogawala Z, Mansfield FL, Borges LF. Spinal radiation before surgical decompression adversely affects outcomes of surgery for symptomatic metastatic spinal cord compression. Spine. 2001;26(7):818–24.
37. Singh H, Vogel RW, Lober RM, Doan AT, Matsumoto CI, Kenning TJ, et al. Intraoperative neurophysiological monitoring for endoscopic endonasal approaches to the skull base: a technical guide. Scientifica (Cairo). 2016;2016:1751245.
38. Kalkman CJ, Been H. Ongerboer de Visser BW. Intraoperative monitoring of spinal cord function: a review. Acta Orthop Scand. 1993;64(1):114–23.
39. Stener B, Gunterberg B. High amputation of the sacrum for extirpation of tumors. Principles and technique. Spine. 1978;3(4):351–66.
40. Althausen PL, Schneider PD, Bold RJ, Gupta MC, Goodnight JE, Khatri VP. Multimodality management of a giant cell tumor arising in the proximal sacrum: a case report. Spine. 2002;27(15):E361–5.
41. Sciubba DM, Petteys RJ, Garces-Ambrossi GL, Noggle JC, McGirt MJ, Wolinsky JP, et al. Diagnosis and management of sacral tumors. J Neurosurg Spine. 2009;10:244–56.
42. Bydon M, De la Garza-Ramos R, Bettegowda C, Suk I, Wolinsky JP, Gokaslan ZL. En bloc resection of a giant cell tumor in the sacrum via a posterior-only approach without nerve root sacrifice: technical case report. Neurosurgery. 2015;11(Suppl 3):E472–8.
43. Zhang HY, Thongtrangan I, Balabhadra RS, Murovic JA, Kim DH. Surgical techniques for total sacrectomy and spinopelvic reconstruction. Neurosurg Focus. 2003;15(2):E5.
44. Newman CB, Keshavarzi S, Aryan HE. En bloc sacrectomy and reconstruction: technique modification for pelvic fixation. Surg Neurol. 2009;72(6):752–6.
45. Terterov S, Diaz-Aguilar D, Scharnweber R, Tucker A, Niu T, Woodard J, et al. Surgical nuances of partial sacrectomy for chordoma. Surg Neurol Int. 2017;8:277.
46. Gunterberg B, Romanus B, Stener B. Pelvic strength after major amputation of the sacrum: an experimental study. Acta Orthop Scand. 1976;47:635–42.
47. Hays RP. Resection of the sacrum for benign giant cell tumor. Ann Surg. 1953;138:115–20.
48. Cybulski GR. Methods of surgical stabilization for metastatic disease of the spine. Neurosurgery. 1989;25:240–52.
49. Li D, Guo W, Qu H, Yang R, Tang X, Yan T, et al. Experience with wound complications after surgery for sacral tumors. Eur Spine J. 2013;22(9):2069–76.
50. Kim JE, Pang J, Chirstensen JM, Coon D, Zadnik PL, Wolinsky JP, et al. Soft-tissue reconstruction after total en bloc sacrectomy. J Neurosurg Spine. 2015;22(6):571–81.
51. Ahmed AK, Goodwin CR, Sciubba DM. Sacral metastases. In: Marco RAW, editor. Metastatic spine disease: a guide to diagnosis and management. New York; Springer; 2018.

Technique of Oncologic Sacrectomy

23

Peter S. Rose and Daniel M. Sciubba

Introduction

Sacrectomy is considered in the curative treatment of patients with primary sacral malignancies. In addition, select patients with locally invasive visceral malignancies with no evidence of metastases are considered for this procedure. Because of the magnitude of these surgeries and their unavoidable neurologic sacrifice, these procedures are rarely, if ever, indicated for the treatment of metastatic disease. Those patients are better treated with stereotactic radiotherapy or ablation procedures. Lesser/intralesional modifications of the procedures described here may be employed for benign conditions which arise in this anatomic area (e.g., giant-cell tumors, locally advanced osteomyelitis, select metastases) [1].

A wide oncologic margin is necessary for curative treatment of sacral chordomas and sarcomas [2–5]. As such, surgery should only be undertaken with a clear anatomic plan to obtain a wide margin. Coincident with this, patients must be accepting of the functional consequences of surgery before proceeding. An accepted working definition of a wide margin in this area includes 1 cm of histologically normal cancellous bone, intact (uninvolved) cortical bone with overlying periosteum, 2 cm of free tissue (e.g., pyriformis muscle), or an intact fascial boundary (e.g., Waldeyer's fascia ventrally) (Fig. 23.1).

Traditional sacral resections may be classified into low sacrectomies (resection at or below the S3 foramen), mid-sacrectomies (resections above this level but less than total sacrectomies), and total sacrectomies (Fig. 23.2) [6]. The majority of patients who preserve bilateral S3 nerve roots will regain functional bowel, bladder, and sexual capacity [7–10]. As such, the long-term morbidity of low sacrectomies is usually modest. Patients undergoing mid-sacrectomies will have variable preservation of these functions depending on the extent of neurologic sacrifice. Most patients in whom both S2 and a single S3 nerve root are preserved will regain functional (not necessarily normal) bowel, bladder, and sexual capacity; those with loss of both S3 roots and/or loss of one S2 root have variable functions. Patients undergoing total sacrectomies can expect loss of bowel, bladder, and sexual function as well as effects on lower extremity function. If both L5 nerve roots can be preserved, patients often have surprisingly near-normal ambulatory (but not athletic) function. If greater sacrifice is needed, patients will usually have the ability to transfer (by locking their knees through preserved femoral nerve function) but rarely can ambulate significant distances. In assessing neurologic sacrifice, it is important to carefully evaluate for extraforaminal involvement of nerves by

P. S. Rose (✉)
Mayo Clinic, Department of Othopaedic Surgery, Rochester, MN, USA
e-mail: rose.peter@mayo.edu

D. M. Sciubba
Department of Neurosurgery, The Johns Hopkins Hospital, Baltimore, MD, USA

D. M. Sciubba (ed.), *Spinal Tumor Surgery*, https://doi.org/10.1007/978-3-319-98422-3_23

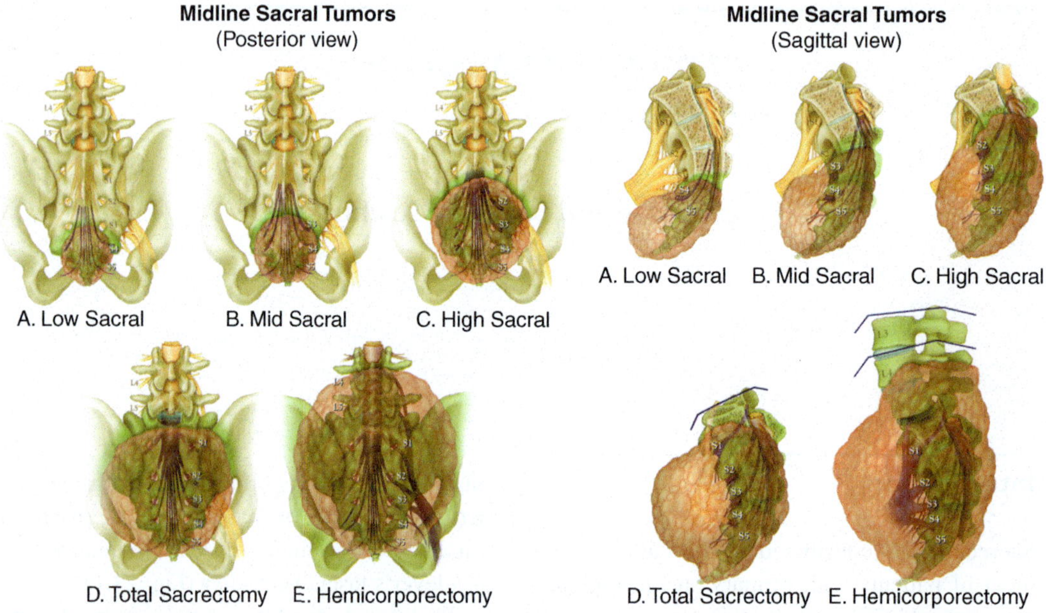

Fig. 23.1 Classification system for primary sacral tumors. (Reprinted with permission from Fourney et al. [6])

tumor. For example, the L5 nerve roots run over the sacral ala. In a patient requiring a total sacrectomy, these roots are often involved by tumor as they traverse the pelvis over the S1 region. As such, the cephalad extent of the tumor only partially predicts the loss of function expected. Similarly, in patients with locally advanced visceral tumors that secondarily involve the sacrum, the presacral involvement of the nerves is often greater than the direct sacral involvement from the tumor.

Patient Presentation

Sacral tumors often initially have poorly localized and non-specific symptoms. Many patients are evaluated for presumed low-lumbar spinal pathology, but many standard imaging protocols of the lumbar spine only include the uppermost sacrum and will fail to diagnose sacral pathologies. Because of the rarity of sacral tumors, the overlapping innervation of the sacral nerve roots, and the large volume of the pelvis, diagnosis is often delayed. At times, this will allow tumors to become quite large with pelvic outlet obstruction (impairment of urination or defecation due to large tumor size). These patients may require a suprapubic catheter and diverting colostomy to prevent visceral rupture, hydronephrosis, and to allow proper evaluation and management of their malignancies (Fig. 23.3).

Patient Evaluation

Patients with sacral malignancies are carefully biopsied to ascertain a certain diagnosis and staged to exclude distant metastases. Core needle biopsy is the preferred method to sample tissue [11]. An ideal biopsy is typically a straight-ahead biopsy performed slightly off midline (Fig. 23.4). This is readily excisable but avoids potential spread of biopsy contamination by epidural veins. Biopsy sites are often marked with methylene blue to facilitate later removal. Transgluteal and transrectal biopsies should be avoided.

Staging classically consists of computed tomography (CT) of the chest, abdomen, and pelvis as well as a bone scan to exclude visceral or bony metastases. In some centers fluorodeoxyglucose-positron emission tomography (FDG-PET) is used

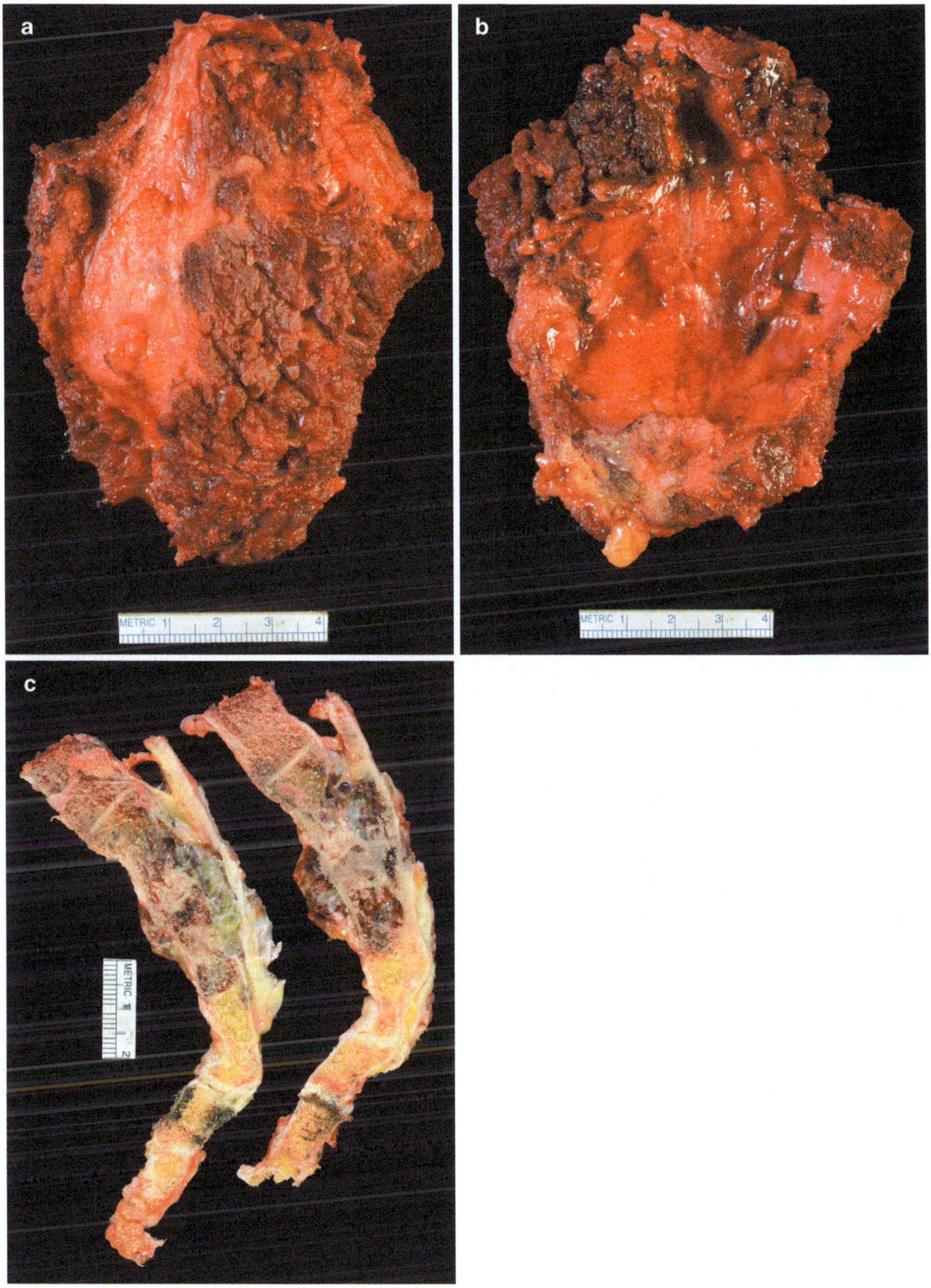

Fig. 23.2 Typical specimen of a sacral malignancy. (**a**, **b**) demonstrate dorsal and ventral views of resected specimen. Note wide margin of soft tissue covering the specimen and Waldeyer's fascia intact in the presacral area. (**c**) cut specimen demonstrating clear cancellous bone margin

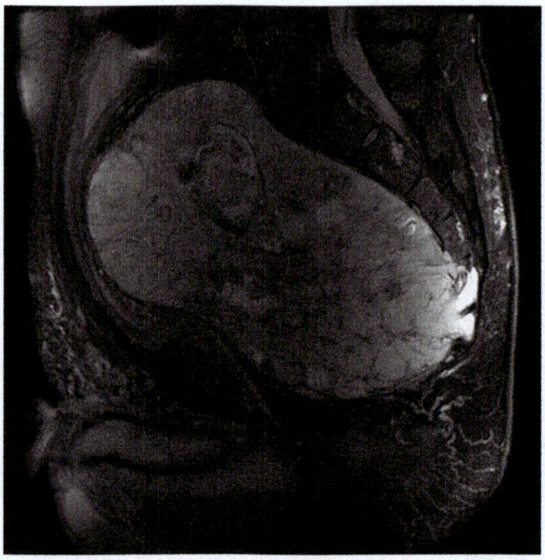

Fig. 23.3 Locally advanced sacropelvic chordoma presenting with obstructive renal failure and impending colon rupture from pelvic outlet obstruction

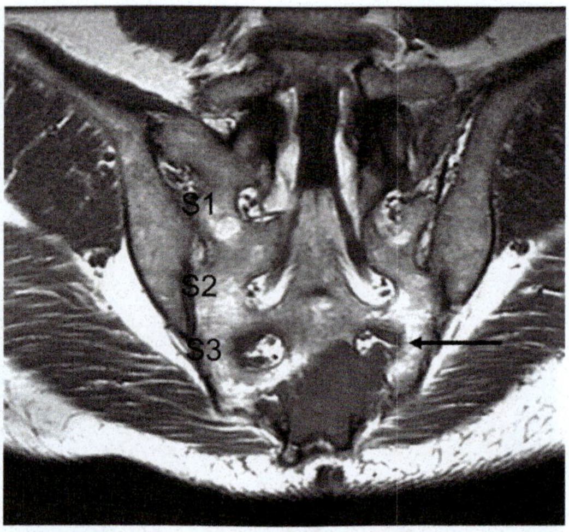

Fig. 23.5 Coronal oblique T1-weighted MR image demonstrates en face view of the sacrum and subtle tumor infiltration into the left S3 foramen

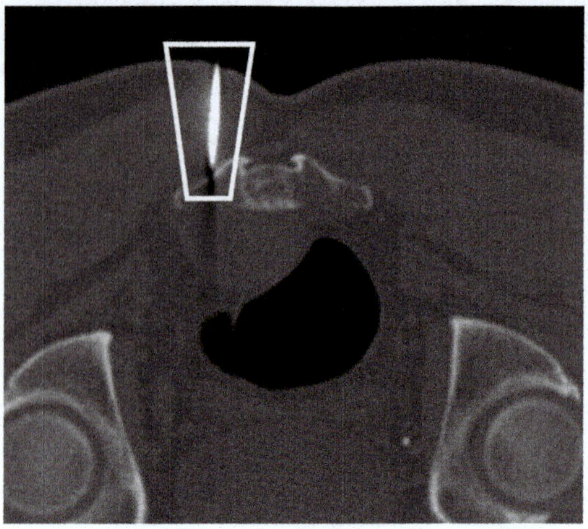

Fig. 23.4 Appropriate needle biopsy of a sacral malignancy. Note the near-midline needle tract is readily excisable and avoids contamination of the epidural space

in place of this protocol. As the sensitivity of PET is influenced by the intrinsic metabolic activity of the tumor, caution should be used while interpreting PET scans of patients with low-grade tumors (e.g., chordoma, low-grade chondrosarcomas) as false negatives can occur.

Magnetic resonance imaging (MRI) provides the best anatomic detail of tumor extent and its relation to neural elements. Our group commonly obtains coronal oblique MR images in addition to traditional axial and sagittal views. These are coronal images in the plane of the sacrum and provide an en face view of the pathologic process (Fig. 23.5). For locally advanced tumors in which vascular or visceral involvement or detail is needed, our group utilizes a three-phase pelvic tumor CT scan. This involves giving a bolus of intravenous (IV) contrast and then obtaining images in the angiographic, venographic, and excretory phases. This allows careful delineation of the pelvic vasculature, rectum, ureters, and bladder in a single scan to establish the visceral involvement of locally advanced tumors (Fig. 23.6).

Note that recent data suggest that a clinically relevant minority of patients presenting with sacral chordomas will have discontiguous lesions elsewhere along the spinal axis [12]. Some chordoma centers obtain a screening MRI of the entire spine as a part of staging in patients with sacral chordomas.

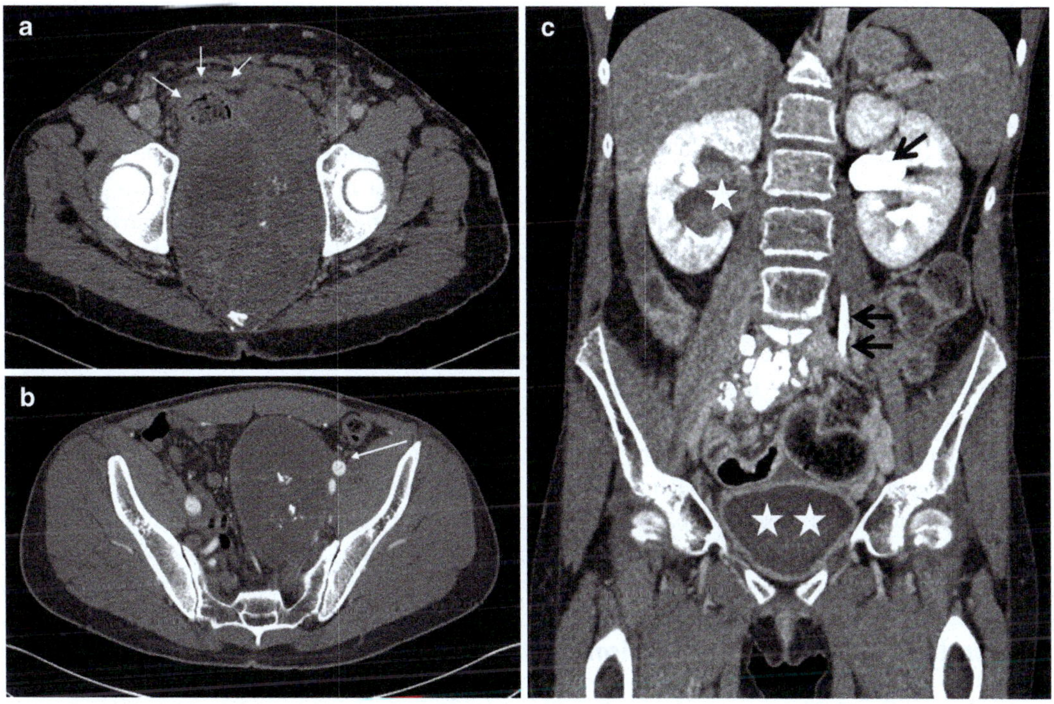

Fig. 23.6 Use of pelvic CT imaging to evaluate surrounding visceral structures. (**a**) rectal invasion by locally advanced chordoma. Note lack of fat plane between tumor and rectum. (**b**) CT angiogram demonstrating dense abutment of left external iliac vessels by tumor. (**c**) Ureteral obstruction from a sacral osteosarcoma. Note dilation with lack of contrast in the right renal pelvis (single star). Left renal pelvis (single arrow) shows contrast with dilation of the left ureter (double arrow). Minimal contrast is present in the bladder (double star). These findings indicate complete occlusion of the right ureter by tumor encasement and significant obstruction of the left ureter

Pre-operative Planning

The primary decision a surgeon makes when planning a sacrectomy is whether to perform a single-stage posterior procedure or an anterior/posterior procedure. An anterior procedure has several advantages. It allows full mobilization of the overlying vascular and visceral structures to minimize the risk of a catastrophic vascular injury to the common or internal iliac vessels from behind. In patients with locally advanced tumors requiring rectal resection or in whom no chance of bowel function exists, it allows for a diverting colostomy to be performed. Additionally, it allows for harvest of a vertical rectus abdominus flap to fill a large soft-tissue defect [13]. These benefits must be balanced against the morbidity of a longer procedure or two separate surgeries that an anterior approach requires.

Unless there is rectal involvement or a very large anticipated soft-tissue defect that requires a rectus abdominus flap, our group will typically perform resections up to the level of mid-S2 level using a single-stage posterior approach. For more proximal resections, we employ a staged anterior/posterior approach and typically perform a diverting colostomy for patients having high or total sacrectomies in which the return of bowel function is not expected. While some authors have advocated performing total sacrectomies through an all-posterior approach [14], we have not favored that for several reasons. First, it is very difficult to confidently stay ventral to Waldeyer's fascia (the presacral fascia that forms the ventral margin of sacral tumor resection) with such an approach. Second, it is difficult to resect through or lateral to the sacroiliac joints in this approach, also commonly necessary to obtain a proper margin. Third, depending on individual anatomy, the common or internal iliac vessels are generally close to the sacral ala and difficult to protect during an all-posterior approach. Fourth, resections of this magnitude have a significant soft-tissue defect that is well served with a rectus abdominus flap. Finally, our group favors colostomy for patients with resections of this magnitude to avoid the wound and quality of life difficulties of a denervated rectum. If a staged approach is used, we typically separate the stages by 48 h and have seen a marked decrease in patient morbidity with this approach [15]. Acknowledging these reasons, other groups have reported reasonable outcomes with an all-posterior approach, and approach decisions remain individualized based on patient factors and institutional practice patterns [16].

General Pre-operative Preparation

All patients receive a mechanical bowel preparation prior to surgery. Patients undergoing anterior/posterior procedures or those of questionable medical fitness undergo a dobutamine stress echocardiogram pre-operatively. Depending on the extent of abnormal anatomy ventrally, temporary ureteral stents may be placed to aid in identification and protection of the ureters. As the spectrum of infecting bacteria for these procedures is broad, piperacillin/tazobactam is used for infectious prophylaxis. We do not perform neurologic monitoring on these cases as neurologic sacrifice is an expected consequence of the tumor resection.

Anterior Approach

Anterior approaches are used in resections above the level of mid-S2, when tumor extension ventrally necessitates visceral resection or if the expected soft-tissue defect requires a rectus abdominus flap [17, 18].

Patients are placed supine on a regular operating room table. A midline transperitoneal approach is performed (a unilateral retroperitoneal approach can be used for unilateral pathology necessitating hemisacrectomy). The visceral structures are mobilized from the tumor or transected as dictated by the oncologic margin needs. Vascular structures are similarly mobilized. While it is generally safe to ligate and transect both internal iliac arteries and veins for locally advanced tumors if the patient is having a colostomy, this does lead to increased bleeding during the posterior approach [19]. The epidural veins (via Batson's plexus) serve as collateral blood returns from the pelvis. Thus, sacrifice of both internal iliac veins will lead to significant epidural engorgement. Additionally, the primary perfusion of the gluteal muscles (which form a portion of the flap closure after sacrectomy) is via the inferior gluteal vessels (branches of the internal iliac arteries). For these reasons we will ligate and divide these vessels only if oncologically necessary. If these vessels are not divided, they must be mobilized fully to avoid inadvertent injury during posterior tumor delivery.

In a similar manner, safe neurologic structures are mobilized as well in this area. This most commonly involves identifying and freeing up the L5 nerve roots as they traverse the sacral ala. If these cannot be freed from the front, they are deliberately transected to avoid avulsion from the dural tube during posterior tumor delivery.

The site of osteotomy is identified using a combination of anatomic landmarks and cross-table lateral fluoroscopy (generally referencing from the superior endplate of S1). A unicortical osteotomy is performed through the ventral cortex of the sacrum. Osteotomy lateral to sacroiliac joints may be performed bicortically. A small screw (typically 10 mm from a standard small fragment set) is placed in the bone just below the osteotomy. This is readily viewable on lateral fluoroscopy during the posterior procedure to guide the surgeon as to the proper site of osteotomy (Fig. 23.7). Note that osteotomies are performed perpendicular to the sacrum (not perpendicular to the operating table). If this distinction is not realized, the osteotomy may traverse more distal than intended into the tumor.

Once these steps are complete, a silastic sheet or sterile sponge is placed between the tumor and the mobilized vessels and visceral

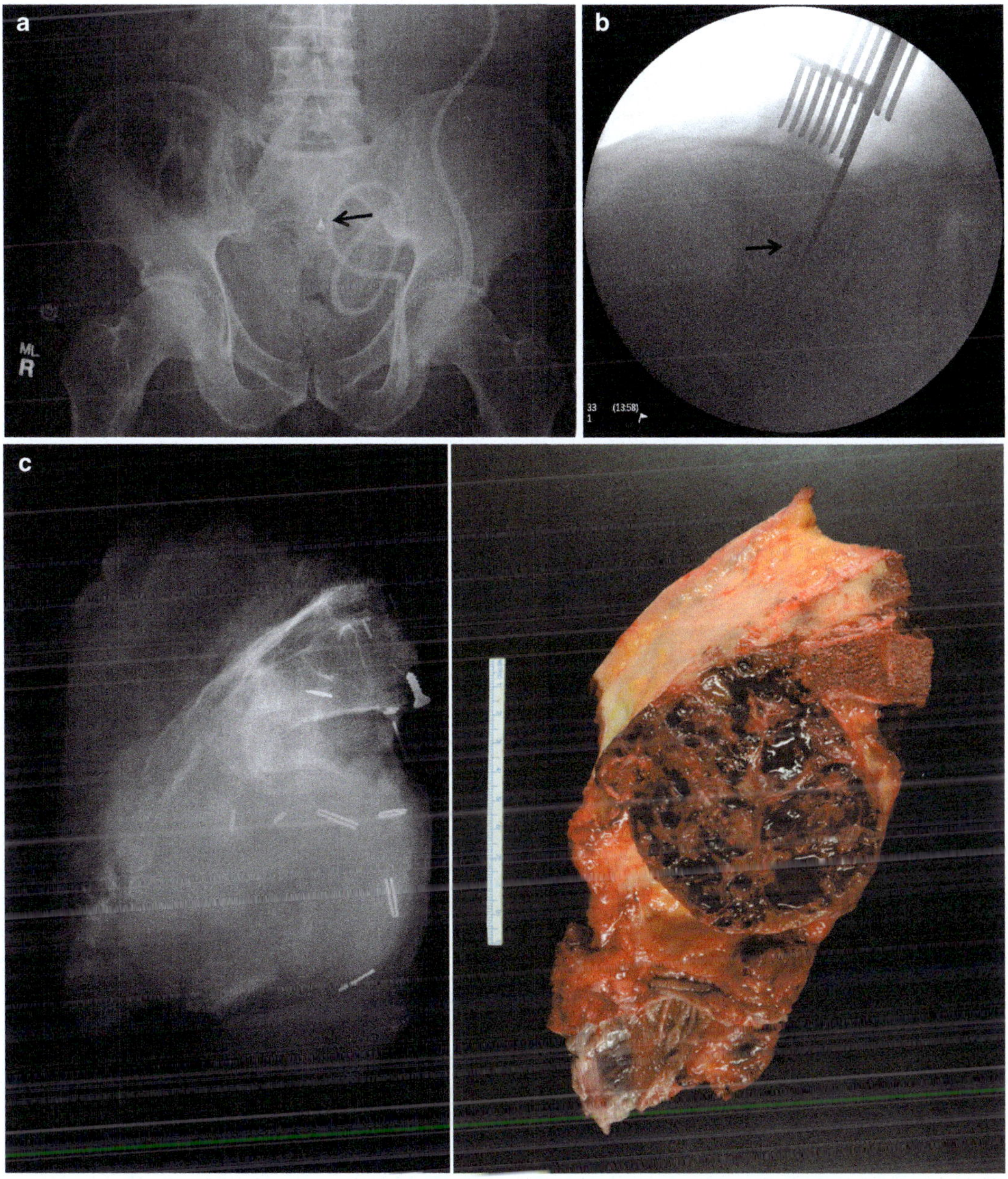

Fig. 23.7 Use of a marker screw during anterior approach. (**a**) Post-operative radiograph demonstrates marker screw placement following anterior approach. (**b**) Screw is readily visualized and guides osteotomy during posterior approach. (**c**) Specimen

structures. A colostomy is performed if indicated, and a vertical rectus abdominus flap is harvested with a skin paddle and tucked into the presacral space just ventral to the silastic sheet or sponge (Fig. 23.8). The rectus abdominus flap is marked for orientation with two sutures to allow it to be brought out without twisting the flap and potentially kinking the pedicle [13]. Wound closure involves interrupted sutures (bearing in mind that the patient will be prone with the abdomen hanging free in 48 h).

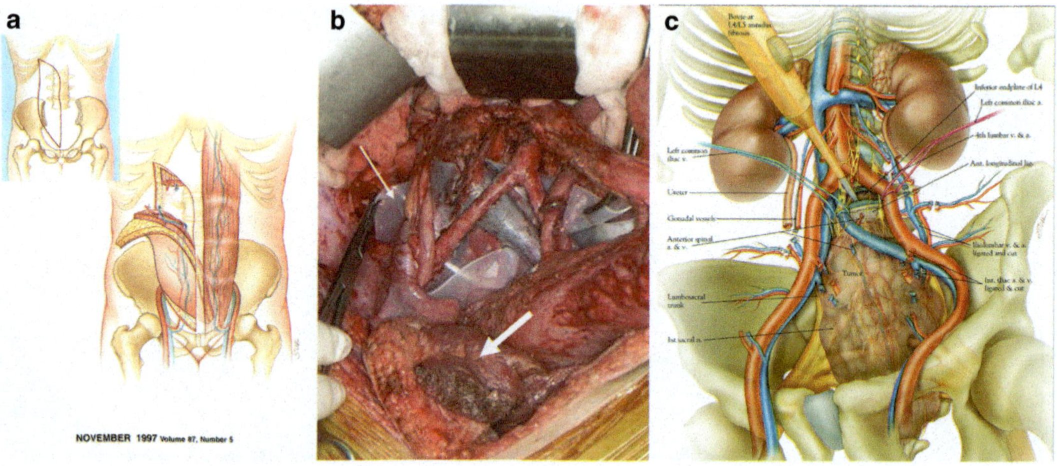

Fig. 23.8 Anterior approach. Note harvested vascularized rectus abdominus muscle (VRAM) flap. (**a**) VRAM artist illustration reprinted with permission from Gokaslan et al. [31]. (**b**) Intraoperative image of VRAM flap tucked into abdomen (large arrow) and silastic sheet placed under dissected vessels (small arrow). (**c**) Artist illustration of anterior release. (Reprinted from Gallia et al. [32], by permission of Oxford University Press)

Patients are usually extubated immediately after the anterior approach and mobilized out of bed to chair that evening or the following day.

Posterior Approach

Patients are positioned prone on a radiolucent table for the posterior approach. If no spinopelvic instrumentation is anticipated, they are placed on a Wilson frame to maximize exposure of the sacrum (if instrumentation is anticipated, they are positioned prone in a standard fashion to avoid instrumenting in relative kyphosis at the lumbopelvic junction). The anus is temporarily sewn shut with a purse-string stitch and draped into the field only if rectal resection is planned. Draping is very wide laterally to allow for mobilization of gluteal advancement flaps. We prefer to use skull tongs to suspend the head and rely primarily on lateral fluoroscopy for intraoperative imaging. Prospectively studied, excellent surgical access and relatively little positioning-related morbidity were observed using this setup [20] (Fig. 23.9).

A midline incision is performed with an ellipse around the biopsy tract. Dissection begins well proximal to the area of suspected tumor, with spot fluoroscopy verifying the location to avoid inadvertent tumor violation. If an anterior approach has been performed, localization is very efficiently done by viewing the marker screw which was placed. Otherwise, the sacral neuroforamen are reliable landmarks that can be viewed fluoroscopically and marked on the operative field (Fig. 23.10). In very heavy patients with low tumors (in which fluoroscopy may be unreliable), a pre-operative fiducial marker may be placed using CT guidance (Fig. 23.11).

Lateral dissection of the parasacral gutters is then performed, with care taken to know the lateral extent of tumor and stay wide of it. The sacrospinous and sacrotuberous ligaments (which separate the greater and lesser sciatic foramen) are divided, usually in the mid-substance or at their pelvic insertions; if tumors have wide lateral extension, the ischial spine may be osteotomized off the pelvis. The pudendal neurovascular bundle is identified between the sacrospinous and sacrotuberous ligaments and preserved if possible (Fig. 23.12). Distal to the sacrotuberous ligament, the coccygeus muscle is divided and the ischiorectal fossa is entered bluntly with a finger. Proximal to these ligaments, the pyriformis muscles are divided. Surgeons are cautioned to be

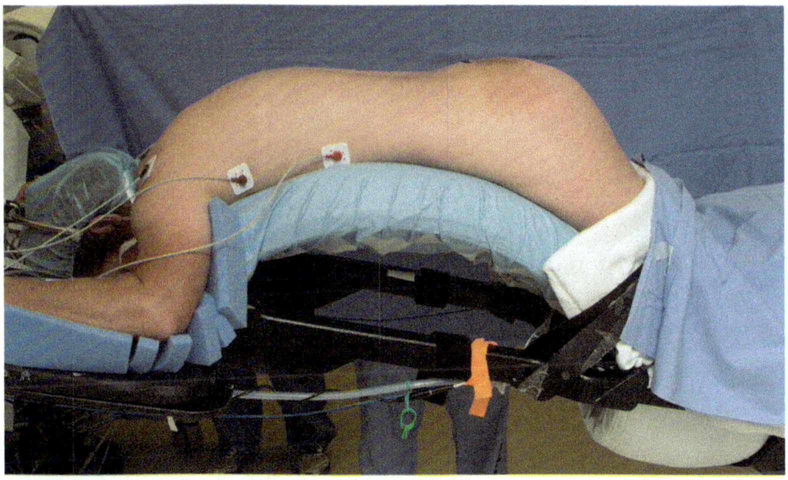

Fig. 23.9 Use of a radiolucent table and Wilson frame to position for sacrectomy

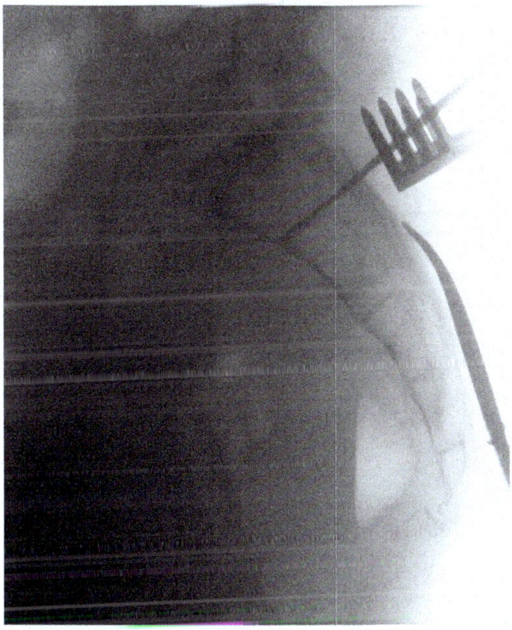

Fig. 23.10 Localization during dorsal sacral resection using lateral fluoroscopy and a blunt probe placed in the neuroforamen safely above the tumor. In this example, the S1 foramen is identified

particularly careful at the roof of the sciatic notch where the superior gluteal vein runs 1–1.5 cm lateral to the caudal sacroiliac joint. Having done this, the surgeon should be able to place his or her finger into the presacral space on either side.

Once this is done, a laminectomy proximal to the level of osteotomy is performed to identify the dural tube and neurologic elements. The tube is ligated with a silk suture and divided. Following this, an osteotomy is performed through the sacrum at the appropriate level. We have found that a 5-mm-round coarse diamond burr works well for this purpose. It can rapidly create a trough through the cancellous bone down to the ventral cortex of the sacrum, with relatively little bony bleeding or tendency to wrap up soft tissue. If the anterior cortex was not breached during an anterior procedure, a 3-mm Kerrison rongeur fits well in the kerf of the burr to allow final delicate extension through the anterior cortex. If a total sacrectomy is performed, the medial quadratus lumborum muscle is released from the posterior ilium, and an osteotomy through the ilium lateral to the sacroiliac joint is performed. The iliolumbar ligaments are preserved between the L5 transverse processes and the medial ilium if possible.

The specimen is delivered proximal to distal, with the last remaining nerve roots being traced and preserved. If the rectum is preserved, dissection is deliberately performed through the mesorectum (ventral to Waldeyer's fascia) to maintain a proper oncologic margin (Fig. 23.13). If an anterior approach was performed, the silastic sheet or sponge marks when the surgeon has reached the proper plane of dissection.

Oncologic margins are verified before proceeding further. The technique of spinopelvic reconstruction is described later separately. If no bony reconstruction is needed, the posterior

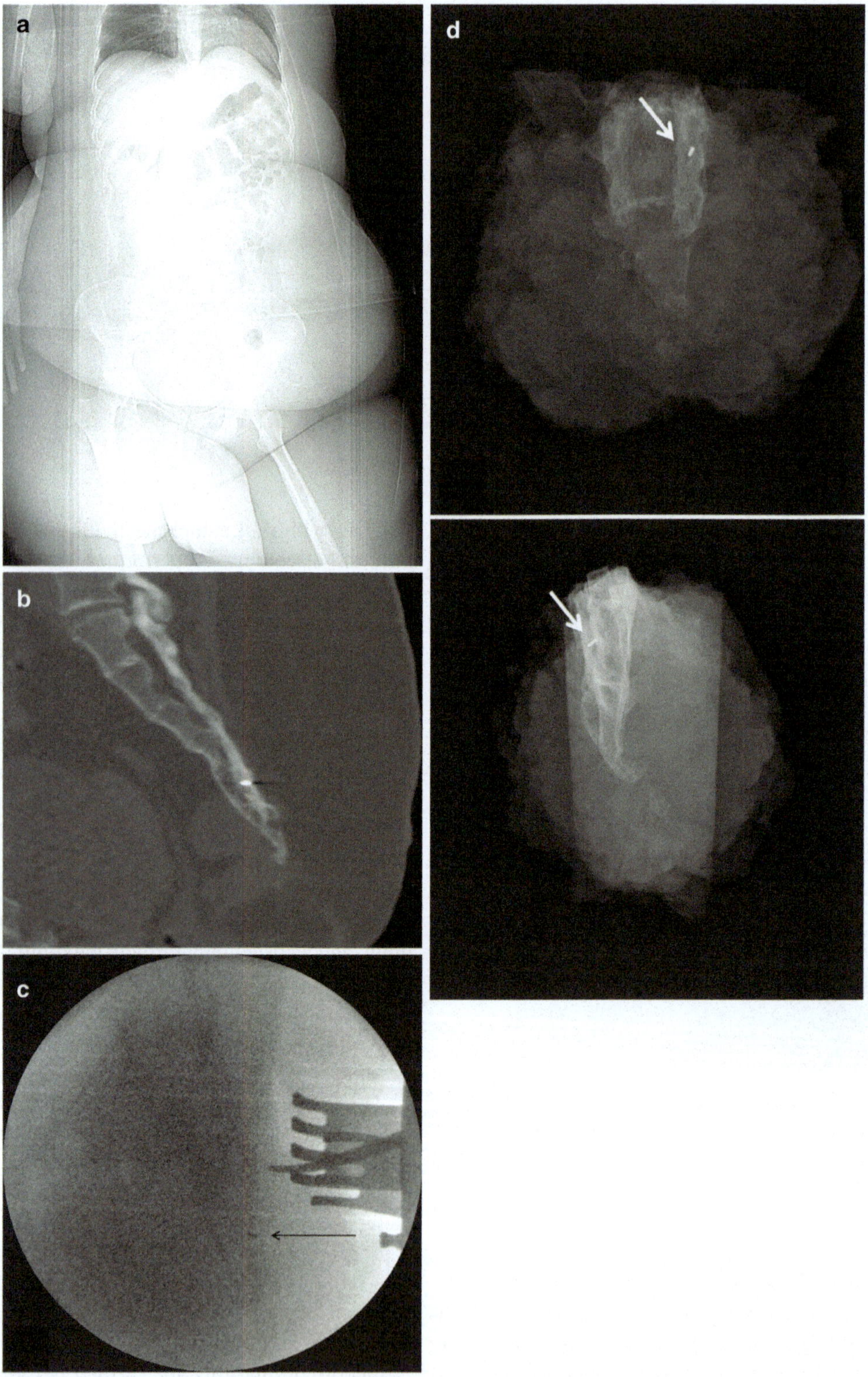

Fig. 23.11 Use of a fiducial marker when fluoroscopy is unreliable. (**a**) Scout CT scan demonstrating body habitus in a woman with a low sacral chordoma. This situation precludes accurate fluoroscopic localization. (**b**) Pre-operative scan showing location of fiducial marker in sacrum. (**c**) Intraoperative lateral fluoroscopy allows identification of marker and proper osteotomy location. (**d**) Specimen

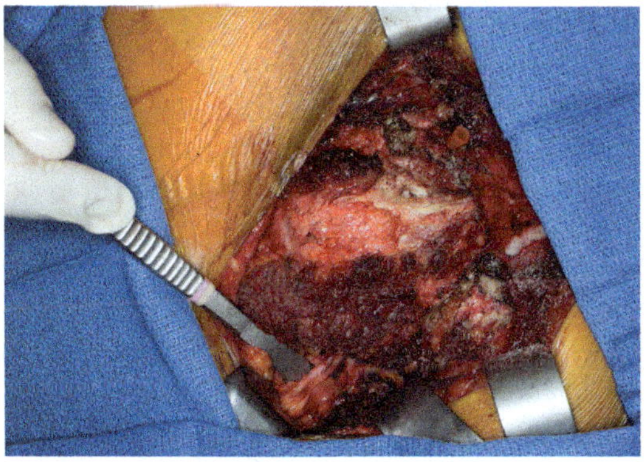

Fig. 23.12 Identification of the pudendal nerve in the parasacral gutter after the sacrospinous and sacrotuberous ligaments have been divided

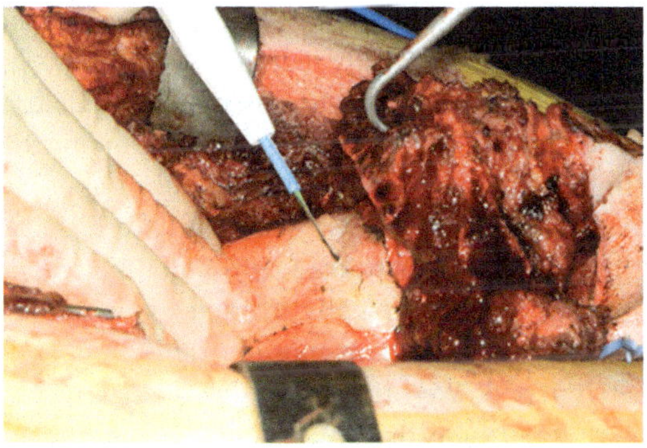

Fig. 23.13 Delivery of specimen proximal to distal with dissection through the mesorectum to stay ventral to Waldeyer's fascia

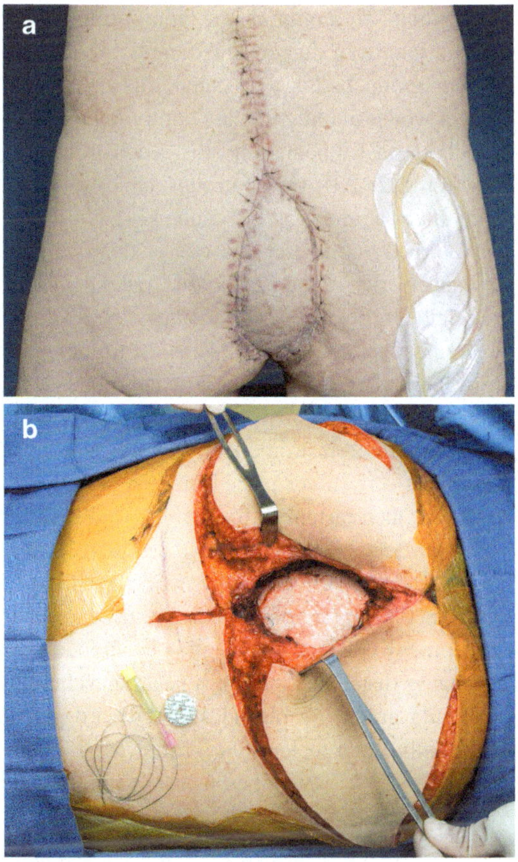

Fig. 23.14 Posterior wound closure options. (**a**) Vertical rectus abdominus flap inset following a staged anterior/posterior procedure. (**b**) Gluteal V–Y advancement flaps over a mesh posterior abdominal wall reconstruction. Note epidural catheter in place for post-operative pain control

abdominal wall is reconstructed in one of two ways. If a rectus abdominus flap is harvested, its bulk will generally reconstruct this area with the fascia of the flap sewn into the fascia of the gluteal muscles on each side. Care should be taken in delivering this so as to not lose orientation and inadvertently rotate it or avulse its vascular pedicle. If no rectus abdominus flap is harvested, bilateral gluteal V–Y advancement flaps are created. A mesh reconstruction of the posterior abdominal wall is performed and covered with the gluteal flaps (Fig. 23.14).

An epidural catheter is introduced through the skin proximal and lateral to the wound edge and inserted into the epidural space under direct vision prior to final closure. An incisional wound vacuum device is placed to protect the wound from soilage and shear stress.

Spinopelvic Reconstruction

Instrumented spinopelvic reconstruction is performed in two situations. First, in the event of total sacrectomy, spinopelvic reconstruction is used to recreate spinopelvic continuity. Second, in near-total sacrectomies performed above the level of the S1 foramina, clinical experience and biomechanical studies have demonstrated a high risk of subsequent fracture of the remaining sacrum [21]. Spinopelvic reconstruction is performed to augment the remaining native bone strength in this circumstance.

Our group favors the "cathedral" reconstruction in which fibula grafts are combined with spinopelvic instrumentation to reconstruct this junction [22, 23]. Other groups have utilized a trans-iliac bar and graft technique [24]. No studies have directly compared the two or demonstrated the superiority of one technique over the other. The cathedral reconstruction is described below.

In most patients, pedicle screw instrumentation is placed into L3, L4, and L5 using aggressively long screws to maximize purchase. In large patients, more proximal instrumentation levels are used. Dual iliac screws are placed in each side. Fibula grafts are then fashioned to span the area between the supra-acetabular ilium and the caudal level of the spine. In extensive bony resections or if the L5 or S1 nerve root is preserved, it can be difficult sometimes to place a fibula in this location, and an alternative distal docking site is near the ischium.

Fibula grafts are placed and rods are placed and compressed to lock the grafts (as shown in Fig. 23.15). We have taken to using two rods on each side whenever practical to minimize the risk of catastrophic failure from a single-rod breakage [25]. It is deceptively easy to fix the spine to the pelvis in relative kyphosis by allowing the distal lumbar spine to drift posteriorly (up into the wound) prior to fixing it in place. If a subtotal sacrectomy is performed and the reconstruction is being used to augment the remaining native strength, true compression across the fibula grafts is not possible. In this circumstance, they are doweled into their docking sites in the pelvis and slotted into the remaining sacrum, with a "biscuit" of bone (either allograft or a piece of iliac crest autograft) used to hold them in place.

Our group has experience using fibula allografts and vascularized autografts for these reconstructions (Fig. 23.16). A recent analysis demonstrated far superior union with the use of vascularized grafts, and this is now our default approach to these patients [26, 27].

Post-operative Care

Patients recover on a specialty air mattress to minimize pressure sites on their wounds. Patients undergoing single-stage posterior resections are typically extubated immediately following the procedure and may go to the regular floor or a monitored ("step-down") unit as clinically indicated for monitoring and pain control. Patients undergoing the second stage of a two-stage procedure are usually extubated the same day if no spinopelvic reconstruction is performed. If a spinopelvic reconstruction is performed (particularly if vascularized fibula grafts are used), the added operative time in the prone position usually results in intubation overnight to allow facial edema to resolve. These patients all go either to a monitored step-down unit or to an intensive care unit (ICU) as clinically indicated.

Patients are allowed to assume any position of comfort on their specialty bed (including sitting up as the bed allows—usually to approximately 40 degrees). We wait until we feel that local swelling has peaked until mobilizing them further. This is typically marked by an autodiuresis that is noted on approximately post-operative day 3. We often use a low-dose (1–2 mg/hr) furosemide drip to encourage diuresis but avoid any bolus furosemide in diuretic naïve patients to avoid any sudden swings in blood pressure that could compromise flap or fibula perfusion.

Beginning approximately on post-operative day 3, patients are allowed to stand and walk as much as possible and to sit on a paraplegic seating cushion (ROHO cushion). We typically have patients sit 20 min at a time the first day, 30 min at a time the second day, and then progress in a similar fashion while the wound is monitored. The epidural catheter dose is halved on day 3 and then removed on day 4 or 5. Prophylactic anticoagulation is begun immediately after surgery with unfractionated heparin.

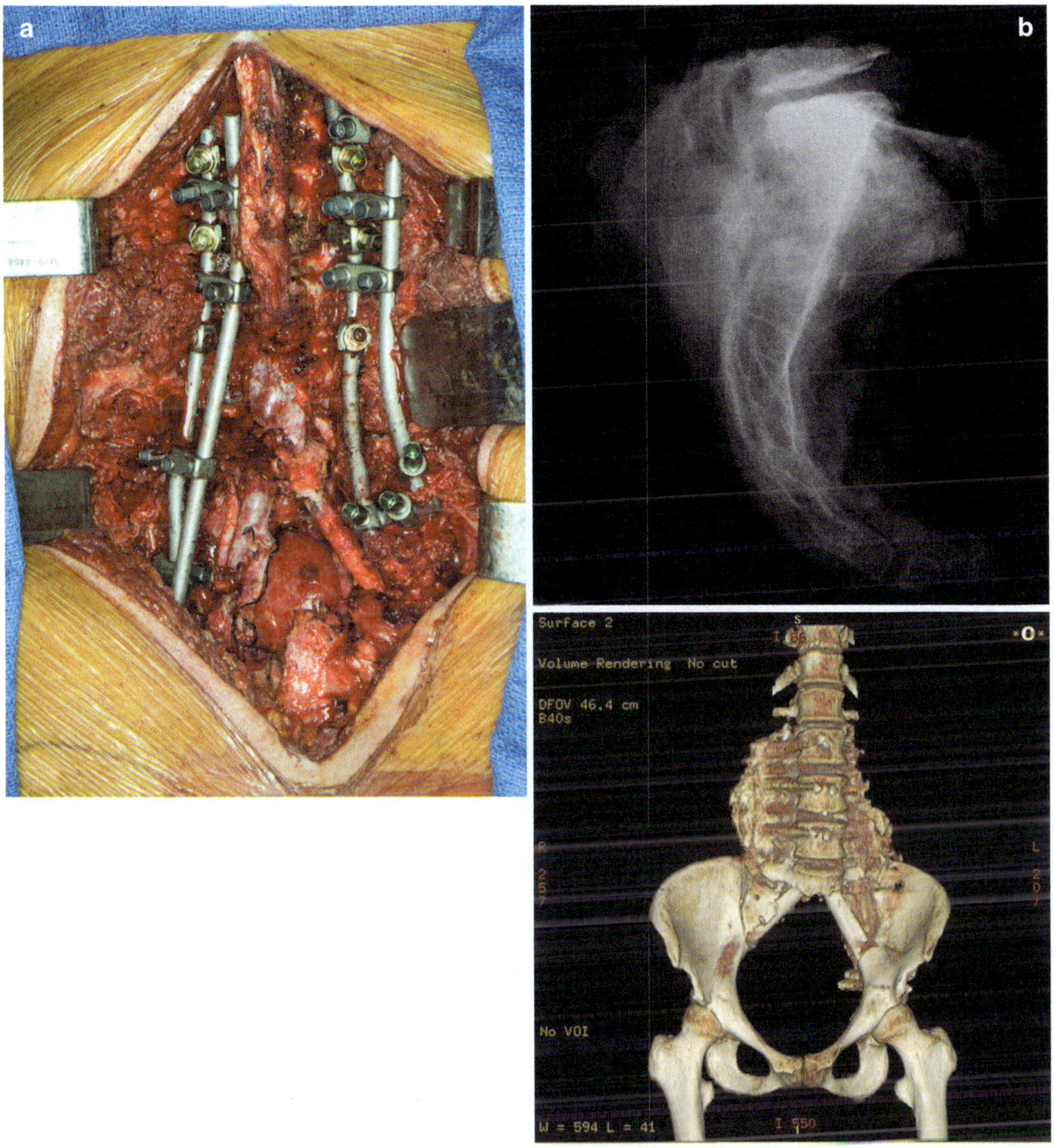

Fig. 23.15 (**a**) Intraoperative photograph of cathedral reconstruction with vascularized fibula grafts following total sacrectomy. (**b**) Specimen radiograph. (**c**) CT demonstrating reconstruction of the spinopelvic junction

Complications

The anatomic complexity of this procedure exposes patients to many potential complications. A general or colorectal surgeon assists with the ventral dissection in patients undergoing anterior/posterior resections to minimize the risk of visceral or vascular injury. Ureteral stents are used if there is any concern for distorted anatomy near the ureters' paths. We have found that separating the anterior and posterior procedures by ~48 h in large spinopelvic resections significantly decreases ICU stay, time of intubation, and morbidity [15].

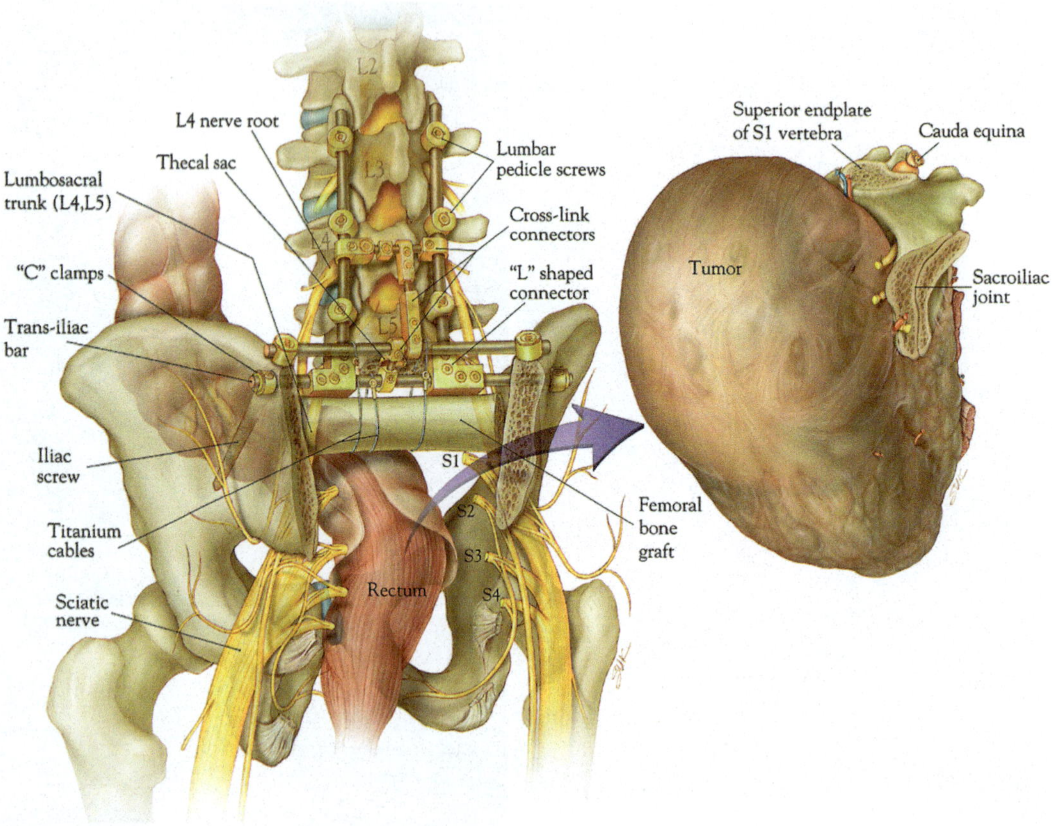

Fig. 23.16 Artist illustration of post-sacrectomy reconstruction with trans-iliac bar and femoral bone graft. (Reprinted from Gallia et al. [32], by permission of Oxford University Press)

Infection and wound dehiscence (really two expressions of the same process) are the most common complications encountered [3, 28]. The magnitude and length of the surgery as well as the anatomic location contribute to this risk. Piperacillin/tazobactam is commonly used for infectious prophylaxis. If no bowel transection is performed, this is given for 24 h around the surgical procedure(s). If a bowel transection is performed during the anterior procedure, this is continued through 72 h after the second procedure. The reasoning behind this approach is that there is inevitably some spillage of bacteria with the bowel transection that could infect the mesh or instrumentation placed in the second-stage procedure. Seventy-two hours of piperacillin/tazobactam is standard antibiotic treatment for heavily contaminated (e.g., barnyard injury) open fractures at our institution. While we have not fully avoided post-operative infections with this regimen, almost all infections have been associated with initial flap dehiscence (i.e., "outside-in" infections). Pre-operative radiotherapy has been shown to greatly increase the risk of infectious and wound complications [29].

Pseudoarthrosis and rod breakage are a recognized risk in patients requiring reconstruction. We have realized the greatly improved healing potential of vascularized fibula grafts in our practice experience [26, 27]. Additionally, the use of dual rods on each side has been shown biomechanically to increase the rigidity of the construct and mitigate the risk of catastrophic rod failure [25].

We have also recognized the importance of reconstructing the posterior abdominal wall with a mesh or rectus abdominus flap. Absent this, when patients Valsalva, they are prone to posterior prolapse of their pelvic viscera. This can lead to functional problems with voiding or defecation even when sphincter innervation remains intact.

Outcomes

Oncologic outcomes are dominated by the histology under study and the surgical margin which is achieved. While the histology is not modifiable, the surgical margin is under the operative team's control. A wide surgical margin in sacral chordomas and spinal chondrosarcomas, for example, has been shown to be the greatest predictor of disease-free survival in patients [2–5]. In a large group of patients who were evaluated for quality of life and other patient-related outcomes after sacrectomy, physical function varied with the level of resection but overall quality of life remained very high. Loss of the S3 root correlated statistically with decreased health-related quality of life in a multi-institutional study of 74 patients undergoing oncologic sacral resections [30].

Case Presentation 1

This 14-year-old female presented with low sacral pain due to a lytic lesion involving S3–S5, with involvement of the S5 nerve roots (Fig. 23.17). CT-guided biopsy confirmed the diagnosis of aneurysmal bone cyst. To treat the lesion and the patient's symptoms, it was determined the best course of action would be a mid-level sacrectomy without instrumentation.

The patient was placed prone on a Jackson table, and x-ray was taken for localization. A midline skin incision and subperiosteal dissection were performed. Laminectomies were performed at S3, S4, and S5, accompanied by soft-tissue dissection around the distal sacrum. The S3, S4, and S5 nerve roots were identified and followed distally. Due to the involvement of the S5 roots with the tumor, these were sacrificed, with preservation of S3 and S4 bilaterally. The tumor was identified, and an ultrasonic blade was utilized to perform a sacrectomy superior to the lesion. This included taking the sacrum and coccyx from S3 down. Meticulous hemostasis was maintained, and intraoperative monitoring was stable throughout the case.

Complex wound closure was performed by plastic and reconstructive surgery. The paraspinal muscles were identified, and the right-sided paraspinal muscle was elevated. An incision was fashioned in the fascia, lateral to the fascial attachment to the thoracolumbar fascia. The left paraspinal muscle was elevated over this, and a

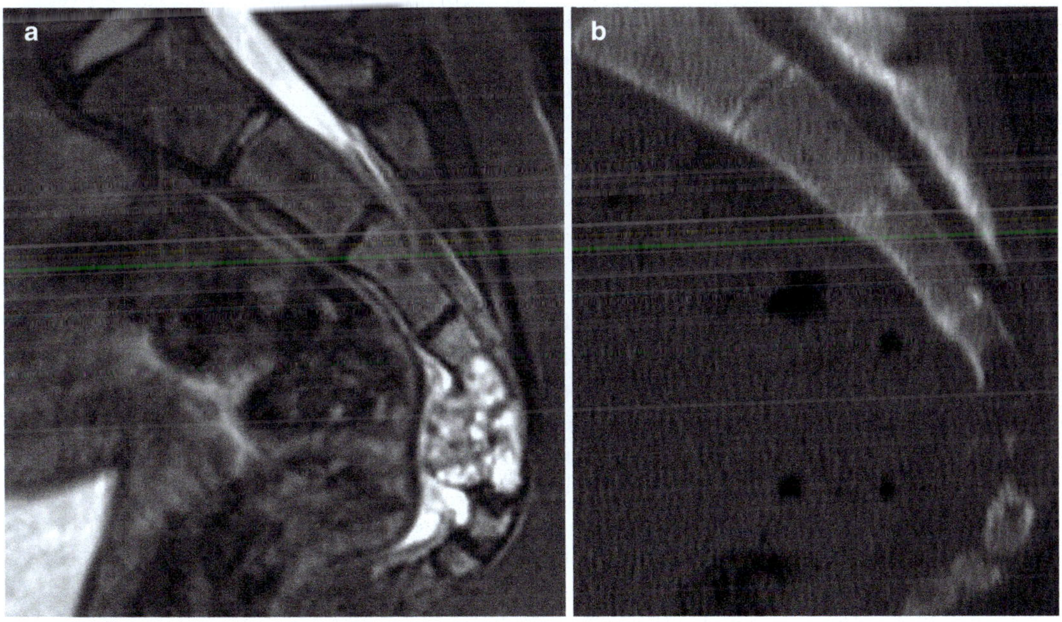

Fig. 23.17 Case presentation 1 pre-operative imaging of distal sacral lesion. (**a**) Sagittal T2-weighted MRI. (**b**) Sagittal CT

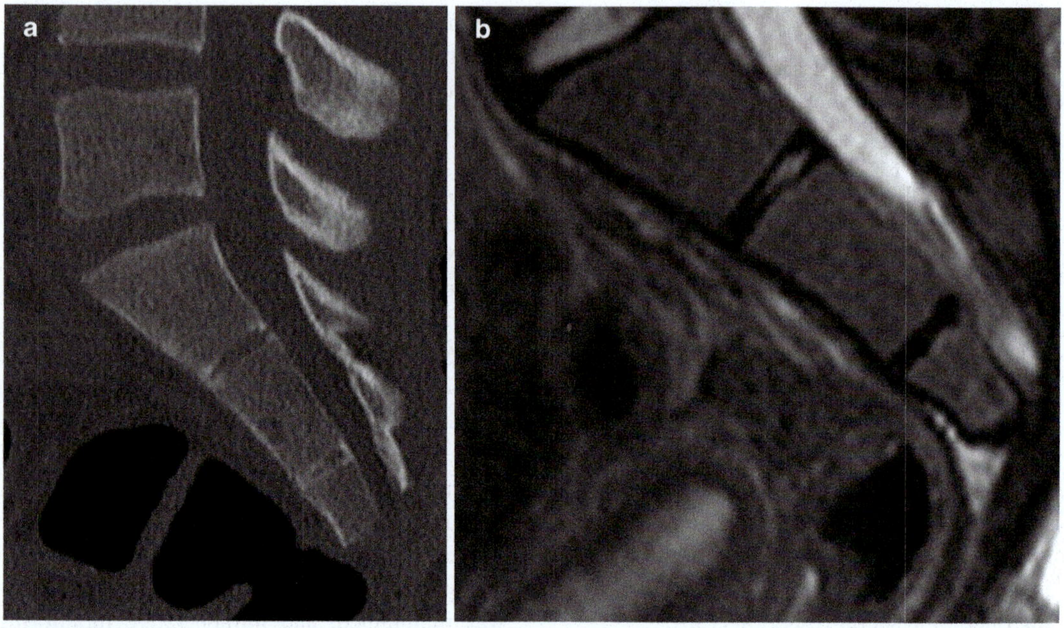

Fig. 23.18 Case presentation 1 post-operative imaging of mid-level sacrectomy. (**a**) Sagittal CT. (**b**) Sagittal T2-weighted MRI

fascial incision was made laterally in the left paraspinal muscle over the central portion of the wound. A 15-French subfascial drain was placed, and the fascia was closed with 0 Vicryl suture. The superficial fascia was closed with interrupted 2–0 Vicryl and dermis closed with 3–0 Vicryl. The subcuticular layer was closed with 4–0 Monocryl. The patient was doing well 8 months post-operatively, with relief of her sacral pain and no evidence of recurrence (Fig. 23.18).

Conclusion

Oncologic sacrectomy represents a spectrum of procedures which can be undertaken in the curative treatment of patients with localized malignancies. Surgeons can plan operations to properly achieve a negative oncologic margin. Local tumor requirements will dictate whether patients require a single posterior or a staged anterior/posterior approach. Patient-reported quality of life after sacrectomy is surprisingly well maintained given the nature of these procedures.

References

1. Du Z, Guo W, Yang R, Tang X, Ji T, Li D. What is the value of surgical intervention for sacral metastases? PLoS One. 2016;11:e0168313.
2. Fuchs B, Dickey ID, Yaszemski MJ, Inwards CY, Sim FH. Operative management of sacral chordoma. J Bone Joint Surg Am. 2005;87:2211–6.
3. Hsieh PC, Xu R, Sciubba DM, McGirt MJ, Nelson C, Witham TF, et al. Long-term clinical outcomes following en bloc resections for sacral chordomas and chondrosarcomas: a series of twenty consecutive patients. Spine. 2009;15:2233–9.
4. Ruggieri P, Angelini A, Ussia G, Montalti M, Mercuri M. Surgical margins and local control in resection of sacral chordomas. Clin Orthop Relat Res. 2010;468:2939–47.
5. Angelini A, Pala E, Calabro T, Maraldi M, Ruggieri P. Prognostic factors in surgical resection of sacral chordoma. J Surg Oncol. 2015;112:344–51.
6. Fourney DR, Rhines LD, Hentschel SJ, Skibber JM, Wolinsky JP, Weber KL, et al. En bloc resection of primary sacral tumors: classification of surgical approaches and outcome. J Neurosurg Spine. 2005;3(2):111–22.
7. Gunterberg B, Kewenter J, Petersen I, Stener B. Anorectal function after major resections of the sacrum with bilateral or unilateral sacrifice of sacral nerves. Br J Surg. 1976;63:546–54.

8. Gunterberg B, Norlen L, Stener B, Sundin T. Neurologic evaluation after resection of the sacrum. Investig Urol. 1975;13:183–8.
9. Todd LT Jr, Yaszemski MJ, Currier BL, Fuchs B, Kim CW, Sim FH. Bowel and bladder function after major sacral resection. Clin Orthop Relat Red. 2002;397:36–9.
10. Moran D, Zadnik PL, Taylor T, Groves ML, Yurter A, Wolinsky JP, et al. Maintenance of bowel, bladder, and motor functions after sacrectomy. Spine J. 2015;15:222–9.
11. Mankin HJ, Mankin CJ, Simon MA. The hazards of biopsy revisited. J Bone Joint Surg Am. 1996;78:656–63.
12. Sebro R, DeLaney TF, Hornicek F, Schwab J, Choy E, Nielsen GP, et al. Frequency and risk factors for additional lesions in the axial spine in subjects with chordoma: indications for screening. Spine. 2017;42:E37–40.
13. Glatt BS, Disa JJ, Mehrara BJ, Pusic AL, Boland P, Cordeiro PG. Reconstruction of extensive partial or total sacrectomy defects with a transabdominal vertices rectus abdominus flap. Ann Plast Surg. 2006;56:526–30.
14. McLoughlin GS, Sciubba DM, Witham T, Bydon A, Gokaslan ZL, Wolinsky JP. En bloc sacrectomy performed in a single stage through a posterior approach. Neurosurgery. 2008;63:ONS115–20.
15. Brown MJ, Kor DJ, Curry TB, Warner MA, Rodrigues ES, Rose SH, et al. Sacral tumor resection : the effect of surgical staging on patient outcomes, resource management, and hospital cost. Spine. 2011;26:1570–8.
16. Clarke MJ, Dasenbrook H, Bydon A, Sciubba DM, McGirt MJ, Hsieh PC, et al. Posterior-only approach for en bloc sacrectomy. Neurosurgery. 2012;71:357–64.
17. MacCarty CS, Waugh JM, Mayo CW, Coventry MB. The surgical treatment of presacral tumors : a combined problem. Proc Staff Meet Mayo Clin. 1952;27:73–84.
18. Stener B, Gunteberg B. High amputation of the sacrum for extirpation of tumors : principles and techniques. Spine. 1978;3:351–66.
19. Hata M, Kawahara N, Tomita K. Influence of ligation of the internal iliac veins on the venous plexuses around the sacrum. J Orthop Sci. 1998;3:264–71.
20. Sherman CE, Rose PS, Pierce LL, Yaszemski MJ, Sim FH. Prospective assessment of patient morbidity from prone sacral positioning. J Neurosurg Spine. 2012;16:51–6.
21. Hugate RR Jr, Dickey ID, Phimolsarnti R, Yaszemski MJ, Sim FH. Mechanical effects of partial sacrectomy: when is reconstruction necessary? Clin Orthop Relat Res. 2006;450:82–8.
22. Dickey ID, Higate RR Jr, Fuchs B, Yaszemski MJ, Simg FH. Reconstruction after total sacrectomy: early experience with a new technique. Clin Orthop Relat Res. 2005;438:42–50.
23. Eck JC, Yaszemski MJ, Sim FH. Sacrectomy and spinopelvic reconstruction. Semin Spine Surg. 2009;21:99–105.
24. Gallia G, Haque R, Garonzik I, Witham TF, Khavkin YA, Wolinsky JP, et al. Spinal-pelvic reconstruction after total sacrectomy for en bloc resection of a giant sacral chordoma: technical note. J Neurosurg Spine. 2005;3:501–6.
25. Kelly B, Shen F, Schwab J, Arlet V, Diangelo DJ. Biomechanical testing of a novel four-rod technique for lumbopelvic reconstruction. Spine. 2008;33:E400–6.
26. Ackerman DB, Rose PS, Moran SL, Dekutoski MB, Bishop AT, Shin AY. The results of vascularized-free fibular grafts in complex spinal reconstruction. J Spinal Disord Tech. 2011;24:170–6.
27. McDowell S, Sim F, Rose P, Yaszemski M. Reconstruction of the pelvic ring following surgery for malignancy involving the sacroiliac joint. 19th International Society of Limb Salvage General Meeting. Kanazawa, Japan. 2017.
28. Zileli M, Hoscuskun C, Brastianos P, Sabah D. Surgical treatment of primary sacral tumors: complications associated with sacrectomy. Neurosurg Focus. 2003;15:1–8.
29. Houdek M, Rose P, Schwab P, Yaszemski M, et al. A comparison of outcome of treatment paradigms for sacral chordoma: does pre-operative radiation improve prognosis? Musculoskeletal Tumor Society Annual Meeting. Denver, 2017.
30. Van Wulfften Palthe OD, Houdek MT, Rose PS, Yaszemski MJ, Sim FH, Boland PJ, et al. How does the level of nerve root resection in en bloc sacrectomy influence patient-reported outcomes? Clin Orthop Relat Res. 2017;475:607–16.
31. Gokaslan ZL, Romsdahl MM, Kroll SS, et al. Total sacrectomy and Galveston L-rod reconstruction for malignant neoplasms. Technical note. J Neurosurg. 1997;87(5):781–8.
32. Gallia GL, Suk I. Lumbopelvic reconstruction after combined L5 spondylectomy and total sacrectomy for en bloc resection of a malignant fibrous histiocytoma. Neurosurgery. 2010;67:E498–02.

Part III

Intradural Approaches

Intradural Extramedullary Tumor: Cervical

24

Kyle L. McCormick and Paul C. McCormick

Introduction

Intradural extramedullary tumors of the cervical spine are overwhelmingly benign, noninvasive, biologically indolent lesions that can be safely and effectively managed or cured with microsurgical resection. The vast majority of these tumors are either nerve sheath tumors or meningiomas. Standard exposures and techniques allow for complete resection with preservation or recovery of neurological function in most cases. Appropriate patient selection and preoperative evaluation; choice and execution of an operative approach that provides safe, secure, and adequate exposure; and appropriate microsurgical techniques of tumor dissection and removal to protect neurological structures and function are long-standing principles of neurosurgical treatment of these tumors. Nevertheless, there are so many factors and variables that must be considered and addressed that each case should be considered unique. Patient condition and co-morbidities, tumor size, axial and sagittal location, vascularity, consistency, origin and attachments, as well as surgeon experience and preferences must be incorporated into each treatment plan. In this chapter, we address both general principles and specific factors and considerations of the surgical management of these tumors.

K. L. McCormick · P. C. McCormick (✉)
Neurosurgery Department, Columbia University Medical Center, New York, NY, USA
e-mail: pcm6@cumc.columbia.edu

Patient Selection

Due to the slow growth of most intradural extramedullary tumors, many of these lesions can be moderately large before the onset of neurological signs or symptoms. Increasingly, however, due to the availability and use of magnetic resonance imaging (MRI), many patients are diagnosed with minimal, nonspecific, or no neurological symptoms.

Management recommendations for asymptomatic or minimally symptomatic patients can be difficult and must be balanced by patient factors and preferences, surgical risks, both current and future, and tumor biology. Small and moderate incidental tumors are often followed over time with annual imaging and clinical evaluation. The onset of symptoms, substantial growth, spinal cord compression, and patient preferences are common circumstances for the recommendation of surgery in these patients. Many of these tumors, however, are very indolent and show little or even negligible growth over long time frames, thereby mitigating the need for intervention. The threshold for surgical treatment is variable in these patients but is clearly appropriate once neurological symptoms commence. In these patients, standard preoperative evaluations are performed to optimize patient condition for surgery.

D. M. Sciubba (ed.), *Spinal Tumor Surgery*, https://doi.org/10.1007/978-3-319-98422-3_24

Operative Planning and Approach

A fundamental key to successful surgical treatment of these lesions is to achieve safe, secure, adequate exposure that is maintained throughout the surgical procedure. For most tumors, this can be achieved through a posterior midline exposure [1–4]. Minimally invasive or mini-open exposures can be utilized in appropriate cases, but it's important to recognize that most of the risks and morbidities are related to the intradural component of the surgery, not the incision, soft-tissue dissection, or bone removal [5]. Following routine induction and endotracheal intubation, the patient is placed in a prone position with the head immobilized in a Mayfield frame.

Intraoperative monitoring and nerve stimulation are utilized but, in our experience, are of limited practical value. The neck and cervical spine are positioned as parallel to the floor as possible with a "military-prone" position with a Mayfield head frame (Fig. 24.1). This optimizes visualization under the operating microscope. The arms are tucked at the side, and the abdomen is free from any pressure. A midline incision and subperiosteal muscle dissection are performed. Meticulous hemostasis is crucial because the surgical field (i.e., intradural space) is at the bottom of the surgical exposure. Thus, any ongoing blood loss from skin, muscle, bone, or epidural space will invariably contaminate the surgical field and violate the principle of secure operative exposure.

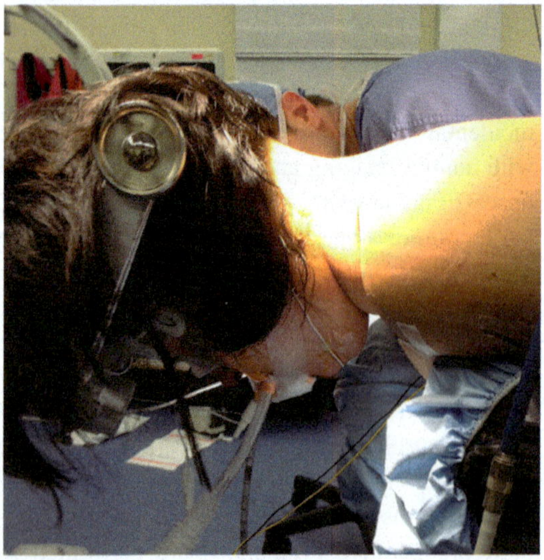

Fig. 24.1 Intraoperative photograph shows "military-prone" position with a Mayfield head frame

Either a standard laminectomy or osteoplastic laminoplasty may be performed. An osteoplastic laminectomy is considered in younger patients and for longer exposures (i.e., more than two spine segments). A unilateral laminectomy is considered for unilateral small or moderate tumors that do no cross the midline. In most cases, optimization of the surgical exposure includes bony removal that extends beyond the tumor margins. This allows for a dural opening that allows both visualization and access just beyond the longitudinal and transverse margins of the tumor. Intraoperative ultrasound is useful prior to dural opening to assure that adequate bone removal has been performed. The dura is then opened in the midline and tented laterally to the paraspinal muscles with suture. The suture should engage the most ventral aspect of the paraspinal muscle in order to evert the dura to both maximize intradural exposure and minimize any epidural venous bleeding into the surgical field. If possible, it is preferable to leave the arachnoid intact during the dural opening. This prevents early cerebrospinal fluid (CSF) drainage, which may obscure the operative field and promote epidural bleeding.

Modifications, Pearls, Pitfalls, and Specific Considerations

The vast majority of tumors are adequately accessed and exposed via a standard posterior approach. Even tumors that arise ventrally or are predominantly ventral to the dentate ligaments can usually be safely accessed via the posterior midline approach because in most cases, the spinal cord has been rotated or displaced to one side to allow access to the ventral spinal canal. Exceptions do exist for purely ventral tumors that displace the spinal cord dorsally without rotation or lateral displacement. This is more likely with meningiomas but is occasionally encountered with nerve sheath tumors arising from the ventral nerve roots. In these cases, a ventral approach may need to be considered since more posterolateral exposure is limited in the cervical spine [6, 7].

In most cases, the dura is opened longitudinally and in the midline. A more eccentric opening may be utilized for eccentric lesions or for dorsal midline meningiomas.

Intradural Exposure/Dissection

Once adequate intradural exposure has been secured, the focus is placed on tumor removal. Again, there are numerous, often interrelated, factors to be considered in terms of how to proceed and sequence the technical and strategic aspects of safe tumor removal. Tumor size, origin, relationship to the spinal cord, vascularity, and consistency are important aspects in this regard. These factors are assessed as part of the initial surgical field inspection, prior to any tumor resection. First, the tumor surface is explored in its most visible location. This requires dissection of the superficial arachnoid membrane from off the tumor surface. For more ventrally located tumors, divisions of one or more of the dentate ligament attachments improve ventral access. Mild suture retraction on the release dentate ligament may slightly elevate and rotate the spinal cord to enhance ventral exposure. The surface dissection is carried out both rostrally and caudally just beyond the tumor poles. Often a small cottonoid is placed just beyond each tumor pole to demark the margins of the tumor and limit any blood leakage into the subarachnoid space. Since both the techniques and strategies are variable for meningiomas and nerve sheath tumors, they are discussed separately.

Nerve Sheath Tumors

Nerve sheath tumors are well-defined encapsulated tumors that arise from either the dorsal or ventral nerve root (Fig. 24.2) [2, 3]. They can be solid or cystic with variable vascularity. The key to resection is identification of the nerve root of origin. For most nerve sheath tumors, a section of the afferent and efferent nerve root of origin allows for sufficient release of the tumor for en bloc removal. The nerve root origin may not be immediately apparent on initial tumor inspection. Gentle rotation of the tumor allows for additional tumor visualization. If the nerve root of origin is not apparent, then the dorsal tumor surface is cauterized and incised for internal decompression with an ultrasonic aspirator. Any cystic components of the tumor are also drained to reduce tumor volume and allow for identification of the nerve root of origin. Once the nerve root of origin is identified, it is helpful to determine if it is the afferent or efferent component. This is usually self-evident based on the relationship to the tumor. More often than not the afferent nerve root is more swollen, as it often has enlarged veins on its surface (Fig. 24.3). The nerve root of origin is typically neither functional nor salvageable and typically can be divided with minimal risk of neurological deficit. However, this is not always the case, especially for smaller tumors.

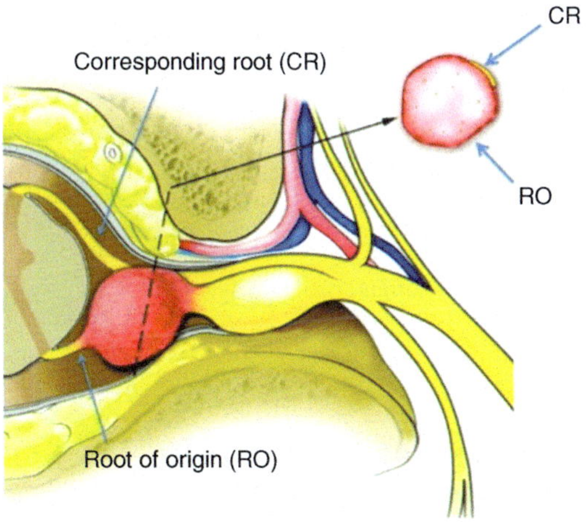

Fig. 24.2 Artist's drawing depicts an intradural schwannoma originating from the dorsal nerve root (RO = root of origin). The corresponding ventral root (CR) is initially separate from the dorsal root and then is tightly applied to the tumor capsule within a common arachnoid sheath. (Figure courtesy of Dr. Paul C. McCormick)

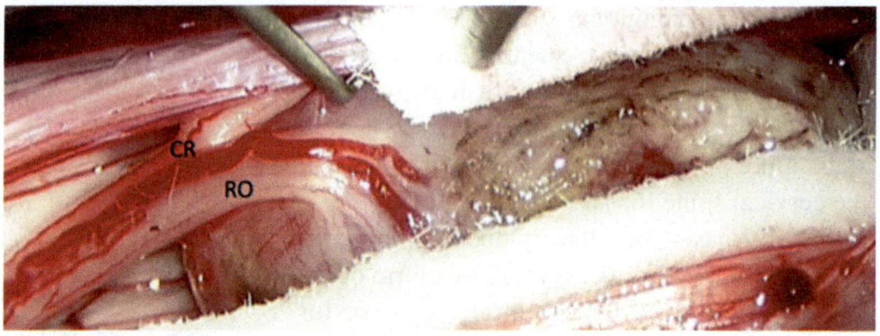

Fig. 24.3 Intraoperative photograph of intradural schwannoma. The afferent (i.e., proximal) root of origin (RO) and corresponding nerve root (CR) are labeled. Note the vascularity on the surface of the afferent root of origin

Modifications, Pearls, Pitfalls, and Specific Considerations

It is important to recognize that there are both the nerve root of origin, more commonly the dorsal nerve root, and a corresponding nerve root, usually the ventral nerve root (see Fig. 24.2). While the corresponding nerve root may run in close proximity to the tumor, sometimes even tightly applied to the tumor capsule in a common arachnoid sheath, it is both functional and salvageable (see Fig. 24.3). The key to preservation of this nerve root is performing the dissection right on the tumor capsule. Thus, any arachnoid that is attached to the tumor capsule should be dissected.

Ventral nerve sheath tumors usually arise from the motor root. These tumors can be challenging because they may be predominantly ventral to the spinal cord, obscure the afferent root of origin to prevent mobilization of the tumor, and present a higher risk for significant postoperative motor nerve root deficit, especially at the C5 and C8 levels. For ventral tumors at these levels, we use nerve root stimulation. If we are able to stimulate the nerve, then only a subtotal resection with preservation of the nerve root is performed. Fortunately, most ventral tumors will rotate or displace the spinal cord to allow adequate ventral visualization and access. Section of the dentate ligament with gentle suture retraction can improve ventral exposure (Fig. 24.4). Generous internal decompression followed by gentle traction directly on the tumor capsule can assist in developing the plane between the tumor and ventral spinal cord and delivering the ventral into the surgical field. Eventually the afferent root will be visualized and can be cauterized and divided.

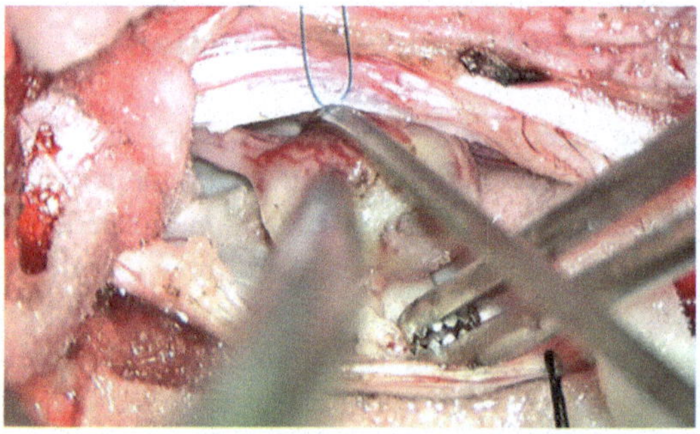

Fig. 24.4 Intraoperative photograph of C3 schwannoma arising from the ventral root. Note the blue prolene suture in the detached dentate ligament that is used to provide mild rotation and elevation on the spinal cord for enhanced ventral access. Gentle traction on the now-mobilized tumor delivers the ventral component of the tumor into the surgical field and provides visualization of the afferent nerve root, which is then cauterized and divided to allow complete tumor resection

Dumbbell Tumors

About 5–10% of nerve sheath tumors are dumbbell tumors, with tumor components in both the intraspinal and extraspinal space. The size, distribution of tumor components, nerve root origin, and surgical strategies are diverse. In general, most can be managed with a single-stage extended posterior approach. It is performed with the patient in a prone position through a midline incision (Fig. 24.5a, b) [2, 8].

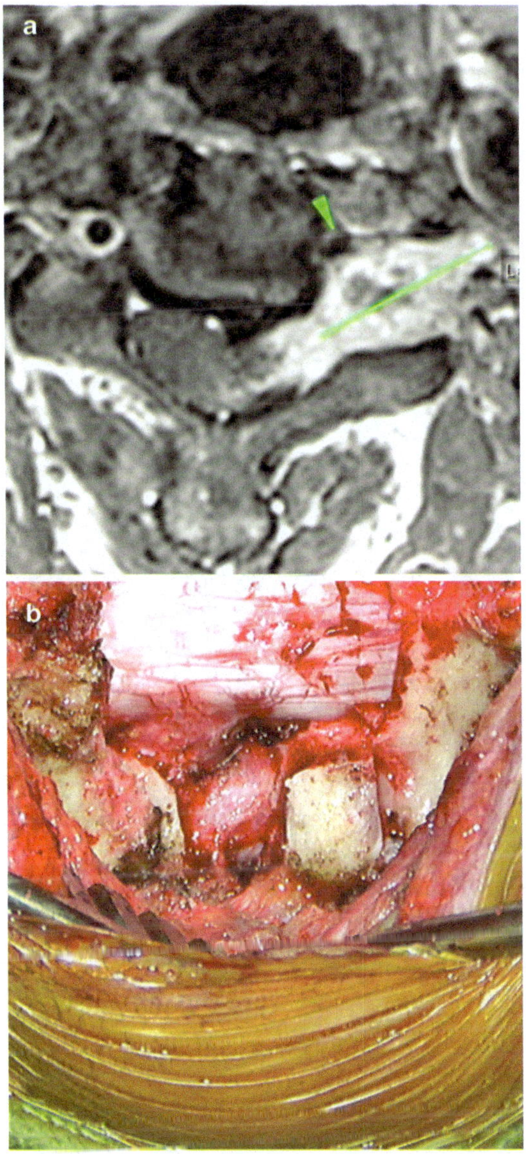

Fig. 24.5 (a) T1-weighted contrast-enhanced cervical MRI shows large left-sided dumbbell tumor at the C3–C4 level. Note that the vertebral artery (arrowhead) is displaced anteromedially by the tumor. (b) Intraoperative photograph shows bilateral C3–C4 laminectomy with complete unilateral left facetectomy to allow access for complete removal of dumbbell schwannoma

The lateral dissection is taken just past the facet joint on the affected side. A unilateral laminectomy is performed if the tumor does not cross the midline. Access to the foraminal and extraforaminal tumor component is achieved via complete facetectomy. This provides access 2–2.5 cm ventrolateral to the dural margin. Tumor extension beyond this may require an additional anterior operation or a radiosurgical procedure for residual tumor. The occiput–C1 and C1–C2 levels are an exception since the joints are ventral and do not require resection for extraforaminal exposure.

Once the spinal canal and foraminal exposure is achieved, the extradural foraminal and extraforaminal tumor component is resected first. It is important that the dissection remains directly on the tumor capsule both to limit bleeding from the foraminal veins and to avoid injury to the vertebral artery. These tumors neither invade nor encase the vertebral artery but usually displace it antero-laterally (see Fig. 24.5a). Tumor capsule incision and internal decompression create space into which the more peripheral aspects of the tumor can be delivered. It is highly unlikely that the nerve of origin can be salvaged in dumbbell tumor cases, especially when there is an intradural component. However, in cases where the origin of the tumor is in the epidural foraminal or paraspinal region that grows centrally into the spinal canal in the epidural space, the nerve may be both functional and preservable. Once the epidural component of the tumor is resected, the dura is opened in the midline for resection of the intradural component. The afferent root origin is identified and divided, and the tumor is dissected away from surrounding tissues to the foramen. It is sometimes useful to sequentially work on both the inside and outside of the dura to remove the foraminal component, often circumferentially excising the dura at the root exit margin. Once tumor resection is complete, the foraminal dural defect is closed with suture, either from inside or outside of the dura. A small muscle patch graft is often utilized. The longitudinal dorsal dural defect is closed separately.

Due to the facetectomy, instrumented fusion is performed following tumor resection below C1–C2. This is generally performed with lateral mass screws one level above and below the laminectomy. Autologous bone from the laminectomy with allograft as needed is used for contralateral lamina and facet fusion.

Modifications, Pearls, Pitfalls, and Specific Considerations

Bleeding tends to be one of the most challenging aspects of the foraminal and extraforaminal tumor dissection. This is best controlled by maintaining dissection directly on the tumor capsule. Often the foraminal veins are tightly applied to the tumor capsule and appear to represent the actual capsule. It is important to keep dissecting through these layers, like peeling an onion, until the true tumor capsule is identified. This greatly reduces bleeding and more safely allows dissection to continue directly on the tumor surface, especially beyond the margins of direct visualization. Direct traction on the tumor capsule while developing the tumor plane can be quite useful. Bleeding from newly developed margins can be managed with gentle packing with small cottonoid pledgets.

Controlled traction on the tumor capsule directed away from the spinal cord is very helpful in delivering aspects of the tumor into the surgical field. One must be careful, however, not to use too much pressure since it may be transmitted to the spinal cord through the afferent limb of the nerve root of origin.

While most nerve sheath tumors arise from the root of origin separate from the spinal cord, some arise very proximally and even seem to elevate the pia at the root entry zone and appear to be subpial or even extend into the spinal cord. For these cases, the tumor is amputated just distal to the root entry zone, and any remaining tumor is removed piecemeal.

Meningiomas

Meningiomas are less common than schwannomas and arise more frequently in adult women. Most originate from, and are attached to, the dura. They occur throughout the spine and tend to be more common in the upper cervical spine and foramen magnum (Fig. 24.6). Patient evaluation, surgical indications, and technical aspects of

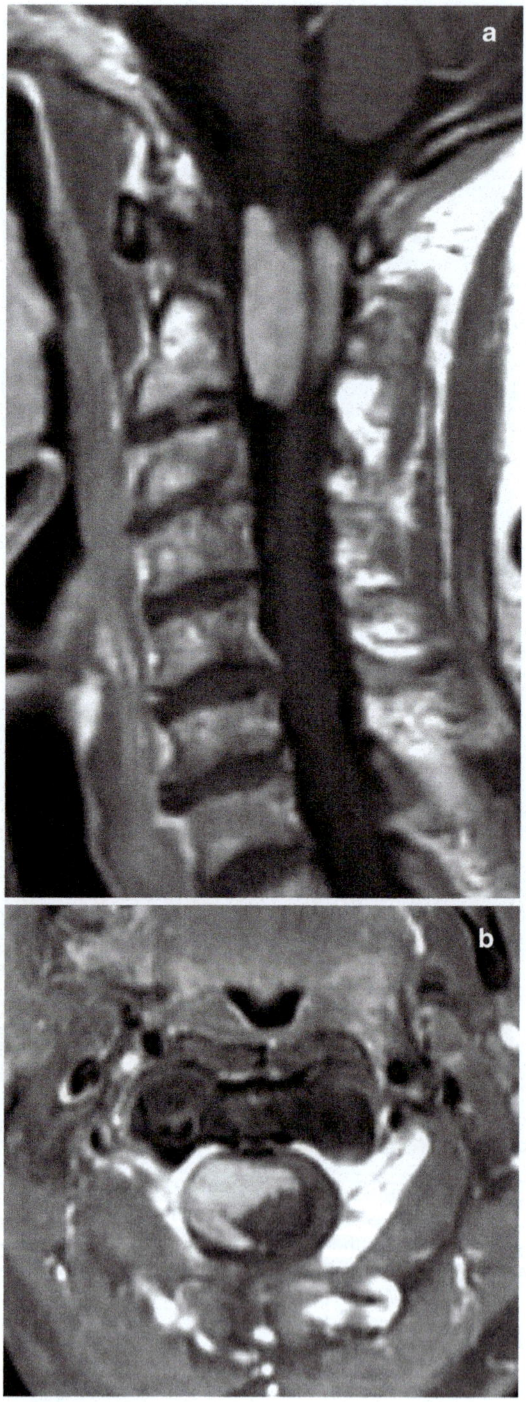

Fig. 24.6 T1-weighted contrast-enhanced sagittal (**a**) and axial (**b**) cervical MRI shows uniformly enhancing mass of the upper cervical spine with broad-based dural attachment consistent with a spinal meningioma

patient positioning and exposure are similar to nerve sheath tumors. Safe secure exposure that allows adequate visualization and access for tumor resection is the cornerstone of effective surgical management of these lesions. For most spinal meningiomas, this can be accomplished with a standard posterior midline approach as previously described for schwannomas. The dura is usually opened in the midline but may have to be altered to one side or the other for meningiomas arising from or near the dorsal midline. Principles of exposure and removal are similar for schwannomas except for the management of the tumor origin. Adequate exposure beyond the tumor poles, maintaining dissection directly on the tumor capsule, internal decompression to allow delivery of tumor, and gentle traction on the tumor capsule are standard techniques for safe removal of most intradural extramedullary tumors. More ventrally located meningiomas usually also either rotate or displace the spinal cord to one side, thereby providing an access to the ventral spinal canal (Fig. 24.7). A section of one or two dentate ligaments can improve ventral access. For large ventral tumor components, it is often useful to thoroughly debulk the lateral aspect of the tumor. If possible, it can be helpful to detach the tumor from its dural origin. This leaves a loose tumor component that can be more easily dissected away from the ventral spinal cord. Key to this dissection is to make sure that the dissection is directly on the tumor capsule, not a thin overlying layer of arachnoid. A small Penfield or slightly curved micro-dissector can be carefully advanced on the tumor surface to allow gentle development of the ventral spinal cord/dorsal tumor capsule dissection plane even if it can't be directly visualized (see Fig. 24.4).

Management of the dural origin of meningiomas varies based on factors such as location, size, and consistency of the dural origin. In most cases of dorsal, lateral, or ventrolateral discrete dural tumor origins, cauterization and detachment of the dural origin is performed flush with the dura. Any small remnants of tumor are sharply peeled off the inner dural surface to complete the resection. The dura is a highly laminated collagen structure, and scraping the inside layers with a sharp Rhoton dissector effectively removes the tumor while leaving the dura intact (Simpson Grade II). This avoids the need for dural patch grafting. Purely ventral or en bloc tumors may not allow for a complete removal of the dural origin (Simpson Grade III) and may be associated with a slightly higher degree of recurrence.

Modifications, Pearls, Pitfalls, and Specific Considerations

High cervical and foramen magnum meningiomas can be challenging due to their often large size and location. Injury to both the spinal accessory and hypoglossal nerves may occur with ventral and lateral lesions. Care must be taken to identify and protect these nerves during dissection and tumor removal. The spinal accessory nerve is also at risk in the mid-cervical spine as it is comprises rootlets from C1 to C5 and ascends closely applied to the spinal cord just dorsal to the dentate ligaments.

Pure ventral meningiomas are rare but difficult to safely remove, especially if they are calcified or highly mineralized. Posterolateral access is not as effective as it is in thoracic and lumbar regions due to the anatomy of the neck and presence of the vertebral artery. A ventral approach is considered for purely ventral meningiomas that do not rotate or laterally displace the spinal cord.

Wound Closure and Postoperative Management

Following tumor resection, the subarachnoid space is copiously irrigated with warm saline solution. Meticulous hemostasis is achieved with irrigated cautery, Floseal (Baxter, Franklin Lakes, NJ, USA), and small Surgicel (Ethicon Inc., Johnson and Johnson, Somerville, New Jersey, USA) pledgets. The dura is closed with a running non-locked 4–0 silk suture. Valsalva to 40 mmHg is performed to ensure as close to a water-tight closure as possible. Floseal is squirted into the lateral epidural gutters. A thin layer of Duragen (Integra Lifesciences, Plainsboro, New Jersey,

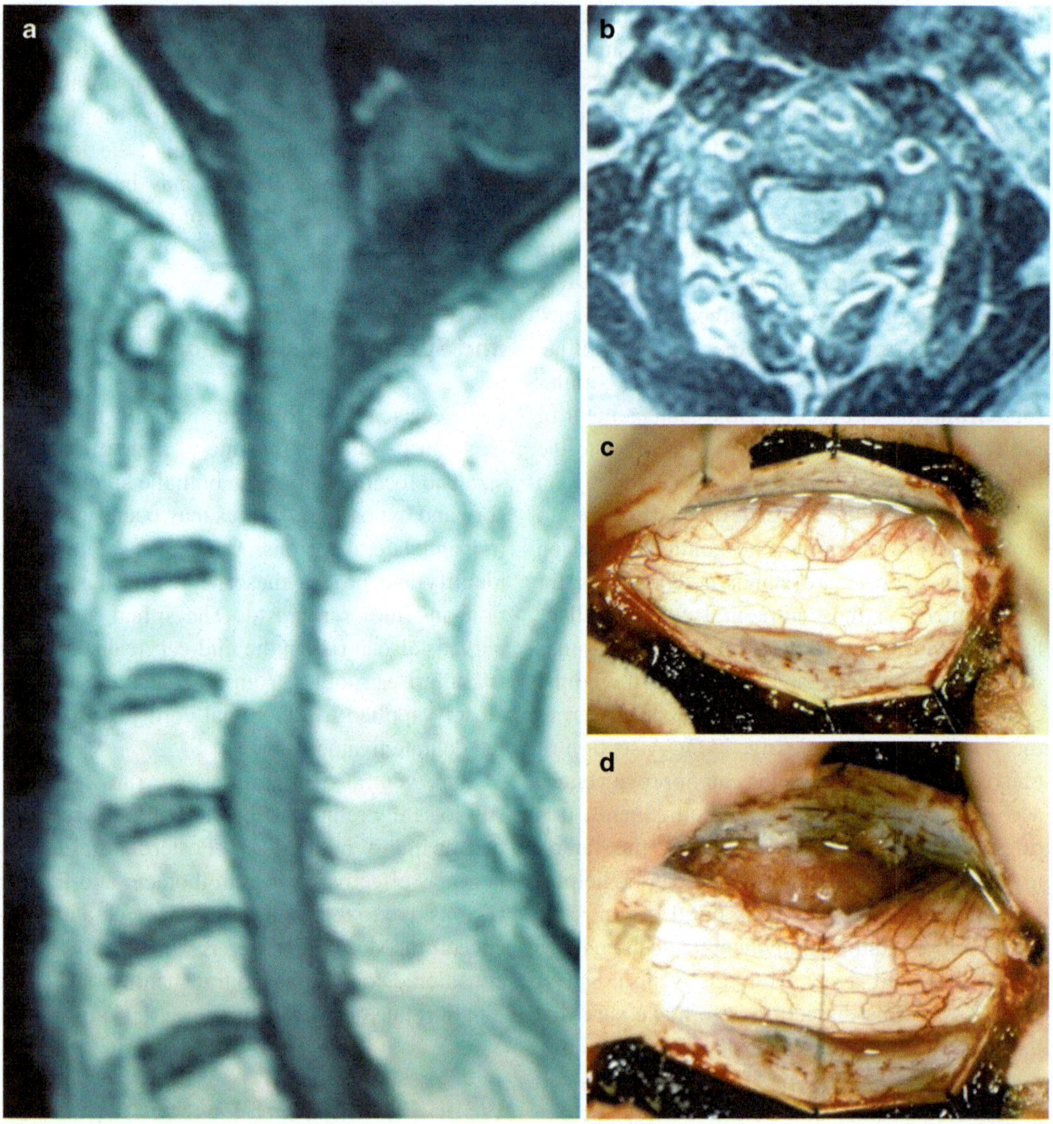

Fig. 24.7 T1-weighted contrast-enhanced sagittal (**a**) and axial (**b**) cervical MRI shows predominantly ventral broad-based uniformly enhancing tumor consistent with meningioma. While completely ventral to the dentate ligaments, the tumor is eccentric to the right and produces some spinal cord rotation to allow ventral access through a posterior lateral corridor. (**c**) Intraoperative photograph demonstrates that the tumor is nearly completely obscured by the overlying spinal cord. (**d**) Following release and gentle suture distraction on the dentate ligaments, a corridor is provided that allows access to the ventral tumor, which can now be seen and safely removed

USA) is placed over the suture line, and this is covered with gelfoam (Pfizer, New York, New York, USA). The epidural space is then compartmentalized by placement of a large cottonoid (Codman, Johnson and Johnson, Raynham, Massachusetts, USA) over the gelfoam. The retractors are removed, and the wound is copiously irrigated with warm saline solution. Hemostasis is secured with bipolar cautery, Floseal, and bone wax under the microscope. The cottonoid is removed and a hemovac drain is placed. The wound is then closed in layers with Biocin and Vicryl. The skin is closed with a running non-locked 2–0 nylon.

The patient remains at bed rest until the morning of postoperative day 2 (POD 2). At that point, ambulation is commenced with physical therapy. Venodynes (EcoLab, Saint Paul, Minnesota, USA), incentive spirometer, and isometrics muscle exercises are encouraged. Most patients are discharged on POD 4, either to their home or to inpatient rehab for those with substantial preoperative deficit. Skin sutures are removed on POD 14.

Modifications, Pearls, Pitfalls, and Specific Considerations

Duraseal and/or sutured muscle grafts can be useful for re-operations or situations where a good multi-layer closure is not possible, especially at the dural level. While small pseudomeningoceles can be tolerated and will usually resolve over time, any CSF leakage through the skin is problematic and should be treated expeditiously. Sterile skin suture, bed rest, or even a spinal drain can be considered. If these methods are not successful, then return to the operating room (OR) for repair should be performed in a timely manner.

The anticipated outcomes following successful resection are usually quite gratifying [9–13]. Most patients experience preservation or return of neurological function. Long-standing or more severe established deficits, however, are less likely to improve, especially spasticity and gait and/or fine motor control deficits. This underscores the importance of timely intervention. Postoperative surveillance is tailored to the patient. Postoperative imaging at 6 weeks and 1 year suffices for most schwannoma patients following complete resection, but longer annual follow-up may be appropriate in some patients, especially meningioma patients following Simpson Grade III or IV resection.

Conclusion

Surgical resection of intradural extramedullary spinal cord tumors is one of the most effective and gratifying neurosurgical procedures. Long-term tumor control or cure with preservation or return of neurological function can be achieved in the vast majority of patients with these benign lesions. Proper patient selection, safe and effective exposure, knowledge of surgical anatomy, and standard microsurgical techniques should be applied in each case in order to optimize the outcome for each patient.

References

1. Agrawal BMBB, McCormick PC, Resnick DK. Intradural extramedullary spinal lesions. In: Benzel EC, editor. Spine surgery – techniques, complication avoidance, and management. 3rd ed. New York: Churchill Livingstone; 2012. p. 991–8.
2. McCormick PC. Surgical management of dumbbell tumors of the cervical spine. Neurosurgery. 1996;38:294–300.
3. Safavi-Abbasi S, Senoglu M, Theodore N, Workman RK, Gharabaghi A, Feiz-Erfan I, et al. Microsurgical management of spinal schwannomas: evaluation of 128 cases. J Neurosurg Spine. 2008;9:40–7. https://doi.org/10.3171/spi/2008/9/7/040.
4. Setzer M, Vatter H, Marquardt G, Seifert V, Vrionis FD. Management of spinal meningiomas: surgical results and a review of the literature. Neurosurg Focus. 2007;23:E14. https://doi.org/10.3171/foc-07/10/e14.
5. Zhu YJ, Ying GY, Chen AQ, Wang LL, Yu DF, Zhu LL, et al. Minimally invasive removal of lumbar intradural extramedullary lesions using the interlaminar approach. Neurosurg Focus. 2015;39:E10. https://doi.org/10.3171/2015.5.focus15182.
6. Angevine PD, Kellner C, Haque RM, McCormick PC. Surgical management of ventral intradural spinal lesions. J Neurosurg Spine. 2011;15:28–37. https://doi.org/10.3171/2011.3.spine1095.
7. O'Toole JE, McCormick PC. Midline ventral intradural schwannoma of the cervical spinal cord resected via anterior corpectomy with reconstruction: technical case report and review of the literature. Neurosurgery. 2003;52:1482–5. discussion 1485-1486.
8. McCormick PC. Resection of a cervical dumbbell schwannoma with stabilization through a single stage extended posterior approach. Neurosurg Focus. 2014;37:Video 2. https://doi.org/10.3171/2014.v3.focus14257.
9. Celli P. Treatment of relevant nerve roots involved in nerve sheath tumors: removal or preservation? Neurosurgery. 2002;51:684–92. discussion 692.
10. Klekamp J, Samii M. Surgical results for spinal meningiomas. Surg Neurol. 1999;52:552–62.
11. Lot G, George B. Cervical neuromas with extradural components: surgical management in a series of 57 patients. Neurosurgery. 1997;41:813–20. discussion 820-812.

12. Seppala MT, Haltia MJ, Sankila RJ, Jaaskelainen JE, Heiskanen O. Long-term outcome after removal of spinal schwannoma: a clinicopathological study of 187 cases. J Neurosurg. 1995;83:621–6. https://doi.org/10.3171/jns.1995.83.4.0621.
13. Solero CL, Fornari M, Giombini S, Lasio G, Oliveri G, Cimino C, Pluchino F. Spinal meningiomas: review of 174 operated cases. Neurosurgery. 1989;25:153–60.

Intradural Extramedullary Tumor: Thoracic

25

Christian B. Theodotou, Ian Côté, and Barth A. Green

Spinal cord tumors are exceedingly rare, comprising only 4–16% of all central nervous system tumors and intradural extramedullary tumors, accounting for only 54% of these lesions [1]. Tumors are typically divided based on their location within the spinal canal: extradural, intradural–extramedullary, intramedullary, dumbbell, or intra- and extramedullary. The most common histologic types for thoracic intradural lesions include schwannoma (68.5%) and meningiomas (20.7%) [1]. This chapter focuses on intradural–extramedullary lesions of the thoracic spine as well as the surgical strategies and technologies available to treat and remove these lesions.

Schwannomas

Schwannomas are benign, intradural (although 30% may have extradural extension), sometimes cystic neoplasms of the nerve sheath which cause local compression of neural elements often leading to pain, weakness, and myelopathy [2, 3]. The annual incidence of these tumors has been reported as 0.3–0.4 per 100,000 patients with no male or female predominance. They typically present between age 40 and 50 [3].

C. B. Theodotou · I. Côté (✉) · B. A. Green
Jackson Memorial Hospital/University of Miami Hospital, Department of Neurological Surgery, Miami, FL, USA
e-mail: icote@med.miami.edu

The ideal treatment for schwannomas is gross total resection; however, subtotal resection may be the best choice in certain cases, especially when high risk of neurological damage accompanies a total resection. Sohn et al. evaluated cases of residual schwannomas after subtotal resections and found that regrowth only occurred in 29.6% of cases with the authors noting that the Ki-67 index was statistically higher in patients who experience a regrowth of their lesion [2]. Radiotherapy can also be used in cases where a subtotal resection is performed or in cases of multiple lesions or if the patient is not a reasonable surgical risk [4].

Meningiomas

Spinal canal meningiomas occur at a rate of 0.33 per 100,000 people [5]. They are generally benign tumors which are slow growing and typically present later in life (75% occurring between age 50 and 70 years) and have a clear female predominance with up to 82% of patients being female [5, 6]. Up to 84% of spinal meningiomas are located in the thoracic spine and in this area, there is an even higher female predominance (87%) than in the spine as a whole [6, 7]. These lesions are most often found intradurally, with 90% completely intradural and 5% both intra- and extradural [6].

The goal of surgery as in schwannomas is the decompression of neural elements and gross total

D. M. Sciubba (ed.), *Spinal Tumor Surgery*, https://doi.org/10.1007/978-3-319-98422-3_25

resection of the lesion, but in contrast to schwannoma, surgery also includes resection of its dural attachment (sometimes referred to as a Simpson Grade I resection) [8]. This classification system was specifically developed by Donald Simpson in 1957 for predicting the recurrence rates of intracranial meningiomas after various levels of resection but has since been applied by some authors to spinal meningiomas as well [7, 8]. However, even when a Grade I or II resection is achieved, recurrence rate has been reported as high at 9.7% overall and 30% for Grade II resection [9]. Surgical resection is not without risk—cerebrospinal fluid (CSF) leak occurs in up to 4% of patients and permanent neurologic deterioration occurs in 6% of patients [7, 10]. Radiotherapy has been used in some cases, particularly in higher-grade meningiomas and cases of subtotal resection, or in patients who are unable to tolerate an operation. However, these indications are not clearly defined, and close follow-up for recurrence is needed in such cases to detect recurrence early [7, 11]. It is not rare to encounter a calcified meningioma which may not be easily removed by using a Cavitron or pituitary rongeur. These lesions often require a biting instrument such as a micro-Kerrison or, even in some cases, a small precision drill. The most challenging of the meningiomas to surgically resect are the en plaque lesions which may not be resectable due to dural attachments which can extend to the posterior longitudinal ligament and vertebrae. They are also frequently associated with spinal cord compression, tethering, and either myelomalacia or cystic changes within the spinal cord.

Surgical Technique

Posterior/Laminectomy (Fig. 25.1)

The standard approach for treating intradural–extramedullary lesions in the thoracic spine involved an open approach with midline posterior incision and full laminectomy [3, 12, 13]. The extent of the laminectomy is determined both preoperatively and intraoperatively. Based on the magnetic resonance imaging (MRI) with gadolinium enhancement, the bony opening should extend the entire tumor length and at least one-half of the laminar level above and below. Once this initial step has been completed, a trans-dural intraoperative ultrasound should be performed to confirm if adequate exposure has been obtained. It will also permit planning of the dural opening which can be midline or paramidline, depending on the eccentricity of the lesion. This approach is effective in lesions which are posterior or lateral to the spinal cord; however, anterior lesions present a unique challenge as the spinal cord must be retracted, increasing the likelihood of neurologic injury. In these cases, a posterior approach may still be feasible by sectioning the dentate ligaments, performing gentle static or dynamic retraction, using pial sutures or simply using various types of micro-retractors. Use of intraoperative ultrasound is quite helpful to minimize the chance of neural injury by better establishing the anatomical relationships between the spinal cord, nerve roots, adjacent meninges, and bony structures in real time. This can also clarify if any residual tumor mass exists in surrounding tissues of the surgical site. Continuous somatosensory-evoked potential (SSEP) monitoring and serial

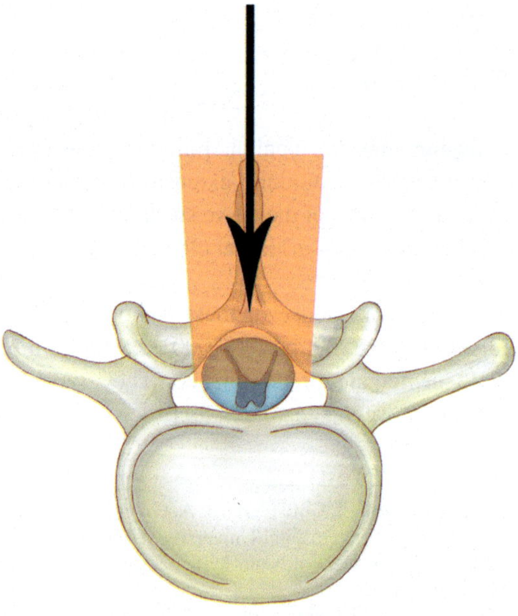

Fig. 25.1 Posterior laminectomy approach

motor-evoked potential (MEP) monitoring are also of significant advantage. Comparing the most current values to baseline values (accounting for other variables such as blood pressure, oxygenation, and anesthesia level), the surgeon can detect early electrophysiological changes and predict potentially reversible neurological compromise. Increases in latency and decreases in amplitude are the key signs that there is "trouble in paradise." This should result in immediate cessation of surgical activity, allowing both the surgeon and anesthesiologist to do a rapid analysis of blood pressure, oxygenation, temperature, anesthesia level, retraction level, etc., and make any necessary adjustments. If a neurological injury is detected, immediate response includes not only cessation of surgical intervention and retraction but also the intravenous administration of a booster dose of steroids and further rapid dropping of the patient's temperature toward a modest hypothermia therapeutic level of 33 °C. This can be accomplished most rapidly by the administration of chilled intravenous saline. The authors remind the readers that these neuroprotective interventions and response to changes in evoked responses do not represent evidence-based medicine but rather the experience of primarily the senior author who preemptively uses a baseline 35 °C temperature before beginning removal of any neoplastic or vascular lesion from the spinal cord or when performing tethered cord or syringomyelia surgery. This level of hypothermia can be achieved by the anesthetic team by making small adjustments in room temperature or by surface cooling in addition to the use of chilled saline as previously mentioned. However, most patients drop their body temperature by 1–2 °C as part of a physiological response to anesthesia and exposure to the operating room environment. If the senior author suspects an extremely high risk of neural damage, he will often percutaneously insert an intravenous femoral catheter into the groin or neck and connect it to a hypothermia machine such as the Icy® lower-body catheter connected to the Thermogard XP Temperature Management System (Zool®, Chelmsford, MA) which can closely regulate temperature and achieve a 33 °C body temperature prior to opening the dura. Regarding high-dose intravenous steroids, there is no evidence to support their use in spinal cord tumors although they are commonly used in brain tumor surgery. The rationale for use or non-use in spinal cord surgery is beyond the scope of this chapter.

It may be technically advantageous for the primary surgeon to stand on the ipsilateral side of paramedian tumors and to create a wider laminectomy on the side of tumor predominance, sparing the integrity of the pars interarticularis so as not to increase instability. Using an "airplane" technique, the anesthesia team can roll the table sideways using the planar rotation function to optimize not just the visualization but the bisection of tumors that are laterally placed. One can then more easily get to the midline and even further without neural damage. Once the tumor has been visualized, the capsule can be coagulated with the micro-bipolar. Biopsy for pathological analysis can then be performed simultaneously with debulking. This should always be done with the illumination and magnification of an operating microscope aided by either suction and irrigating micro-bipolar, ultrasonic aspirator, laser, or other technologies now available for this purpose. For teaching purposes, it is most useful to record this procedure which later can be edited and lessons learned can be shared with others who are not present during the procedure.

Other factors dictating the aggressiveness of the dissection and tumor removal include the patient's age, premorbid conditions, and the stability of intraoperative physiological parameters including MEPs/SSEPs. WHO grade of the lesion and composition of the lesion may also be important factors to consider. A Simpson Grade I resection in the case of a meningioma or a total resection of a dumbbell schwannoma may be of certain value in younger patients; however, obtaining this result may place the patient at a higher risk of complications, including CSF leak. Difficulty can also arise from calcified lesions and rarer malignant lesions which can have poor dissection planes. Schwannomas can also hemorrhage preoperatively which often causes greater adhesions to the surrounding tissue, particularly if the hemorrhage has broken through the tumor capsule. Preoperative computed tomography (CT) confirms the degree and extent of calcification and has important strategic value. Repair of dural defects depends directly on the size and location of the tumor.

Schwannomas generally originate from a sensory nerve fascicle from the dorsal rootlet but, less commonly, can encompass multiple fascicles or arise from a ventral rootlet motor fascicle. Again, the goal is to obtain a gross total resection. It is important to first identify an electrically silent perineurium overlying the tumor capsule using a nerve stimulator with 0.5–2 mA of current. Next, the perineurium should be coagulated parallel to the exiting nerve fibers using bipolar forceps and opened in the same direction with a #15 blade, peeling away each layer until the tumor's true capsule is identified. Similar to meningiomas, intralesional debulking can be done in a piecemeal fashion or using an ultrasonic aspirator. Micro-cottonoids can be used to maintain the developing plane between surrounding fascicles/endoneurium and the tumor capsule, eventually obtaining a circumferential dissection. The tumor should be followed proximally and distally to identify the fascicle or fascicles of origin. They should then be separated from neighboring fibers, coagulated, and sharply sectioned using micro-scissors. Persistent ooze from feeding blood vessels can be controlled using dry or thrombin-soaked GelFoam® (Pfizer Inc.), or similar. Although this micro-dissection technique may seem optimal, it is the senior author's experience that resection of the entire dorsal rootlet does not result in any significant motor or sensory deficits.

It has also been the senior author's experience that, prior to dural closure, spinal cord untethering should be accomplished to prevent development of a tethered cord associated with chronic neuropathic pain and progressive cystic or myelomalacic myelopathy. This should be done by circumferentially releasing the subdural space by removing arachnoid adhesions that develop from chronic compression and cord displacement. This is especially important on the contralateral side to the tumor, that is, where the spinal cord is plastered to the dura and arachnoid.

A complete resection with total removal of dural attachment must be balanced against the challenges of reconstruction of a water-tight dural lining. This is particularly true of ventral and en plaque calcified meningiomas. There are multiple structural options for repair including autograft (fascia lata, percranium), onlay dural substitutes (Duraform®—Depuy Synthes Companies, DuraGen®—Integra LifeScience), xenograft (bovine pericardium), and allografts (cadaveric dura or Alloderm®—LifeCell Corporation). It is the senior author's preference to suture in the latter using 6–0 Prolene® polypropylene suture (Ethicon US, LLC—Johnson Johnson) and then cover the dural repair with a layer of DuraGen®. The repair is most successful if the case is preceded by a percutaneous placement of lumbar cerebrospinal fluid drainage system for postoperative cerebrospinal fluid diversion, usually starting 6–8 h postop with a volume of 5–10 cc per hour for a 3 to 5 day period. The drain can be removed earlier if the CSF is totally cleared of blood products and debris which can otherwise cause chronic arachnoiditis and spinal cord tethering.

The same reconstruction technique following dural-based meningioma removal can be used in dumbbell schwannoma cases. However, there is often a much larger dural defect, commonly lateral at the site of the exiting nerve root and involving its sleeve. Depending on the level, closure can be facilitated by sacrificing the entire intercostal nerve. Care has to be taken to look for the artery of Adamkiewicz which is usually found eccentric to the left side between T9 and L1, accounting for individual anatomic variants. If included in the resection, it can result in either complete paraplegia or more commonly incomplete paraplegia in the form of an anterior cord syndrome.

Other Approaches (Figs. 25.2, 25.3, 25.4 and 25.5)

In the senior author's experience, less than 5% of intradural–extramedullary tumor cases involve large midline anterior lesions that may not be

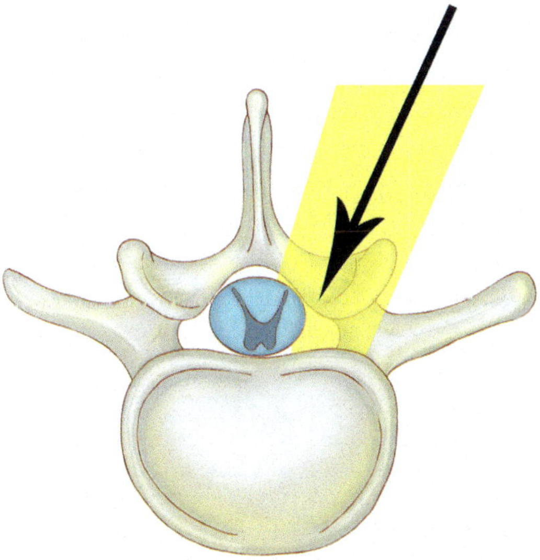

Fig. 25.2 Transpedicular approach

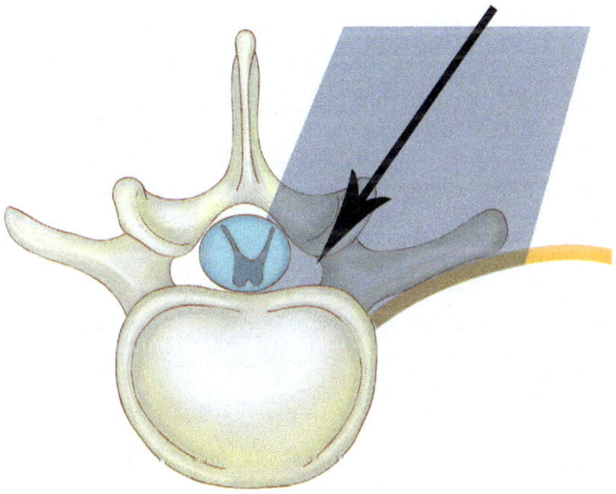

Fig. 25.3 Costotransversectomy approach

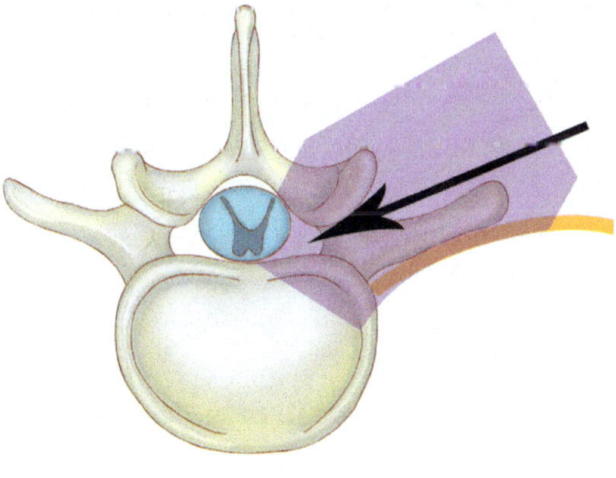

Fig. 25.4 Lateral extracavitary approach

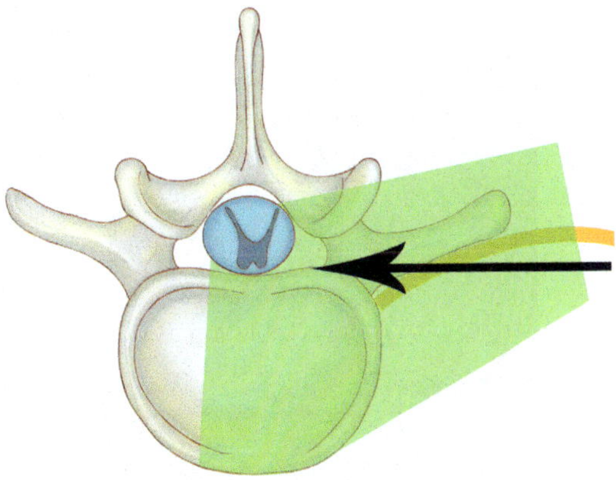

Fig. 25.5 Transthoracic approach

easily accessed from the posterior approach described earlier. In these cases, there are several other options, including transpedicular, costotransversectomy, extracavitary, and transthoracic, which are traditional approaches to the spine and are well documented in the references of this chapter [14–17]. All of these are associated with a higher degree of morbidity and mortality and are rarely, if ever, indicated. They also often require in tandem insertion of spinal stabilization instrumentation because structural components must be removed to access these rare tumors.

Case Presentation 1

A 43-year-old female with no prior cancer history presented with progressive pain over her thoracic spine and weakness in her lower extremities bilaterally. She tolerated these symptoms for several months prior to admission until she became paraparetic and unable to walk. On physical examination, the patient had 3/5 motor strength and 3+ reflexes in the lower extremities bilaterally.

MRI revealed a well-circumscribed 1.8 × 0.8 × 0.8 cm contrast-enhancing mass at the level of T5–T6. The mass was anterior to the spinal cord and slightly eccentric to the right, with displacement of the spinal cord to the left (Fig. 25.6).

The patient was taken to the operating room for a T5–T6 laminectomy. After the laminae were removed, intraoperative ultrasound was

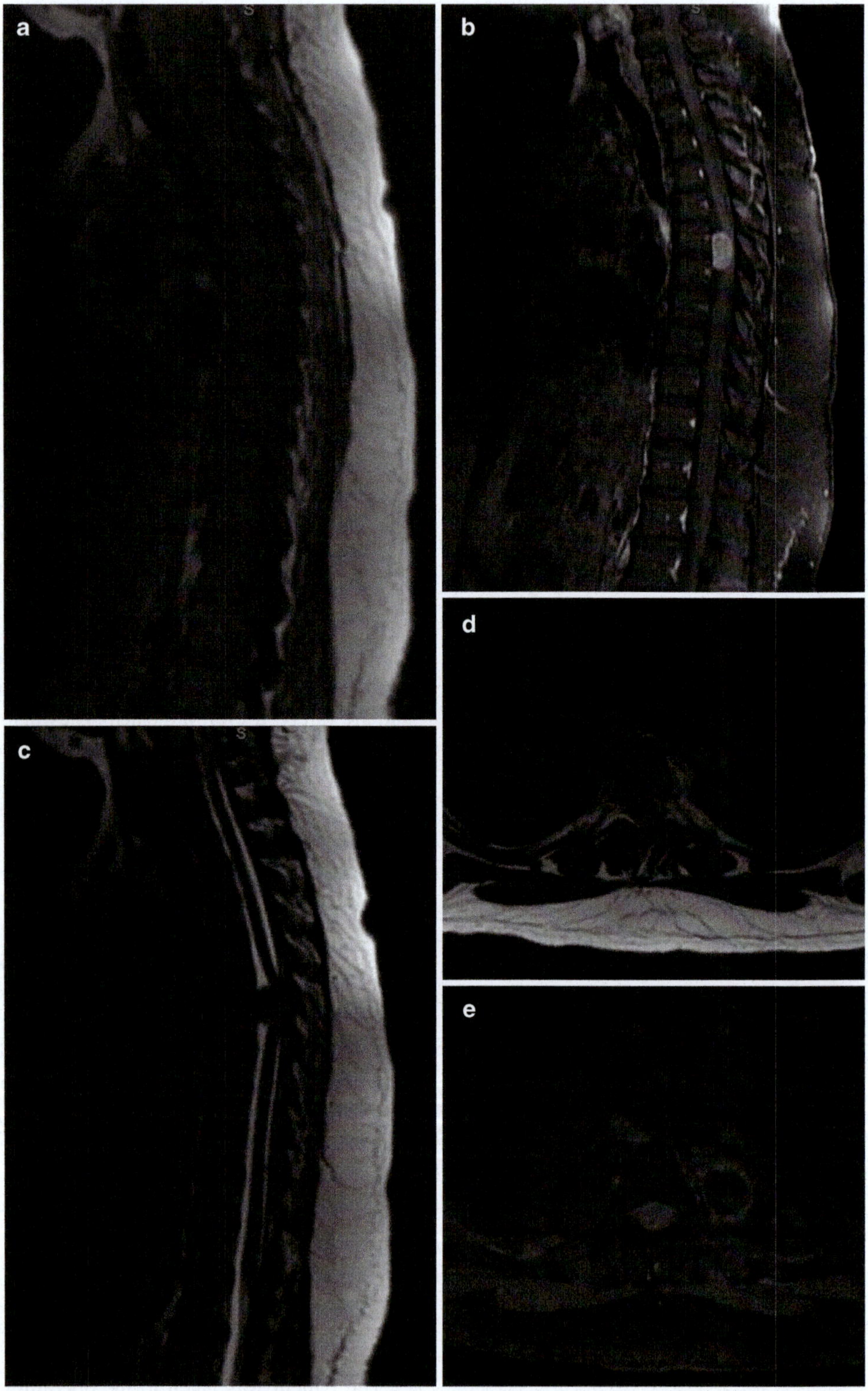

Fig. 25.6 MRI of thoracic spine showing T5–T6 meningioma. (**a**) Mid-sagittal T1 image showing isointense intradural extramedullary lesion anterior to the spinal cord causing posterior displacement. (**b**) Mid-sagittal T1 image with gadolinium contrast showing homogeneous enhancement. (**c**) Mid-sagittal T2 image showing spinal cord myelomalacia. (**d**, **e**) Axial T1 without and with contrast showing dural-based lesion

used to localize the lesion and plan the durotomy (Fig. 25.7). A midline durotomy was done exposing the posterior columns. The lesion was slightly eccentric to the right and seen on the anterior surface of the dentate ligaments. These were sectioned using an arachnoid knife and micro-scissors, exposing the lateral aspect of the tumor capsule. Using gentle dynamic retraction from a Rhoton 6 micro-dissector and a PMT® suction (PMT Corporation), intralesional debulking was carried out using an ultrasonic aspirator (Fig. 25.8). The ventral dural attachment was identified and resected sharply, obtaining a gross total resection with Simpson 1 result. The dura was reconstructed using AlloDerm, which was placed between the cord and the dura, covering the defect. Polypropylene suture was used to keep the graft in place. Throughout the procedure, SSEPs and MEPs were monitored and showed gradual improvement from baseline.

Postoperatively, however, the patient experienced a transient worsening of neurological function. She was placed in the intensive care unit with mean arterial blood pressure artificially maintained above 90 mmHg for 3 days with corporal cooling to 35 °C. Beginning on the second postoperative day, the neurological function gradually improved from a baseline of 0/5 up to 3/5 at discharge to spinal cord injury rehab. Pathology eventually showed a WHO Grade I meningioma. At 2 months post-surgery, the patient's strength had improved to 4/5 and she was able to stand independently. By 6 months the patient was ambulating almost normally.

The case illustrates several points. First, despite the lesion being anterior to the spinal cord, a posterior approach can be utilized with great care. While the costotransversectomy and other approaches may be more ideal for these anterior lesions, a tumor with soft consistency can be removed piecemeal and safely. An important point of this case is that one cannot rely solely on neuro-monitoring as this did show improving signals while the patient's exam was found to be worse postoperatively. A causative factor was a transient period of hypotension during the emergence phase of anesthesia which may have caused relative ischemia in the upper thoracic watershed

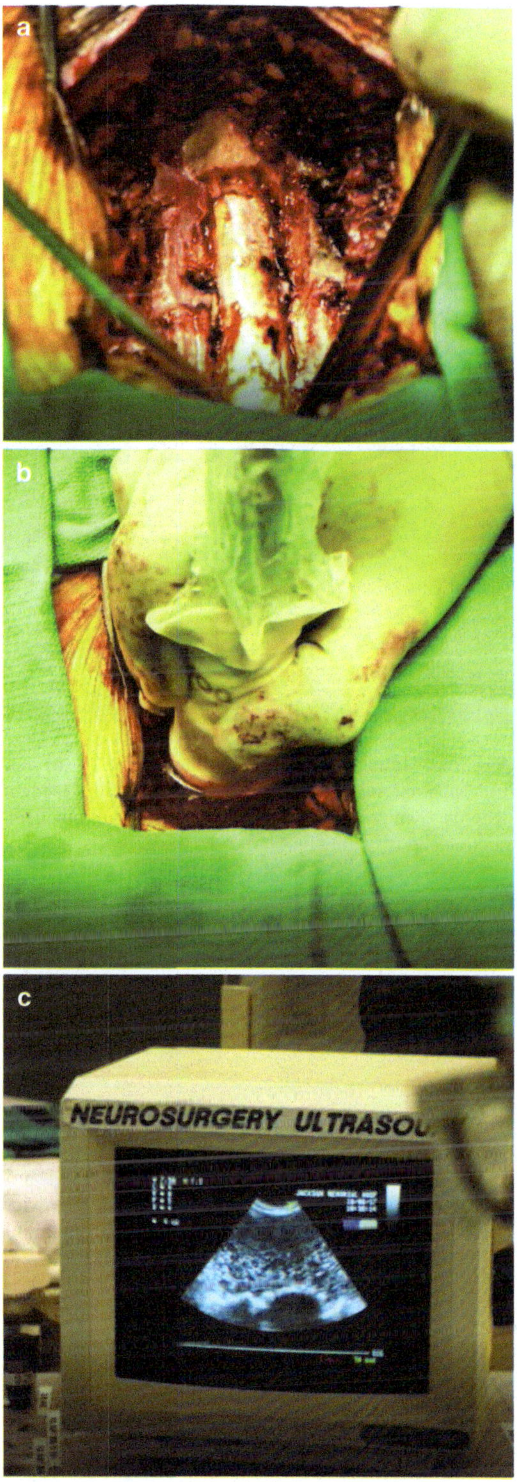

Fig. 25.7 Intraoperative picture showing (**a**) thoracic 5–6 laminectomy, (**b**) use of sterile intraoperative ultrasound probe, and (**c**) ultrasound localization of ventral intradural–extramedullary lesion

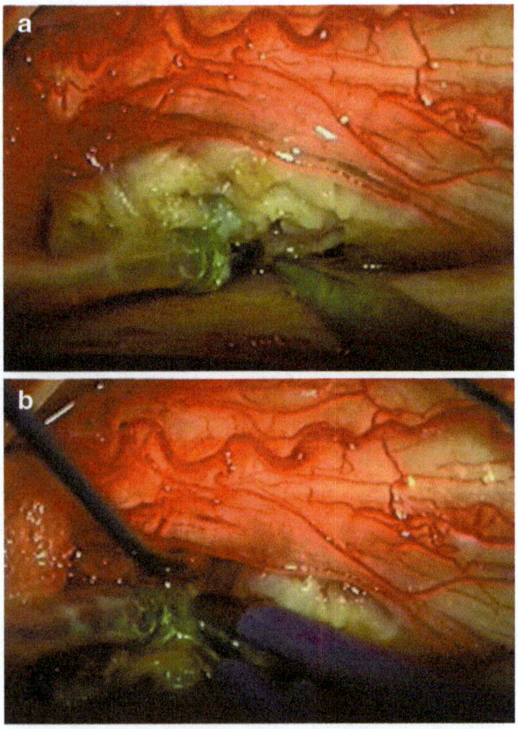

Fig. 25.8 Intraoperative microscope picture of (**a**) ventral meningioma and (**b**) dynamic retraction using a Rhoton 6 micro-dissector for lesional debulking using suction and irrigating bipolar

zone of spinal cord vascularization. Aggressive perioperative management and extensive rehabilitation resulted in an excellent outcome with the patient having minimal residual deficits.

References

1. Hirano K, Imagama S, Sato K, Kato F, Yukawa Y, Yoshihara H, et al. Primary spinal cord tumors: review of 678 surgically treated patients in Japan. A multicenter study. Eur Spine J. 2012;21(10):2019–26.
2. Sohn S, Chung CK, Park SH, Kim ES, Kim KJ, Kim CH. The fate of spinal schwannomas following subtotal resection: a retrospective multicenter study by the Korea spinal oncology research group. J Neuro-Oncol. 2013;114(3):345–51.
3. Seppala MT, Haltia MJ, Sankila RJ, Jaaskelainen JE, Heiskanen O. Long-term outcome after removal of spinal schwannoma: a clinicopathological study of 187 cases. J Neurosurg. 1995;83:621–6.
4. Kufeld M, Wowra B, Muacevic A, Zausinger S, Tonn JC. Radiosurgery of spinal meningiomas and schwannomas. Technol Cancer Res Treat. 2012;11(1):27–34.
5. Kshettry VR, Hsieh JK, Ostrom QT, Kruchko C, Benzel EC, Barnholtz-Sloan JS. Descriptive epidemiology of spinal Meningiomas in the United States. Spine (Phila Pa 1976). 2015;40(15):E886–9.
6. Solero CL, Fornari M, Giombini S, Lasio G, Oliveri G, Cimino C, et al. Spinal meningiomas: review of 174 operated cases. Neurosurgery. 1989;25(2):153–60.
7. Ravindra VM, Schmidt MH. Management of spinal meningiomas. Neurosurg Clin N Am. 2016;27(2):195–205.
8. Simpson D. The recurrence of intracranial meningiomas after surgical treatment. J Neurol Neurosurg Psychiatry. 1957;20(1):22–39.
9. Nakamura M, Tsuji O, Fujiyoshi K, Hosogane N, Watanabe K, Tsuji T, et al. Long-term surgical outcomes of spinal meningiomas. Spine (Phila Pa 1976). 2012;37(10):E617–23.
10. Westwick HJ, Yuh SJ, Shamji MF. Complication avoidance in the resection of spinal meningiomas. World Neurosurg. 2015;83(4):627–34.
11. Sun SQ, Cai C, Ravindra VM, Gamble P, Yarbrough CK, Dacey RG, et al. Simpson grade I-III resection of spinal atypical (World Health Organization Grade II) Meningiomas is associated with symptom resolution and low recurrence. Neurosurgery. 2015;76(6):739–46.
12. Wong AP, Lall RR, Dahdaleh NS, Lawton CD, Smith ZA, Wong RH, et al. Comparison of open and minimally invasive surgery for intradural-extramedullary spine tumors. Neurosurg Focus. 2015;39(2):E11.
13. Raygor KP, Than KD, Chou D, Mummaneni PV. Comparison of minimally invasive transspinous and open approaches for thoracolumbar intradural-extramedullary spinal tumors. Neurosurg Focus. 2015;39(2):E12.
14. Ito K, Aoyama T, Miyaoka Y, Seguchi T, Horiuchi T, Hongo K. Surgery for ventral intradural thoracic spinal tumors with a posterolateral transpedicular approach. Acta Neurochir. 2016;158(8):1563–9.
15. Lubelski D, Abdullah KG, Mroz TE, Shin JH, Alvin MD, Benzel EC, et al. Lateral extracavitary vs. costotransversectomy approaches to the thoracic spine: reflections on lessons learned. Neurosurgery. 2012;71(6):1096–102.
16. Lubelski D, Abdullah KG, Steinmetz MP, Masters F, Benzel EC, Mroz TE, et al. Lateral extracavitary, costotransversectomy, and transthoracic thoracotomy approaches to the thoracic spine. J Spinal Disord Tech. 2013;26(4):222–32.
17. Wiggins GC, Mirza S, Bellabarba C, West GA, Chapman JR, Shaffrey CJ. Perioperative complications with costotransversectomy and anterior approaches to thoracic and thoracolumbar tumors. Neurosurg Focus. 2001;11(6):1–9.

Intradural Extramedullary Tumor in the Lumbar Spine

26

Luis M. Tumialán

Introduction

When Love described the resection of intradural extramedullary tumors in the lumbar spine in 1966, he was working in an era where the diagnosis was made in large part with a neurological examination alongside an injection of intrathecal contrast and a radiograph for a rudimentary form of myelography [1]. Localization in the operating room was performed with cross-table lateral radiographs and with direct exposure at times of the first non-rib-bearing vertebra or the sacrum to confirm the operative level. It is no surprise to read that Love's technique recommended resection of three spinous processes and three laminae prior to opening the dura. Such wide exposure affords the surgeon some element of adjustment in the event the operative level was off by one segment. For decades, Love's approach was the basis for resection of intradural extramedullary lesions. However, the extensive disruption of the posterior tension band raised concern that in the years and decades after a successful resection in a patient, kyphosis and scoliosis would be the inevitable result [4–9]. Seeing the untoward effects of such wide exposures, surgeons began to explore less invasive means of addressing these lesions.

In 1983, Eggert and colleagues [10] described a unilateral approach for the resection of intradural extramedullary lesions. Illustrative images (Fig. 26.1) from that initial publication demonstrate their bone work to access the central spinal canal. A unilateral approach to the spinal canal was a significant departure from Love's description of the removal of three spinous processes and three laminae. Eggert and colleagues reported their results on 39 patients in whom the unilateral hemilaminectomy approach was used for resection of the lesion; 2 of the 39 patients had lesions in the lumbar spine. The bone work shown in Fig. 26.1 bears a striking resemblance to the exposures eventually made possible by modern minimal access ports.

In 1991, Yaşargil and colleagues [3] published their experience with the unilateral laminotomy approach for intradural extramedullary lesions, which corroborated the experience of Eggert's group. In 1997, Foley and Smith [11] described a paramedian transmuscular approach to the lumbar spine for management of herniated lumbar discs. The paradigm shift of looking at the spine in three dimensions, with the spinous process not considered to be an obstacle to the central spi-

Electronic Supplementary Material The online version of this chapter (https://doi.org/10.1007/978-3-319-98422-3_26) contains supplementary material, which is available to authorized users.

L. M. Tumialán (✉)
Department of Neurosurgery, Barrow Neurological Institute, St. Joseph's Hospital and Medical Center, Phoenix, AZ, USA
e-mail: Neuropub@barrowneuro.org

D. M. Sciubba (ed.), *Spinal Tumor Surgery*, https://doi.org/10.1007/978-3-319-98422-3_26

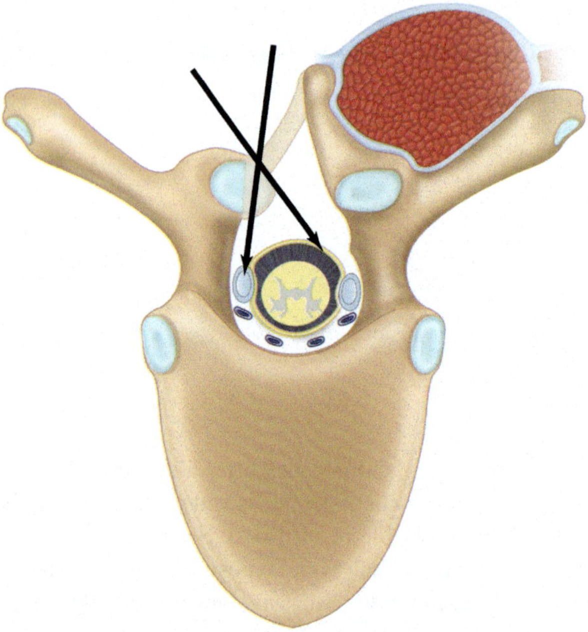

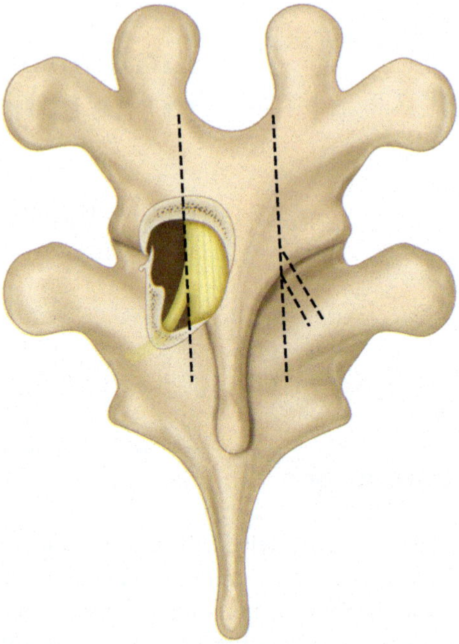

Fig. 26.1 Illustrations based on the original artwork from Eggert et al.'s 1983 publication on unilateral approaches to the central canal. (**a**) Axial illustration demonstrating the capacity to access the central canal from a unilateral approach. (**b**) Posterior view of the spine demonstrating the limited bone work required for resection of a lesion. These illustrations bear a striking resemblance to an exposure that would be offered by a minimally invasive approach. (Modified from Eggert et al. [10]. With permission of Springer)

nal canal, continued to evolve. Soon thereafter, Schwender et al. [12] described paramedian transmuscular lumbar fusions. As minimally invasive platforms became increasingly available to spine surgeons at the turn of the century, the experience gained from the minimally invasive management of degeneration of the spine allowed surgeons to apply that skill set to the management of intradural extramedullary lesions.

In 2006, Tredway et al. [13] published their experience with a paramedian minimally invasive approach for resection of intradural extramedullary lesions. Since that description, several minimally invasive series have been published [14–16]. The paramedian minimally invasive technique described in this chapter embraces the principles of a focal exposure and limits disruption of the spine, thereby representing the inevitable evolution of a technique that began with Love and was continually modified throughout the decades by Eggert, Yaşargil, and Fessler.

Anatomical Basis

The thoughtful deconstruction of the lumbar spine becomes possible only with knowledge of the canal dimensions that establish the anatomical basis for the resection of an intradural extramedullary lesion. Whether the resection is performed using a paramedian minimally invasive approach or a midline approach, command of the canal dimensions lays the foundation for the necessary bone work to access the lesion. In 1992, Panjabi and colleagues [17] presented a quantitative dimensional analysis of the lumbar spine that offers a sophisticated understanding of the lumbar spinal canal and establishes the anatomical basis of a minimally invasive resection of an intradural extramedullary lesion in the lumbar spine.

The width of the central canal ranges from 23 mm at L1 to 27 mm at L5, with a gradual increase of about 1 mm with each level. The

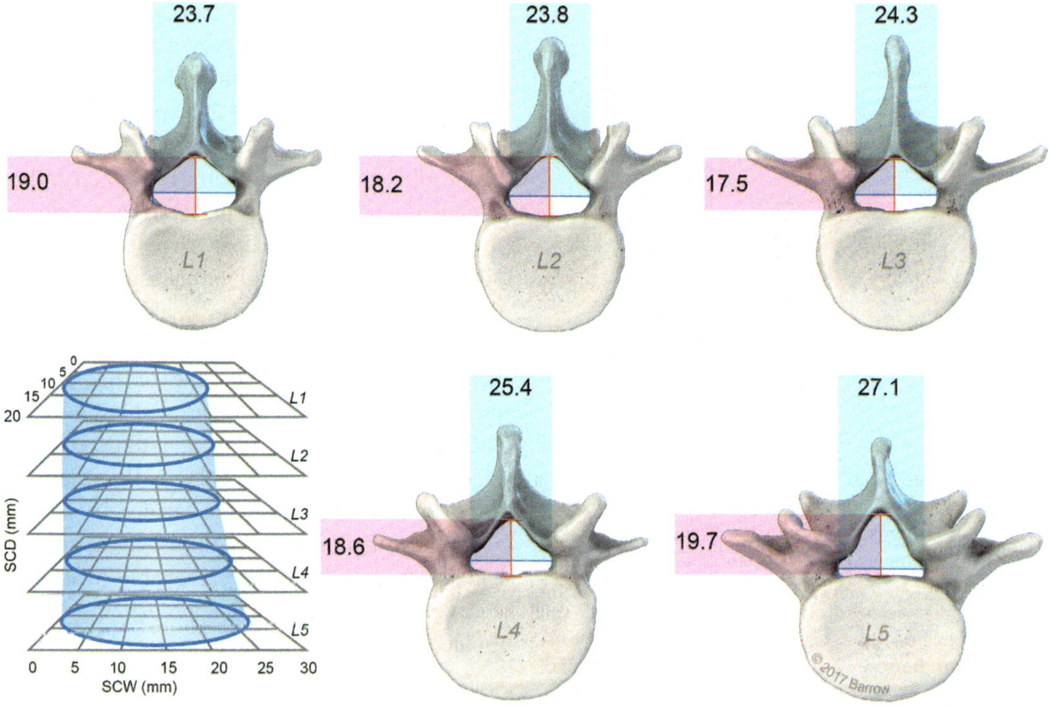

Fig. 26.2 A graphical representation of the dimensions of the lumbar canal as reported by Panjabi et al. (Used with permission from Barrow Neurological Institute, Phoenix, Arizona)

depth (anteroposterior [AP] dimension) of the canal is comparable at L1 and L5, and it actually tapers at L3. At L1, the depth measures 19.0 mm, then it decreases to 17.5 mm at L3 before enlarging to 19.7 mm at L5 [17]. Figure 26.2 provides a graphical representation of the dimensions of the lumbar canal based on the measurements by Panjabi et al. Intradural extramedullary lesions tend to match the dimensions of the lumbar spine since patients typically come to medical attention only after they become symptomatic. The slow growth of these lesions makes them clinically silent until they reach the proverbial tipping point. That tipping point is when the lesion has grown enough to reach the dimensions of the canal and compress the neural elements, thereby causing symptoms. The only variable is the rostral–caudal dimension, which is the only dimension not bound by the spinal canal. However, with the exception of the myxopapillary ependymomas, which can grow considerably in the rostral–caudal dimension before radiographic diagnosis, intradural lesions such as schwannomas and meningiomas tend to have a rostral–caudal dimension of less than 30 mm, making them especially amenable to a minimally invasive resection [18, 19].

The dimensions of the lumbar canal are the inherent limit of an intradural extramedullary lesion. Recognizing that a lumbar lesion will have the maximum dimensions of 20 × 27 × 30 mm in the AP, lateral, and rostral–caudal dimensions, respectively, would suggest that bone work measuring slightly more than these dimensions will be adequate for complete resection of the lesion. These dimensions are well within the capacity of an expandable minimal access port (Fig. 26.3).

Preoperative Considerations

Preoperative AP and lateral radiographs are essential to confirm five non-rib-bearing vertebrae. These preoperative studies are the essential

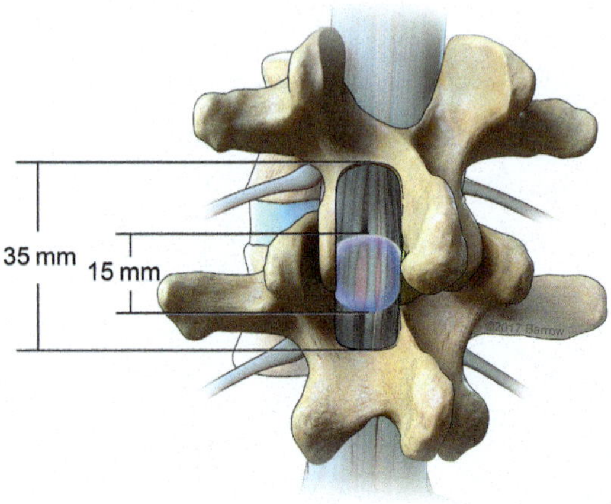

Fig. 26.3 The bone work needed for resection of a 15-mm lumbar intradural extramedullary lesion. Illustration demonstrating the 20 × 35-mm dimensions at the L2–L3 segment. Whether performed through a minimally invasive access port or midline approach, this exposure provides the necessary access to the canal for safe and complete resection of the lesion. (Used with permission from Barrow Neurological Institute, Phoenix, Arizona)

first step in the localization process that will be completed at the time of surgery. Prior to surgery, patients should undergo surveillance magnetic resonance imaging (MRI) of the brain, cervical spine, and thoracic spine to exclude the possibility of an additional lesion elsewhere in the central nervous system [20].

Careful review of the MRI should exclude the possibility of a vascular lesion. Typically, an intradural extramedullary lesion has a classic homogeneous enhancing pattern and would seldom be misconstrued for a vascular lesion. The presence of flow voids should prompt concern for a vascular lesion. Any such concern should be put to rest with either magnetic resonance angiography (MRA) or spinal angiography.

The dimensions of the lesion should be carefully assessed to determine the capacity of a minimally invasive technique. Unlike the various neoplastic processes of the thoracic spine that seldom exceed a rostral–caudal dimension of 30 mm, lumbar lesions have the capacity to grow considerably in the rostral–caudal dimension before causing symptoms that lead the patient to seek an evaluation that ultimately yields a diagnosis. Schwannomas and meningiomas in the lumbar spine tend to grow circumferentially and seldom exceed 30 mm in the rostral–caudal dimension. The reality is that patients become symptomatic only after the lesion reaches the canal dimensions. In contrast, myxopapillary ependymomas have the capacity to cause patients to present after the lesions have grown extensively in the rostral–caudal dimension. Although these lesions may not be amenable to resection via a minimal access port, the principles of hemilaminectomy without sacrifice of the spinous process, as espoused by Eggert and Yaşargil, can still be applied. Even with a midline incision, there is no need to sacrifice the midline elements to reach the lesion within the canal.

Lesions that are 30 mm or less in the rostral–caudal dimension will be amenable to a minimally invasive paramedian approach. For lesions greater than 30 mm in the rostral–caudal dimension, hemilaminectomies that encompass 1 cm above and below the lesion will be adequate for exposure and resection. Larger lesions may be outside the access corridor provided by minimal access ports but still do not require sacrifice of the spinous processes or bilateral laminae for resection.

Surgical Technique

Operating Room Setup

The paramedian minimally invasive approach requires the surgeon to select a side. Although intradural extramedullary lesions tend to occupy the entire canal (Fig. 26.4a), there tends to be a laterality to the symptoms or, at minimum, a laterality to the displacement of the thecal sac as shown in Fig. 26.4b, where the T1-weighted MRI with gadolinium contrast demonstrates displacement to one side. The side selected for approaching the canal should obviously be the same side as that of the symptoms, which typically corresponds with the displacement of the thecal sac. The operating microscope is positioned on the side of the approach, and the fluoroscope is positioned opposite the microscope. The patient will be positioned

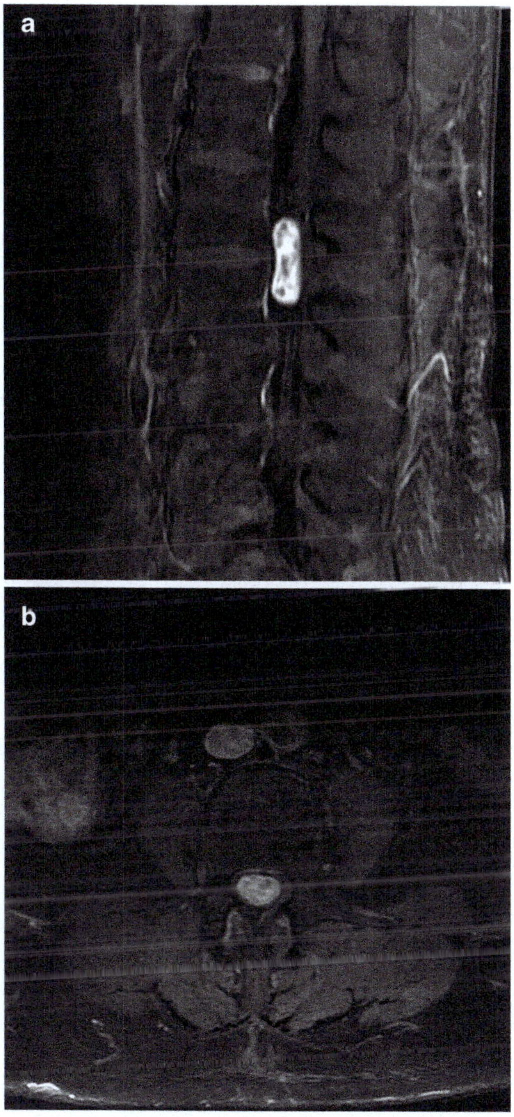

Fig. 26.4 Lumbar ependymoma. (**a**) Sagittal T1-weighted magnetic resonance image with gadolinium contrast demonstrating an intradural extramedullary lesion. After resection, histologic results showed the lesion to be an ependymoma. The rostral–caudal dimension was measured as 28 mm. As the only dimension not bound by the bony canal, the rostral–caudal dimension is almost without exception the largest dimension. (**b**) Axial T1-weighted MRI with gadolinium demonstrating the AP dimension of 10 mm and lateral dimension of 12 mm. These dimensions are well within the capacity of a minimal access port. (Used with permission from Barrow Neurological Institute, Phoenix, Arizona)

on a Jackson table or Wilson frame atop a Jackson table. The operating room team secures the clamp for the table-mounted frame on the same side as the surgeon in preparation for the table-mounted arm that will secure the access port. Having these elements in place prior to the incision will create a seamless transition between localization, dilatation, securing the access port, and beginning the work under the operating microscope. It is also essential to have microsurgical instruments and an ultrasonic aspirator available.

Before positioning the patient for the procedure, I prefer to place a lumbar drain for the lumbar lesion. During the postoperative course, the lumbar drain continues to drain whatever blood products enter the thecal sac from the surgery. It further protects the dural repair, thereby mitigating the potential for a cerebrospinal fluid leak.

Localization and Positioning

A precise, focal, and limited exposure is the central goal of minimally invasive resection of an intradural extramedullary lesion. Therefore, localization of the level becomes the most important component of planning the incision. To that end, confirmation of the segment should be performed by counting up from the sacrum on a lateral fluoroscopic image and down from the last rib-bearing vertebra on AP fluoroscopic imaging. The patient may be positioned on a Wilson frame atop a Jackson table or simply on a Jackson table. A Wilson frame has the capacity to open the intralaminar space, which can offer greater access to the central canal with the same amount of bone work. However, unlike lesions in the thoracic spine which are typically associated with a nerve root that anchors them in position, lumbar lesions are associated with a nerve root of the cauda equina and thus are more susceptible to migration. In my experience, migration of a lesion within the canal by several millimeters has the capacity to shift the lesion away from where it appeared on the MRI. Such migration can limit access to the rostral and caudal poles after the dural opening has been made. Consequently, I prefer to position patients similar to how they were positioned for their preoperative MRIs. A Jackson table without a Wilson frame closely mimics the position a patient assumed for the MRI and thereby limits the potential for migration of a lesion within the central canal.

Planning the Incision

Palpation of the anterior superior iliac crest allows for approximation of the L4–L5 level and a preliminary mark. Further palpation of the spinous processes relative to the initial preliminary L4–L5 mark allows for an approximation of the segment with the lesion. Whether at L1, L2, or L3, an additional preliminary mark is helpful. The skin is prepped before docking a spinal needle onto the lamina that harbors the lesion. Figure 26.5 demonstrates a lateral fluoroscopic image with a spinal needle in position for localization. The sacrum will be included in the first image to ensure that the segments can be counted. If the sacrum and the spinal needle cannot be included within the same field of view, it may be necessary to place an additional confirmatory spinal needle at the L4 lamina. After the segment has been confirmed in the AP and lateral projections, a 35-mm-long incision 30 mm lateral to the spinous process is marked, prepped, and draped (Fig. 26.6).

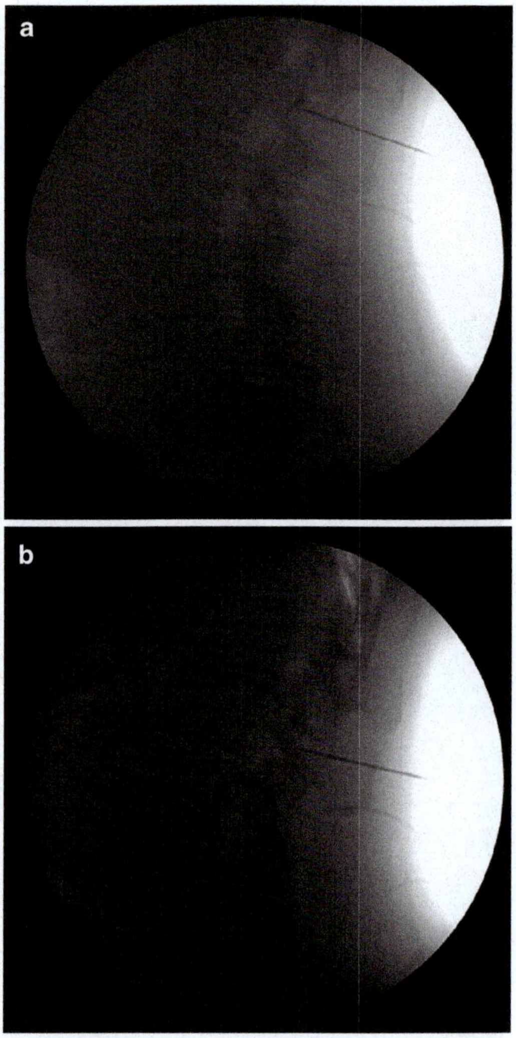

Fig. 26.5 Preliminary lateral fluoroscopic images demonstrating needle localization. (**a**) Lateral fluoroscopic image including the sacrum in the field of view for the preliminary count. In this circumstance, the L1–L2 segment has a characteristic appearance and becomes the reference segment when (**b**) the fluoroscopy unit is moved to center on the L2–L3 segment. On the basis of the lateral image, the incision can be planned and prepped and the patient can be draped. (Used with permission from Barrow Neurological Institute, Phoenix, Arizona)

Incision and Exposure

After unequivocal confirmation of the segment on AP and lateral fluoroscopic images, a 35-mm-long incision is made, the fascia is divided with cautery, and dilatation of the muscle begins. The first dilator should be secured up against the lamina and directed to the geometric center of the canal, where the lesion resides. A 25- to 30-degree angle of convergence is necessary to be able to undercut the spinous process and lamina, which will secure access to the entire canal (Fig. 26.7).

Wanding with each sequential dilator up against the lamina will establish a plane of dissection. Sequential dilatation to a diameter of 22 mm allows for placement of an expandable access port. As discussed in the anatomical basis

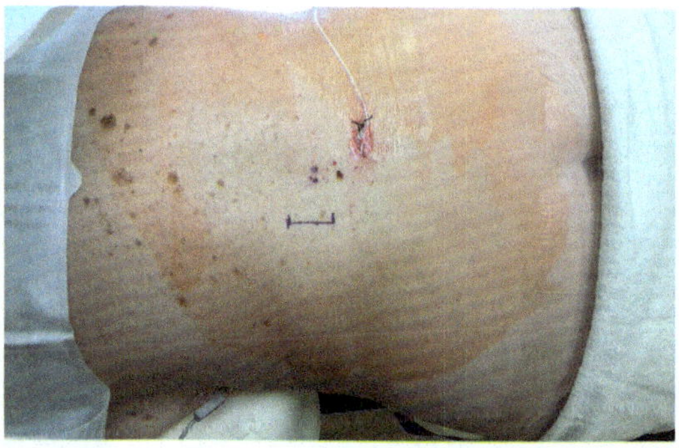

Fig. 26.6 Intraoperative photograph of a planned incision site for resection of an L2 intradural extramedullary lesion. Note the preoperative placement of the lumbar drain. The incision is planned to be approximately 35 mm long with placement 30 mm from the midline. (Used with permission from Barrow Neurological Institute, Phoenix, Arizona)

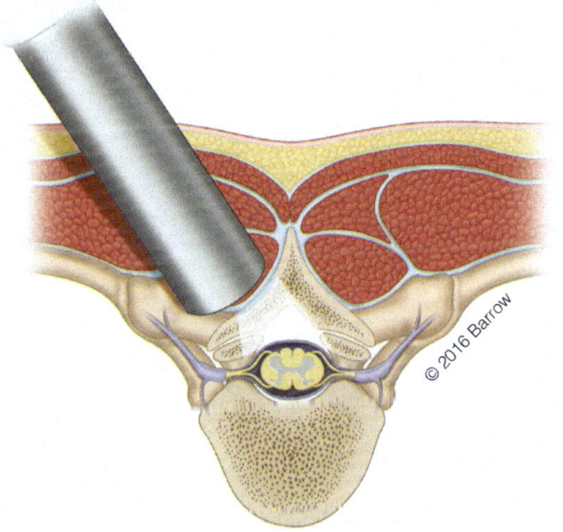

Fig. 26.7 Angle of convergence. Illustration of the angle of convergence onto the lamina. An incision 3 cm lateral to the spinous process with 25–30 degrees of angulation will allow for convergence onto the lamina with the diameter of the access port encompassing the entire spinal canal. (Modified with permission from Barrow Neurological Institute, Phoenix, Arizona)

section earlier, the lumbar canal dimensions do not exceed 27 mm in the lateral dimension and 20 mm in the AP dimension. Downward pressure on the minimal access port is maintained while the surgical assistant or scrub technician secures it to the table-mounted frame to optimize the interface of the port with the lamina as demonstrated in the fluoroscopic sequence in Fig. 26.8. After the minimal access port is secured in position, the operating room team can bring in the operating microscope.

Exposure and Laminectomy

The entire exposure offered by the minimal access port will be needed for the operation. Invariably, a film of muscle tissue will remain over the top of the lamina, which has to be exposed in its entirety. Before beginning the laminectomy, it is essential to ensure that there is a full 35 mm of rostral–caudal exposure in addition to clear visualization of the base of the spinous process. Undercutting the spinous process will allow for complete exposure of the central canal (see Fig. 26.7). Rotating the bed approximately 15 degrees away from the surgeon is essential to enable the surgeon to reach the contralateral recess and access the entire canal.

A laminectomy with a medial facetectomy is performed using a drill with a minimally invasive curved drill attachment. The subtle curvature of a minimally invasive attachment optimizes the visualization at the tip of the drill and is ideal for working through a minimal access port. The focus should be on undercutting the spinous process and drilling into the underside of the contralateral lamina. Accomplishing those two tasks will optimize access to the entire central canal. The bone work extends almost to the extent of the entire exposure, for a full 35 mm of rostral–caudal exposure and resection of the ligamentum flavum. I prefer to confirm the rostral–caudal exposure with a ruler trimmed to 35 mm. Only after the breadth of exposure is confirmed should the dura be opened.

Dural Opening

At times the lesion becomes evident beneath the dura. In my experience, the heat from the light of the microscope can sometimes make the previously white dura more diaphanous. A window into the intradural contents becomes evident

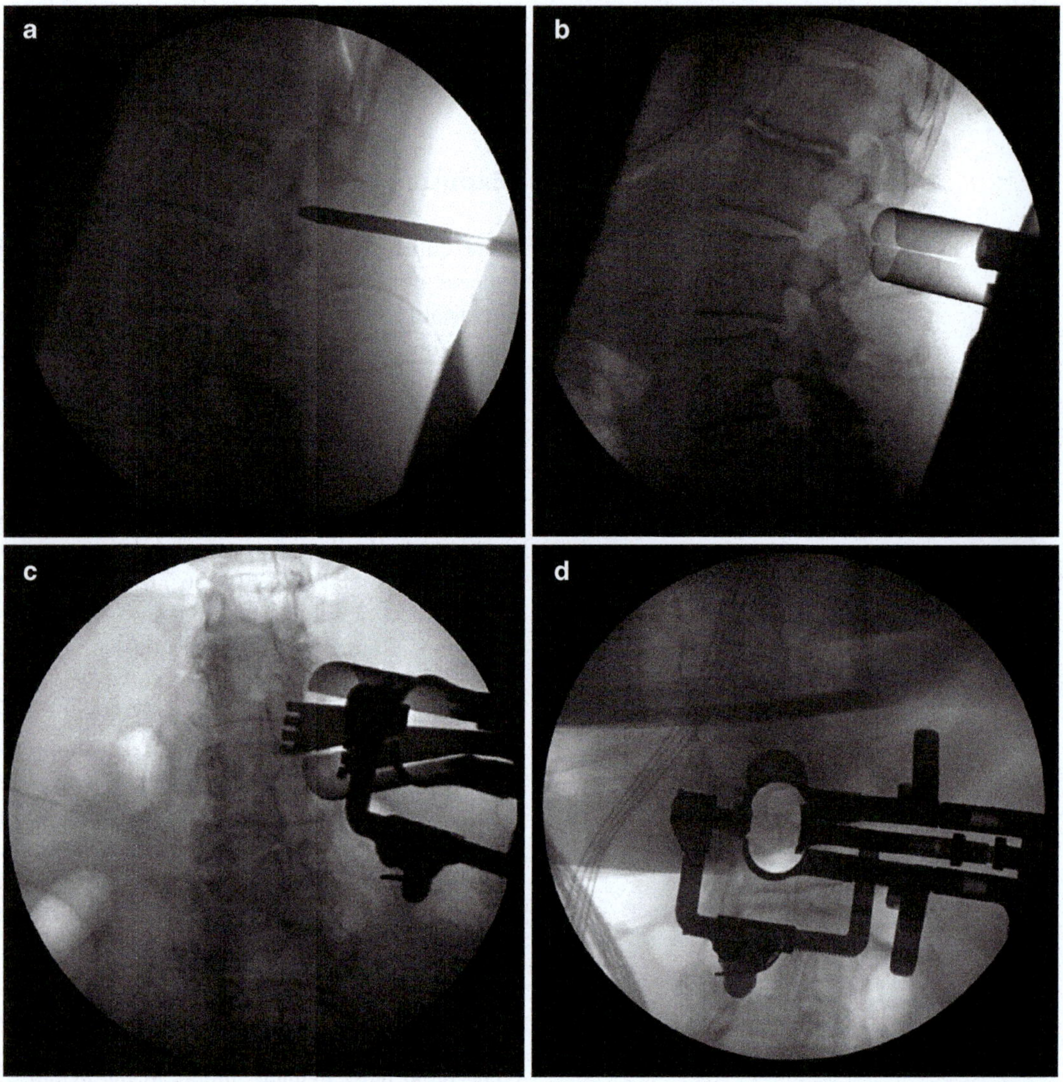

Fig. 26.8 Securing the minimal access port. (**a**) Lateral fluoroscopic image demonstrating the first dilator secured onto the lamina of L2. (**b**) Lateral fluoroscopic image with the minimal access port secured into position. (**c**) True anteroposterior image with the minimal access port in position after a preliminary exposure. A medial–lateral component has been added to optimize the medial exposure. (**d**) Oblique lateral fluoroscopic view into the minimal access port. The field of view is 35 mm in the rostral–caudal dimension and 25 mm in the lateral dimension. (Used with permission from Barrow Neurological Institute, Phoenix, Arizona)

through the now-transparent dura. An encouraging sensation overcomes the surgeon when a perfect sphere can be seen pulsating among the nerve roots of the thecal sac. However, a translucent dura does not always afford visualization of the lesion. In some cases, the dura remains opaque and does not offer an intradural view. When the lesion is visualized, the dura is definitively opened immediately over the top of the lesion extending above and below its rostral and caudal poles. When the lesion cannot be seen, the dura is opened slightly off the midline. A No. 11 blade on a bayonet knife handle can be used to score the dura. Opening the dura while keeping the arachnoid membrane intact is an art requiring both patience and meticulous technique. A 6.0 Prolene (polypropylene) suture can be used as a tack-up suture on each side of the opening.

After a limited opening, microdissectors displace the nerve roots and allow identification of the lesion. Unlike lesions in the thoracic spine, which seem anchored to a nerve root and are found precisely where the MRI demonstrated the lesion would reside, lesions in the lumbar spine will often drift rostral. For lesions associated with a freely mobile lumbar nerve root of the cauda equina, migration is always a possibility. For this reason, a preliminary opening in the dura should be made when the lesion is not directly visible to allow the lesion to be found before widening the dural opening. On more than one occasion, I have found it necessary to close the dura and extend the bone work further rostral to completely expose the lesion.

Direct visualization of the lesion allows you to decide in which direction to continue the dural opening or in which direction to extend the bone work. The criterion for an adequate dural opening is simultaneous visualization of the rostral and caudal poles of the lesion. Once the dural opening extends above and below the lesion, the dura can be tacked up with 6.0 Prolene sutures on either side. Microdissection and resection of the lesion can now begin.

Resection of the Lesion

At this point in the operation, there is little, if any, difference between a traditional midline approach with complete laminectomy and a minimally invasive approach with hemilaminectomy. Despite the spinous processes having been preserved in the minimally invasive technique, the exposures at high magnification of the operating microscope will appear indistinguishable. After all, the entire canal will have been exposed in either case. Therefore, the same principles of microsurgical resection for a midline approach apply to a minimally invasive approach.

Identification of the rostral and caudal poles remains the first priority. Shrinking the lesion with bipolar cautery is a helpful preemptive maneuver to decrease bleeding. Adequate mobilization of the lesion precedes internal debulking. After the entire lesion has been visualized and freed from the surrounding nerve roots, a sample should be sent for an immediate frozen section to confirm pathology. The diagnosis of a meningioma prompts careful consideration of adherence to the dura and may even prompt resection of a section of dura and the need for a dural patch to repair the defect. The diagnosis of a myxopapillary ependymoma on frozen section necessitates resection of the filum terminale. Cauterization above and below the filum should be completed first, with division of the rostral filum to prevent migration of the lesion outside the surgical field. The filum terminale has an unmistakable appearance that distinguishes it from the surrounding nerve roots of the cauda equina. First, a zigzagging tortuous vessel is typically seen atop the filum, which is not seen on the surrounding nerve roots. Second, ligamentous-appearing strands course within the filum, giving it a distinctly non-neural appearance. In addition to these characteristics of the filum terminale, neurophysiological monitoring can be helpful in identifying it. Stimulating the nerve and recording anal sphincter electromyography build confidence when the filum is being prepared for division and resection. The goal of surgery is gross-total resection, regardless of the histology of the lesion.

Closure of the Dura

Several authors have commented on the difficulty of dural closure in minimally invasive approaches. In my experience, a dural closure in the lumbar spine is not a particularly facile task, whether performed through a minimally invasive access port or a traditional midline approach. Regardless, bayonet microsurgical needle drivers and bayonet pick-ups are essential. A running 6.0 Prolene suture begun at either end of the dural opening and secured in the middle will provide a water-tight closure. Dural sealant is applied to the repair before removal of the minimal access port. If a dural patch is needed because of adherence to the dura by a meningioma that required resection, the patch is cut to the precise dimensions and secured with a series of interrupted 4.0 Nurolon (nylon) sutures. Securing a 0 Vicryl (polyglactin 910) suture on a UR-6 needle in an interrupted fashion approximates the fascia. The 5/8 circle offered by the UR-6 needle is of great value when approximating fascia in a constrained incision. Interrupted 2.0 Vicryl sutures on an X-1 needle approximate the subcutaneous tissues, and 3.0 Vicryl, Mastisol (liquid adhesive), and Steri-Strips (wound closure strips) bring the skin edges together.

Case Presentation

Clinical History and Neurological Examination

A 64-year-old woman presented with a 2-year history of neurogenic claudication, right greater than left radicular leg pain, and urinary urgency. After an exhaustive urological and orthopedic evaluation, an MRI of the lumbar spine was obtained. On examination, the patient had decreased sensation on the right anterior thigh (the remaining lumbosacral dermatomes were intact to pinprick and light touch examination), patellar and Achilles reflexes were absent bilaterally, but the patient had remarkably preserved strength in the proximal and distal muscle groups of the lower extremities when at rest. However, with any degree of ambulation, the patient experienced profound claudication and weakness.

Radiographic Studies

Unenhanced MRI of the lumbar spine suggested an intradural extramedullary lesion at the level of the L2 vertebral body (Fig. 26.9). Gadolinium-enhanced MRI demonstrated an intradural extramedullary lesion that was 14 × 13 mm in the AP and lateral dimensions and 15 mm in the rostral–caudal dimension (Fig. 26.10).

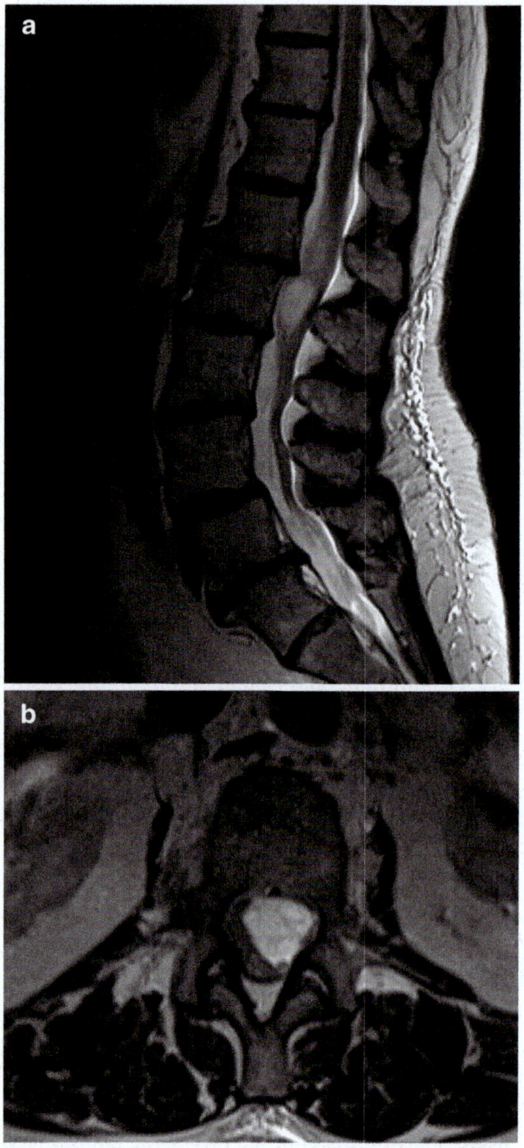

Fig. 26.9 Unenhanced magnetic resonance image (MRI) suggestive of an intradural lesion. (**a**) Sagittal T2-weighted MRI demonstrating a lesion isointense with cerebrospinal fluid at the level of the L2 vertebral body (transitional anatomy). (**b**) Axial T2-weighted MRI demonstrating displacement of the caudal equina to the right. With the lesion off to the left, a left paramedian approach would afford the exposure needed for resection. (Used with permission from Barrow Neurological Institute, Phoenix, Arizona)

Preoperative Considerations

In my experience, the more spherical geometry of this lesion is more suggestive of a nerve sheath lesion or a meningioma than an ependymoma, which characteristically grows considerably in the rostral–caudal dimension (see Fig. 26.4). However, no firm conclusion may be drawn purely from imaging, and definitive histological analysis is always required. In this case, the lesion resides

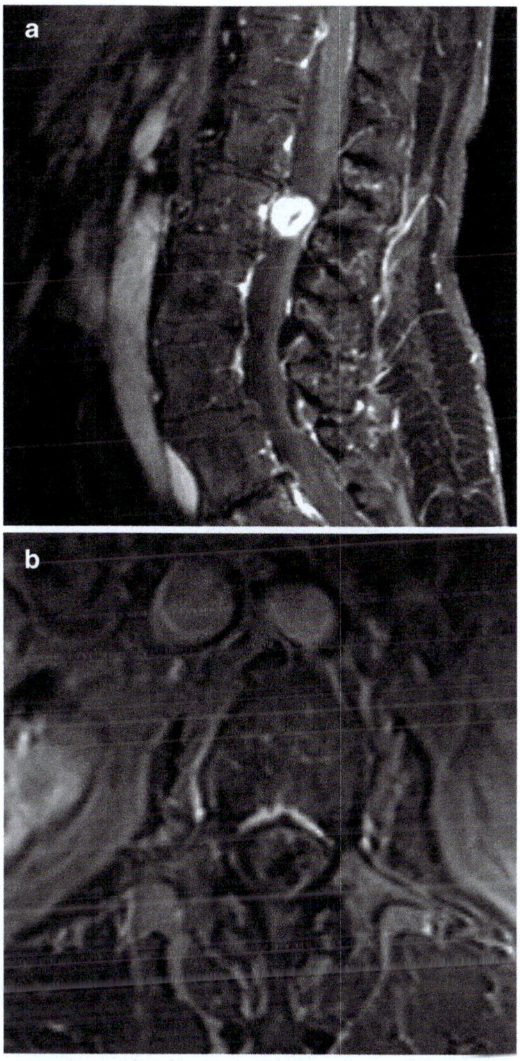

Fig. 26.10 MRI with gadolinium contrast demonstrating an intradural extramedullary lesion. (**a**) Sagittal gadolinium-enhanced MRI demonstrating a 14 × 13 × 15-mm lesion in the anteroposterior, lateral, and rostral–caudal dimensions, respectively. It is common for the rostral–caudal dimension of a lesion, as the only dimension not bound by the bony canal, to be the largest dimension of the lesion. (**b**) Axial T1-weighted MRI with gadolinium contrast demonstrates that the lesion is occupying nearly the entire canal on this axial cut. (Used with permission from Barrow Neurological Institute, Phoenix, Arizona)

at the level of the L2 vertebral body based on a counting scheme that incorporates transitional anatomy. The axial images (see Figs. 26.9b and 26.10b) clearly demonstrate the lesion displacing cauda equina to the right. Thus, a left paramedian approach onto the lamina of L2 would offer an ideal corridor for approaching the lesion.

With regard to the dimensions of the lesion, a 14 × 13 × 15-mm lesion lends itself especially well to a minimally invasive approach. With 35 mm of rostral–caudal exposure and a complete hemilaminectomy over the lesion, a generous corridor for resection of the lesion is offered by an expandable minimal access port. All the while, the spinous process and the contralateral lamina are preserved.

Surgical Technique

A lumbar drain was placed before the patient was positioned on a Jackson table for surgery. An incision was planned 30 mm lateral to the midline and 35 mm long on the left and was confirmed with the localization process described earlier (Fig. 26.11). The microscope was positioned on the left side of the patient, and the fluoroscope was positioned on the right side. Intraoperative neurophysiological monitoring with anal sphincter electromyography was set up, and baseline measurements were obtained.

An incision was made with a No. 15 blade, and cautery was used to divide the fascia. Sequential dilatation over the top of the lamina of L2 to a 22-mm diameter allowed for placement of a minimal access port onto the lamina with a 25 to 30-degree angle of conversion (as demonstrated in Fig. 26.7). The exposure of 35 mm of lamina includes L2, the interlaminar space, and the inferior part of L1. It is preferable to expose slightly rostral to the lesion than caudal because of the tendency for untethered lumbar lesions to migrate rostral.

The operative video demonstrates that the removal of bone encompasses nearly the entire exposure provided by the minimal access port (Video 26.1). As seen in the operative footage, there is a particular focus in undercutting the spinous process and drilling the contralateral lamina beneath the spinous process. It will be the removal underside of the contralateral lamina and the underside of the spinous process that will provide access to the entire canal. After the liga-

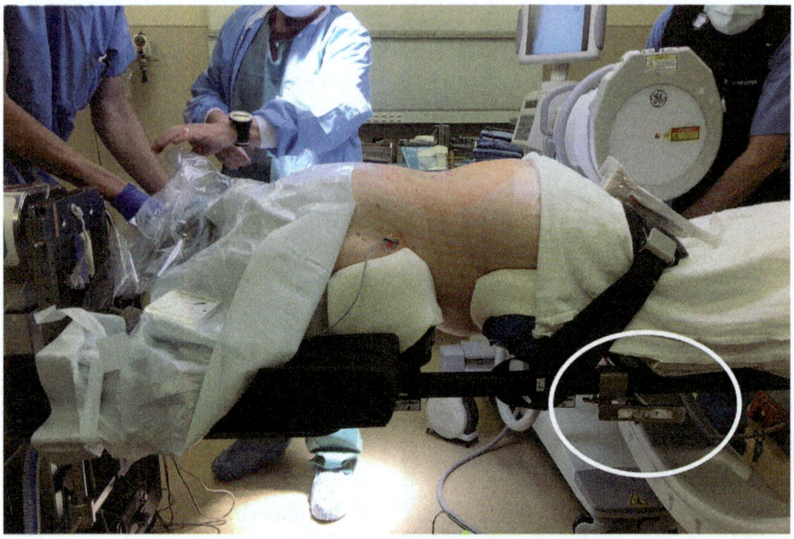

Fig. 26.11 Intraoperative photograph showing the position of the patient. The lumbar drain has already been placed. The fluoroscope is placed opposite the side of the incision, and the microscope is placed on the side of the incision (not shown). Note the attachment (circle) where the clamp for the retractor arm will be secured to hold the minimal access port in position. (Used with permission from Barrow Neurological Institute, Phoenix, Arizona)

mentum flavum is widely exposed and resected, the epidural veins are cauterized and an attempt is made to peer through the translucent dura to identify the lesion. Regardless of whether the lesion can be seen, confidence in the localization process allows for the dura to be opened with a No. 11 blade. The dural edges are tacked up with a series of 6.0 Prolene sutures and the lesion is identified and resected. The dura is closed in a water-tight fashion, the retractor is removed, and the lumbar fascia, subcutaneous tissues, and skin edges are brought together in a multilayered fashion (Fig. 26.12).

Postoperative Course

The patient had lumbar drainage of 10–15 mL per hour for 48 h, after which the cerebrospinal fluid became clear. The lumbar drain was clamped, and the patient ambulated without experiencing positional headache. The lumbar drain was removed, and the patient was discharged home on the morning of the third postoperative day. Postoperative MRI demonstrated gross-total resection (Fig. 26.13).

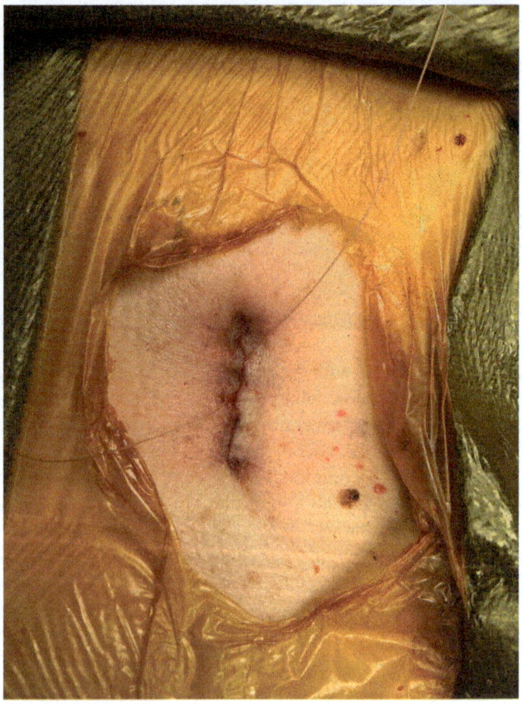

Fig. 26.12 Intraoperative photograph of a 35-mm incision for resection of the L2 intradural lesion. The final pathologic finding was Grade I meningioma. (Used with permission from Barrow Neurological Institute, Phoenix, Arizona)

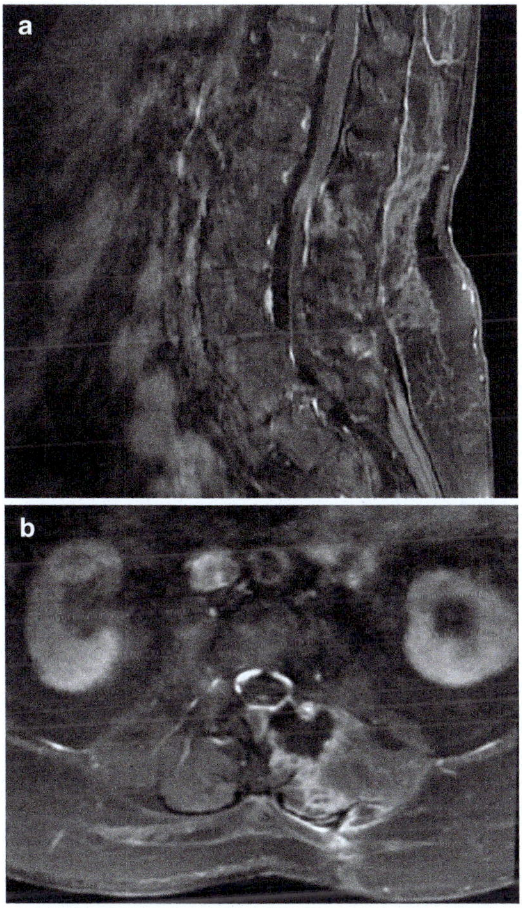

Fig. 26.13 Postoperative MRI. (**a**) Sagittal T1-weighted MRI with gadolinium contrast demonstrating a gross-total resection of the Grade I meningioma. (**b**) Axial T1-weighted MRI with gadolinium contrast demonstrating the left paramedian access corridor. (Used with permission from Barrow Neurological Institute, Phoenix, Arizona)

Complications and Strategies for Complication Avoidance

Cerebrospinal Fluid Leak

My preference is to place lumbar drains in patients with lumbar intradural extramedullary lesions and to refrain from placing lumbar drains in patients with cervical or thoracic lesions in whom the hydrostatic pressure at the level of the repair would be considerably less. The placement of a lumbar drain protects the dural repair during the immediate postoperative period and has virtually eliminated any issues with delayed pseudomeningoceles.

Localization of the Lesion

As mentioned in the positioning section, since lumbar lesions are associated with an untethered nerve root, migration of the lesion after positioning is common. The limited corridor of a minimally invasive exposure requires precise positioning over the top of the lesion. For this reason, one should avoid the use of a Wilson frame, which opens the interlaminar space but also has an unpredictable effect on the location of the lesion. Turel and Rajshekhar [21] took the possibility of lesion migration a step further by placing the patient in the MRI gantry in a position that mimicked the position during surgery. MRI markers were placed on the skin of the lumbar spine to help further localize the lesion in the surgical position. Although I have not used this particular technique, there may be potential value in such a preoperative study. In my experience, the lesion consistently migrates rostral. Thus, the rostral exposure should always be more generous than the caudal exposure at the outset and then be modified after the lesion is identified.

Conclusion

The resection of a lumbar intradural extramedullary lesion through a minimally invasive approach is the culmination of the decades of work toward an evolving surgical technique alongside advancing technology. Advances in imaging and refinements in localization have allowed for a focused exposure that, when coupled with a sophisticated understanding of the canal dimensions, allows for a precise and minimal exposure. Given the limited size of these lesions, there is no real need for extensive exposures, removal of the spinous process, or removal of bilateral lamina. With the realization that the spinal canal can be viewed in three dimensions, one can see that the midline structures, specifically the spinous process and lamina, need not be considered barriers to access and complete resection of these lesions. Preservation of these structures maintains the stability of the spine in the years and decades after a successful operation and may prevent iatrogenic scoliosis and kyphosis. Equally important is the decrease in the postoperative discomfort from a smaller incision and minimal disruption of the native spine.

Acknowledgments The author thanks the staff of Neuroscience Publications at Barrow Neurological Institute for assistance with manuscript preparation.

Disclosures The author is a consultant for Medtronic, plc, and DePuy-Synthes.

Financial Support None

References

1. Love JG. Laminectomy for the removal of spinal cord tumors. J Neurosurg. 1966;25(1):116–21. https://doi.org/10.3171/jns.1966.25.1.0116.
2. Chiou SM, Eggert HR, Laborde G, Seeger W. Microsurgical unilateral approaches for spinal tumour surgery: eight years' experience in 256 primary operated patients. Acta Neurochir. 1989;100(3–4):127–33.
3. Yasargil MG, Tranmer BI, Adamson TE, Roth P. Unilateral partial hemi-laminectomy for the removal of extra- and intramedullary tumours and AVMs. Adv Tech Stand Neurosurg. 1991;18:113–32.
4. Ahmed R, Menezes AH, Awe OO, Mahaney KB, Torner JC, Weinstein SL. Long-term incidence and risk factors for development of spinal deformity following resection of pediatric intramedullary spinal cord tumors. J Neurosurg Pediatr. 2014;13(6):613–21. https://doi.org/10.3171/2014.1.PEDS13317.
5. Kelley BJ, Johnson MH, Vortmeyer AO, Smith BG, Abbed KM. Two-level thoracic pedicle subtraction osteotomy for progressive post-laminectomy kyphotic deformity following resection of an unusual thoracolumbar intradural extramedullary tumor. J Neurosurg Pediatr. 2012;10(4):334–9. https://doi.org/10.3171/2012.7.PEDS11526.
6. McGirt MJ, Chaichana KL, Atiba A, Bydon A, Witham TF, Yao KC, et al. Incidence of spinal deformity after resection of intramedullary spinal cord tumors in children who underwent laminectomy compared with laminoplasty. J Neurosurg Pediatr. 2008;1(1):57–62. https://doi.org/10.3171/PED-08/01/057.
7. de Jonge T, Slullitel H, Dubousset J, Miladi L, Wicart P, Illes T. Late-onset spinal deformities in children treated by laminectomy and radiation therapy for malignant tumours. Eur Spine J. 2005;14(8):765–71. https://doi.org/10.1007/s00586-004-0778-1.
8. Otsuka NY, Hey L, Hall JE. Postlaminectomy and postirradiation kyphosis in children and adolescents. Clin Orthop Relat Res. 1998;354:189–94.
9. Albert TJ, Vacarro A. Postlaminectomy kyphosis. Spine (Phila Pa 1976). 1998;23(24):2738–45.
10. Eggert HR, Scheremet R, Seeger W, Gaitzsch J. Unilateral microsurgical approaches to extramedullary spinal tumours: operative technique and results. Acta Neurochir. 1983;67(3–4):245–53.
11. Foley KT, Smith MM. Microendoscopic discectomy. Tech Neurosurg. 1997;3(4):301–7.
12. Schwender JD, Holly LT, Rouben DP, Foley KT. Minimally invasive transforaminal lumbar interbody fusion (TLIF): technical feasibility and initial results. J Spinal Disord Tech. 2005; 18(Suppl):S1–6.
13. Tredway TL, Santiago P, Hrubes MR, Song JK, Christie SD, Fessler RG. Minimally invasive resection of intradural-extramedullary spinal neoplasms. Neurosurgery. 2006;58(1 Suppl):ONS52–8. discussion ONS-8.
14. Zhu YJ, Ying GY, Chen AQ, Wang LL, Yu DF, Zhu LL, et al. Minimally invasive removal of lumbar intradural extramedullary lesions using the interlaminar approach. Neurosurg Focus. 2015;39(2):E10. https://doi.org/10.3171/2015.5.FOCUS15182.
15. Turel MK, D'Souza WP, Rajshekhar V. Hemilaminectomy approach for intradural extramedullary spinal tumors: an analysis of 164 patients. Neurosurg Focus. 2015;39(2):E9. https://doi.org/10.3171/2015.5.FOCUS15170.
16. Nzokou A, Weil AG, Shedid D. Minimally invasive removal of thoracic and lumbar spinal tumors using a nonexpandable tubular retractor. J Neurosurg Spine. 2013;19(6):708–15. https://doi.org/10.3171/2013.9.SPINE121061.
17. Panjabi MM, Goel V, Oxland T, Takata K, Duranceau J, Krag M, et al. Human lumbar vertebrae: quantitative three-dimensional anatomy. Spine (Phila Pa 1976). 1992;17(3):299–306.
18. De Verdelhan O, Haegelen C, Carsin-Nicol B, Riffaud L, Amlashi SF, Brassier G, et al. MR imaging features of spinal schwannomas and meningiomas. J Neuroradiol. 2005;32(1):42–9.
19. Kucia EJ, Maughan PH, Kakarla UK, Bambakidis NC, Spetzler RF. Surgical technique and outcomes in the treatment of spinal cord ependymomas: part II: myxopapillary ependymoma. Neurosurgery. 2011;68(1 Suppl Operative):90–4.; discussion 4. https://doi.org/10.1227/NEU.0b013e3181fdf912.
20. Iunes EA, Stavale JN, de Cassia Caldas Pessoa R, Ansai R, Onishi FJ, de Paiva Neto MA, et al. Multifocal intradural extramedullary ependymoma: case report. J Neurosurg Spine. 2011;14(1):65–70. https://doi.org/10.3171/2010.9.SPINE09963.
21. Turel MK, Rajshekhar V. Magnetic resonance imaging localization with cod liver oil capsules for the minimally invasive approach to small intradural extramedullary tumors of the thoracolumbar spine. J Neurosurg Spine. 2014;21(6):882–5. https://doi.org/10.3171/2014.9.SPINE14199.

Intradural, Intramedullary Tumor

27

Mari L. Groves and George Jallo

Introduction

Primary spinal cord tumors account for approximately 2–4% of all central nervous system neoplasms and about 15% of adult intradural tumors [1, 2] Roughly two-thirds of these lesions are extramedullary, while one-third are intramedullary. In adults, the overwhelming majority of IMSCTs are gliomas (80–90%), of which 60–70% are ependymomas with 30–40% being astrocytomas [3, 4]. In the pediatric population, astrocytomas are the most common intramedullary lesion, followed by gangliogliomas and mixed gliomas [1, 5]. Certain subpopulations are particularly susceptible to development of IMSCT, including patients with neurofibromatosis and von Hippel-Lindau (VHL) disease. The reported incidence of IMSCT in the total neurofibromatosis population is approximately 19% [6]. Neurofibromatosis type 1 (NF1) predisposes patients to development of astrocytomas and intradural extramedullary nerve sheath tumors, whereas patients with neurofibromatosis type 2 (NF2) are more closely associated with development of ependymomas [6]. Patients with VHL are predisposed to the development of hemangioblastomas.

Surgery for IMSCT has been well established in the modern surgical age but in the last several decades has become a cornerstone in the treatment for these low-grade lesions. The introduction of magnetic resonance imaging (MRI), operative microscope, bipolar coagulation, and intraoperative neuromonitoring and the use of an ultrasonic aspirator have made surgery safer. Technical advancements have also allowed surgeons to perform more aggressive resections and still achieve good functional outcomes with lower rates of morbidity.

Operative Treatment

Surgical goals include tissue diagnosis, maximum safe tumor removal, and maintaining a stable or improving neurologic function. Operative planning includes attention to tumor location, preoperative deficits, and presumed pathology. Ependymomas are generally more benign lesions and as such tend to have a more distinct tumor/spinal cord interface [7]. These tumors are typically more amenable to gross total resection regardless of the size or radiological features. Astrocytomas are typically more infiltrative, non-encapsulated tumors that have less well-defined borders [8]. Separation from normal anatomical structures can be challenging unless there

M. L. Groves (✉)
Johns Hopkins Hospital, Department of Neurosurgery, Baltimore, MD, USA
e-mail: mgroves2@jhmi.edu

G. Jallo
Johns Hopkins All Children's Hospital, Department of Neurosurgery, St. Petersburg, FL, USA

D. M. Sciubba (ed.), *Spinal Tumor Surgery*, https://doi.org/10.1007/978-3-319-98422-3_27

is a clear pseudocapsule. High-grade lesions, whether ependymoma or astrocytoma, portend a poor prognosis regardless of surgical resection and additionally have limited adjuvant treatment options. These tumors are more infiltrative into the surrounding cord parenchyma and are less amenable to surgical resection without causing significant neurological deficits [9]. Safe surgical management of IMSCT relies on the surgeon's meticulous technique in order to prioritize good functional outcomes and progression-free survival [1].

Surgical Anatomy

Safe surgical technique is grounded in a thorough understanding of the spinal cord anatomy. Better appreciation of the cross-sectional surgical anatomy will help delineate safe surgical corridors to the infiltrative process. Even IMSCTs that are not well encapsulated will have some borders and typically displace normal spinal cord tissue. Appreciation of anatomical zones within a fully formed spinal cord is rooted in an understanding of embryological formation of the spinal cord. With neural tube formation, embryonically distinct sets of commissural and association neurons differentiate in the dorsal half of the spinal cord, and motor neurons and ventral interneurons develop in the ventral half of the neural tube [10]. Thus, in a generalized fashion, the white matter consisting of ascending and descending fibers is located in the dorsal spinal cord, with gray matter and anterior horn cells being located within the ventral aspect of the spinal cord (Fig. 27.1).

Similar to cerebral anatomy, the spinal cord is split into symmetrical halves by a shallow posterior median sulcus and a deeper anterior median fissure. The anterior median fissure is a pial border that houses the anterior spinal artery. The posterior median sulcus is typically identified by midline venous drainage and can be identified by serial diving vessels into the pial surface. The posterolateral sulcus and anterolateral sulcus are where dorsal and ventral nerve roots are attached to the spinal cord, respectively. This is more typically a shallow groove that can be identified where the nerve roots dive into the spinal cord itself [10].

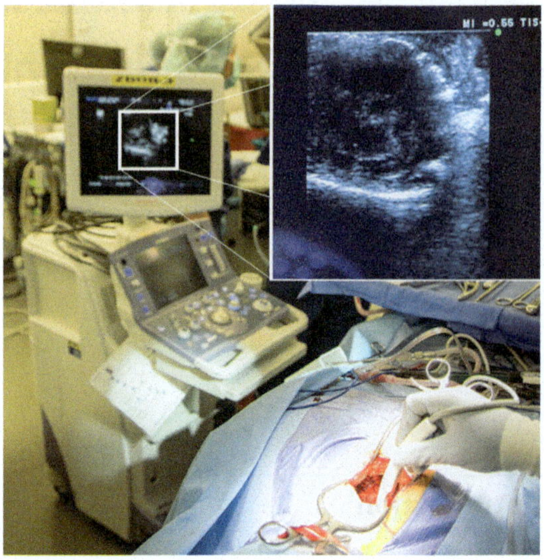

Fig. 27.1 Intraoperative ultrasound may be used to confirm adequate exposure prior to durotomy. Tumor borders and any adjacent cyst or syrinx can be seen and correlated with preoperative imaging

Operative Technique

Once appropriate patient selection has been made, the patients are taken to the operating room. The most typical approach is posterior, even for more ventrally situated tumors (Fig. 27.2). Patients are given perioperative steroids as well as standard prophylactic antibiotics. Blood pressure parameters should also be discussed prior to induction as any fluctuation can lead to hypoperfusion of the spinal cord, with potential neuromonitoring changes that could alter intraoperative decision-making as well as postoperative recovery. Patients with cervical or high thoracic lesions are secured with a three-point Mayfield clamp (Integra LifeSciences, Plainsboro, NJ). Prone positioning with care emphasizes on minimizing venous hypertension while maintaining neutral spinal alignment. Intraoperative neurophysiological monitoring (IONM) should include continuous somatosensory evoked potentials (SSEPs), motor evoked potentials (MEPs), and epidural

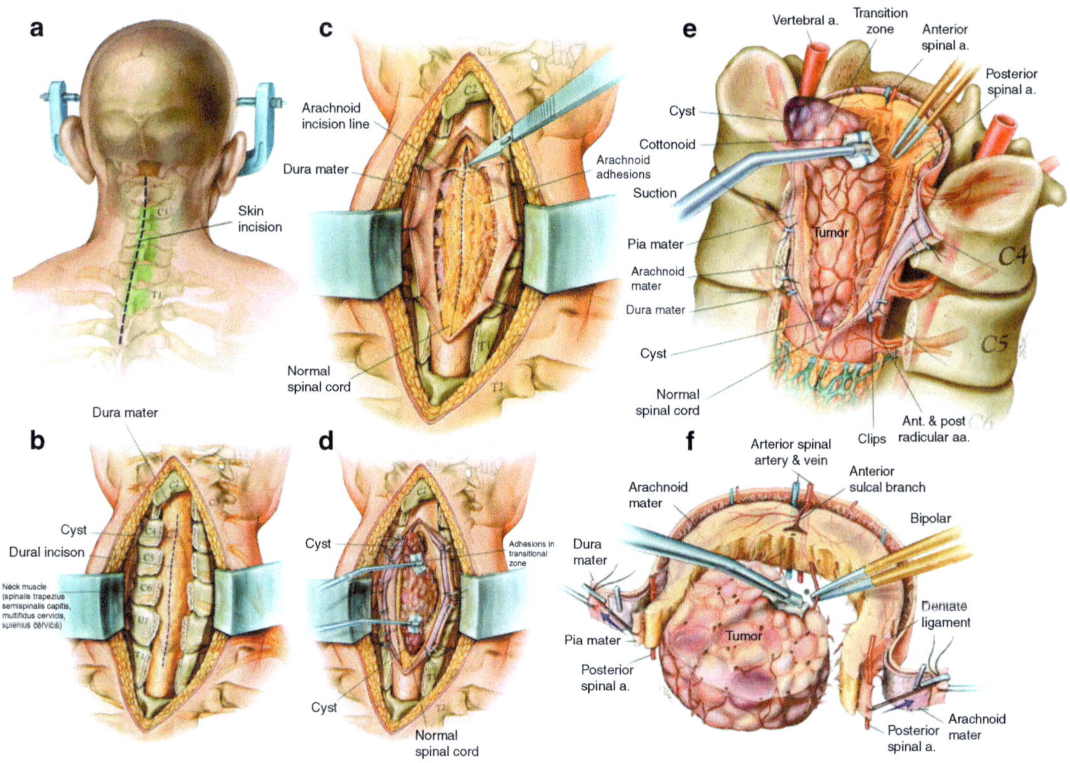

Fig. 27.2 Artist illustration of operative steps for intramedullary spinal cord tumor resection. Midline skin incision and laminectomy (**a**, **b**). Dural opening and dorsal midline myelotomy to enter the spinal cord (**c**). Meticulous detachment of tumor from transitional zone adhesions with careful hemostasis (**d**, **e**). Complete tumor removal (**f**). Reprinted from Hanbali et al. [11], by permission of Oxford University Press

continuous motor (D-wave), when possible, which is discussed in more detail later in this chapter. Anesthetic planning should be discussed to minimize any non-surgical disruption in signals [2, 12] as well as to establish blood pressure parameters. The appropriate spinal level selection is confirmed via intraoperative radiographs or ultrasound. Intraoperative ultrasound can help determine the margins of the tumor as well as any cystic structures or hyperechogenic areas that might correlate with areas of significant contrast enhancement (see Fig. 27.1).

A standard, posterior midline incision is made, and paraspinal muscles are dissected away in a subperiosteal manner (Fig. 27.3). Dissection and exposure should take care to preserve the lateral ligamentous attachments and facet joints to help minimize postoperative instability and the development of future deformities [2, 13, 14]. If patients have a significant spinal deformity preoperatively, a fusion procedure at the time of resection may be considered. However, this may be staged if there is concern for any residual that needs to be followed with imaging. A laminectomy or laminoplasty may also be used to provide bony decompression or revision of the posterior elements [15]. While there is no consensus, a laminoplasty may provide anatomical boundaries that can be helpful for future resections as well as perhaps slow the progress of spinal deformities. Laminectomies should be considered if patients are presenting with significant pain and concern for a higher grade of malignancy, as a bony decompression in addition to a standard duraplasty may provide some decompression for pressure on the spinal cord. We prefer the ultrasonic osteotome (BoneScalpel by Aesculap Central Valley, PA) for the laminectomy of the dorsal spinal elements as this provides a safe, effective way to remove the bone (Fig. 27.4) [16].

Prior to the durotomy, hemostasis from the muscular layer and bony decompression should be obtained. This helps minimize any rundown of blood products into the intradural space which can technically complicate surgical resection. Hemostasis may be obtained through a mixture

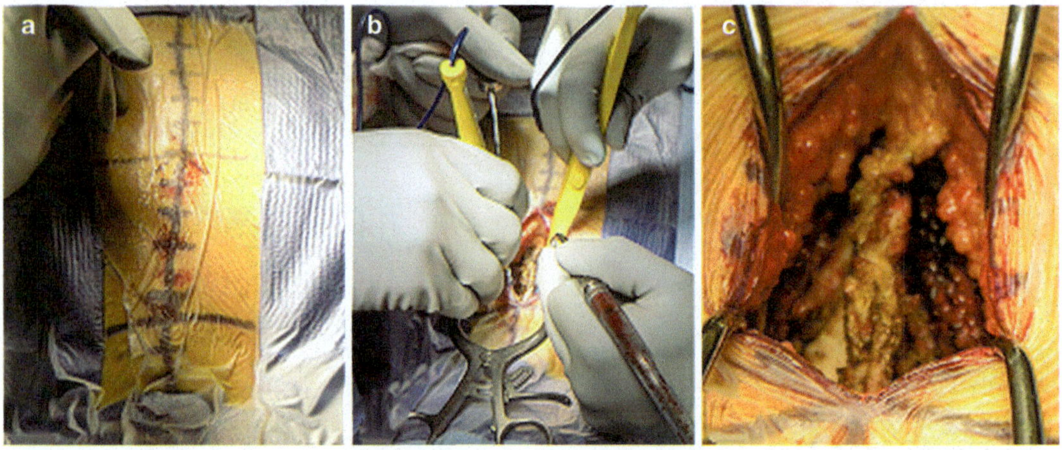

Fig. 27.3 A standard, posterior midline incision is made (**a**) and paraspinal muscles are dissected away in a subperiosteal manner (**b**). Dissection and exposure should take care to preserve the lateral ligamentous attachments and facet joints to help minimize postoperative instability and the development of future deformities (**c**)

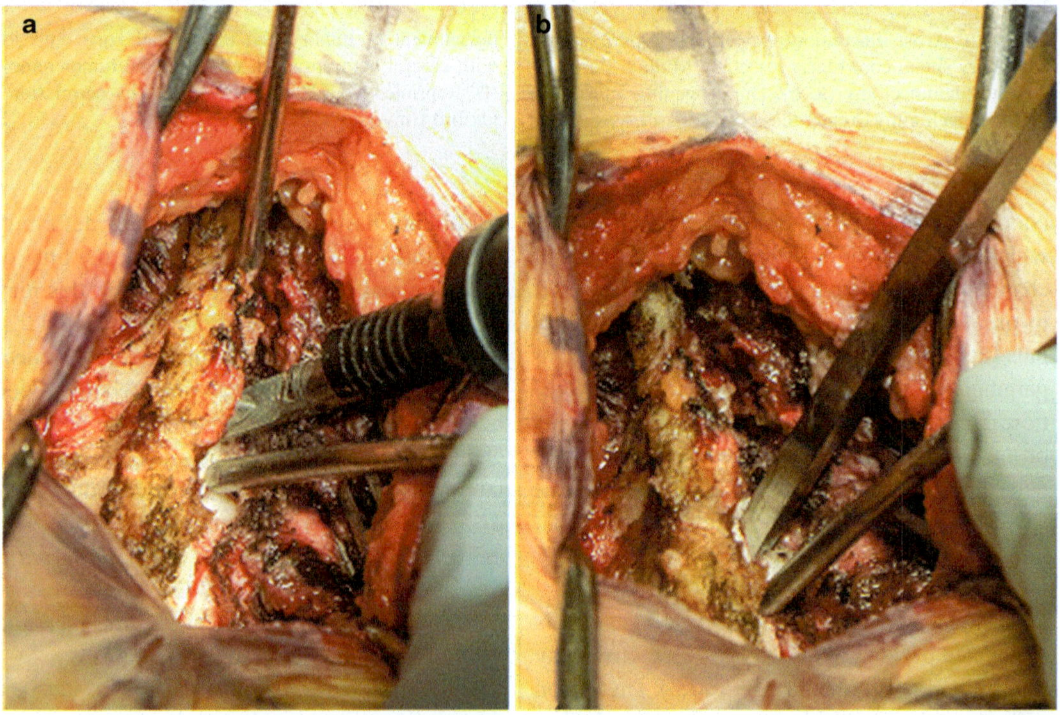

Fig. 27.4 A laminectomy or laminoplasty may also be used to provide bony decompression or revision of the posterior elements. We prefer the ultrasonic osteotome (BoneScalpel by Aesculap Central Valley, PA) for the laminectomy of the dorsal spinal elements as this provides a safe, effective way to remove the bone (**a**). The bony cuts are thin and allow precise osteotomies. (**b**) The depth and complete release of the laminar cuts may be confirmed using a thin osteotome to provide tactile confirmation that all bony attachments have been cut. The laminectomy may then be removed in an en bloc fashion

of Gelfoam, Gelfoam slurry, and bone wax to help tamponade bony bleeding. Cotton strips may also be placed in the lateral gutters to help limit epidural run down. The operative microscope should be prepared at this time. Epidural leads to provide D-wave monitoring should also be placed when possible both rostral and caudal to the lesion. Rostral epidural leads may not be possible in the high cervical spine. In addition, caudal epidural electrode is not helpful beyond the level of the conus.

A midline dural incision is made, with care to maintain the arachnoid plane if possible. This will limit cerebrospinal fluid (CSF) escape and prevent inadvertent damage to the spinal cord. Significant preoperative pain and obliteration of the CSF space on imaging due to engorgement of the spinal cord can be markers for raised intraspinal pressure and potential cord herniation. In these patients, an extended durotomy should be planned to minimize cord herniation and occlusive pressure upon opening. Once the dura is widely opened, the dural edges may be retracted and tacked up laterally. These retraction sutures may be accomplished through suturing into the surrounding paraspinal muscles or through hanging stay sutures (Fig. 27.5).

Appropriate myelotomy should be fashioned to enter the spinal cord in a way to minimally disrupt normal-functioning spinal tissue. If the tumor is diffuse, a standard midline approach is typically preferred which helps split the dorsal columns. If the tumor is more laterally situated, the dorsolateral sulci can be accessed safely. Normal anatomical planes may be altered due to the underlying tumor, causing rotation. The posterior median sulcus may most commonly be estimated by identifying bilateral dorsal root entry zones and the convergence of midline vessels that then dive into the median sulcus. Typical anatomical

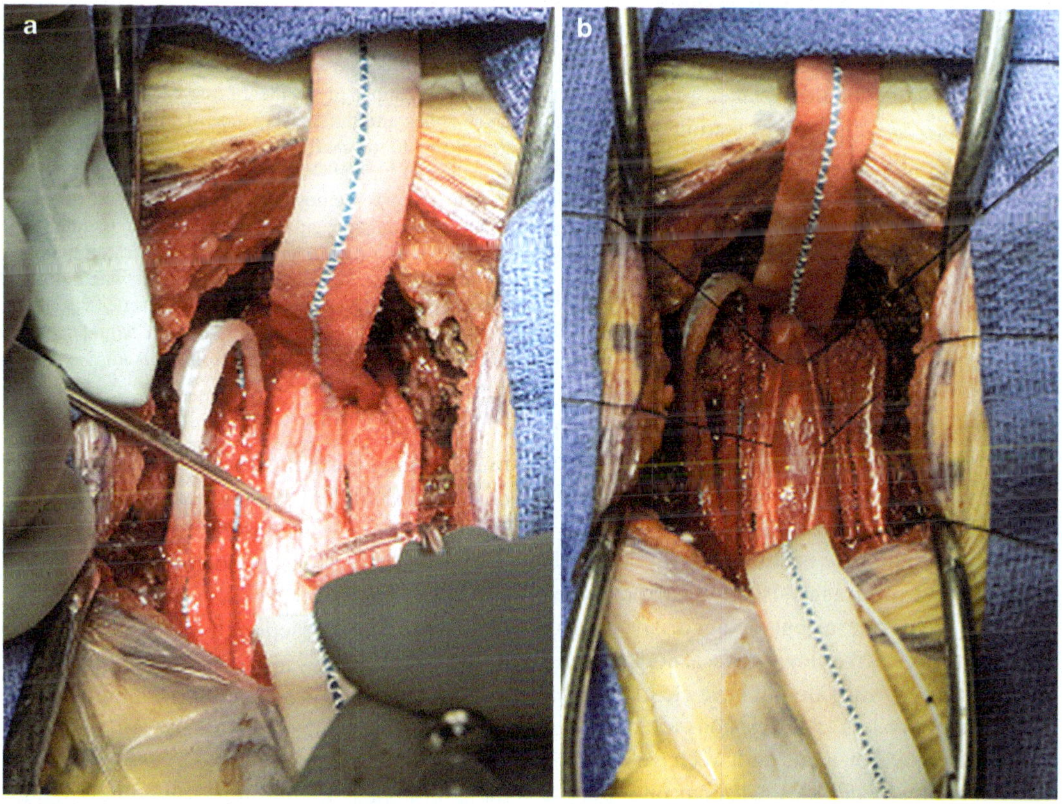

Fig. 27.5 Durotomy is performed using a No.15 blade and may be widened using a nerve hook (**a**), sharp dissection over an instrument or microscissors. Following dural opening, the dural edges should be retracted using stay sutures (**b**) that may be hung over the surgical edge or sutured into the surrounding tissue to provide adequate retraction

markers may be difficult to identify when the spinal cord is swollen or abnormal in configuration. However, exiting small veins from the posterior median sulcus draining into a larger dorsal vein may be used to help identify the midline posterior median sulcus. These veins can be mobilized and pushed laterally to help fully expose the sulcus. Some posterior spinal veins may be sacrificed, and centers have used intraoperative indocyanine green videoangiography (ICG-VA) to help judge the importance of venous circulation [17]. We do not routinely find this necessary, but it can be a helpful adjunct to identify important vascular structures. Dorsal column mapping may also be helpful to identify the midline. Furthermore, identification of the bilateral posterolateral sulcus can be used to help determine the degree of spinal cord rotation.

Many techniques exist to split the pial surface via individualized surgical preference, including the arachnoid knife, microscissors, and CO_2 laser (Fig. 27.6). All techniques should take care to help preserve hemostasis and minimize bleeding. When using bipolar electrocautery within the spinal cord, care should be taken to only cauterize necessary vessels at a low setting to minimize current spread to surrounding normal spinal tissue. Small pial vessels can be safely cauterized, whereas larger vessels should be dissected and retracted laterally by myelotomy. Pial sutures may be implemented to provide countertraction, but this can also provide constant tension to the spinal cord, which if too vigorous may result in higher level of postoperative neurological compromise. We favor intermittent retraction using plated forceps to help improve visualization while minimizing continual retraction on the spinal cord.

Once the tumor is visualized, a sample should be sent for frozen analysis. Surgical pathology can help guide the extent or aggressiveness of resection. Infiltrative, low-grade lesions such as astrocytoma typically do not have clearly demarcated tumor borders. These lesions are often difficult to remove in total, and we have found it safer to internally debulk the lesions until normal spinal tissue is visualized or there is a concern for decrease in IONM. Gross total resections of these lesions are not typically advocated at the cost of neurological dysfunction. Better encapsulated lower grade lesions such as ependymomas may often have a capsule or pseudocapsule that can be circumferentially delineated. It is possible to provide countertraction through plated forceps or microinstruments along the tumor–spinal cord interface. If there is a concern for a higher grade pathology, surgical goals are for debulking and diagnosis only as these patients are susceptible to neurological compromise and often require close transition to additional treatment strategies through radiation and/or chemotherapy.

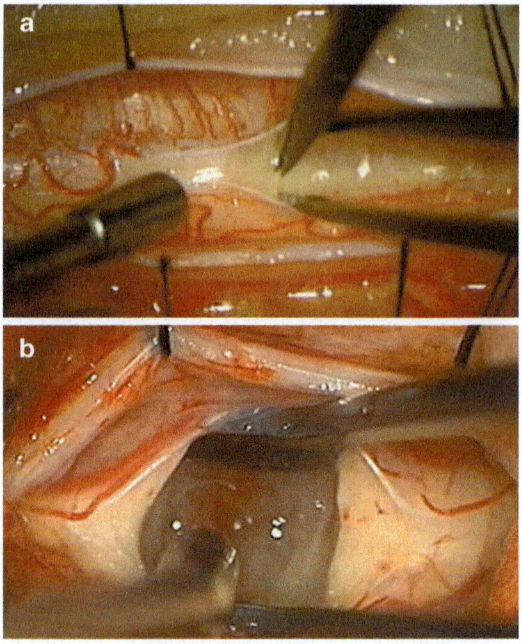

Fig. 27.6 (**a**) Appropriate myelotomy should be fashioned to enter the spinal cord in a way to minimally disrupt normal-functioning spinal tissue. Normal anatomical planes may be altered due to the underlying tumor, causing rotation. The posterior median sulcus may most commonly be estimated by identifying bilateral dorsal root entry zones and the convergence of midline vessels that then dive into the median sulcus. Many techniques exist to split the pial surface via individualized surgical preference to help preserve hemostasis and minimize bleeding. (**b**) Traditional microcoagulation of the tumor tissue in combination with suction or ultrasonic aspirator can help shrink the tumor. With serial debulking, the lateral tumor–spinal cord interface can sometimes be better visualized. It is possible to provide intermittent countertraction through plated forceps or microinstruments along the tumor–spinal cord interface

Debulking can be done through a variety of methods to help relieve pressure on the surrounding spinal cord tissue. Traditional microcoagulation of the tumor tissue, in combination with suction or ultrasonic aspirator, can help shrink the tumor. With serial debulking, the lateral tumor–spinal cord interface can sometimes be better visualized. This can result from partial devascularization during the debulking that allows the abnormal tumor to become more readily apparent in comparison to the surrounding normal spinal cord tissue. The ultrasonic aspirator can also be utilized for internal debulking in larger masses or masses with a more fibrous consistency.

Hemangioblastomas are typically well-encapsulated masses that arise on the dorsal or dorsolateral pial surface. These are most often accessed directly and require meticulous attention to the surface vessels feeding the tumor. Vascular control should be obtained prior to complete resection, and care should be taken to preserve draining veins if possible. A clear dissection plane is usually able to be established, and gross total resection is often possible.

Hemostasis can typically be maintained through serial tamponading with cotton products. We generally avoid direct cauterization of vessels within the tumor capsule or during the resection until we are clear these are tumor vessels, as heat can sometimes be transmitted through bipolar cautery. Care should be taken along the ventral and lateral borders as well, as motor fibers typically run in this area and the blood supply to these nerves is through the anterior spinal artery.

Tumor removal is guided by surgical planes as well as neuromonitoring. The tumor–spinal cord interface at all borders may not be visualized in all cases. In these instances, if there is a decrement in the neuromonitoring that is concerning for neurological compromise, then surgical resection is halted. Hemostasis following tumor resection is often obtained through a series of thrombin and Gelfoam-type devices with targeted use of the bipolar electrocautery. Once the surgical bed is examined and irrigated and hemostasis is attained, attention is then turned toward a watertight dural closure. We have not routinely found it necessary to reapproximate the spinal cord edges with suture. If there is any concern for dural retraction or if a significant debulking was not able to be accomplished, a dural patch graft should be considered. Most often a primary closure is obtained using a non-braided monofilament suture and tested using a held Valsalva (Fig. 27.7). If no CSF leak is visualized, it is safe to cover with fibrin glue to help prevent leakage or the formation of a pseudomeningocele.

Patients with concern for still significant spinal cord compression should not proceed with a laminoplasty. However, if a laminoplasty is deemed appropriate, this may be reattached using small craniofacial plating systems (Fig. 27.8). Systems with significant bulk and longer screw lengths are typically more structurally sound than thin, low-profile plates. Sutures can be additionally used to help recreate the posterior tension band. If laminoplasty is reapplied, one should ensure that there is no significant fibrin layer, which can sometimes be a mass occupying lesion that can cause subsequent neurological compromise. The plates should be large and strong enough to inhibit rotational movement of the lamina because if the plates loosen, this can also cause progressive spinal cord compression and neurological damage.

Meticulous hemostasis should be applied to minimize epidural rundown following decompression of the CSF space. Following several rounds of irrigation, the paraspinal muscles can be reattached to the laminoplasty through a multilayered approach to help reduce the amount of dead space. Postoperative drains, both suprafascial and subfascial, are controversial. If adequate hemostasis has been obtained, we prefer not to leave a drain as this can increase the risk of CSF fistula formation. However, if there is any question of ongoing bleeding that is difficult to control, a subfascial drain can be left in place that is either on a lower suction or to straight drain to help decompress the epidural space and to minimize postoperative seroma formation.

Additional techniques have been described including minimally invasive approaches using tubular retractors or through a mini-open approach. Most approaches favor either intralaminar spreading or a hemilaminectomy to

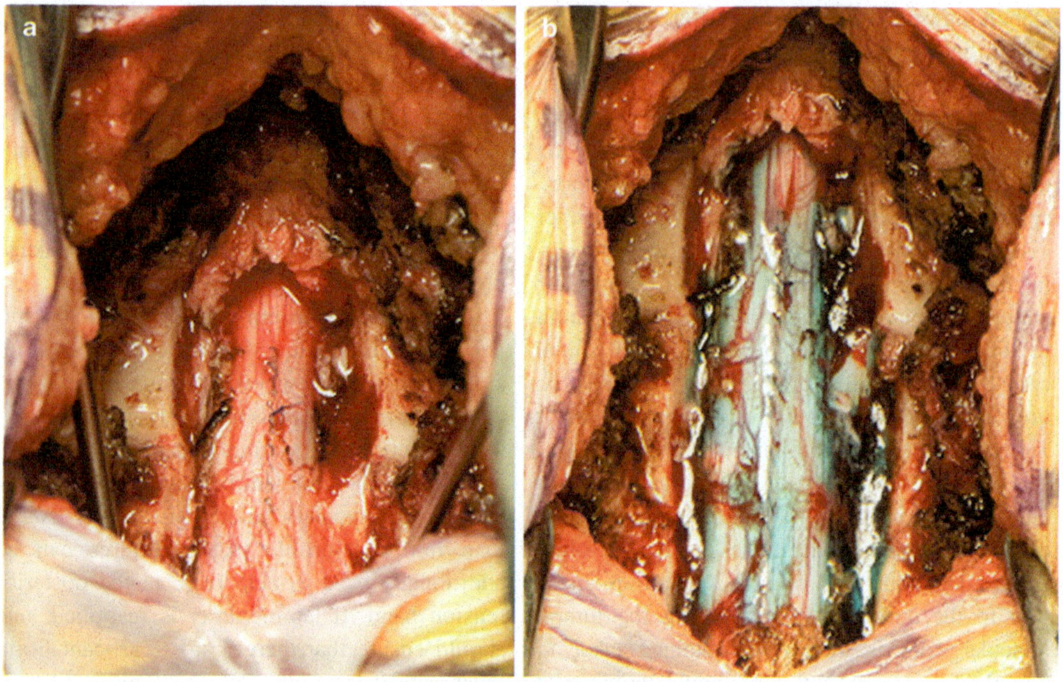

Fig. 27.7 (a) Most often a primary closure is obtained using a non-braided monofilament suture and tested using a held Valsalva. (b) If no CSF leak is visualized, it is safe to cover with fibrin glue to help prevent leakage or the formation of a pseudomeningocele

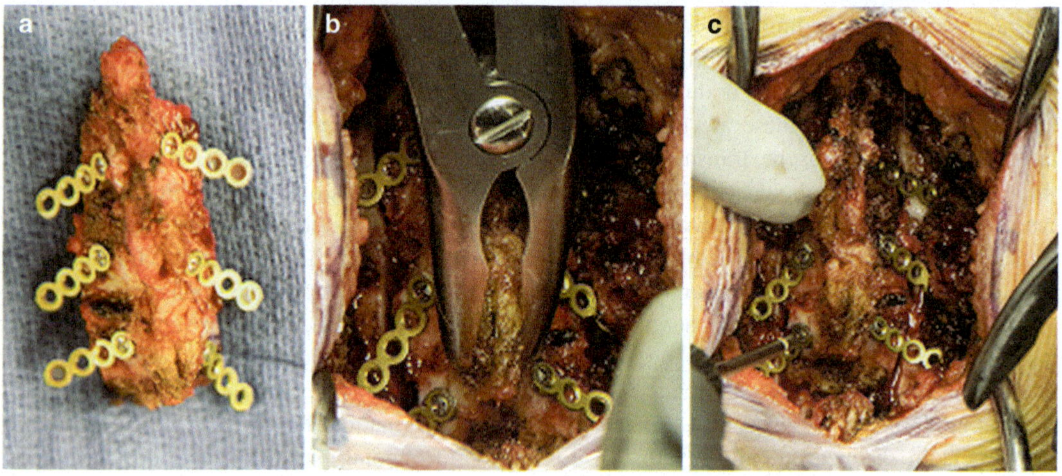

Fig. 27.8 (a) Laminoplasty following plating with a craniofacial plating system. Plates should be affixed to the laminectomy block of bone prior to inserting into the surgical bed (b). Care should be taken not to affix the plates within the joint or through the facet. The laminectomy should be attached (c) using at least two-point fixation, and care should be taken to ensure there is little to no movement following reattachment. Bony edges are well approximated following fixation

reduce trauma and destabilization of the posterior tension band. Given the ability for adequate tumor exposure, this technique is only appropriate for the minority of patients as in one recent series only 5.3% of IMSCTs could be accessed in this way [18].

Postoperatively, several precautions can be put into place to minimize complications. In order to minimize formation of pseudomeningoceles and to alleviate pressure on the dural repair, patients with cervical or cervicothoracic lesions should have an elevated head of bed. Conversely, patients with thoracolumbar or lumbosacral lesions should be kept flat for 24–48 h following surgery [19]. Perioperative steroids may be considered to help with vasogenic edema following tumor resection. Some swelling from cord manipulation and transection through normal spinal cord tissue is to be expected, and steroids can help mitigate these symptoms. Patients will typically benefit from evaluation and ongoing physical therapy, as the most common postoperative deficit in patients is some degree of proprioceptive loss or dysfunction [20]. Sphincter dysfunction may also be exacerbated, given the use of catheterization as well as narcotic medications. As such, monitoring for any ongoing difficulty with bowel or bladder dysfunction is imperative, and intermittent catheterization may be indicated for a short period of time.

Intraoperative Neuromonitoring

IONM has allowed more aggressive surgical resections for intramedullary spinal cord lesions. While not absolute, IONM has allowed real-time monitoring of possible spinal cord compromise, which is critical in tumors that may not have adequate dissection planes to help minimize excessive spinal cord manipulation. SSEPs, which measure sensory pathways running through the posterior column of the spinal cord, and transcranial MEPs, which provide information on the descending corticospinal tracts through stimulation of the cerebral cortex, have gained widespread use. SSEPs are less reliable for intra medullary tumor resection, as most dissection planes enter from a dorsal approach and disrupt the ascending sensory fibers. SSEPs may also be influenced by anesthetic changes, and care should be taken to avoid certain anesthetic agents. Furthermore, recordings within the periphery can be obtained from end muscles via electromyography (EMG) from direct stimulation of the spinal cord through D-wave EMPS. With the adoption of MEPs, however, several studies have indicated a correlation between MEP waveform changes and postoperative motor deficits [21–24].

Transcranial MEPs are typically set up with needle electrodes within the distal muscles and are run every several minutes. Myogenic MEPs measure waveforms from the muscles and are typically categorized into three patterns: polyphasic, biphasic, or absent. Changes from polyphasic to biphasic waveforms may suggest disruption within the descending motor pathways. Amplitude changes can also predict motor function after surgery, and most centers will use changes of 50% as an indicator of permanent motor weakness postoperatively [21–23]. D-wave fibers indicate activation of the fast axonal fibers that make it possible to monitor motor pathways in real time as they are more sensitive to detect early injury of the spine. Recordings can also compare the rostral electrode with the caudal electrode. Traditionally, studies have shown that with less than 50% change in D-wave amplitude, even with a complete loss of MEP, there is typically transient paraplegia. If D-waves are lost intraoperatively, then patients typically have permanent paraplegia [21–24].

A combined monitoring approach allows a broader array of information to help guide IMSCT surgery. Both methods of monitoring target different spinal cord anatomies and have different thresholds for signal change and together help improve sensitivity and specificity [23]. Intraoperative factors such as operative time, blood pressure, and anesthetic agents may influence IONM and, as such, intraoperative changes must be interpreted within the surgical context.

Operative Complications

Despite optimal surgical techniques, IMSCT removal remains technically challenging. Operative complications may occur immediately during the perioperative period with resulting neurologic or vascular compromise or CSF leak. Other more common perioperative complications include hematoma formation, wound dehiscence, and infection. Delayed complications such as spinal deformity, arachnoiditis, or tumor recurrence should also be monitored closely.

Early Complications

CSF leakage with resultant pseudomeningocele or frank CSF leak may occur if watertight closure of the dura is not obtained. Patients who require duraplasty, given spinal cord swelling, may be at higher risk of formation of a CSF leak [19]. Clinical symptoms such as formation of a pseudomeningocele, postural headaches, nausea, or emesis might lead one to suspect concern for a CSF leak. This can be further confirmed with MRI across the surgical bed as well as with computed tomography (CT) myelogram. If a surgical drain is left in place, this can be tested for beta-2 transferrin, which would indicate presence of CSF. While surgical drains might increase the risk for development of a CSF fistula, the primary objective of a surgical site drain is to help prevent outward leakage of CSF past the skin. Despite development of a pseudomeningocele following healing of the skin, we believe that patients are better able to resorb their pseudomeningocele over the infectious risk of a CSF leak. A watertight fascial closure is imperative because even if the dural edges are not able to be fully closed in a watertight fashion, this can prevent further migration of CSF toward the skin. If the patient is symptomatic, a re-exploration may be indicated. Fixing a dural leak might require finding the area of faulty closure and reinforcing this area or the addition of a patch if unable to be primarily closed. Attention to a multi-layered closure as well as elimination of dead space is critical to aid with closure. If the patient has had previous surgeries or radiation treatment, consideration for involvement of a plastic surgeon might aid with local muscle flap advancements. This might also be augmented by use of a lumbar drain if there is concern for additional CSF leakage.

Postoperative neurological deterioration is not an unusual finding following resection of IMSCT lesions. The etiology may result from direct surgical manipulation and tension that is placed on traversing spinal parenchyma. In addition, vascular compromise or insult may also contribute to functional decline. Neurological worsening within the initial perioperative period may be seen in approximately 9–34% of patients [25, 26]. However, 25–41% of these patients will revert to their preoperative baseline within 6 months of surgery [25, 26]. Most commonly, patients will have abnormalities with proprioception or discriminative touch. Gait difficulties may also be present in the initial perioperative period.

Intraoperative changes in motor evoked potentials and increasing age of the patient are both risk factors for worsening neurological condition immediately following surgery [27]. If there is concern for loss of intraoperative monitoring signals, this will help guide discussions with patients regarding the prognosis for improvement in their neurological status. Blood pressure augmentation within the perioperative period as well as steroid administration both preoperatively and within the perioperative period should be considered in cases of significant neurological changes or loss. Patients with good preoperative functional status as well as a localized tumor burden are more likely to have improved outcomes.

Delayed Complications

Development of spinal deformity is a complication that has been reported in 16–100% of pediatric patients following resection of IMSCT [28, 29]. Post-laminectomy deformity is more common in the pediatric population than in adults. The presence of preoperative deformity has also been associated with a higher risk of progressive postoperative deformity. Other risk factors that can contribute to the development of progressive spinal deformity include neurogenic or paralytic deformity, post-radiation effects on bone marrow and bony growth, and post-laminectomy deformity. In addition, studies have shown that increasing the number of levels involved also increases the likelihood of developing instability. Other predictors of progressive postoperative deformity requiring fusion include involvement of the thoracolumbar junction, the presence of a tumor associated syrinx, and the need for multiple resections. Care should be taken to avoid exposing the lateral joints during the initial dissection. Patients should be followed with standing films if there is concern for ongoing deformity, as these patients may eventually require some intervention. Spinal hardware can impact our ability to follow tumor recurrence, and so the timing of spinal instrumentation should be carefully considered.

Postoperative neuropathic pain or worsening myelopathy over time without evidence of tumor recurrence may be related to postoperative tethering. Postoperative cord tethering can be observed in up to 37% of postoperative imaging studies [30], although only 10% of these patients become symptomatic. Radiographical evidence of tethering may be decreased from 51.7% to 19.6% with pial closure. Untethering procedures should be reserved only for patients who have progressive deterioration in neurological symptoms.

Neuropathic pain syndromes may also affect up to 19–27.4% [30, 31] of patients. These syndromes are more common in patients who present with syringomyelia as the syrinx may affect the posterior horns preferentially over the central part of the cord. Other risk factors include surgery during growth periods, preoperative presence of neuropathic pain, high spinal level, as well as presence of a syrinx [32].

Conclusion

While challenging, surgical resection of IMSCT lesions has evolved into a mainstay of treatment for benign intramedullary spinal lesions. Goals of surgery should weigh the maintenence or improvement in neurological function with long-term tumor control and the extent of resection. Surgical morbidity has improved with the addition and improvement of MRI as a method of diagnostic imaging, surgical tools and microsurgical technique, ultrasonic aspirator, and intraoperative neuromonitoring. Adherence to meticulous surgical technique can achieve both acceptable surgical and functional outcomes

References

1. Constantini S, Miller DC, Allen JC, Rorke LB, Freed D, Epstein FJ. Radical excision of intramedullary spinal cord tumors: surgical morbidity and long-term follow-up evaluation in 164 children and young adults. J Neurosurg. 2000;93(2 Suppl):183–93.
2. Sciubba DM, Liang D, Kothbauer KF, Noggle JC, Jallo GI. The evolution of intramedullary spinal cord tumor surgery. Neurosurgery. 2009;65(6 Suppl):84–91. discussion 91-2.
3. Boström A, von Lehe M, Hartmann W, Pietsch T, Feuss M, Boström JP, Schramm J, Simon M. Surgery for spinal cord ependymomas: outcome and prognostic factors. Neurosurgery. 2011;68(2):302–8.
4. Parsa AT, Lee J, Parney IF, Weinstein P, McCormick PC, Ames C. Spinal cord and intradural-extraparenchymal spinal tumors: current best care practices and strategies. J Neuro-Oncol. 2004;69(1–3):291–318.
5. Yang I, Parsa AT. Intramedullary spinal cord tumors. In: Gupta N, Banerjee A, Haas-Kogan D, editors. Pediatric CNS tumors. Berlin, Heidelberg: Springer; 2010. p. 187–204.
6. Lee M, Rezai AR, Freed D, Epstein FJ. Intramedullary spinal cord tumors in neurofibromatosis. Neurosurgery. 1996;38(1):32–7.
7. Kucia EJ, Bambakidis NC, Chang SW, Spetzler RF. Surgical technique and outcomes in the treatment of spinal cord ependymomas, part 1: intramedullary ependymomas. Neurosurgery. 2011;68(1 Suppl operative):57–63.
8. Ardeshiri A, Chen B, Hütter BO, Oezkan N, Wanke I, Sure U, Sandalcioglu IE. Intramedullary spinal cord astrocytomas: the influence of localization and tumor extension on resectability and functional outcome. Acta Neurochir. 2013;155(7):1203–7.
9. Liu A, Sankey EW, Bettegowda C, Burger PC, Jallo GI, Groves ML. Poor prognosis despite aggressive treatment in adults with intramedullary spinal cord glioblastoma. J Clin Neurosci. 2015;22(10):1628–31. https://doi.org/10.1016/j.jocn.2015.05.008. Epub 2015 Jun 30.
10. Waxman SG. Correlative neuroanatomy. 23rd ed. Stamford: Appleton & Lange; 1996. p. 43–68.
11. Hanbali F, Fourney DR, Marmor E, et al. Spinal cord ependymoma: radical surgical resection and outcome. Neurosurgery. 2002;51(5):1162–72.
12. Vaccaro AR, Albert TJ. Spine surgery: tricks of the trade. 2nd ed. New York: Thieme; 2008.
13. de Jonge T, Slullitel H, Dubousset J, Miladi L, Wicart P, Illes T. Late-onset spinal deformities in children treated by laminectomy and radiation therapy for malignant tumours. Eur Spine J. 2005;14:765–71.
14. Papagelopoulos PJ, Peterson HA, Ebersold MJ, Emmanuel PR, Choudhury SN, Quast LM. Spinal column deformity and instability after lumbar or thoracolumbar laminectomy for intraspinal tumors in children and young adults. Spine (Phila Pa 1976). 1997;22:442–51.
15. Hersh DS, Iyer RR, Garzon-Muvdi T, Liu A, Jallo GI, Groves ML. Instrumented fusion for spinal deformity after laminectomy or laminoplasty for resection of intramedullary spinal cord tumors in pediatric patients. Neurosurg Focus. 2017;43(4):E12. https://doi.org/10.3171/2017.7.FOCUS17329.
16. Parker SL, Kretzer RM, Recinos PF, Molina CA, Wolinsky JP, Jallo GI, Recinos VR. Ultrasonic BoneScalpel for osteoplastic laminoplasty in the resection of intradural spinal pathology: case series and technical note. Neurosurgery. 2013;73(1

Suppl Operative):ons61–6. https://doi.org/10.1227/NEU.0b013e318283c98b.
17. Takami T, Yamagata T, Naito K, Arima H, Ohata K. Intraoperative assessment of spinal vascular ow in the surgery of spinal intramedullary tumors using indocyanine green videoangiography. Surg Neurol Int. 2013;4:135.
18. Mende KC, Krätzig T, Mohme M, Westphal M, Eicker SO. Keyhole approaches to intradural pathologies. Neurosurg Focus. 2017;43(2):E5.
19. Jallo GI, Kothbauer KF, Epstein FJ. Intrinsic spinal cord tumor resection. Neurosurgery. 2001;49(5):1124–8.
20. Woodworth GF, Chaichana KL, McGirt MJ, Sciubba DM, Jallo GI, Gokaslan Z, et al. Predictors of ambulatory function after surgical resection of intramedullary spinal cord tumors. Neurosurgery. 2007;61(1):99–105.
21. Sala F, Palandri G, Basso E, Lanteri P, Deletis V, Faccioli F, et al. Motor evoked potential moni- toring improves outcome after surgery for intramedullary spinal cord tumors: a historical control study. Neurosurgery. 2006;58:1129–43. [discussion: 1129-1143].
22. Jin SH, Chung CK, Kim CH, Choi YD, Kwak G, Kim BE. Multimodal intraoperative monitoring during intramedullary spinal cord tumor surgery. Acta Neurochir. 2015;157:2149–55.
23. Muramoto A, Imagama S, Ito Z, Ando K, Tauchi R, Matsumoto T, et al. The cutoff amplitude of transcranial motor evoked potentials for transient postoperative motor deficits in intra- medullary spinal cord tumor surgery. Spine. 2014;39:E1086–94.
24. Kothbauer KF, Deletis V, Epstein FJ. Motor- evoked potential monitoring for intramedullary spinal cord tumor surgery: correlation of clinical and neurophysiological data in a series of 100 consecutive procedures. Neurosurg Focus. 1998;4:e1.
25. Eroes CA, Zausinger S, Kreth FW, Goldbrunner R, Tonn JC. Intramedullary low grade astrocytoma and ependymoma. Surgical results and predicting factors for clinical outcome. Acta Neurochir. 2010;152:611–8.
26. Garcés-Ambrossi GL, McGirt MJ, Mehta VA, Sciubba DM, Witham TF, Bydon A, et al. Factors associated with progression-free survival and long-term neurological outcome after resection of intramedullary spinal cord tumors: analysis of 101 consecutive cases. Clinical article. J Neurosurg Spine. 2009;11:591–9.
27. Cristante L, Herrmann HD. Surgical management of intramedullary spinal cord tumors: functional outcome and sources of morbidity. Neurosurgery. 1994;35(1):69–74. discussion 74-6.
28. Albert TJ, Vacarro A. Postlaminectomy kyphosis. Spine (Phila Pa 1976). 1998;23:2738–45.
29. McGirt MJ, Chaichana KL, Atiba A, Bydon A, Witham TF, Yao KC, Jallo GI. Incidence of spinal deformity after resection of intramedullary spinal cord tumors in children who underwent laminectomy compared with laminoplasty. J Neurosurg Pediatr. 2008;1:57–62.
30. Klekamp J. Treatment of intramedullary tumors: analysis of surgical morbidity and long-term results. J Neurosurg Spine. 2013;19(1):12–26. https://doi.org/10.3171/2013.3.SPINE121063.
31. Fischer G, Brotchi J. Intramedullary spinal cord tumors. Stuttgart: Thieme; 1996.
32. McGirt MJ, Chaichana KL, Atiba A, Attenello F, Yao KC, Jallo GI. Resection of intramedullary spinal cord tumors in children: assessment of long-term motor and sensory de cits. J Neurosurg Pediatr. 2008;1:63–7.

Minimally Invasive Intradural Tumor Resection

28

Hani Malone and John E. O'Toole

Introduction

Intradural spinal tumors represent a relatively rare clinical entity, with an annual incidence of approximately 1 in 10,000 [1]. However, the increasing availability of advanced diagnostic imaging has brought greater numbers of these lesions to surgical attention. Historically, and indeed currently, most intradural tumors are resected using a traditional midline incision, subperiosteal muscle dissection, and bilateral laminectomies. This dissection has been shown to cause denervation and devascularization of the paraspinal musculature leading to significant loss of axial muscle strength [2]. By comparison, minimally invasive surgical (MIS) techniques utilize a tubular retractor system through a paramedian approach, sparing the midline ligaments, and minimizing damage to the paraspinal musculature.

The microsurgical resection of intradural spinal tumors can be one of the more technically challenging procedures in neurosurgery. Accordingly, some have avoided implementing MIS techniques due to the learning curve associated with performing this already difficult procedure through a tubular retractor system. Nevertheless, minimally invasive approaches to spinal tumors have evolved rapidly over the past 10–15 years as more surgeons become facile with MIS techniques and seek to avoid the morbidity associated with traditional open surgery [3–15]. This evolution was driven, in part, by the morbidity and significant complication rates associated with traditional surgical approaches to spinal tumors, particularly for metastatic disease [16–19]. There is a growing body of evidence that minimally invasive approaches can be used to reduce the morbidity associated with the resection of intradural spinal tumors, without compromising extent of resection or safety [3–15].

In this chapter, we discuss the technical details of using a minimally invasive approach for the resection of intradural spinal tumors, including patient selection, surgical set-up, MIS exposure, dural closure, and postoperative considerations. A case example with an accompanying video is provided to illustrate the procedure. When properly performed, MIS techniques should aim to reduce operative time, blood loss, pain, postoperative immobilization, and length of hospital stay. These benefits should ultimately translate into faster recovery and cost reduction. The available evidence supporting these proposed benefits in intradural extramedullary (IDEM) tumor surgery is also discussed.

Electronic Supplementary Material The online version of this chapter (https://doi.org/10.1007/978-3-319-98422-3_28) contains supplementary material, which is available to authorized users.

H. Malone
Scripps Clinic, Division of Neurosurgery, San Diego, CA, USA

J. E. O'Toole (✉)
Rush University Medical Center, Department of Neurosurgery, Chicago, IL, USA
e-mail: john_otoole@rush.edu

D. M. Sciubba (ed.), *Spinal Tumor Surgery*, https://doi.org/10.1007/978-3-319-98422-3_28

Patient Selection: Indications, Advantages, and Disadvantages

The indications and limitations of minimally invasive spine surgery for degenerative disease continue to evolve, as advances in MIS instrumentation and surgical navigation expand spine surgeons' armamentarium. This evolution has led to corollary advances in MIS surgery for intradural spinal tumors [3–15]. Successful MIS resection of well-circumscribed intramedullary spinal tumors has been reported [20, 21]. The ligation of spinal vascular malformations has also been shown to be safe and effective through a tubular retractor system [22, 23]. However, minimally invasive approaches to intradural spinal pathology are most commonly used for intradural extramedullary spinal tumors, which will be the focus of this chapter.

There are a number of definitive advantages to traditional open surgical approaches to intradural tumors. Midline approaches provide a wide exposure and large surgical corridor. This exposure may be necessary for large lesions that span multiple segments. Dural closure is also more facile when a large surgical corridor is created. However, this exposure comes at the cost of a larger excision with greater soft-tissue destruction, blood loss, and recovery time [4–6].

Open surgical approaches also sacrifice the support provided by posterior midline structures, specifically the interspinous ligaments. Compromise of this posterior tension band may predispose patients to segmental instability and/or postoperative kyphosis, necessitating instrumented fusion. The risk of postoperative kyphosis may be particularly significant following surgery for intradural tumors [16, 24, 25]. By comparison, MIS techniques generally utilize a unilateral paramedian approach that preserves the posterior tension band, mitigating the risk of postoperative instability and kyphosis [16].

The fundamental advantages of minimally invasive spine surgery (reduced soft-tissue destruction, blood loss, mobilization, and hospital stay) have been reproducible in series of patients with intradural tumors treated through an MIS approach [3–15]. There is also evidence that MIS approaches limit the risk of postoperative cerebrospinal fluid (CSF) leak following intended durotomies, which in turn reduces the risk of wound breakdown and postoperative infection [6, 7, 26]. This is most likely due to the relatively small amount of dead space that remains following removal of an MIS tubular retractor, compared to traditional midline approaches.

The appropriateness of an MIS approach to IDEM tumors is largely dictated by a preoperative assessment of the space required to remove the lesion. For example, tumors that lie purely ventral to the spinal cord may not be amenable to an MIS approach. These lesions often require a larger dural opening to facilitate sectioning of the dentate ligaments and slight mobilization of the spinal cord. By comparison, dorsal and lateral intradural lesions are candidates for MIS surgery. Good visualization of these lesions can be achieved using a tubular retractor from a paramedian approach (Video 28.1) [3]. Size is not necessarily a contraindication, as rather large lesions (up to 4 cm) can be removed with the use of expandable retractors [3]. Nevertheless, MIS approaches generally are best for intradural lesions that are one or two spinal segments in length [15, 16].

There is a learning curve associated with all minimally invasive techniques. This may be particularly true for intradural tumors, and some repetition is necessary to become facile with dural closure in a limited corridor [26]. However, as minimally invasive surgery for degenerative spine pathology becomes more ubiquitous and is increasingly incorporated into residency training, more neurosurgeons are likely to consider MIS approaches to IDEM pathology.

Preoperative Assessment and Planning

The evaluation of any patient with a known or suspected spinal tumor begins with a detailed history and neurologic exam. Compared to patients with epidural disease or tumors of the vertebral column, those with intradural lesions are relatively less likely to present with severe radicular or axial back pain. However, these patients may develop neurologic deficits from ongoing compression of the spinal cord or nerve roots [27]. Magnetic resonance imaging (MRI) is the primary imaging modality used to evaluate intradural spinal tumors.

T1-weighted sequences with gadolinium contrast are useful to define the extent and margins of intradural pathology. Although the degree of enhancement on post-contrast sequences may vary considerably for intramedullary pathology, commonly encountered IDEM lesions, such as schwannomas, nerve sheath tumors, and meningiomas, tend to avidly enhance. T2-weighted sequences are useful for determining nature and extent of cord deformation and/or nerve impingement, as well as cord edema and syrinx formation. For patients with pacemakers, pain pumps, or other metallic foreign bodies precluding MRI, computed tomography (CT) myelography can be used as an alternative modality.

When reviewing imaging for intradural pathology and considering a minimally invasive approach, special attention must be paid to the space required to remove the lesion. It is critical that the MIS retractor used allows for adequate visualization of the full length of the tumor. In ideal conditions, normal (non-pathologic) tissue rostral and caudal to the lesion should also be visualized to allow for accurate identification of tumor margins [28]. Inadequate visualization of IDEM tumors may lead to piecemeal and subtotal resection of lesions that could otherwise be removed en bloc [3, 28]. It is important to consider that adjustment of the tubular retractor system is limited after making a durotomy, and any attempt to do so may introduce blood into the subarachnoid space or risk injury to exposed neural tissue. Some have advocated that the retractor used should be 5–10 mm larger than the planned length of the dural incision, in order to ensure enough length to reliably obtain a watertight dural closure [3, 28]. It is also important to consider that the length of the durotomy should generally be 5–10 mm longer than the underlying intradural pathology to ensure adequate visualization.

When counseling patients with intradural pathology, expectations and operative goals must be frankly discussed prior to formulating a surgical plan. For intramedullary lesions, the nature of the pathology and the presence or absence of a safe dissection plane often limit extent of resection, making diagnosis the primary goal of surgery. Conversely, for intradural extramedullary tumors, surgical resection is often curative. Accordingly, careful surgical planning is critical to ensure maximal resection and definitive treatment when possible. Like all spinal tumor surgeries, the primary goals for IDEM tumor surgery are pathologic diagnosis, symptomatic relief, tumor resection/source control, and decompression of the spinal cord and/or roots. The operating surgeon must be confident that these goals can be effectively addressed through an MIS approach before attempting a minimally invasive operation.

Surgical Technique

Positioning and Anesthesia

General anesthesia is recommended for all minimally invasive approaches to intradural pathology. We use intraoperative neurophysiologic monitoring with continuous somatosensory evoked potentials (SSEPs), evoked and free-running electromyography (EMG), and, when indicated, motor evoked potentials. Open communication between the anesthesia and neuro-monitoring teams is critical to achieve the appropriate balance between muscle relaxation and accurate neurophysiologic recording. Prepositioning potentials may be necessary when intradural pathology has led to significant deformation of the spinal cord but is generally not necessary.

Following the induction of anesthesia, the patient is placed in the prone position on a standard radiolucent spine table, such as a Jackson table (Mizuho OSI I Union City, CA). A Wilson frame (Mizuho OSI I Union City, CA) may be used to open the interlaminar space at lumbar levels but at thoracic levels may limit anteroposterior (AP) fluoroscopy and complicate localization. In the thoracic spine, we generally use a combination of standard radiolucent chest, hip, and thigh pads for this reason. With the patient positioned, fluoroscopy is used to identify the appropriate spinal level and mark the intended incision and site of dilation.

Exposure

An approximately 3-cm paramedian skin incision is made, typically 2–3 cm lateral to the midline. The position of the lesion in the spinal canal dictates the lateral extent of the incision, which can be measured on MRI preoperatively. An incision made too medial will prevent angulation of the tubular retractor and limit exposure of the midline and contralateral canal. Following skin incision, the opening is carried through the subcutaneous fat with monopolar cautery, achieving hemostasis and leaving the thoracolumbar fascia intact. The fascia can be cut sharply prior to dilation or traversed upon dilation with the K-wire and tubular dilators. The former technique is preferred for cervical spine cases.

Dilation with the tubular retractor system then takes place in a stepwise fashion. The initial dilator should target the laminofacet junction (Fig. 28.1). Dilators of increasing caliber are then passed over each other to pass deep to the fascia. Lateral fluoroscopic guidance is used to ensure correct depth at the level of the joint. Once the planned dilator width has been achieved and the depth of dilation measured, the corresponding tubular retractor can be placed and secured to the system's table-mounted articulating arm. Fluoroscopy should be used judiciously during minimally invasive surgery, given the cumulative risk of radiation exposure to the operating surgeon and ancillary staff. However, optimal retractor placement is paramount to success in MIS surgery for IDEM lesions, and fluoroscopy should be used as needed until this can be confidently achieved.

The choice of tubular retractor should be based on the location and size of the IDEM tumor, with the retractor diameter ideally 5–10 mm larger than the length of the lesion. We have experience using fixed diameter tubes ranging from 18 to 26 mm for intradural pathology, which are significantly larger than the standard 18-mm diameter tubes commonly used for lumbar microdiscectomy. Expandable retractors can be used for larger lesions, which are capable of providing over 4 cm of longitudinal exposure. Once the retractor is secured in place, the microscope is brought into position and focused to the

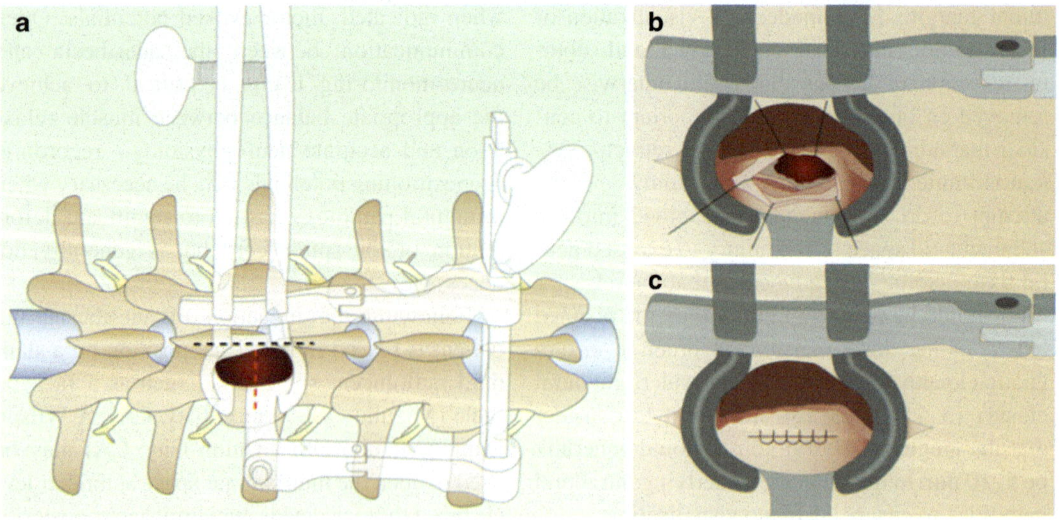

Fig. 28.1 (**a**–**c**) Artist illustration of minimally invasive intradural tumor resection. (Reprinted with permission from Mende et al. [35])

depth of the operative site. We prefer a minimum working distance of 350 mm to allow for facile passing of instruments in and out of the tubular dilator without interference from the operative microscope.

At the depth of the tubular retractor, a soft-tissue muscle plug is circumferentially sectioned and removed with monopolar cautery, exposing the underlying lamina and medial facet joint. Using a high-speed burr, a standard ipsilateral hemi-laminectomy is performed, exposing the underlying ligamentum flavum which is preserved. With the ligament serving as a protective barrier to the dura, the tubular retractor is then redirected medially. The high-speed burr can then be used to undercut the spinous process. The inner cortex of the contralateral lamina is then removed with a combination of drilling and the use of a Kerrison punch until the contralateral pedicle is visualized. This approach provides access to both the ipsilateral and contralateral sides of the spinal canal while maintaining the integrity of the spinous process, interspinous ligaments, and posterior tension band.

Next, the ligamentum flavum, which has served as a barrier to the dura during drilling, can be efficiently removed. A straight curette can be used to separate the two bellies of the ligament in the midline, establishing an epidural plane. The ligament can then be freed from its rostral and caudal laminar attachments using a ball-tip probe, angled curette, and Kerrison punch, exposing the underlying dura.

Tumor Resection

Prior to initiating the dural opening, it is important to ensure that meticulous hemostasis is achieved to prevent blood running into the operative field and subarachnoid space. We use a long-handled no. 11 blade scalpel to initiate the durotomy in the midline and then extend the opening rostrally and caudally using a nerve hook. The dural edges are then tacked up using 4–0 Nurolon or silk sutures.

Following the dural opening, tumor resection begins with careful dissection of the arachnoid layers overlying the mass and adjacent neural elements. At this stage in the operation, standard microsurgical techniques are used to remove the lesion. We most frequently utilize micro-scissors and Rhoton dissectors to create a plane around the mass. When addressing tumors in the thoracic and cervical spine, microdissection must free extramedullary tumors from the spinal cord and exiting nerve roots. In the lumbar spine, microsurgical technique must be similarly used to dissect the tumor free from the nerves of the cauda equina (Fig. 28.2).

Once an IDEM tumor has been dissected from adjunct neural tissue, the size and location of the mass dictate how it can be safely and efficiently resected. Large extramedullary lesions that deform the adjacent spinal cord, such as large thoracic meningiomas, generally have to be debulked prior to removal to avoid any additional physical stress to the spinal cord. In some cases, an ultrasonic aspirator with an MIS attachment can be used to perform debulking. Importantly, the ultrasonic aspirator must be used on low-power settings to minimize the risk of collateral mechanical injury to the adjacent cord. Although piecemeal tumor removal is less efficient and may increase the likelihood of subtotal resection, it is occasionally necessary to avoid cord injury and neurologic deficit.

Conversely, schwannomas and other nerve sheath tumors at the level of the cauda equina can often be safely removed en bloc, without internal debulking [27]. For these lesions, microsurgical dissection is used to isolate the tumor and its associated afferent and efferent fascicles from all other roots in the thecal sac. Special care should be taken to ensure that no traversing roots are adherent to the ventral side of the mass, which may be originally difficult to identify. Once isolated, direct stimulation with a unipolar probe is applied to both the afferent and efferent nerve fascicles associated with the mass.

In the case of schwannoma, direct stimulation will produce a motor response in only rare cases. If a motor response is recorded, it is often because the nerve stimulated was not the nerve fascicle truly associated with the tumor but rather a traversing nerve adherent to the mass. If there is

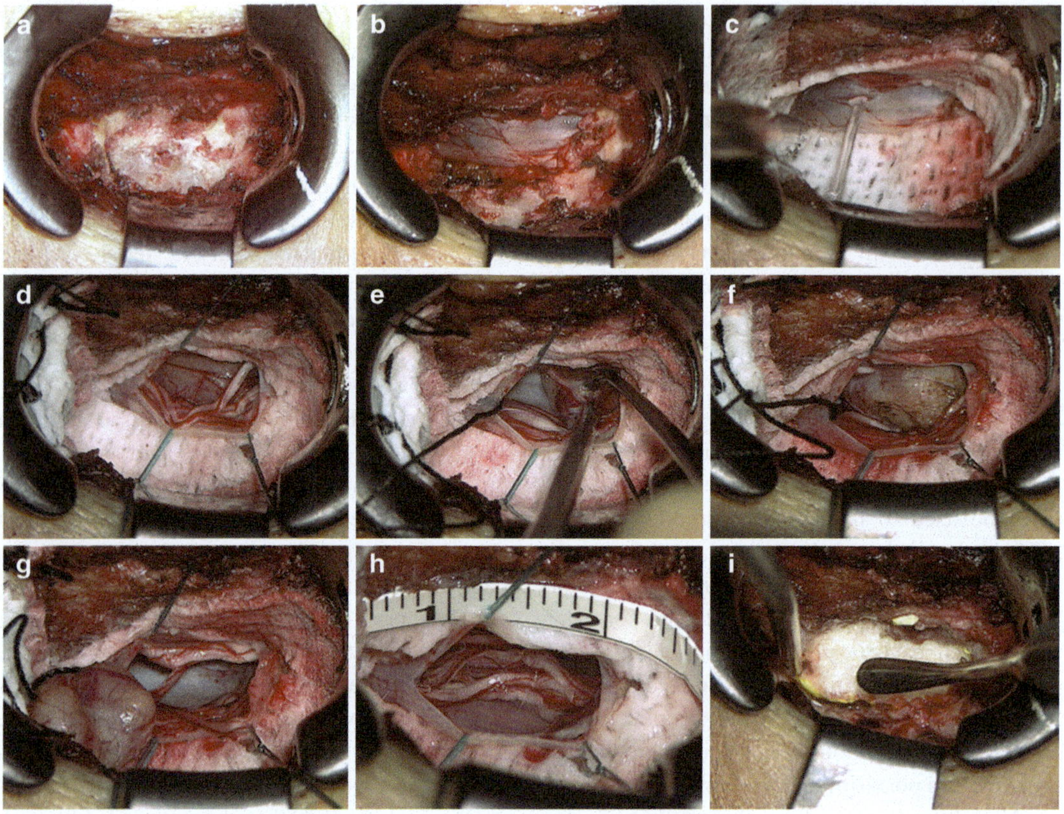

Fig. 28.2 Intraoperative imaging and surgical technique of minimally invasive intradural tumor resection. (**a–c**) Laminectomy and midline dural incision. (**d, e**) Dural retraction and blunt dissection of intradural lesion. (**f, g**) Gentle mobilization and complete resection of intradural extramedullary tumor. (**h, i**) Reapproximation of dural edges with watertight closure and fibrin matrix sealant. (Reprinted with permission from Mende et al. [35])

no motor response, the afferent nerve is sectioned first and then the efferent nerve. This is to prevent rostral rebounding of the tumor mass above the dural opening from rostral nerve tension. Once the afferent and efferent roots are coagulated and sectioned, the mass can be removed en bloc. While performing microsurgery, surgeons accustomed to using the operating microscope may observe fewer differences than anticipated between MIS and open approaches, even as the operation is reduced to a small corridor.

Dural Closure

Dural closure represents one of the more technically challenging components of minimally invasive surgery for intradural tumors. As with open surgery, a watertight dural closure is paramount to avoiding CSF leakage, pseudomeningocele formation, infection, and wound breakdown in the postoperative period. Prior to closing the dura, it is again critical to ensure that hemostasis is achieved, as the drainage of CSF during surgery precipitates bleeding from stretched epidural veins. Although a number of dural closure devices have been developed [29], we prefer to repair the dura with a running stitch. With elongated instruments adapted for use through an MIS tubular retractor, dural closure can be performed in a manner similar to open techniques. A Valsalva maneuver is performed at the end of the closure to evaluate for any defects in the suture line and to ensure a watertight closure. Hydrogel or fibrin-based dural sealants can be used as an adjunct to reinforce the suture line. At the conclusion of the case, the retractor system is removed slowly, taking care to identify and cauterize any sites of bleeding. The fascia and subcutaneous layers are closed with absorbable sutures. We close the skin with a topical adhesive glue.

Postoperative Care and Concerns

CSF leakage is the primary postoperative concern specific to intradural spine tumor surgery. To reduce the amount of pressure on the healing durotomy closure, patients have historically been kept flat on bedrest following surgery. Traditionally, open surgery postoperative protocols recommend that patients be kept flat and immobilized until postoperative day 2. Following minimally invasive surgery, this may not be necessary [26]. Compared to open intradural surgery, the minimal epidural dead space following MIS surgery reduces the risk of postoperative CSF leakage [4, 6, 26]. We occasionally keep patients on bed rest the day of surgery but mobilize them no later than first thing in the morning on postoperative day 1.

Case Presentation (Video 28.1)

The patient is a 55-year-old man who presents with 4 weeks of progressive lower back and left lower extremity pain in an L5 distribution. His physical examination reveals diminished sensation in the left L5 dermatome. MRI reveals a right paramedian intradural lesion that is hyperintense on T2 with significant gadolinium enhancement on T1 post-contrast sequences, suggestive of a schwannoma. Of note, there is also a left paramedian lumbar disk herniation at L4/5, causing significant lateral recess stenosis at the affected level (Fig. 28.3). Given the patient's clinical presentation and imaging findings, his symptoms are thought to be due to a combination of the two pathologies. The decision is made to address the herniated disk first and then resect the intradural tumor through one minimally invasive approach.

The patient is brought to the operating room and prepped and positioned using standard MIS techniques as described earlier. A 3-cm paramedian incision is made approximately 2 cm to the left of midline at the level of the L4/5 joint. This is approximately 1 cm more lateral than would be used for a standard lumbar microdiscectomy, facilitating a more lateral to medial trajectory to access and resect the tumor. A 26-mm tubular retractor is docked at L4/5 and used to dilate the paraspinal musculature. A soft-tissue muscle plug is circumferentially dissected and removed as described earlier, exposing the underlying lamina and medial portion of the L4/5 facet joint. Using a high-speed burr, a standard laminectomy and medial facetectomy are performed, exposing the underlying ligamentum flavum. Under routine conditions, the ligament would be preserved to act as a dural barrier while undercutting the spinal process and contralateral lamina. However, in this case the ipsilateral ligamentum flavum is removed to facilitate the discectomy. With the ligament removed, the underlying dura and nerve root are brought into site. The nerve root and thecal sac are gently retracted medially and the microdiscectomy performed in standard fashion.

Upon completion of the microdiscectomy, a concerted effort is made to ensure reliable hemostasis so that blood does not run into the subarachnoid space during the intradural stage of the case. The MIS tubular retractor is then redirected medially, revealing the undersurface of the spinous process, which is drilled with the high-speed burr, exposing midline, the contralateral lamina, and the entire dorsal thecal sac. A low-profile MIS needle driver is used to place the initial tenting stich and tack up sutures. A no. 11 blade is used to initiate the durotomy, which is rostrally and caudally extended with a nerve hook.

Tumor dissection begins with careful splitting of the arachnoid layers overlying the tumor. Standard microsurgical techniques are used to carefully separate the mass from the adjacent nerve roots of the cauda equina. Once the tumor is isolated and exposed, slight traction is used to herniate the mass partially through the dural opening to facilitate easier manipulation and avoid trauma to the other roots of the cauda equina.

Direct stimulation is applied to both the afferent and efferent nerve fascicles, with no motor

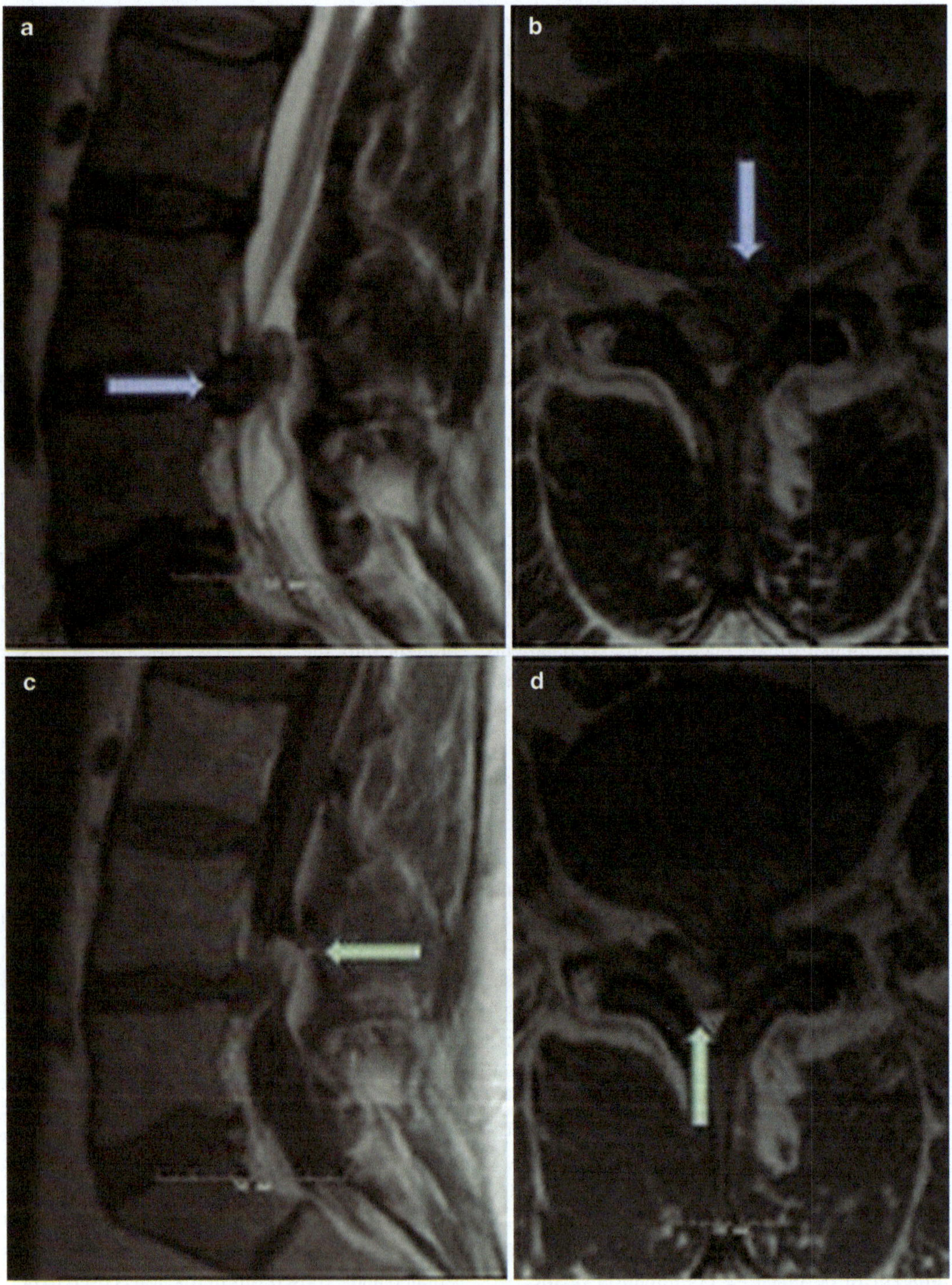

Fig. 28.3 Magnetic resonance imaging of a patient with a concurrent herniated lumbar disc and intradural extramedullary lesion. The hypointense herniated disc (blue arrows) on the left at L4–L5 can be well appreciated on T2-weighted sagittal (**a**) and axial (**b**) images. The intramedullary lesion enhances avidly (green arrows), seen here on sagittal (**c**) and axial (**d**) T1 post-contrast images

response elicited. In most cases, the afferent nerve is sectioned first and then the efferent nerve. As mentioned above, this is to prevent rostral rebounding of the tumor above the durotomy from rostral nerve tension. However, in this case, exposure of the afferent fascicle is limited, and the tumor mass does not appear to be under tension rostrally. Accordingly, the efferent fascicle is sectioned first, followed by the afferent fascicle. The tumor is then rolled, exposing its ventral surface and facilitating lysis of any remaining arachnoid adhesions. With the mass dissected free, it can be removed en bloc without the need for internal debulking.

Once hemostasis is achieved, dural closure commences. A 6–0 running Gore-Tex suture is used with adapted MIS instruments. The assistant stays actively involved by helping advance each suture throw down to the knot. A dural sealant is then placed prior to removal of the tubular dilator. Adjacent soft tissue collapses upon removal of the tubular dilator, effectively obliterating the epidural dead space and reducing the risk of pseudomeningocele formation and CSF leak. Several stitches are placed to close the fascia and subcutaneous tissue. Finally, the skin edges are sealed with topical adhesive glue.

The patient's left lower extremity radiculopathy improved immediately after surgery. He was kept on bedrest overnight but mobilized the next morning. His postoperative course was uncomplicated, and he was discharged home in stable condition. Final pathology confirmed a diagnosis of schwannoma.

Discussion

Since first reported by Treadway and colleagues in 2006, a growing body of evidence has demonstrated the safety and efficacy of minimally invasive surgery for intradural extramedullary spinal tumors [3–15]. Neurosurgeons who have become facile using MIS retractors for degenerative disease may be well-equipped to adapt MIS techniques for intradural tumors. However, success is contingent on an understanding of the proper indications and advantages/disadvantages related to these techniques. MIS approaches work particularly well for well-circumscribed dorsal and lateral extramedullary tumors. Lesions that lie ventral to the spinal cord or span more than two spinal segments may be better approached with traditional open surgery.

In properly selected patients, minimally invasive surgery for IDEM tumors has been shown to offer a number of potential benefits over open surgery. These benefits are well summarized in a recent meta-analysis by Pham and colleagues in which data for 114 patients were pooled from 9 retrospective studies and analyzed [4]. Compared to open surgery, patients receiving MIS surgery for IDEM tumors experienced reduced CSF leakage, blood loss, length of hospital stay, and postoperative pain without an increased incidence of complications [4].

The most common complication in this MIS meta-analysis was CSF leakage and/or pseudomeningocele formation, occurring in 5.3% of patients [4, 30]. Yet compared to open surgery, MIS approaches are generally protective against CSF-related complications [9, 15, 16]. This is due to a reduction in tissue destruction and displacement that allows for re-expansion of the paraspinal musculature upon removal of the tubular retractors. This re-expansion obliterates much of the dead space that remains following open surgery and creates a physical barrier to CSF leakage. In a retrospective series directly comparing MIS to open surgery for IDEM tumors, Wong and colleagues report a significant difference in the number of postoperative CSF leaks between patients treated with MIS (one patient, 3.7%) versus open approaches (three patients, 16.7%) (6). In a study similarly comparing MIS to open surgery for IDEM lesions, Raygor et al. report that 1 of 25 (4%) MIS patients had a CSF leak or pseudomeningocele, while 3 of 26 (11.5%) patients in the open cohort experienced CSF leaks [7]. In our own retrospective study of 23 consecutive patients with an MIS dural closure following intended durotomy, we did not experience any cases of CSF leakage or symptomatic pseudomeningocele [26]. All patients were allowed full activity less than 24 h after surgery in this study, further suggesting that prolonged bed rest after successful primary dural closure appears unnecessary after MIS surgery.

Reports of MIS approaches to IDEM lesions have also consistently found reductions in estimated blood loss (EBL) compared to open surgery. In the meta-analysis conducted by Pham et al., blood loss from MIS cohorts ranged from 134 to 153 ml, while EBL in open surgeries ranged from 320 to 558 ml [6, 7, 31]. In the comparative series by Wong and colleagues, three open surgery patients required blood transfusions but no MIS patients did [6]. Similarly, in the study by Raygor et al., three patients in the open group received a blood transfusion compared to one MIS patient [7]. This difference can be attributed to the decreased muscle cutting and soft-tissue destruction caused by an MIS approach, as well as the tamponading effect of muscle re-expansion in the surgical cavity following retractor removal.

This reduction in dead space may also contribute to lower infection rates in MIS intradural surgery, as the volume of hematomas and seromas that may act as an infectious nidus is minimized. There is evidence suggesting that MIS surgery for degenerative spinal conditions may reduce postoperative wound infections as much as ten-fold [32]. In their meta-analysis, Pham and colleagues found evidence of a postoperative infection in only 1 of the 114 patients analyzed (0.88%), a significantly lower rate compared to previous studies of open surgery for IDEM lesions [4, 33].

One of the primary reported benefits of minimally invasive surgery is reduced length of hospital stay (LOS), which often translates into cost reduction [34]. There is evidence that these benefits can be achieved when MIS techniques are applied to intradural spinal tumors. In a comparison between MIS and open surgery for IDEM tumors, Lu and colleagues reported shorter hospital stays for patients in the MIS cohort (4.9 days vs. 8.2 days, $p = 0.003$) [31]. Wong and colleagues similarly found patients undergoing MIS resection to have a shorter LOS compared to patients receiving open surgery (3.9 vs. 6.1 days, $p < 0.01$) (6). However, Raygor et al. found no significant difference between MIS and open groups (6.2 vs. 6.0 days, $p = 0.78$) [7]. In our own cohort of patients with IDEM lesion, LOS and time spent in intensive care were both significantly reduced in the MIS cohort compared to patients receiving open surgery [5]. This shortened length of stay and intensive care unit (ICU) time helped account for a nearly 30% reduction in cost in the MIS group [5]. As the emphasis on cost control in our healthcare systems continues to grow, the cost efficacy of MIS approaches to IDEM lesions may become increasingly important.

Conclusion

The use of minimally invasive retractor systems in the resection of intradural spinal tumors has been shown to be both safe and effective. There is increasing evidence from retrospective data that MIS techniques can be used to reduce the morbidity and cost of IDEM tumor resection, without compromising extent of resection or safety. Due to the growth of minimally invasive spine surgery in residency training and an ever-increasing emphasis on cost effectiveness, more neurosurgeons are likely to adopt MIS techniques for IDEM pathology in the future.

References

1. Kurland LT. The frequency of intracranial and intraspinal neoplasms in the resident population of Rochester, Minnesota. J Neurosurg. 1958;15(6):627–41.
2. Sasaoka R, Nakamura H, Konishi S, Nagayama R, Suzuki E, Terai H, et al. Objective assessment of reduced invasiveness in MED. Compared with conventional one-level laminotomy. Eur Spine J. 2006;15(5):577–82.
3. Snyder L, Clark J, Nakaji P, Tumialán L. Minimally invasive surgical techniques for intradural extramedullary lesions of the thoracic spine. Barrow Q. 2016;26(1):20–5.
4. Martin H, Pham K-EC, Liu JC, Hsieh PC. Minimally invasive surgery for intradural extramedullary spinal tumors: a comprehensive review with illustrative clinical cases. World Spinal Column J. 2016;7(2):84–96.
5. Fontes RB, Wewel JT, O'Toole JE. Perioperative cost analysis of minimally invasive vs open resection of intradural extramedullary spinal cord tumors. Neurosurgery. 2016;78(4):531–9.
6. Wong AP, Lall RR, Dahdaleh NS, Lawton CD, Smith ZA, Wong RH, et al. Comparison of open and minimally invasive surgery for intradural-extramedullary spine tumors. Neurosurg Focus. 2015;39(2):E11.

7. Raygor KP, Than KD, Chou D, Mummaneni PV. Comparison of minimally invasive transspinous and open approaches for thoracolumbar intradural-extramedullary spinal tumors. Neurosurg Focus. 2015;39(2):E12.
8. Afathi M, Peltier E, Adetchessi T, Graillon T, Dufour H, Fuentes S. Minimally invasive transmuscular approach for the treatment of benign intradural extramedullary spinal cord tumours: Technical note and results. Neurochirurgie. 2015;61(5):333–8.
9. Nzokou A, Weil AG, Shedid D. Minimally invasive removal of thoracic and lumbar spinal tumors using a nonexpandable tubular retractor. J Neurosurg Spine. 2013;19(6):708–15.
10. Gandhi RH, German JW. Minimally invasive approach for the treatment of intradural spinal pathology. Neurosurg Focus. 2013;35(2):E5.
11. Lee B, Hsieh PC. Minimally invasive lumbar intradural extramedullary tumor resection. Neurosurg Focus. 2012;33(Suppl 1):1.
12. Dahlberg D, Halvorsen CM, Lied B, Helseth E. Minimally invasive microsurgical resection of primary, intradural spinal tumours using a tubular retraction system. Br J Neurosurg. 2012;26(4):472–5.
13. Mannion RJ, Nowitzke AM, Efendy J, Wood MJ. Safety and efficacy of intradural extramedullary spinal tumor removal using a minimally invasive approach. Neurosurgery. 2011;68(1 Suppl Operative):208–16. discussion 16.
14. Dakwar E, Smith WD, Malone KT, Uribe JS. Minimally invasive lateral extracavitary resection of foraminal neurofibromas. J Clin Neurosci. 2011;18(11):1510–2.
15. Tredway TL, Santiago P, Hrubes MR, Song JK, Christie SD, Fessler RG. Minimally invasive resection of intradural-extramedullary spinal neoplasms. Neurosurgery. 2006;58(1 Suppl):ONS52–8. discussion ONS-8.
16. O'Toole JE, Eichholz KM, Fessler RG. Minimally invasive approaches to vertebral column and spinal cord tumors. Neurosurg Clin N Am. 2006;17(4):491–506.
17. Klimo P Jr, Kestle JR, Schmidt MH. Treatment of metastatic spinal epidural disease: a review of the literature. Neurosurg Focus. 2003;15(5):E1.
18. Weigel B, Maghsudi M, Neumann C, Kretschmer R, Muller FJ, Nerlich M. Surgical management of symptomatic spinal metastases. Postoperative outcome and quality of life. Spine (Phila Pa 1976). 1999;24(21):2240–6.
19. Ghogawala Z, Mansfield FL, Borges LF. Spinal radiation before surgical decompression adversely affects outcomes of surgery for symptomatic metastatic spinal cord compression. Spine (Phila Pa 1976). 2001;26(7):818–24.
20. Haji FA, Cenic A, Crevier L, Murty N, Reddy K. Minimally invasive approach for the resection of spinal neoplasm. Spine (Phila Pa 1976). 2011;36(15):E1018–26.
21. Ogden AT, Fessler RG. Minimally invasive resection of intramedullary ependymoma: case report. Neurosurgery. 2009;65(6):E1203–4. discussion E4.
22. On Tsang AC, Hang Tse PY, Ting Ng GH, Kit Leung GK. Minimal access microsurgical ligation of spinal dural arteriovenous fistula with tubular retractor. Surg Neurol Int. 2015;6:99.
23. Patel NP, Birch BD, Lyons MK, DeMent SE, Elbert GA. Minimally invasive intradural spinal dural arteriovenous fistula ligation. World Neurosurg. 2013;80(6):e267–70.
24. Fassett DR, Clark R, Brockmeyer DL, Schmidt MH. Cervical spine deformity associated with resection of spinal cord tumors. Neurosurg Focus. 2006;20(2):E2.
25. McGirt MJ, Chaichana KL, Atiba A, Bydon A, Witham TF, Yao KC, et al. Incidence of spinal deformity after resection of intramedullary spinal cord tumors in children who underwent laminectomy compared with laminoplasty. J Neurosurg Pediatr. 2008;1(1):57–62.
26. Tan LA, Takagi I, Straus D, O'Toole JE. Management of intended durotomy in minimally invasive intradural spine surgery: clinical article. J Neurosurg Spine. 2014;21(2):279–85.
27. Tan LA, Kasliwal MK, Wewel J, Fontes RB, O'Toole JE. Minimally invasive surgery for synchronous, same-level lumbar intradural-extramedullary neoplasm and acute disc herniation. Neurosurg Focus. 2014;37(Suppl 2). Video 16.
28. Tan LA, O'Toole JE. Tubular retractor selection in minimally invasive spinal tumor resection. J Neurosurg Spine. 2014;20(5):596–7. author reply 7-8.
29. Park P, Leveque JC, La Marca F, Sullivan SE. Dural closure using the U-clip in minimally invasive spinal tumor resection. J Spinal Disord Tech. 2010;23(7):486–9.
30. Hoover JM, Clarke MJ, Wetjen NM, Mandrekar J, Puffer RC, Krauss WE. Complications necessitating a return to the operating room following intradural spine surgery. World Neurosurg. 2012;78(3–4):344–7.
31. Lu DC, Chou D, Mummaneni PV. A comparison of mini-open and open approaches for resection of thoracolumbar intradural spinal tumors. J Neurosurg Spine. 2011;14(6):758–64.
32. O'Toole JE, Eichholz KM, Fessler RG. Surgical site infection rates after minimally invasive spinal surgery. J Neurosurg Spine. 2009;11(4):471–6.
33. Omeis IA, Dhir M, Sciubba DM, Gottfried ON, McGirt MJ, Attenello FJ, et al. Postoperative surgical site infections in patients undergoing spinal tumor surgery: incidence and risk factors. Spine (Phila Pa 1976). 2011;36(17):1410–9.
34. Wang MY, Lerner J, Lesko J, McGirt MJ. Acute hospital costs after minimally invasive versus open lumbar interbody fusion: data from a US national database with 6106 patients. J Spinal Disord Tech. 2012;25(6):324–8.
35. Mende KC, Krätzig T, Mohme M, Westphal M, Eicker SO. Keyhole approaches to intradural pathologies. Neurosurg Focus. 2017;43:E5.

Index

D. M. Sciubba (ed.), *Spinal Tumor Surgery*, https://doi.org/10.1007/978-3-319-98422-3

The manufacturer's authorised representative in the EU is Springer Nature Customer Service Centre GmbH, Europaplatz 3, 69115 Heidelberg, Germany. If you have any concerns regarding our products, please contact ProductSafety@springernature.com

Printed and bound by CPI Group (UK) Ltd, Croydon, CR0 4YY
30/09/2026
02225593-0020